Clinical Assessment
in Respiratory Care

Clinical Assessment in Respiratory Care

ROBERT L. WILKINS, M.A., R.R.T.

Associate Professor
Associate Chairman and Program Director
Department of Respiratory Therapy
School of Allied Health Professions
Loma Linda University
Loma Linda, California

SUSAN JONES KRIDER, R.N., M.S., C.C.R.N.

Clinical Director
Loma Linda International Heart Institute
Loma Linda University Medical Center
Loma Linda, California

RICHARD L. SHELDON, M.D., F.A.C.P., F.C.C.P.

Clinical Professor of Medicine
Loma Linda University School of Medicine
Medical Director, School of Respiratory Care
Crafton Hills College
Beaver Medical Clinics, Inc.
Redlands, California

THIRD EDITION

With 206 illustrations
Illustrations by Nathan Lindsey and Anna-Marie Fletcher

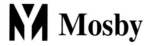 Mosby

St. Louis Baltimore Berlin Boston Carlsbad Chicago London Madrid
Naples New York Philadelphia Sydney Tokyo Toronto

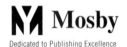
Mosby
Dedicated to Publishing Excellence

Editor: James F. Shanahan
Developmental Editor: Jennifer Roche
Project Manager: Mark Spann
Senior Production Editor: Jerry Schwartz
Design Manager: Dave Zielinski
Designer: Duncan Dickinson
Manufacturing Supervisor: Betty Richmond

THIRD EDITION

Printed in the United States of America
Composition by Carlisle Communications, Ltd.
Printing/binding by Von Hoffmann Press

Mosby-Year Book, Inc.
11830 Westline Industrial Drive
St. Louis, Missouri 63146

Library of Congress Cataloging-in-Publication Data

Wilkins, Robert L.
    Clinical assessment in respiratory care / Robert L. Wilkins, Susan
Jones Krider, Richard L. Sheldon ; illustrations by Nathan Lindsey
and Anna-Marie Fletcher. — 3rd ed.
      p.   cm.
    Includes bibliographical references and index.
    ISBN 0-8151-9334-3
    1. Respiratory insufficiency—Diagnosis.   2. Respiratory
therapists.   3. Cardiopulmonary system—Diseases—Diagnosis.
I. Krider, Susan Jones. II. Sheldon, Richard L. III. Title.
    [DNLM: 1. Respiratory Tract Diseases—diagnosis. 2. Critical
Care. 3. Physical Examination.   WF 141 W684c 1995]
RC776.R4W55 1995
616.2'4—dc20
DNLM/DLC
for Library of Congress
             94-35037
             CIP

95 96 97 98 99 / 9 8 7 6 5 4 3 2 1

Contributors

RICHARD BRANSON, R.R.T.
Clinical Instructor, Department of Surgery
College of Medicine
University of Cincinnati Medical Center
Cincinnati, Ohio

KENNETH I. BURKE, Ph.D., R.D.
Professor/Associate Chairman, Department of
   Nutrition and Dietetics
School of Allied Health Professions
Loma Linda University
Loma Linda, California

LINDA W. CHU, M.D.
Clinical Director, Department of Pathology
Kettering Medical Center
Kettering, Ohio
Assistant Clinical Professor of Pathology
Wright State University, School of Medicine
Dayton, Ohio

GERILYNN L. CONNERS, R.C.P., R.R.T., B.S.
Co-Director, Pulmonary Rehabilitation
Clinical Coordinator, Nicotine Intervention Program
St. Helena Hospital
Deer Park, California

DOUGLAS D. DEMING, M.D.
Assistant Professor of Pediatrics, School of Medicine
Loma Linda University
Medical Director, Neonatal Respiratory Care
Loma Linda University Medical Center
Loma Linda, California

JAMES R. DEXTER, M.D., F.C.C.P.
Associate Professor, School of Medicine
Loma Linda University
Loma Linda, California

RALPH DOWNEY III, Ph.D.
Assistant Professor of Medicine and Pediatrics
Diplomate, American Board of Sleep Medicine
Director, Loma Linda Sleep Disorders Center
School of Medicine, Loma Linda University
Loma Linda, California

PATRICK J. DUNNE, M.Ed., R.R.T.
Managing General Partner
Southwest Medical Mart
Fullerton, California

TOM MALINOWSKI, B.S., R.R.T., R.C.P.
Clinical Director, Department of Respiratory Care
Loma Linda University Medical Center
Loma Linda, California

KENNETH D. McCARTY, M.S., R.R.T.
Director of Clinical Education, Department of
   Respiratory Therapy
School of Allied Health Professions
Loma Linda University
Loma Linda, California

SUSAN L. McINTURFF, R.R.T.
Clinical Director
Bay Area Home Health Care
Novato, California

KATHLEEN V. MORRIS, R.N., M.S., R.R.T.
Co-Director, Pulmonary Rehabilitation
St. Helena Hospital
Deer Park, California

JAMES A. PETERS, M.D., D.H.Sc., M.P.H., R.R.T.,
   R.D.
Medical Director, Smoking Cessation Program
Assistant Medical Director, Respiratory Care
   Department
St. Helena Hospital and Health Center
Deer Park, California

MARSHALL WOOLNER, R.N., C.C.R.N.
Educator, Nursing Staff Development
Loma Linda University Medical Center
Loma Linda, California

Preface

Patient assessment continues to be a vital part of health care. With this in mind, the goals of this third edition are the same as previous editions: to educate respiratory care students about patient assessment and to further develop the skills of practitioners. Students in nursing, medicine, and other health professions as well as practitioners will find this text helpful if they are to care for patients with cardiopulmonary disease. All chapters have been updated, but the more significant changes in this edition are the following:

1. A new chapter at the beginning of the text, "Preparing for the Patient Encounter." This chapter introduces the reader to the important issues of bedside manner.
2. A new and separate chapter entitled "Vital Signs." This chapter helps emphasize the importance of vital signs and makes the information more manageable.
3. Two new chapters in section III, "Assessment of the Home Care Patient" and "Assessment of the Pulmonary Rehabilitation Patient." This information reflects the more recent emphasis on outpatient care for the patient with cardiopulmonary disease.

4. Chapter objectives at the beginning of each chapter to clarify the important points.
5. A glossary of assessment terms and abbreviations at the end of the text for easy reference.
6. A companion *Quick Reference Guide to Clinical Assessment in Respiratory Care* that summarizes key concepts related to patient assessment. It is intended to assist the student or new clinician with patient assessment at the bedside. The Quick Reference Guide contains updated and revised information on synopsis of pulmonary disorders previously found in the last chapter of the first and second editions. We believe that the format of the Quick Reference Guide is a pragmatic place for the tables summarizing clinical findings in common cardiopulmonary disorders.

Patient assessment is the foundation upon which quality patient care is built. We hope that you find the additions and updates for the third edition of *Clinical Assessment in Respiratory Care* useful in your care of patients with cardiopulmonary diseases.

RLW, SJK, RLS

To
OUR SPOUSES
Kris, Judy, and Terry
and
OUR CHILDREN
Tyler, Nicholas, Kirsten,
Karl, Christopher, and Michael

Acknowledgments

We would like to express our gratitude to all those who helped in developing this third edition. The reviewers of the manuscript provided many suggestions that helped shape the final product. We especially want to thank George Hicks and Bud Spearman for their suggestions and words of wisdom. Audrey Romero, Sharon Dietrich, and Chris Kilburn, who provided clerical and word-processing assistance, deserve special mention. Finally, we want to thank our students whose feedback and input has proved invaluable.

RLW, SJK, RLS

Contents

SECTION TWO

ADVANCED ASSESSMENT TECHNIQUES

Fundamentals of Respiratory Assessment

Chapter 1

Preparing for the Patient Encounter

Robert L. Wilkins

Chapter Overview

The purpose of this chapter is to help you develop an appropriate bedside manner, which is vitally important to the process of patient assessment. As a bedside clinician you must be capable of efficient and accurate assessments and must conduct yourself in a professional manner during all patient encounters. This chapter will help you understand some of the important issues related to professionalism at the bedside of patients needing medical care.

Working with the hospitalized patient represents a unique challenge for health care providers. In some cases the patient will be feeling anxious, angry, or depressed, or all of these. You must be sensitive to these and other possible feelings and do all you can to help the patient feel as comfortable as possible under the circumstances. A professional bedside manner is the foundation upon which each assessment and all quality patient care are built.

Stages of Patient-Clinician Interaction

The Preinteraction Stage

The majority of patient encounters begin with a review of the patient's chart to identify details such as the name, age, gender, chief complaints, history of present illness (see Chapter 2), and the physician's initial orders. You can use this information when you introduce yourself to the patient and for making an initial assessment of the patient. This stage should only take a few minutes but is well worth the time and effort. Finally, clarify in your mind what your role will be with regard to caring for the patient you are about to encounter.

The Introductory Stage

This is the stage in which you enter the patient's room and introduce yourself. Your initial introduction should take place in the social space, which is about 4 to 12 ft from the patient (see Use of Space). This introduction sets the tone for the rest of the visit. You should introduce yourself by greeting the patient using his or her formal name. This is to be followed by a brief description of the purpose of your visit and your role in caring for the patient during the hospitalization. This type of formal introduction is to be used in most clinical settings. Even the comatose patient unable to respond deserves this type of respect. An exception would be made for the critically ill patient in need of emergency care such as cardiopulmonary resuscitation.

The introductory stage is important in establishing a rapport between you and the patient. A positive rapport is necessary to obtain the patient's cooperation with assessment and treatment procedures. Patients usually appreciate and respond positively to a warm, friendly introduction done in a professional manner. Be careful to avoid overly friendly or jovial statements as they may be irritating to those patients who are depressed or upset as a result of their illness. For example, stating "Isn't it a wonderful day?" to a patient dying from lung cancer is likely to be received poorly. Be friendly, but avoid extremes.

During the introductory phase look for signs of resistive behavior in the patient. This may be seen as crossed arms, refusal to make eye contact, or very brief responses to your questions. These responses represent clues that the patient is not likely to be cooperative

or accepting of your suggestions and may not be listening carefully to your questions and instructions. In such cases you will need to make an extra effort to establish a rapport with the patient and improve communication. Other techniques for establishing a rapport and demonstrating genuine concern are discussed later in this chapter.

The Initial Assessment Stage

This stage actually overlaps with the introductory stage since you can easily begin visual inspection of the patient during your introduction. Take time to note the patient's general appearance, attitudes, and responses to your statements and questions as mentioned above. Formal assessment of the patient with a brief interview regarding chief complaints at admission can now take place (see Chapter 2). The interview is followed in most cases by a brief physical examination to determine the pretreatment status of the patient (see Chapters 3 and 4). Your goal at this point is to determine the condition of the patient and to make sure the prescribed treatment ordered by the physician is appropriate. Occasionally, you may evaluate the patient whose condition has abruptly changed recently and who is now in need of different treatment. In fact, the prescribed treatment may be contraindicated. If you skip the initial assessment stage you will be blindly following orders that may result in inappropriate and possibly harmful treatment. Contacting the head nurse and the attending physician is necessary when your initial assessment reveals a need for different treatment.

The Treatment and Monitoring Stage

Following your initial assessment of the patient you are now ready to administer treatment. During the treatment stage you will need to continue to use your assessment skills to evaluate the effects of the treatment. Occasionally the patient may develop side effects from the treatment, or the therapy may not result in the expected beneficial response. Your ability to identify and document the positive and negative effects of the therapy is crucial to the patient's care. Therapy should be stopped immediately when side effects occur. The respiratory care supervisor, head nurse, and the attending physician need to be notified in such cases.

The Follow-up Stage

You should take a minute to communicate with the patient once the treatment or bedside procedure is completed. Note any changes in symptoms, attitudes, alertness, and so forth, and document your findings. Let the patient know when you will return and how to contact you if the need arises. Make sure the patient is

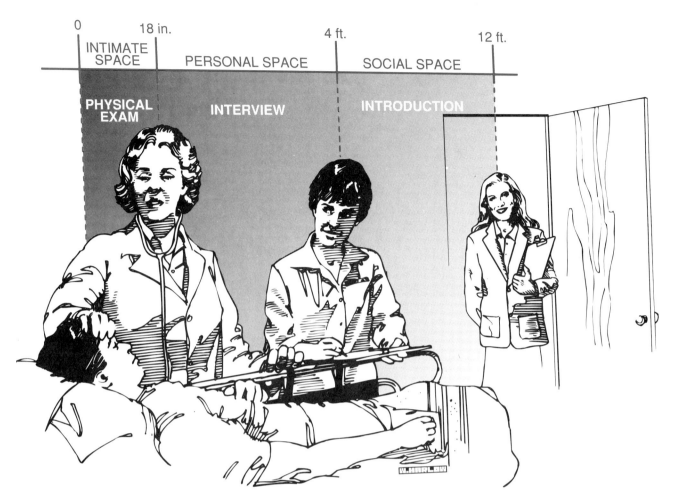

Fig. 1–1 *Illustration of the social, personal, and intimate spaces of the patient needing health care.*

as comfortable as possible and ask if there is anything you can do to help the patient before exiting the room. This brief stage is useful in developing your rapport with the patient and in building a positive attitude in the patient toward you and your employer.

Use of Space

An important, but often overlooked, issue related to interaction with patients is the appropriate use of the space surrounding each patient. Proper use of the three zones described below adds to professionalism of all bedside clinicians.

Social Space (4–12 ft)

This zone is useful for your introduction to the patient and is where you begin to establish rapport (Fig. 1–1). At this distance you can see the "big picture" and gain an appreciation for the whole patient and his or her environment. Vocalizations are limited to the more formal issues, and

personal questions are to be avoided in this space as others in the room can easily overhear the conversation.

Personal Space (18 in.–4 ft)

This space is most useful for the interview, especially when more personal questions are to be asked. For example, some patients are uncomfortable when answering questions about their daily sputum production or smoking habits. Answers to such personal questions are more likely to be accurate and detailed when the questions are asked from the personal space. In addition, providing privacy by pulling the bedside curtain may be useful in making the patient feel more comfortable about answering questions. The personal space is best entered only after a rapport with the patient has been established in the social space previously described.

The interview is not only useful for gathering information but also for further development of the rapport between you and the patient. The rapport you have with the patient becomes more important when you invade his or her intimate space, as described below, and when you begin therapeutic procedures. Attention to details regarding your professional appearance are important in the personal space. The patient will often feel more comfortable and confident with you if your appearance is neat, clean, and professional. Appropriate use of eye contact is needed in the personal space as this will increase the patient's trust in you.

Intimate Space (0–18 in.)

In most cases invasion of the intimate space is done only after your introduction in the social space and brief interview in the personal space. These initial steps in establishing a rapport with the patient make invasion of the patient's intimate space more comfortable for both of you. Additionally, invasion of the intimate space should be preceded by a request for permission to do so. This communicates your respect for the patient as a person and also lets the patient know that he or she has a say in the medical care. Permission to invade the patient's intimate space is often obtained simply by requesting permission to listen to breath sounds or check vital signs.

The intimate space is reserved primarily for physical examination of the patient and for therapeutic procedures. Minimal or no eye contact is used in this space. Verbal communication with the patient should be limited to brief commands or simple questions such as "Please take a deep breath."

Invasion of the patient's intimate space is often met with a variety of responses. Gender, age, race, physical appearance, health status, and cultural background represent a few of the many factors that may influence the comfort level of the patient when you enter the intimate space. Be aware that some patients may respond poorly to your invasion of their space and be prepared to move more slowly and communicate very carefully in such cases.

Territoriality

Most patients lay claim to all items within a certain boundary around their bed. For patients in a private room the boundary will extend to the walls of the room. Removing items from the patient's "territory" should only occur after permission has been obtained. For example, when borrowing a bedside chair from the bedside of Mr. Jones for use at the bedside of Mr. Smith, you should ask Mr. Jones for permission to borrow his bedside chair. Although technically the majority of bedside items are owned by the hospital they temporarily "belong" to the patient while he or she is hospitalized. Being aware of the territoriality issue

will improve your bedside manner and may avoid upsetting a patient.

Expressing Genuine Concern

Working in a hospital setting requires a sincere demonstration of concern or empathy toward your patients. Phony attempts at empathy are easily detected by patients and usually have a very negative impact on the patient's attitude. Expressing empathy can be awkward for some clinicians, especially when new to the hospital setting. For this reason several general techniques for expressing genuine concern are listed below. Use them only when you feel comfortable with the technique described. The list represents only a few of the more commonly used techniques. You may discover other techniques by watching more experienced clinicians. Learning to use any of the techniques associated with demonstrating empathy will require practice to become more effective.

Face the Patient Squarely

This simple maneuver, used during all conversations with the patient, tells the patient that he or she has your undivided attention. It suggests that you are interested in what the patient has to say and allows you to better visualize the patient.

Use Eye Contact Appropriately

This represents one of the most important and powerful techniques for demonstrating true concern for the patient. Appropriate use of eye contact conveys your interest in the patient and in his or her comments. Eye contact is particularly important when the patient is speaking to you and when you are asking questions of the patient. Equally important is the avoidance of extremes with eye contact. For example, staring at the patient or out the window during conversation is inappropriate. Looking out the window while the patient is speaking sends a message to the patient that you are not interested in what he or she has to say.

Maintain an Open Posture

An open posture means sitting or standing in a relaxed manner with your arms at your side. This relaxed position creates a more comfortable setting for the patient and represents nonverbal communication that says you accept the patient and want to help. Sitting or standing with your arms crossed sends a signal of unacceptance.

Consider Appropriate Use of Touch

Touch also can be a powerful tool for communicating genuine concern to the patient. It is, however, the most difficult technique to use appropriately. Touch to communicate empathy should only be used in those patients with whom you have established a solid rapport. Even then its use should be reserved for those patients in whom you feel it will be received positively.

Only certain sites on the patient are acceptable for you to touch as an empathic gesture. The patient's hand, arm, or shoulder are acceptable sites for most patients. For example, a gentle pat or squeeze of the patient's shoulder or hand just prior to exiting the room while reassuring the patient you will return later is an effective way to communicate genuine empathy. Keep in mind that cultural background, gender, age, and so forth are factors that may influence how receptive a patient will be to the use of touch. If you sense that your patient is demonstrating verbal or nonverbal signs of resistive behavior, touch is probably not likely to be well received.

Be an Active Listener

Listening carefully to what the patient has to say is another technique that communicates true concern. Clues that you are not listening carefully are often demonstrated by repeating questions that you asked just minutes ago or by lack of eye contact when the patient is making statements or asking questions. If the patient senses that you are not carefully listening you are not likely to get his or her attention when you need it and the patient's responses to your questions will become progressively more brief. Additionally, patients often interpret poor listening as a general lack of concern for their well-being. Active listening takes practice to become proficient. Good eye contact, asking for clarification on certain points, and brief note taking demonstrate active listening. Active listening can lead to more accurate assessments when all details are noted.

Universal Precautions

The Centers for Disease Control recommends that all clinicians who may come into contact with the body fluids of their patients wear protective gear. This recommendation is based on the fact that it is often not clear which patients are infected with transmittable diseases. As a result, the term *universal precautions* is used for the precautionary measures that clinicians should take to protect themselves against possible exposure to the body fluids of patients.

The assessment process often calls for bedside clinicians to draw blood from the patient or obtain sputum samples for analysis. Rubber gloves are needed in all situations in which you may contact the blood, saliva, or sputum of your patient. In addition, if splashes or airborne droplets of the patient's body fluids are possible, masks and protective eyewear are needed.

Accidental needle sticks with a contaminated needle represent one of the most common ways in which health care workers are exposed to transmissible diseases. For this reason all hospital and clinic workers must be extra careful when handling used needles. Needles should not be recapped, manipulated, or removed from the syringe after use on a patient. Used needles must be discarded into appropriate puncture-resistant containers usually located in all patient care areas. Thorough handwashing before and after each patient contact is equally important in reducing the incidence of transmissible diseases.

REVIEW QUESTIONS

1. The preinteraction stage is useful in which of the following ways?
   a. to determine the effect of the therapy
   b. for clarifying the patient's history and your role in the therapy
   c. for establishing rapport with the patient
   d. to allow the patient to evaluate the clinician's abilities

2. What is the appropriate distance of the social space?
   a. 0-18 inches
   b. 18 inches-4 feet
   c. 4-12 feet
   d. 6-18 feet

3. In which of the following spaces is patient introduction properly performed?
   a. social
   b. personal
   c. intimate
   d. all of the above

4. In which of the following spaces is the interview properly performed?
   a. social
   b. personal
   c. intimate
   d. all of the above

5. T F Eye contact is appropriate in the intimate space during patient-clinician interaction.

6. In which of the following spaces is rapport best established?
    a. social
    b. personal
    c. intimate
    d. a and b

7. T   F   A clinician who, during the patient encounter, stands with his arms crossed and avoids eye contact is conveying a lack of concern for the patient.

8. T   F   Asking for permission to use an article within the patient's room acknowledges the patient's territorial rights while conveying respect for the patient.

9. T   F   The practice of universal precautions presumes that all patients are potentially infective.

10. Which of the following pieces of personal protective equipment are required when splattering of blood and body fluids is likely?
    a. gown
    b. gloves
    c. eye shield
    d. mask
    e. all of the above

BIBLIOGRAPHY

Hirschmann JV: Infection control and isolation procedures in respiratory care. In Pierson DJ and Kacmarek RM, editors: *Foundations of respiratory care,* New York, 1992, Churchill Livingstone.

Judge RD, Zuidema GD, and Fitzgerald FT: *Clinical diagnosis: a physiologic approach,* ed 4, Boston, 1982, Little, Brown.

Kozier, B, Erb G, and Olivieri R: *Fundamentals of nursing: concepts, process, and practice,* ed 4, Redwood City, Calif, 1991, Addison-Wesley.

Malasanos L, Barkauskas V, and Stoltenberg-Allen K: *Health assessment,* ed 4, St Louis, 1990, Mosby.

Pierson DJ and Wilkins RL: Clinical skills in respiratory care. In Pierson DJ and Kacmarek RM, editors: *Foundations of respiratory care,* New York, 1992, Churchill Livingstone.

Scanlon C, Spearman CB, and Sheldon RL: *Egan's fundamentals of respiratory care,* ed 5, St Louis, 1990, Mosby.

Chapter 2

Interviewing and Respiratory History

Susan Jones Krider

LEARNING OBJECTIVES

Upon completion of this chapter, the reader should be able to accomplish the following:

1. *Describe the importance of properly obtaining and recording a patient history.*

2. *Recognize factors which can influence communication between the patient and clinician during the interview.*

3. *Describe techniques for structuring the interview.*

4. *Describe the techniques used to facilitate conversational interviewing.*

5. *Recognize alternate sources that are available for the patient history.*

6. *Describe or recognize the components of a complete health history.*

7. *Recognize the definition, cause(s), characteristics, and typical diseases associated with the following pulmonary symptoms:*
   a. *cough*
   b. *shortness of breath (including orthopnea, paroxysmal nocturnal dyspnea, and platypnea)*
   c. *sputum production*
   d. *fever*
   e. *hemoptysis*
   f. *chest pain*
   g. *dependent edema*

Chapter Outline

Interviewing the Patient
Principles of Communication
Structuring the Interview
Questions and Statements Used to Facilitate
   Conversational Interviewing
Alternative Sources for a Patient History

Pulmonary History

Comprehensive Health History
Chief Complaint
History of Present Illness
Past History
Family History
Occupational and Environmental History
Nursing Assessment Standards for Adult Patients with
   Pulmonary Dysfunction

Common Symptoms of Pulmonary Disorders

Coughing
Shortness of Breath (Dyspnea)
Sputum Production
Hemoptysis
Chest Pain
Noisy Breathing
Hoarseness or Voice Changes
Dizziness and Fainting (Syncope)
Swelling of the Ankles (Dependent Edema)
Long Bone, Joint, and Muscle Pain
Fever, Chills, and Night Sweats
Headache, Altered Mental Status, and Personality
  Changes

Chapter Overview

The history is the foundation of comprehensive assessment. It is a written picture of the patient's perception of his or her past and present health status and how health problems have affected both personal and family life style. Properly recorded, it provides an organized, unbiased, detailed, and chronologic description of the development of symptoms that caused the patient to seek health care. The history guides the rest of the assessment process: physical examination, x-ray and laboratory studies, and special diagnostic procedures. When skillfully done, the history often provides sufficient information for an accurate diagnosis. It has been said that at least 75% of the time a diagnosis can be made after the history has been taken and before the physical examination begins.

Traditionally, the task of obtaining a patient's complete history has belonged to the physician, and only sections of the history were taken by other members of the health care team. Today, however, complete health histories are taken by nurses and physician's assistants. Physical therapists, social workers, dietitians, and respiratory care practitioners working in rehabilitation, home care, or pulmonary function laboratories complete histories, placing emphasis on information pertaining to their specialty.

Regardless of whether a student or clinician is expected to obtain and write a comprehensive history, each must be able to locate and interpret historical information recorded in the medical record. The information is used with other assessment data to develop or alter a plan of care. In addition, obtaining *subjective data*—that which the patient reports, feels, or experiences that cannot be perceived by an observer—is an important part of assessing the effects of therapeutic intervention. Those involved in direct patient care obtain subjective data from patients each day through interview and general conversation. The same techniques are used to identify, clarify, and communicate subjective and historical information.

This chapter highlights interviewing principles and the types of questions used in history taking; describes the content of the comprehensive health history, emphasizing specific information needed for assessment of the patient with pulmonary complaints; and discusses the most common pulmonary symptoms.

Interviewing the Patient

Principles of Communication

Communication is a process of imparting a meaningful message. If the receiver does not understand the message, communication has not occurred. Multiple personal and environmental factors affect the way both patients and health care professionals send and receive messages. Figure 2–1 shows the multiple factors that can influence communication during an interview. Attention to the potential effects each of these components may have on communication makes the difference between an effective and ineffective interview.

Each person brings to an interchange with another individual attitudes and values developed by previous experiences, cultural heritage, religious beliefs, level of education, and self-concept. These internal forces alter the way a message is sent as well as the interpretation of an incoming message. Messages can be sent in a variety of ways and at times without awareness. Body movement, facial expression, touch, and eye movement are all types of *nonverbal communication*. Combined with voice tone, body language (nonverbal communication) frequently says more than words. Since one of the purposes of the interview is to establish a trusting relationship (rapport) with the patient, the interviewer must make a conscious effort to send signals of compassion, empathy, and professionalism.

Messages are also altered by feelings, language barriers (jargon as well as foreign languages), listening habits, comfort with the situation, and preoccupation. Patients experiencing pain or difficulty in breathing have a hard time concentrating on the content of an interview until their comfort is restored. The temperature, lighting, noise, and privacy of the environment, to say nothing of the patient's attire (or lack thereof), also contribute greatly to comfort. Patients may communicate their discomfort nonverbally. Sighing, restlessness, looking into space, and avoiding eye contact may be clues that the patient is experiencing physical or psychologic discomfort. In one case, a trip to the bathroom may reestablish communication; in another,

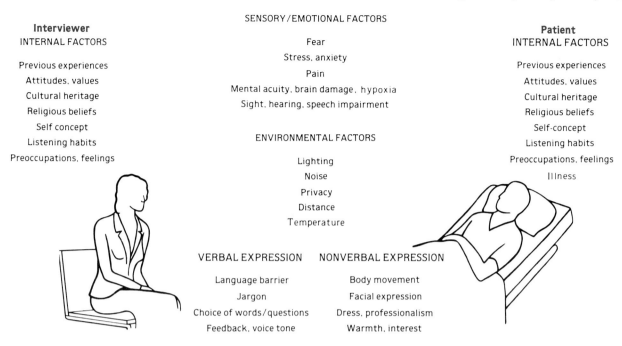

Fig. 2-1 *Factors that influence communication.*

changing the current topic of the interview may solve the problem.

Structuring the Interview

The ideal interview, whether a 5-minute assessment of therapy or a 50-minute history, is one in which the patient feels secure and free to talk about important personal things. Interviewing is an art that takes time and experience to develop. It is a skill as useful in daily patient care as it is to the person obtaining a comprehensive history. Keeping the following points in mind facilitates an effective interaction with the patient.

1. *Your ability to project a sense of undivided interest in the patient is the key to a successful interview and patient rapport.*
   - Provide for privacy. Don't permit interruptions.
   - Review records or new information and prepare equipment and charting materials before entering the room.
   - Listen and observe carefully. Avoid worrying about what to say next while the patient is talking. Rather, be attentive and respond to the patient's priorities, concerns, feelings, and comfort.
2. *Your introduction establishes your professional role, asks permission to be involved in the patient's care, and conveys your interest in the patient.*
   - Dress and groom professionally.
   - Enter with a smile and unhurried manner.

- Make immediate eye contact and, if the patient is well enough, introduce yourself with a firm handshake.
- State your role and the purpose of your visit, and define the patient's involvement in the interaction.
- Call the patient by name. A person's name is one of the most important things in the world to that person; use it to identify the patient and establish the fact that you are concerned with the patient as an individual. Address adult patients by title—Mr., Mrs., or Ms.—and their last name. Occasionally patients will ask to be called by their first name or nickname, but that is the patient's choice and not an assumption to be made by the health care professional. Keep in mind that by using the more formal terms of address you alert the patient to the importance of the interaction.
3. *Professional conduct shows your respect for the patient's beliefs, attitudes, and rights and enhances patient rapport.*
   - Be sure the patient is appropriately covered.
   - Position yourself so that eye contact is comfortable for the patient. Ideally, patients should be sitting up with their eye level at or slightly above yours, which suggests that their opinion is important too. Avoid positions that require the patient to look directly into the light.

- Avoid standing at the foot of the bed or with your hand on the door while you talk with the patient. This may send the nonverbal message that you do not have time for the patient.
- Ask the patient's permission before moving any personal items or making adjustments in the room (see Chapter 1).
- Remember, the patient's dialogue with you and the medical record are *confidential.* The patient expects and the law demands that this information be shared only with other professionals directly involved in the patient's care. When a case is discussed for teaching purposes, the patient's identity should be protected.
- Be honest. Never guess at an answer or information you do not know. Remember too that you have neither the obligation nor the right to provide information beyond your scope of practice. Providing new information to the patient is the privilege and responsibility of the attending physician.
- Make no moral judgments about the patient. Set your values for patient care according to the patient's values, beliefs, and priorities. Belittling or laughing at a patient for any reason is unprofessional and intolerable.
- Expect a patient to have an emotional response toward illness and the health care environment and accept it. *Listen,* then clarify and teach, but *never argue.* If you are not prepared to explore the issues with the patient, contact someone who is.
- Adjust the time, length, and content of the interaction to your patient's needs. If the patient is in distress, obtain only the information necessary to clarify immediate needs. It may be necessary to repeat some questions again later, to schedule several short interviews, or to obtain the information from other sources.

4. *A relaxed, conversational style on the part of the health care professional with questions and statements that communicate empathy encourages patients to express their concerns.*
   - Expect and accept some periods of silence in a long or first interview. Both you and the patient need short periods to think out the correct responses.
   - Close even the briefest interview by asking if there is anything else the patient needs or wants to discuss and tell the patient when you will return.

Questions and Statements Used to Facilitate Conversational Interviewing

An interview made up of one direct question followed by an answer and another direct question is mechanical, monotonous, and anxiety-producing. This type of interview usually takes longer and acquires less pertinent information than a conversational interview; however, it is a characteristic pattern for people who are anxious about interviewing. A rambling discussion is also inefficient and frustrating. Using a conversational style by mixing the types of questions and responses described below encourages spontaneous descriptions by the patient while giving enough direction to clarify, quantify, and qualify details.

1. *Open-ended questions* encourage patients to describe events and priorities as they see them and thereby help bring out concerns and attitudes and promote understanding. Questions such as "What brought you to the hospital?" or "What happened next?" encourage conversational flow and rapport while giving patients enough direction to know where to start.
2. *Closed questions* such as "When did your cough start?" or "How long did the pain last?" focus on specific information and provide clarification.
3. *Direct questions* can be either open-ended or closed questions and always end in a question mark. Though they are used to obtain specific information, a series of direct questions or frequent use of the question "Why?" can sound intimidating.
4. *Indirect questions* are less threatening because they sound like statements: "I gather your doctor told you to take the treatments every four hours." Inquiries of this type also work well to confront discrepancies in the patient's statements: "If I understood you correctly, it is harder for you to breathe now than it was before your treatment."
5. *Neutral questions and statements* are preferred for all interactions with the patient. "What happened next?" and "Tell me more about . . ."are neutral open-ended questions. A neutral closed question might give a patient a choice of responses while focusing on the type of information desired: "Would you say there was a teaspoon, a tablespoon, or a half cup?" By contrast, leading questions such as "You didn't cough up blood, did you?" should be avoided because they imply a desired response.
6. *Reflecting* (echoing) is repeating words, thoughts, or feelings the patient has just stated and is a successful way to clarify and stimulate the patient to elaborate on a particu-

lar point. However, overuse of reflecting can make the interviewer sound like a parrot.

7. *Facilitating phrases* like "yes" or "umm" or "I see," used while establishing eye contact and perhaps nodding your head, show interest and encourage patients to continue their story, but do not overuse this type of phrase.

8. *Communicating empathy (support)* with statements like "That must have been very hard for you" shows your concern for the patient as a human being. Showing the patient that you really care about how life situations have caused stress, hurt, or happiness tells the patient it is safe to risk being honest about real concerns. Other techniques for showing empathy were described in Chapter 1.

Alternative Sources for a Patient History

Various factors affect the patient's ability or willingness to provide an accurate history. Age, alterations in level of consciousness, language and cultural barriers, emotional state, ability to breathe comfortably, and the acuteness of the disease process may alter a patient's ability to communicate. For instance, the patient suffering an acute asthma attack or someone just admitted to an intensive care unit may be unable to give even the most brief history. Patients with longstanding chronic disease may have become so accustomed to the accompanying symptoms or their lives may have changed so gradually that they may minimize and even deny symptoms. In such cases family members, friends, work associates, previous physicians, and past medical records often can provide a more accurate picture of the history and progression of symptoms. Keeping these possibilities in mind, most hospital histories begin with a one- or two-sentence description of the current state of the patient, the source of the history, and a statement of the estimated reliability of the patient.

Pulmonary History

Abnormalities of the respiratory system are frequently manifestations of other systemic disease processes. Additionally, alterations in pulmonary function may affect all body systems. Therefore, pulmonary assessment cannot be limited to the chest; a comprehensive evaluation of the patient's entire health status is essential. A detailed discussion of all aspects of obtaining and recording such a health history is beyond the scope of this text but has been well covered by other authors.[1-4] This section provides an overview of the content of complete health histories and discusses specifically (in their classic order) chief complaint, history of present illness, past history, family history, and occupational and environmental history.

Comprehensive Health History

Health (medical) histories vary in length, organization, and content depending on the preparation and experience of the interviewer, the patient's age, the reason for obtaining the history, and circumstances surrounding the visit or admission. A history taken for a 60-year-old person complaining of chronic and debilitating symptoms is much more detailed and complex than that obtained for a summer camp applicant or a school physical. Histories recorded in emergency situations are usually limited to describing events surrounding the patient's immediate condition, with hours and sometimes days before a name, much less a complete history, can be obtained. Nursing histories emphasize the effect of the symptoms on activities of daily living and the identification of the unique care, teaching, and emotional support needs of the patient and family. Histories done by physicians emphasize making a diagnosis. Since diagnosis and initial treatment may be done before there is time to dictate or record the history, the experienced physician may record data obtained from a combination of the history, physical examination, laboratory tests, and x-ray films rather than the more traditional history outlined in the accompanying box. Although these variations in recording styles do exist, all histories contain the same types of information: general background, screening, and description of present health status or illness.[5,6]

Background information tells the interviewer who the patient is and what types of diseases are likely to develop. It also provides a basic understanding of the patient's previous experiences with illness and health care and the patient's current life situation, including the impact of culture, attitudes, relationships, and finances on health. Knowing the level of education, patterns of health-related learning, past health care practices, and reasons for compliance or noncompliance with past courses of therapy gives insight into patients' ability to comprehend their current health status. This may predict their willingness or ability to participate in learning and therapy. From the free discussion used to obtain background information, the interviewer may also get a clue as to patients' reliability and to possible psychosocial implications of their disease.

Conversely, *screening information* is designed to uncover problem areas the patient forgot to mention or omitted. This information is classically obtained by a head-to-toe review of all body systems but may also be obtained by a review of common diseases or from a description of body functions. Experienced examiners usually elicit the *review of systems (ROS)* in conjunction with the system-by-system physical examination; however, the two must not be confused. The physical examination provides *objective data:* that which can be seen, felt, smelled, or heard by the examiner, commonly

OUTLINE OF A COMPLETE HEALTH HISTORY

1. **Demographic data** (usually found on first page of chart)
   Name, address, age, birth date, place of birth, race, nationality, marital status, religion, occupation, source of referral
2. **Date and source of history,** estimate of reliability of historian
3. **Brief description of patient's condition at time of history or patient profile**
4. **Chief complaint:** reason for seeking health care
5. **History of present illness** (chronologic description of each symptom):
   Onset: time, type, source, setting
   Frequency and duration
   Location and radiation
   Severity (quantity)
   Quality (character)
   Aggravating/alleviating factors
   Associated manifestations
6. **Past history or past medical history**
   Childhood diseases and development
   Hospitalizations, surgeries, injuries, accidents, major illnesses
   Allergies
   Drugs and medications
   Immunizations
   Habits
   General health and sources of previous health care
7. **Family history**
   Familial disease history
   Family history
   Marital history
   Family relationships
8. **Social and environmental history**
   Education
   Military experience
   Occupational history
   Religious and social activities
   Living arrangements
   Hobbies and recreation
   Satisfaction/stress with life situation, finances, relationships
   Recent travel or other event that might affect health
9. **Review of systems** (Fig. 2–2)
10. **Signature**

only to the patient and cannot be perceived by an observer or is no longer present for the observer to see and therefore can only be described by the patient. Subjective manifestations of disease are termed *symptoms*.

The review of systems is a recording of past and present information that may be relevant to the present problem but might otherwise have been overlooked. It is grouped by body or physiologic systems to guarantee completeness and to assist the examiner in arriving at a diagnosis. Fig. 2–2 is an example of a review of systems checklist that may be completed by a patient before an interview or by an examiner. It provides for recording both positive and negative responses so that when the documentation is later reviewed, there is no doubt as to which questions were asked. Negative responses to important questions asked at any time during the interview are termed *pertinent negatives;* affirmative responses are termed *pertinent positives.*

All histories contain a *description of the patient's current health or illness.* Chief complaint (CC) and history of present illness (HPI) are the most commonly used headings, although reason for visit and current health status may be seen in some outpatient records. Since it is this information that most concerns the patient, the interview and recording of the history begin with this information.

Chief Complaint

The chief complaint is a brief notation explaining why the patient sought health care. It is the answer to such open-ended questions as "What brought you to the hospital?" or "What is bothering you the most?" Each symptom is recorded separately with its duration or date of initial occurrence. Ideally, symptoms are written in the patient's own words. They should not be diagnostic statements, someone else's opinion, or vague generalities. At times, more directed questions such as "Could you describe what you mean by not enough air?" or "In what ways don't you feel well?" are necessary to clarify the changes in perceptions or body functions experienced by the patient.

Asking the patient to recount the sequence of symptoms and then closing this section of the interview with a question such as "What else is bothering you?" often elicits problems the patient forgot to mention or was too uncomfortable to mention earlier. Now the interviewer is left with two types of problems: (1) those related to the chief complaint and (2) those that are important to the patient but may have little or no relationship to the present illness. The interviewer must now group the problems and decide how to proceed with the interview. Problems not related to the illness are usually incorporated with an appropriate section of background data when the history is written. The symptoms relating the current illness are listed as the chief complaint and then investigated one by one and described in detail under history of present illness.

referred to as *signs*. On the other hand, the review of systems provides *subjective data:* that which is evident

Have you recently had the following. Circle 'yes' or 'no'; if in doubt, leave blank

General
- Tire easily, weakness — yes no
- Marked weight change — yes no
- Night sweats — yes no
- Persistent fever — yes no
- Sensitivity to heat — yes no
- Sensitivity to cold — yes no

Skin
- Eruptions (rash) — yes no
- Change in color — yes no
- Change in hair — yes no
- Change in nails — yes no

Eyes
- Trouble seeing — yes no
- Eye pain — yes no
- Inflamed eyes — yes no
- Double vision — yes no
- Worn glasses — yes no

Ears
- Loss of hearing — yes no
- Ringing in ears — yes no
- Discharge — yes no

Nose
- Loss of smell — yes no
- Frequent colds — yes no
- Obstruction — yes no
- Excess discharge — yes no
- Nosebleeds — yes no

Mouth
- Sore gums — yes no
- Soreness of tongue — yes no
- Dental problems — yes no

Throat
- Postnasal drainage — yes no
- Soreness — yes no
- Hoarseness — yes no

Breasts
- Lumps — yes no
- Discharge — yes no

Cardio-Respiratory System
- Cough, persisting — yes no
- Sputum (phlegm) — yes no
- Bloody sputum — yes no
- Wheezing — yes no
- Chest pain or discomfort — yes no
- Pain on breathing — yes no
- Shortness of breath — yes no
- Difficulty breathing while lying down — yes no
- Swelling of ankles — yes no
- Bluish fingers or lips — yes no
- High blood pressure — yes no
- Palpitations — yes no
- Vein trouble — yes no

Digestive System Indicate average food selection each meal:

Breakfast _____

Lunch _____

Dinner _____

- Change in appetite — yes no
- Difficulty swallowing — yes no
- Heartburn — yes no
- Abdominal distress — yes no
- Belching or excess gas — yes no
- Abdominal enlargement — yes no
- Nausea — yes no
- Vomiting — yes no
- Vomiting of blood — yes no
- Rectal bleeding — yes no
- Tarry stools — yes no
- Dark urine — yes no
- Jaundice — yes no
- Constipation — yes no
- Diarrhea — yes no
- Hemorrhoids — yes no
- Need for laxatives — yes no

Genitourinary System
- Increase in frequency of urination (day) — yes no
- Increase in frequency of urination (night) — yes no
- Feel need to urinate without much urine — yes no
- Unable to hold urine — yes no
- Pain or burning — yes no
- Blood in urine — yes no
- Albuminuria — yes no
- Impotence — yes no
- Lack of sex drive — yes no
- Pain with intercourse — yes no

Endocrine
- Thyroid trouble — yes no
- Adrenal trouble — yes no
- Cortisone treatment — yes no
- Diabetes — yes no

Locomotor
- Muscle cramps — yes no
- Muscle weakness — yes no
- Pain in joints — yes no
- Swollen joints — yes no
- Stiffness — yes no
- Deformity of joints — yes no

Nervous System
- Headaches — yes no
- Dizziness — yes no
- Fainting — yes no
- Convulsions or fits — yes no
- Nervousness — yes no
- Sleeplessness — yes no
- Depression — yes no
- Change in sensation — yes no
- Memory loss — yes no
- Poor coordination — yes no
- Weakness or paralysis — yes no

GYN-OB

Started menstruating at age _____ Date of last PAP test _____

Interval between periods _____ days   Duration _____ days

Flow: light   normal   heavy   Date of last period _____

Pain with periods   yes   no   duration _____

Number of pregnancies _____   Number of miscarriages _____

Number of births _____

Wt. of babies at birth _____

Fig. 2–2 *Review of systems form that can be completed by patient or examiner.*

Once written, the chief complaint should express the patient's, not the examiner's, priorities; provide a capsule account of the patient's illness; and guide the collection of the history of present illness.

The symptoms most commonly associated with problems of the respiratory system include coughing with or without sputum production (expectoration), breathlessness (dyspnea), chest pain, and wheezing, commonly described as chest tightness. Other symptoms associated with respiratory problems include coughing up blood (hemoptysis), hoarseness, voice changes, dizziness and fainting (syncope), headache, altered mental status, and ankle swelling. These symptoms are discussed at the end of this chapter. Some pulmonary symptoms like bluish discoloration of the nail beds, especially with exertion (cyanosis), can also be seen by the examiner; therefore they can be both a sign and a symptom. Common pulmonary signs are discussed in Chapter 4.

Patients with pulmonary problems may also have any of the so-called *constitutional symptoms*, those commonly occurring with problems in any of the body systems. Constitutional symptoms include chills and fever, excessive sweating, loss of appetite (anorexia), nausea, vomiting, weight loss, fatigue, weakness, exercise intolerance, and altered sleep patterns. Hay fever, allergies, acute sinusitis, postnasal discharge, and frequent bouts of colds or "flu" are upper respiratory tract symptoms commonly associated with pulmonary disease.

History of Present Illness

The history of present illness is the narrative portion of the history that describes chronologically and in detail each symptom listed in the chief complaint and its effect on the patient's life. It is the most difficult portion of the history to obtain and record accurately, but it is the information that guides the physical examination and diagnostic testing to follow. All caregivers should be familiar with the history of present illness for each of their patients.

Encouraging the patient to talk freely about each problem allows maximal information to be obtained. The patient is first asked to describe the progression of symptoms from the first occurrence to the present. Occasionally, patients are unable to recall the first occurrence of the symptom, and the chronologic picture must then be developed by working backward from the most recent event. Once a rough chronologic picture is outlined, the interviewer obtains a description of each symptom by using an open-ended approach like "Now tell me about your . . . (cough, chest pain, etc.)." Using silence, nonverbal clues (like leaning forward expectantly), and facilitative expressions such as "Yes," "hmm," and "Tell me more about . . . ," or restating or summarizing what the patient just said shows interest and encourages the patient to continue talking. When the patient exhausts the spontaneous description of each symptom, directed questions are used to elicit whatever additional information is necessary. Questions that can be answered with yes or no and leading questions are avoided. For example, "What brings on your cough?" encourages more accurate information than a question like "The only time you cough is when you first get up in the morning, isn't it?" Since most patients want to please the interviewer, they are likely to agree with a leading question rather than report the specific information needed.

When the patient's descriptions and the interviewer's clarifying questions are complete, the following information should have been gathered for each symptom listed in the chief complaint and each additional symptom identified during the interview:

1. *Description of onset:* date, time, type (sudden or gradual)
2. *Setting:* cause, circumstance, or activity surrounding onset
3. *Location:* where on the body the problem is located and whether or not it radiates
4. *Severity:* how bad it is; how it affects activities of daily living
5. *Quantity:* how much, how large an area, or how many

6. *Quality:* what it is like, character or unique properties such as color, texture, odor, composition, sharp, viselike, throbbing
7. *Frequency:* how often it occurs
8. *Duration:* how long it lasts, constant or intermittent
9. *Course:* if it is getting better, worse, or staying the same
10. *Associated symptoms:* symptoms from the same body system or other systems that occur before, with, or following the problem
11. *Aggravating factors:* things that make it worse such as position, weather, temperature, anxiety, exercise
12. *Alleviating factors:* things that make it better such as position, hot, cold, rest

Various listings and mnemonic devices have been suggested to help the novice remember all of the information necessary to fully describe a symptom. One such mnemonic device is PQRST.[7,8]

P Provocative/palliative: What is the cause? What makes it better? What makes it worse?
Q Quality/quantity: How much is involved? How does it look, feel, sound?
R Region/radiation: Where is it? Does it spread?
S Severity scale: Does it interfere with activities? (Rate on scale of 1 to 10.)
T Timing: When did it begin? How often does it occur? Is it sudden or gradual?

Once all the information is collected, it is written in narrative form with a paragraph given to each time division in the chronologic progression of the symptom(s). The left-hand margin of the page or the first few words of each paragraph are used to identify the applicable date or the time period (days, weeks, months, or years) prior to admission (PTA).

By the time each symptom is reviewed in detail, even a novice is usually able to assign the majority of the symptoms to one body system. The pertinent points of the review of systems, personal history, and family history are reviewed for the applicable body system(s). The pertinent negatives as well as positives are recorded. Usually, when writing the review of systems, the interviewer puts "see HPI" behind the applicable body system rather than restating data previously recorded.

Past History

The past history, also called the *past medical history,* is a written description of the patient's past medical problems. It may include previous experiences with health care, and personal attitudes and habits that may affect both health and compliance with medical treatment plans. Information recorded in the past history includes a chronologic listing of the following:

1. Illnesses and development since birth
2. Surgeries and hospitalizations
3. Injuries and accidents
4. Immunizations
5. Allergies, including a description of the allergic reactions and effective treatment
6. Medications, both prescribed by a physician and over-the-counter (OTC) drugs, vitamins, and "home remedies"
7. Names of physicians and sources and types of previous health care
8. Habits, including diet, sleep, exercise, and the use of alcohol, coffee, tobacco, and illicit drugs
9. Description of general health

PERSONAL HISTORY
Birthplace _____ Date _____
Nationality _____ Religion _____
Marital status _____ Health of spouse _____
Occupations _____

Residence past 5 years: _____
Education through_____grade   Sleep (usual hrs.) ____ Aids to sleep _____
Recreation _____
Exercise _____
Average per day:
    Alcohol (type) _____
    Tobacco (type) _____
    Tea, coffee _____

Medicines taken regularly	Reason	Last Dose

PERSONAL PAST HISTORY

Circle 'yes' or 'no'   Circle 'yes' or 'no'

Have you ever had:			Year	Operations:			Year
Measles	yes	no		Tonsils	yes	no	
Mumps	yes	no		Appendix	yes	no	
Whooping cough	yes	no		Gall bladder	yes	no	
Polio	yes	no		Stomach	yes	no	
Scarlet fever	yes	no		Breast	yes	no	
Diphtheria	yes	no		Uterus and/or ovary	yes	no	
Meningitis	yes	no		Prostate	yes	no	
Infectious mono	yes	no		Hernia	yes	no	
Valley fever	yes	no		Thyroid	yes	no	
Tuberculosis	yes	no		Varicose veins	yes	no	
Exposure to TB	yes	no		Hemorrhoids	yes	no	
Malaria	yes	no		Heart	yes	no	
Hives	yes	no		Other	yes	no	
Cancer	yes	no		Injuries:			
Venereal disease	yes	no		Head	yes	no	
Arthritis	yes	no		Chest	yes	no	
Back trouble	yes	no		Abdomen	yes	no	
Bronchitis	yes	no		Broken bones	yes	no	
Pneumonia	yes	no		Back	yes	no	
Pleurisy	yes	no		Other	yes	no	
Asthma	yes	no		Allergies (are you allergic to):			
Emphysema	yes	no		Tetanus antitoxin	yes	no	
Rheumatic fever	yes	no		Penicillin	yes	no	
High blood pressure	yes	no		Sulfa	yes	no	
Heart disease	yes	no		Other drugs	yes	no	
Anemia	yes	no		List _____			
Bleeding tendency	yes	no					
Blood transfusion	yes	no		Foods	yes	no	
Hepatitis	yes	no		Cosmetics	yes	no	
(yellow jaundice)				Other	yes	no	
Ulcer	yes	no		Immunizations:			
Hemorrhoids	yes	no		Smallpox	yes	no	
Bladder infections	yes	no		Tetanus	yes	no	
Kidney disease	yes	no		Polio shots	yes	no	
Hay fever/sinusitis	yes	no		Polio oral	yes	no	
Glaucoma	yes	no		Other	yes	no	
Nose bleeds	yes	no					

Fig. 2-3 *Form for recording personal history and personal past history (past medical history).*

Forms (Fig. 2–3) may be used by either the patient or the interviewer to record concisely much of the information just listed. It is important to record the dates of accidents, major illnesses, hospitalizations, and immunizations. If past medical records are needed during the patient's hospitalization, the names and addresses of hospitals and physicians that have provided care to the patient in the past should be recorded.

There is a strong link between the use of illicit drugs and respiratory problems; however, an honest history of drug abuse is extremely difficult if not impossible for even the most experienced examiner to obtain. It is often the staff members giving routine daily care who have the first indication that drug abuse may be implicated in the patient's respiratory complaints. The patient should be encouraged to share this information honestly with the primary physician so that the best treatment can be obtained as early as possible. Staff members and students must remember that free dissemination of such information is a breach of confidentiality and may result in losing the patient's trust. Also, concluding too quickly that a drug history is the cause of the patient's problem may result in a missed diagnosis and an improper treatment program.

Because of the strong relationship between smoking and chronic pulmonary diseases, respiratory infections, lung cancer, and cardiovascular diseases, a careful and accurate smoking history is important. It is preferable to ask a patient "What types of tobacco have you used?" rather than "Do you smoke?" Use of pipes, cigars, marijuana, chewing tobacco, or snuff is usually recorded in terms of the amount used daily. The consumption of cigarettes is recorded in "pack-years." A *pack-year* is the number of years the patient has smoked times the number of packs smoked each day. If a patient smoked three packs a day for 10 years, it would be recorded as a 30-pack-year smoking history. It is also important to record the age when the patient began to smoke, variations in smoking habits over the years, the type and length of the cigarettes smoked, the habit of inhaling, the number and success of attempts to stop smoking, and the date when the patient last smoked. Members of the health care team have a professional responsibility to educate patients and their family about the harmful effects of smoking and guide them to programs designed to help people stop smoking.

For patients with pulmonary complaints, it is important to ask about the frequency and treatment of each of the following diseases: pneumonia, pleurisy, fungal diseases, tuberculosis, colds, sinus infections, bronchiectasis, asthma, allergies, pneumothorax, bronchitis, or emphysema. Because of the close relationship between the heart and the lungs, it is also important to know if the patient has a history of heart attack, hypertension (high blood pressure), heart failure, or congenital heart disease. Dates and types of heart or chest surgery and trauma should be recorded. Dates and results of tests that assess pulmonary status, including chest x-ray films, bronchoscopy, pulmonary function tests, and skin tests, should also be documented. Patients' discussion of previous diseases, tests, and treatments gives a good indication of their understanding of the disease process and compliance with medical therapy.

Family History

The purposes of the family history are to learn about the health status of the patient's blood relatives and immediate family, the presence within the family of diseases with hereditary tendencies, and sources of physical, emotional, or economic support or stress within the family structure.

To assess the current health status of the extended family, the patient is asked to describe the present age and state of health of blood relatives for three generations: siblings, parents, aunts and uncles, and grandparents. The resulting information may be recorded in narrative style, drawn schematically as a family tree, or written on a form like the one shown in Figure 2–4. When patients are asked to complete a form before an interview, the responses should be reviewed and notations added as necessary to capture the age and cause of death or current health status for each family member. A notation such as "18 A/W" indicates that the patient listed was 18 years old and alive and well on the day the history was recorded.

The health of the current family of a patient who was adopted is important for identification of communicable and environmentally related diseases; however, a history of the patient's true blood relatives is needed to assess genetically transmitted diseases or illnesses with strong familial relationships.

In addition to documenting the current health status of the family members, a review of diseases with strong hereditary or familial tendencies is also performed. Fig. 2–4 shows a form that permits either the patient or examiner to record the presence or absence of the most frequently reviewed diseases known to occur in the patient's family (pertinent positives) and those denied by the patient (pertinent negatives).

Patients with pulmonary complaints are asked specifically about the following diseases or problems, which have been shown to have a hereditary link with pulmonary disease: chronic allergies, asthma, lung cancer, cystic fibrosis, emphysema, neuromuscular disorders, kyphosis, scoliosis, sleep disturbances and sleep apnea, collagen-vascular diseases (such as lupus erythematosus), alpha$_1$-antitrypsin deficiency, cardiovascular disorders (such as hypertension, heart attack, heart failure, and congenital abnormalities), diabetes, and obesity. Since exposure to family and friends with infections can also result in pulmonary symptoms, the patient is asked about contact with, or family history of, frequent colds, tuberculosis, influenza, pneumonia, and fungal infections.

FAMILY HISTORY — Has any blood relative had any of the following:
Circle 'yes' or 'no' — if so, what relationship:

Anemia	yes	no	
Bleeding tendency	yes	no	
Leukemia	yes	no	
Repeated infections	yes	no	
Crippling infections	yes	no	
Heart disease	yes	no	
Chronic lung disease	yes	no	
Tuberculosis	yes	no	
High blood pressure	yes	no	
Kidney disease	yes	no	
Asthma	yes	no	
Severe allergies	yes	no	
Mental illness	yes	no	
Convulsions or fits	yes	no	
Migraine headaches	yes	no	
Diabetes	yes	no	
Gout	yes	no	
Obesity	yes	no	
Thyroid trouble	yes	no	
Peptic ulcer	yes	no	
Chronic diarrhea	yes	no	
Cancer	yes	no	

	Present Age, or Age at Death	If living, health (good, fair, poor) if deceased, cause of death
Father		
Mother		
Brothers or Sisters		
1.		
2.		
3.		
4.		
5.		
6.		
7.		
Children		
1.		
2.		
3.		
4.		
5.		
6.		
7.		

Fig. 2–4 *Form for recording family history.*

Occupational and Environmental History

An occupational and environmental history[9–12] is particularly important in patients with pulmonary symptoms. The purpose is to elicit information concerning exposure to potential disease-producing substances or environments. Most occupational pulmonary diseases are the result of workers inhaling particles, dusts, fumes, or gases during the extraction, manufacture, transfer, storage, or disposal of industrial substances. However, the hazards of an industrial society are not limited to those working directly with the toxic substances. Other employees working in or near an industrial plant, as well as people living in the surrounding areas, are subject to breathing toxic fumes and dusts. Family members come in contact with contaminated clothing and may develop pulmonary disease years later. Accidental spills of toxic chemicals and gases can endanger and even necessitate evacuation and treatment of large numbers of people.[13]

Though there have been dramatic decreases in exposure to some hazardous materials, exposures to dusts, fumes, and chemicals from indoor as well as outdoor air pollutants continue to increase. Outbreaks of work-related illnesses in buildings not contaminated by industrial processes can be traced to these pollutants or simply to an inadequate provision of fresh air with no identifiable contaminant.[14] The terms *tight building syndrome* or *sick building syndrome* are now used to describe these epidemics in which large numbers of employees complain of symptoms, including runny or stuffy nose, eye irritation, cough, chest tightness, fatigue, headache, and malaise. Additionally, more than 200 agents have been shown to cause allergic occupational asthma. As this number grows, it appears that occupational asthma is becoming the most prevalent occupational lung disease.[15–18]

Reactions to inhalation of toxic substances can occur within minutes to hours (acute) or may take weeks, months, or years to develop (Table 2–1). Inhalation of soluble gases such as ammonia, chlorine, or sulfur dioxide causes sufficient upper airway irritation to warn workers of immediate danger. However, metal fumes and insoluble gases like phosgene and nitrogen dioxide are less irritating to the upper airways. Because they may be inhaled for long periods of time with little discomfort, workers are not warned to escape, and more severe pulmonary damage results.

Hypersensitivity reactions may be acute or delayed and often occur in patterns. Shortness of breath, wheezes, or flulike symptoms usually occur within 4 to 8 hours of exposure. However, symptoms may occur only at night and may recur for several nights following a single exposure. In some cases the most severe symptoms occur at the start of the workweek, and tolerance develops as the week progresses. Such a pattern, often termed *Monday fever,* is commonly seen with inhalation of cotton dust. More commonly, allergic reactions worsen with reexposure and decrease during days off. In subacute forms of hypersensitivity pneumonitis, symptoms occur insidiously over weeks. Most of the chronic occupational pulmonary diseases (pneumoconioses) take 20 years or more to become symptomatic. Whenever there is a delay in the development of pulmonary symptoms, their relationship to occupational and environmental exposure becomes obscure.

The occupational and environmental history therefore must be more than just a chronologic listing of job titles. Questioning may include the occupation of the patient's father and descriptions of childhood residences. Pneumoconiosis resulting from asbestos exposure (asbestosis) has been seen in people who lived near shipyards or asbestos dump sites as children and in people whose fathers were asbestos workers. The patient should be queried about location of schools,

summer jobs, dates and types of military service, and all subsequent full- and part-time jobs. The precise dates, duration, and activities of each job must be delineated. These include materials and processes involved, amount of workspace and type of ventilation, use of protective devices, cleanup practices, and work going on in adjacent areas.

Work or residence near mines, farms, mills, shipyards, or foundries should be clarified. Sources of possible irritants within the home such as humidifiers, air-conditioning systems, woodpiles, insulation, smoking, paints and glues used for hobbies, and household pets must also be reviewed.

It is important to review the various places a patient has lived or visited for any period of time. Certain fungal infections that involve the respiratory system have strong geographic relationships. Histoplasmosis is particularly common in Ohio, Maryland, the central Mississippi Valley, and the Appalachian Mountains, blastomycosis in the southeastern United States, especially Texas and the San Joaquin Valley in California, as well as sections of South America.

When the pulmonary history is written, occupational and environmental histories are usually given specific headings because of the detail recorded. However, in most routine histories this information may be found under general headings such as personal history, social history, psychosocial history, or social-environmental history.

Nursing Assessment Standards for Adult Patients with Pulmonary Dysfunction

The beginning student may be confused by the fact that the patient's medical record contains more than one style of history done on or about the same date. This occurs in teaching institutions because students and residents see the patient, as well as the attending physician. It also occurs because each of the health care professions is responsible for specifying the scope of practice for its practitioners and monitoring the quality of their performance. As a result, there may be patient histories completed by nursing and several allied health professions in addition to those done by physicians. In 1989, the Section on Nursing of the American Thoracic Society adopted specific standards of nursing care for adult patients with actual or potential pulmonary dysfunction.[19] These process and outcome standards are used within the "nursing process" (assessment, diagnosis, goal setting, intervention, and evaluation) to assure that the patient receives an acceptable level of care. The pulmonary history assessment guide from these standards is shown in Table 2–2. Note that in addition to gathering and analyzing the traditional pulmonary history, the nursing assessment is to include additional categories which focus on the

Table 2–1 Occupational Lung Diseases

Inhaled Substance	Occupation or Source	Usual Symptoms and Course	Disease Names
Acute airway or lung reactions			

Irritant gases
  Chlorine, ammonia, sulfur
    dioxide
	Various industries
	Accidental exposure
		Short exposure
		  Eye and airway irritation,
		    productive cough
		Prolonged exposure
		  Dyspnea, wheezing,
		    pulmonary edema	

Insoluble gases and metal fumes
  Nitrogen dioxide
	Filled silos, closed welding spaces, chemical laboratories	Very little airway irritation
		Headache, shortness of breath,
		  cough, chest tightness,
		  pulmonary edema
			Silo-filler's disease

Phosgene	Chemical warfare, heating metals treated with production chlorine and toluene diisocyanate (TDI)	Acute pulmonary edema, pneumonia	

Copper, zinc, iron, nickel, tin,
    antimony, manganese,
    magnesium
	Welders in closed spaces, mining, electroplating	Fever, malaise, nausea, aching
		  muscles, lasting 2–3 days
			Metal fume fever
			Galvanization
			Polymer fume fever

Cadmium, mercury, beryllium		Above with acute pulmonary edema and pneumonia	
Acute or subacute allergic reactions			

Toluene diisocyanate (TDI)
Proteolytic enzymes
  (detergents)
	Plastic and foam production
	Industrial accidents
	Manufacture of detergents
		Allergic reactions include:
		  Immediate or delayed
		    asthma-like reactions usually
		    occur in sensitive persons but
		    may occur in others; fever,
		    chills, malaise, weight loss,
		    nocturnal wheezing, cough,
		    cyanosis, dyspnea at rest
			Hypersensitivity pneumonitis
			Extrinsic allergic alveolitis
			Occupational asthma

Contaminated water	Air conditioners, humidifiers		Air conditioner (humidifier) lung

Droppings/feathers
  Pigeons, parakeets, chickens,
    turkeys
	Bird handlers	Acute reactions within 4–8 hr
		Delayed reactions occur at night
		  after leaving work environment
		In some cases, chronic disease
		  with fibrosis may develop if
		  repeated exposure continues
			Bird fancier's lung, ornithosis
			Pigeon breeder's lung

Pituitary extract/organic dusts
  Paprika, fishmeal, coffee
    bean, weevil-infested flour
	Workers with specific products		Pituitary-snufftaker's lung
			Paprika splitter's–fishmeal-coffee
			  bean–worker's lung
			Wheat-weevil lung

Cotton, hemp, flax
Fungal spores from moldy hay,
  straw, grains, malt, or barley,
  sugar cane (bagasse),
  mushroom compost, maple
  bark, logs, wood pulp (Western
  red cedar)
	Textile and farm workers
	Agriculture and farm workers
		"Monday fever"
		Repeated bouts of pneumonia
		  with symptoms listed and
		  weight loss
			Byssinosis (brown lung)
			Farmer's lung
			Malt-worker's lung
			Bagassosis
			Mushroom-handler's lung

	Wood and paper mill workers		Wood- and paper mill–worker's lung
	Lumbering		Maple bark–stripper's lung
Drugs and chemicals	Antibiotic, pharmaceutical, chemical manufacture		
Chronic Occupational lung diseases			

Crystalline-free silica	Sandblasters in enclosed spaces, manufacture of ceramics and abrasive agents, construction, mines, quarries, foundries: gold, copper, lead, zinc, iron, coal, granite	Acute—1–3 yr of intense
		  exposure
		  Shortness of breath, fever,
		    frequent pulmonary
		    infections
		Chronic—20 yr or more of
		  exposure
		  No symptoms to exertional
		    dyspnea, obstructed
		    breathing, productive cough,
		    reduced exercise tolerance,
		    chest pain, weight loss,
		    hemoptysis with fibrosis
		40+ yr: infection, cor
		  pulmonale
			Silicosis
			  Associated in unknown way
			    with rheumatoid arthritis and
			    scleroderma
			  High incidence of associated
			    tuberculosis and
			    bronchogenic cancer

Continued

Table 2–1	Occupational Lung Diseases—cont'd		
Inhaled Substance	**Occupation or Source**	**Usual Symptoms and Course**	**Disease Names**

Coal	Coal miners	Simple
		  Asymptomatic, cough with
		    smoking
		  Complicated with fibrosis
		    As just listed with black
		    sputum
			Coal-worker's pneumoconiosis
			Coal-miner's lung

Asbestos	Manufacture of fireproofing and
	  insulation, shipbuilding,
	  automobile mechanics (clutch
	  and brake), demolition workers,
	  fire fighters, living/working near
	  dumps or high-use areas
		External dyspnea, clubbing,
		  restricted breathing, rales at
		  lung bases usually appear
		  before x-ray film changes and
		  cancer symptoms approximately
		  20 yr after exposure
			Asbestosis

Other mineral dusts
  Fuller's earth, kaolin (China
  clay), graphite, tin, iron,
  mixed dusts, tungsten
	Quarrying, mining, milling,
	  drying, bagging, and loading
	  minerals
	  Welding and foundries
	  Manufacture of industrial
	  precision instruments
		Vary from asymptomatic with dust
		  retention to same as
		  complicated silicosis
			Pneumoconiosis
			
			Stannosis
			Siderosis

Beryllium	Nuclear physics, manufacture of
	  electronics, ceramics, x-ray tube
	  windows (in past: fluorescent
	  lights)
		Acute
		  Pulmonary edema,
		    pneumonia
		  Chronic granulomatous disease
		    appears years after
		    exposure
		  Dyspnea, dry cough, weakness,
		    weight loss, skin lesions, rales
			Pulmonary granuloma

Paraquat	Agriculture	Inhalation or ingestion may lead to pulmonary fibrosis	

patient's response to interferences with normal respiratory function, self-management capacity, resources, and knowledge of respiratory medications and treatments. Some hospitals are moving toward what is termed the *patient history,* one history per patient per admission, which is used and augmented by all the allied health professionals involved in the patient's care, as well as by physicians.

Common Symptoms of Pulmonary Disorders

The primary symptoms associated with pulmonary disorders are cough, sputum production, shortness of breath (dyspnea), wheezing, hemoptysis, and chest pain. Hoarseness or voice changes; dizziness and fainting; ankle swelling (peripheral edema); fever, chills, and night sweats; and long bone, joint, and muscle pain are frequent but less specific complaints. This section defines terms, briefly discusses causes (etiology), describes normal and abnormal characteristics, and lists related pulmonary symptoms and diseases for each of the symptoms just mentioned.

Coughing

Coughing is the most common symptom in patients with pulmonary disease.[6,20-23] It is a powerful protective reflex arising from stimulation of receptors located in the pharynx, larynx, trachea, large bronchi, and even the lung and the visceral pleura. Coughing can be produced by inflammatory, mechanical, chemical, or thermal stimulation of cough receptors anywhere from the oropharynx to the terminal bronchioles or simply by tactile pressure in the ear canal (Table 2–3).

Impulses generated by stimulation of the cough receptors are carried by efferent pathways of the reflex, primarily the vagus, phrenic, glossopharyngeal, and trigeminal nerves, to the cough center located diffusely in the medulla, separate from the respiratory center. Conduction of the impulses down the efferent pathway of the reflex stimulates the smooth muscles of the larynx and tracheobronchial tree via the vagus nerve and the diaphragm and other respiratory muscles via the phrenic and other spinal motor nerves. The cough mechanism can be divided into three phases.

1. *Inspiratory phase:* Reflex opening of the glottis and contraction of the diaphragm, thoracic, and abdominal muscles cause deep inspiration with a concomitant increase in lung volume accompanied by an increase in the caliber and length of the bronchi.
2. *Compression phase:* Closure of the glottis and relaxation of the diaphragm while the expiratory muscles contract against the closed glot-

Table 2-2 American Thoracic Society's Nursing Assessment Guide for Adult Patients with Pulmonary Dysfunction*

History and Symptoms Profile	Self-Management Capacity

Pulmonary Symptoms†
 Dyspnea
 Cough
 Sputum
 Hemoptysis
 Wheeze
 Chest pain (e.g., pleuritic)
 Extrapulmonary Symptoms†
 Night sweats
 Headaches on awakening *in the morning*
 Weight changes
 Fluid retention
 Nasal stuffiness, discharge
 Fatigue
 Orthopnea, paroxysmal nocturnal apnea
 Snoring, sleep disturbances, daytime drowsiness
 Sinus problems
 Pulmonary Risk Factors
 Smoking history
    Type (cigarettes, cigar, pipe)
    Amount per day
    Duration (yr)
 Childhood emergency diseases/symptoms
 Family history of respiratory disease
 Alcohol and chemical substance abuse
 Environmental exposures
    Location (e.g., home, work, region)
    Type (e.g., asbestos, silica, gases)
    Duration
 Obesity or nutritional depletion
 Compromised immune system function (e.g., IGg deficiency, human immunodeficiency virus (HIV) infection, alpha$_1$-antitrypsin deficiency)
 Previous History
 Pulmonary problems
 Treatments
 Number of hospitalizations
 Medical diagnosis(es)
 Immunizations
	Physical Ability (0-4 scale, 4=dependent)
	 Lower extremity (e.g., walking, stair climbing)
	 Upper extremity (e.g., hair care, meal preparation)
	 Activities of daily living
	    Toileting
	    Hygiene
	    Feeding
	    Dressing
	 Activity pattern during a typical day
	 Patient statement re: management of problems
	 Sensory-perceptual factors (e.g., vision, hearing)
	 Cognitive Ability
	 Mental age
	 Memory
	 Knowledge about diagnosis, treatment, and risk factors of pulmonary disease
	 Judgment
	 Psychosocial-Cultural Factors
	 Self-concept
	    Self-esteem
	    Body image
	    Role(s), changes
	 Value system (e.g., spiritual and health beliefs)
	 Coping mechanisms
	    Displaced anger
	    Anxiety
	    Hostility
	    Dependency
	    Withdrawal
	    Isolation
	    Avoidance
	    Denial
	    Noncompliance
	    Acceptance
	 Socioeconomic Factors
	 Social support system
	    Family
	    Significant others
	    Friends
	    Community resources
	    Government resources
	 Financial situation/health insurance
	 Employment/disability
	 Environmental factors
	 Home
	 Community
	 Worksite
	 Health care setting (e.g., hospital, nursing home)

*Adapted from American Thoracic Society Medical Section of the American Lung Association: Standards of nursing care for adult patients with pulmonary dysfunction, *Am Rev Respir Dis* 144:231, 1991.
†Consider onset, duration, character, precipitating, aggravating, and relieving factors of symptoms.

Table 2-3 Possible Causes of Cough Receptor Stimulation*

Types of Stimulation	Possible Causes
Inflammatory	Infection, lung abscess, drug reaction, allergy, edema, hyperemia, collagen-vascular disease, radiotherapy, pneumoconiosis, tuberculosis
Mechanical	Inhaled dusts
Obstructive	Foreign bodies, aspiration of nasal secretions, tumor or granulomas within or around the lung, aortic aneurysm
Airway wall tension	Pulmonary edema, atelectasis, fibrosis, chronic interstitial pneumonitis
Chemical	Inhaled irritant gases, fumes, smoke
Temperature	Inhaled hot or cold air
Ear	Tactile pressure in the ear canal (Arnold's nerve response) or from otitis media

*Adapted from Schmidt CO: In Conn HF and Conn RB, editors: *Current diagnosis*, ed 6, Philadelphia, 1980, WB Saunders.

tis generate very high intrathoracic pressures and narrowing of the trachea and bronchi.

3. *Expiratory phase:* Opening of the glottis, explosive release of trapped intrathoracic air, and vibration of the vocal cords and mucosal lining of the posterior laryngeal wall, which shakes secretions loose from the larynx, move undesired material out of the respiratory tract.

The cough reflex may be voluntary or involuntary and occurs in almost everyone. The efficiency of the cough (force of the airflow) is determined by the depth of the inspiration and amount of pressure that can be generated in the airways. The effectiveness of a cough is reduced if one or more of the following conditions exist:

1. Weakness of either the inspiratory or expiratory muscles
2. Inability of the glottis to open or close correctly
3. Obstruction, collapsibility, or alteration in shape or contours of the airways
4. Decrease in lung recoil as occurs with emphysema
5. Abnormal quantity or quality of mucus production

Cough may be *acute* (sudden onset, usually severe with a short course), *chronic* (persistent and troublesome for more than 3 weeks), or *paroxysmal* (periodic, prolonged, forceful episodes). An acute self-limiting cough is usually due to the common cold. Chronic persistent cough is most commonly caused by postnasal drip syndrome, followed by asthma, gastroesophageal reflux, chronic bronchitis, bronchiectasis, and other conditions such as left heart failure, bronchogenic cancer, and sarcoidosis. In smokers, chronic cough is usually due to chronic bronchitis. Postnasal drip, asthma, and gastroesophageal reflux account for most chronic coughs in nonsmokers who have a normal chest film and who are not taking angiotensin converting enzyme (ACE) inhibitors. Most patients will have a single cause for their cough; however, in about 25% of patients two or three simultaneous causes may be found for their chronic cough. Frequent, annoying, painful, or persistent cough or cough equivalent, such as throat clearing, is not normal, especially when it is productive.

Cough is not only a symptom of pulmonary problems, it may occur in conjunction with other pulmonary symptoms such as wheezing, stridor, chest pain, and dyspnea. Additionally, cough may cause problems. The vigorous muscular activity and high intrathoracic pressures created by chronic forceful coughing may produce a number of complications in addition to fatigue, including torn chest muscles, rib fractures, disruption of surgical wounds, pneumothorax or pneumomediasti-

num, syncope, arrhythmia, esophageal rupture, and urinary incontinence.

Cough should be described as *effective* (strong enough to clear the airway) or *inadequate* (audible but too weak to mobilize the secretions), *productive* (mucus or other material is expelled by the cough), or *dry* (moisture or secretions are not produced). Since dry coughs often become productive, a chronologic report of the circumstances surrounding the change and a description of the sputum should be recorded.

The quality, time, and setting in which a cough occurs may also provide some clues to the location and type of disorder (Table 2–4). *Barking* (like a seal bark), *brassy* (harsh, dry), and *hoarse* coughs and those associated with *inspiratory stridor* are usually heard when there is a problem with the upper airway; *wheezy* coughs (accompanied by whistling or sighing sounds) suggest bronchial disorders; and *chronic productive* coughs are generally indicative of significant bronchopulmonary disease. *Hacking* (frequent brief periods of coughing or clearing the throat) may be dry and may be the result of smoking, a viral infection, a nervous habit, or difficult-to-move secretions as occur with postnasal drip.

Acute onset or change in a cough is obvious to the patient and family and probably to the interviewer; therefore an accurate history is easily obtained. However, careful inquiry is often required to identify the characteristics of a chronic cough. Because coughing and sputum production are not socially acceptable, patients may deny or minimize their presence or learn to adapt to the extent that they may even be unaware of chronic coughing. Questioning family members or close friends may provide valuable information about the onset, persistence, duration, severity, and factors that precipitate and aggravate the coughing.

Shortness of Breath (Dyspnea)

Dyspnea (*dys,* difficult; *pnea,* breathing) is the patient's unpleasant awareness of difficulty breathing or "shortness of breath" in an inappropriate setting such as at rest or with limited exertion.[6,22–24] Patients may describe the feeling as "breathlessness" or a sensation of air hunger at rest or during exercise. Dyspnea is the most distressing symptom of respiratory disease, frequently causing the patient to cease physical activity and seek medical attention. It is also a cardinal symptom of cardiac disease. Dyspnea frequently impairs the ability to work or exercise and even interferes with the simplest activities of daily living like eating, bathing, speaking, and sleeping.

Dyspnea may be associated with an increase in the work of breathing, neurologic and metabolic disorders, severe anemia, acidosis, neuromuscular disorders, apprehension, and neurosis. In the last two situations, difficult breathing is more often associated with

Table 2-4 Terms Used to Describe Coughing

Description	Possible Causes*
Acute (<3 wks)	Postnasal drip, allergies, and infections, especially viral URI (common cold), bronchitis, laryngitis
Chronic (>3 wks) or recurrent (adults)	Postnasal drip, asthma, gastroesophageal reflux, chronic bronchitis, bronchiectasis, COPD, TB, lung tumor, ACE inhibitors, left heart failure, sarcoidosis, habit
Recurrent (children)	Viral bronchitis, asthma, allergies
Barking	Epiglottal disease, croup, influenza, laryngotracheal bronchitis
Brassy or hoarse	Laryngitis, laryngeal paralysis, laryngotracheal bronchitis, pressure on recurrent laryngeal nerve, mediastinal tumor, aortic aneurysm, left atrial enlargement
Inspiratory stridor	Tracheal or mainstem bronchial obstruction, croup, epiglottitis
Wheezy	Bronchospasm, asthma, cystic fibrosis, bronchitis
Dry	Viral infections, inhalation of irritant gases, interstitial lung diseases, tumor, pleural effusion, cardiac condition, nervous habit, radiation therapy, chemotherapy
Dry progressing to productive	Atypical and mycoplasmal pneumonia, legionnaires' disease, pulmonary embolus and edema, lung abscess, asthma, silicosis, emphysema (late in disease), smoking, AIDS
Chronic productive	Bronchiectasis, chronic bronchitis, lung abscess, asthma, fungal infections, bacterial pneumonias, tuberculosis
Inadequate *too old, too sick*	Debility, weakness, oversedation, pain, poor motivation
Paroxysmal (especially at night) *sudden onset*	Aspiration, asthma, left heart failure
Morning	Chronic bronchitis, smoking
Afternoon and evening	Exposure to irritants during the day
Associated with lying down or position change	Bronchiectasis, left heart failure, chronic postnasal drip or sinusitis, gastroesophageal reflux with aspiration
Associated with eating or drinking	Neuromuscular disease of the upper airway, esophageal problems, aspiration

*AIDS=acquired immunodeficiency syndrome; COPD=chronic obstructive pulmonary disease; TB=tuberculosis; ACE=angiotensin converting enzyme.

"sighing" respirations and irregular but normal respiratory rate and may be relieved by exertion.

Acute dyspnea in children is most frequently associated with asthma, epiglottitis, croup, and bronchiolitis. In adults with dyspnea, pulmonary embolism should be suspected if the patient is in the postoperative period, is pregnant or taking birth control pills, or has a history of prolonged bed rest, phlebitis, or cardiac arrhythmia. Asthma, upper airway obstruction, foreign body aspiration, pneumonia, pneumothorax, pulmonary edema, hyperventilation, and panic disorder may also cause acute dyspnea. The most common cause of *chronic* or *recurrent* dyspnea in children is asthma. Chronic obstructive pulmonary disease (COPD), chronic congestive heart failure, and severe anemia are the most common causes in adults, especially elderly patients. Heavy smoking, obesity, and inactivity are frequently associated with complaints of dyspnea associated with minimal exertion.

The neurophysiologic mechanisms causing dyspnea are not fully understood, but the signals of discomfort may originate from altered length-tension relationships in the respiratory muscles. The increased work of breathing resulting in the feeling of dyspnea is caused by restriction of the lung or chest (making it difficult to expand the lungs) and obstruction of the flow of air into and out of the lungs. In addition, hyperventilation from any cause increases airway resistance, leading to a feeling of dyspnea.

Occurrences of dyspnea should be chronologically recorded, including progression, duration, severity, and relationships to respiratory rate, coughing, wheezing, pain, position, and exertion. Coughing in conjunction with dyspnea occurs with acute or chronic infection, asthma, aspiration, many of the diffuse lung diseases, COPD, and congestive heart failure. Table 2-5 lists diseases commonly associated with dyspnea and the associated symptoms.

Patients may complain of dyspnea occurring at different times of the day or in association with a position or specific phase of the respiratory cycle. *Inspiratory dyspnea* is usually associated with upper airway obstruction, whereas *expiratory dyspnea* occurs with obstruction of smaller bronchi and bronchioles. *Paroxysmal nocturnal dyspnea (PND)* is the sudden onset of difficult breathing that occurs in a sleeping patient in the recumbent position. It is often associated with coughing and is relieved when the patient assumes an upright position. In patients with congestive heart failure, PND usually occurs 1 to 2 hours after lying down. In the patient with COPD, PND usually occurs on lying down and is often relieved by coughing and expectorating sputum. *Orthopnea* is the inability to breathe lying down. It is often described as two- or

Table 2-5 Some Diseases and Symptoms Associated with Dyspnea

Diseases	Dyspnea	Associated Symptoms
Emphysema	Predominant symptom, insidious onset, exertional, recumbent, may be relieved by coughing	Coughing in advanced stages
Asthma	Episodic, may be exertional, may be worse at night, symptom-free between attacks	Wheezing, productive coughing, tightness in chest
Chronic bronchitis	In advanced stages or with infection	Chronic, productive coughing
Upper airway obstruction	Severity is dependent on size of object/tumor, amount of edema	Coughing, possible dull or pleuritic pain
Pulmonary congestion		
Acute	Abrupt, slow regression	Tachypnea, "cardiac wheeze," coughing
Chronic	Gradual onset over time with orthopnea, paroxysmal nocturnal dyspnea	Tachypnea, "cardiac wheeze," coughing
Pneumothorax	Moderate to severe	Sudden and sharp pleuritic pain
Pleural effusion	Usually present	Possible pleuritic dull pain
Chest wall deformities	Only in severe deformities	Chest wall/back pain
Obesity, pickwickian syndrome	Only on exertion	Nighttime snoring, daytime sleepiness
Bacterial pneumonia	Exertional	Productive cough, pleuritic pain
Lung abscess	Frequent	Productive cough, pleuritic pain
Tuberculosis	Advanced cases	Productive cough, pleuritic pain
AIDS	Progressive, severe	Weight loss, fever, night sweats, diarrhea, enlarged lymph nodes
Diffuse lung disease (Hamman-Rich syndrome)	Present	Variable depending on disease; rate of respiration is increased
Pulmonary fibrosis		
Nonchemical (includes dusts, allergens)	Progressive, exertional, may occur 6–8 hr after exposure	Tachypnea, dry cough progressing to productive wheezing, pain
Chemical (drug-induced, toxic fumes)	Onset varies with agent, may be sudden and explosive	Wheezing, coughing, pain

three-pillow orthopnea, depending on the number of pillows the patient must use to elevate the upper portion of the body and obtain relief. PND and orthopnea are most commonly associated with left heart failure but may be seen in patients with other pulmonary problems. *Platypnea,* the opposite of orthopnea, is difficulty breathing while sitting up, which is relieved by recumbency. This rare symptom is usually caused by a right-to-left intracardiac shunt. It has been reported in postoperative pneumonectomy patients[20] and patients with cirrhosis or COPD.

The effects of dyspnea on activities of daily living (dressing, eating, sleeping, walking) must be reviewed. Patients with COPD tend to decrease their exercise progressively to prevent being short of breath until their activities of daily living are compromised out of proportion to their actual cardiorespiratory potential. It is essential to gain a picture of the patient's daily habits and routines as well as the physical, emotional, familial, and occupational environment. The potential for relief of the factors contributing to dyspnea should be assessed and recorded.

Sputum Production

Sputum is the substance expelled from the tracheobronchial tree, pharynx, mouth, sinuses, and nose by coughing or clearing the throat. The term *phlegm* refers strictly to secretions from the lungs and tracheobronchial tree. These respiratory tract secretions may contain a variety of materials including mucus, cellular debris, microorganisms, blood, pus, and foreign particles and should not be confused with saliva. The tracheobronchial tree normally secretes up to 100 mL of sputum each day, which is moved upward by the wavelike motion of the cilia (tiny hairlike structures) lining the larynx, trachea, and bronchi, and is usually swallowed unnoticed. As previously mentioned, sputum may be difficult or impossible for the patient to describe accurately because of social stigma and lack of awareness. Thus collection and inspection of a sample are often necessary.

Sputum should be described as to color, consistency, quantity, time of day, odor, and presence of blood or distinguishing matter. The character may be highly indicative of the underlying disorder (Table 2–6). The amount may vary from scanty (a few teaspoons) to copious (as much as a pint or more), which is seen in chronic bronchial and pulmonary inflammation. The consistency may be described as thin, thick, viscous (gelatinous), tenacious (extremely sticky), or frothy. Color depends on the origin and cause of the sputum production. Other descriptions include *mucoid* (clear, thin, may be somewhat viscid as a result of oversecretion of bronchial mucus), *mucopurulent* (thick, viscous, colored, and often in globs with an offensive odor), and

Table 2-6   Presumptive Sputum Analysis

Appearance of Sputum	Possible Cause
Mucoid	Bronchial asthma (small silicone-like bronchial casts), legionnaires' disease (grayish), pulmonary tuberculosis, emphysema, neoplasms, early chronic bronchitis
Mucopurulent	Above and infection, pneumonia, cystic fibrosis
Purulent	
Yellow or green, copious	Bronchiectasis (separates into layers), advanced chronic bronchitis, *Pseudomonas* pneumonia
Apple-green, thick	*Haemophilus influenzae* pneumonia
Pink, thin, blood-streaked	Streptococcal pneumonia, staphylococcal pneumonia
Red currant jelly	*Klebsiella* pneumonia
Rusty	Pneumococcal pneumonia
Foul odor	Lung abscess, bronchiectasis, anaerobic infections, aspiration
Sand or small stone	Broncholithiasis, aspiration of foreign material
Black	Smoke or coal dust inhalation
Frothy white or pink	Pulmonary edema
Blood-streaked or frankly bloody (hemoptysis)	*Pulmonary:* embolism with infarction, pneumonias, bronchiectasis, neoplasm, tuberculosis, abscess, trauma, arteriovenous malformation, aspiration of a foreign body, pulmonary hypertension *Cardiac:* mitral valve disease, pulmonary edema *Systemic:* coagulation disorders, Wegener's granulomatosis, Goodpasture's syndrome, sarcoidosis *Other:* emesis, oropharyngeal bleed rather than true hemoptysis

Table 2-7   Distinguishing Characteristics of Hemoptysis and Hematemesis

Characteristics	Hemoptysis	Hematemesis
History	Cardiopulmonary disease	Gastrointestinal disease
Patient statement	Coughed from lungs	Vomited from stomach
Blood		
pH	Alkaline	Acid
Color	Bright red	Dark (coffee grounds)
		Clotted
Froth	May be present	Absent
Mixed with	Sputum	Food
Associated symptoms	Dyspnea, pain or tickling sensation in chest	Nausea, pain referred to stomach

blood-tinged. Copious, foul-smelling (*fetid*) sputum that separates into layers on standing and is produced when the patient's position is changed occurs with lung abscess and bronchiectasis. Morning expectoration implies accumulation of secretions during the night and is commonly seen with bronchitis. Nonpurulent, silicone-like bronchial casts are seen with asthma. Sudden large amounts of sputum production may be indicative of development of a bronchopleural fistula.

Hemoptysis

Hemoptysis, expectoration of sputum containing blood, varies in severity from slight streaking to frank bleeding. It is an alarming symptom that may herald serious disease and massive hemorrhage. Differential diagnosis is complex and includes bronchopulmonary, cardiovascular, hematologic, and other systemic disorders (Table 2–7). A history of pulmonary or cardiovascular disease, cigarette smoking, trauma, anticoagulant therapy or bleeding disorders, aspiration of foreign bodies, and travel to areas where fungal infections such as coccidioidomycosis or histoplasmo-

sis are prevalent help to identify the underlying disorder.

The most common causes of streaky hemoptysis are pulmonary infections (chronic bronchitis, bronchiectasis, bacterial pneumonias), lung cancer, and thromboemboli. Massive (gross) hemoptysis (400 mL in 3 hours or more than 600 mL in 24 hours) is seen with carcinoma of the lung, tuberculosis, bronchiectasis, and trauma. It is an emergency condition associated with mortality as high as 75%. Immediate action is required to maintain an adequate airway, and emergency bronchoscopy and surgery may be necessary.

Obtaining a description of the amount and color of blood produced, appearance and odor of accompanying sputum, and acuteness or chronicity of the bleeding and associated symptoms may also provide a clue to the source of bleeding. Hemoptysis associated with sudden onset of chest pain and dyspnea in a patient at risk for venous stasis of the legs must be evaluated for pulmonary embolism and possible infarction. Frothy, blood-tinged sputum associated with paroxysmal cough accompanies cardiac-induced pulmonary edema. Purulent, blood-streaked sputum signifies an infectious process, chronic bronchitis, or bronchiectasis. Hemoptysis without severe coughing suggests a cavitary lesion in the lung or bronchial tumor.

"Spitting up blood," as it is frequently called by patients, may be confused with blood originating in the oropharynx, esophagus, or stomach. Patients can sometimes describe a sensation, often warmth, in the area where the blood originates, but careful questioning and often examination of the bloody sputum are usually required to distinguish hemoptysis from hematemesis (vomited blood) (see Table 2–7). It is important to elicit a detailed sequence of events, since large amounts of blood originating in the respiratory tract may be swallowed and later vomited; likewise, blood that is vomited may be aspirated and later expectorated.

Chest Pain

Chest pain caused by pulmonary disease is usually the result of involvement of the chest wall or parietal pleura (the serous membrane that lines the inner chest wall), both of which are well supplied with pain fibers. Chest wall pain may originate from the intercostal and pectoral muscles (myalgia), ribs and cartilages (chondro-ostealgia), or stimulation of a neural pathway (neuralgia) anywhere along a *dermatome* (skin area innervated by a particular spinal cord segment). It is usually described as a well-localized, constant aching soreness that increases with direct pressure on the area of tenderness and with any arm movement that stretches the thoracic muscles.

Pleuritic pain, often described as inspiratory pain, is the most common symptom of diseases causing inflammation of the pleura (pleurisy). It is sharp, often abrupt in onset, and severe enough to cause the patient to seek medical help (often within hours of onset). It increases with inspiration, a cough, a sneeze, a hiccup, or a laugh; is usually localized to one side of the chest (frequently the lower, lateral aspect); and may be only partially relieved by splinting and pain medication. It also increases with pressure and movement but not to the same degree as pain originating in the outer chest wall. In contrast, the lung parenchyma and the visceral pleura that cover the lungs are relatively insensitive to pain; therefore pain with breathing usually indicates involvement of the parietal pleura.

Chest pain is not limited to pulmonary causes; in fact, it is a cardinal symptom of cardiac disease. Since the thorax contains the heart, great vessels, tracheobronchial tree, and esophagus, chest pain may originate from any of these sources. It may be referred from the abdomen or may result from multiple organ involvement. Patients who experience migraine headaches or hyperventilation with anxiety may also complain of coexisting chest pain. Table 2–8 lists the most common causes of chest pain and its distinguishing characteristics.

Pain is a purely subjective symptom. The perception of pain varies not only with the source of pain but also with previous experience, culture, personality traits, amount of rest, and emotional content of the pain. Since chest pain varies from relatively benign neuromuscular skeletal pain (the most common) to life-threatening angina (caused by a decreased blood supply to the heart muscle), the interviewer must be careful to obtain an accurate and impartial history. The following characteristics must be reviewed in detail: onset, location, radiation, frequency, duration, severity, precipitation and relieving factors, and specific descriptors (e.g., tearing, stabbing, dull, sharp, crushing, burning). Clues to locating the source of chest pain include a history of trauma, surgery, or muscle strain; local tenderness; swelling; and relationship to inhaling, coughing, and position.

Noisy Breathing

Noisy breathing can be described medically as either wheezing or stridor. *Wheezing* is a whistling or musical sound produced by narrowing of the bronchi and bronchioles by spasm, tissue swelling (edema), plugging, or pressure from the surrounding lung. It is heard primarily during expiration but may be heard as well during inspiration in patients having a severe asthma attack. A healthy person can produce a wheeze by forced expiration, but an involuntary wheeze is indicative of a pulmonary disorder. Although wheezes may be audible to the patient and others within the patient's vicinity, they frequently are only heard using a stethoscope (see Chapter 4).

Stridor is a harsh "crowing" or "snoring" sound that can be heard on inspiration or expiration when one of the major airways is obstructed (see Chapter 4). Loud snoring, especially when the patient complains of frequent awakenings during the night and sleepiness during the day, is suggestive of sleep apnea syndrome (see Chapter 16).

The interviewer should help the patient analyze what initiates, accompanies, and follows wheezing and stridor. Do they occur abruptly, with inspiration or expiration, only at night or during sleep, only with exertion or at rest? Do they occur daily, seasonally, or only with exposure to allergens? Are they associated with job or hobbies? Are they better or worse at the end of the workweek? Are they preceded, accompanied, or followed by shortness of breath, cough, increased secretions, tightness in the chest, or fever? What relieves the attacks? Is breathing normal between attacks?

Hoarseness or Voice Changes

Hoarseness occurs when there is irritation or inflammation (swelling) of the vocal cords (as with laryngitis, aspiration, or following removal of an endotracheal tube) or vocal cord paralysis. Congestion and obstruction of the nasal passages also cause voice changes. When there is chronic irritation of the larynx and upper

Table 2-8   Causes and Characteristics of Chest Pain

Condition	Location and Characteristics	Etiology/Precipitating Factors	Associated Findings
Chest wall pain			
Myalgia	Intercostal and pectoralis muscles Localized dull aching Increases with movement Usually long-lasting	Trauma, seizure, nonisometric and isometric exercise, COPD, steroid therapy Persistent severe cough	Usually no visible erythema or ecchymosis with occult trauma
Chondro-ostealgia	Ribs and cartilages, precisely located (chondral pain in sternal area) Increases with pressure to area, movement, respiration, coughing Can be severe and disabling	Trauma (e.g., steering wheel, cardiopulmonary resuscitation), severe coughing, osteoporosis, tumor, myelocytic leukemia, systemic autoimmune disease, Tietze's syndrome, COPD	Rib fractures, chondral dislocations, periostitis, fever with some systemic causes
Neuralgia	Dermatome distribution Superficial tingling to deep burning pain	Thoracic spine disease, metastatic tumor, blunt trauma, herpes zoster (shingles)	Specific changes on x-ray films, fever with infection
Pleuritic and pulmonary pain			
Pleuritis (pleurisy)	Pleura, usually well localized Sharp, stabbing, raw, burning Often rapid onset, increased by inspiration, coughing, laughing, hiccuping	Infection/inflammation of pleura, trauma, autoimmune and connective tissue disease	Fever, productive cough, tachypnea, splinting of affected side
Pulmonary embolus, pulmonary infarction	Usually at base of lung, may radiate to abdomen or costal margins Stabbing, sudden onset, increased by inspiration	Immobilization, obesity, pelvic surgery	Symptoms vary with size of embolus Anxiety to panic Dyspnea, tachypnea, tachycardia, coughing with blood tinged to hemoptic sputum
Pneumothorax	Lateral thorax, well localized Sharp, tearing Sudden onset Increased by inspiration	Interstitial lung disease, bullous emphysema, asthma, idiopathic May follow deep inspiration, Valsalva maneuver, or exercise, or occur at rest	Dyspnea, tachypnea, decreased breath sounds on affected side Mediastinal shift and jugular venous distention if tension pneumothorax develops
Tumors	May be localized or diffuse Constant, sharp, boring, or dull	Invasion of primary or metastatic tumor through parenchyma to parietal pleura, mesothelioma	Symptoms vary with type and location Evidence from x-ray films History of asbestos exposure
Pulmonary hypertension (primary)	Substernal, dull, aching similar to angina Related to stress and exertion	Unknown Seen most commonly in young women	Dyspnea, tachypnea, anxiety, syncope, jugular venous distention
Cardiac pain			
Angina pectoris	Substernal, may radiate to arms, shoulders, neck, and jaw Tightness of dull, heavy pressure-like pain not related to respiration Sudden onset, short duration	Coronary artery blockage or spasm Hot, humid weather, large meals, intense emotion, exertion	Anxiety, feeling of impending doom, dyspnea, sweating, nausea Relieved by nitroglycerin and rest
Myocardial infarction	Substernal, radiating like angina Sudden crushing, viselike pain lasting minutes to hours		As above, diaphoresis, vomiting Not relieved by nitroglycerin or rest
Pericardial pain	Substernal or parasternal radiating to neck, shoulder, and epigastrium (rarely to arms) Sharp, stabbing, intermittent Intensified by respiration and lying on left side	Inflammation of pericardium, infection, metastatic tumor, trauma, irradiation, autoimmune diseases	Pericardial friction rub Tachycardia, distended neck veins, paradoxical pulse with tamponade, dyspnea
Mediastinal pain			
Esophageal	Substernal, retrosternal, epigastric Radiates toward shoulders Deep burning pain Sudden, tearing pain	Esophagitis aggravated by bending over, lying down, smoking, ingestion of coffee, fats, large meals Esophageal spasm Esophageal tear	Regurgitation of sour-tasting acid secretions relieved by antacids or may be relieved by nitroglycerin Hematemesis, shock
Dissecting aortic aneurysm	Tearing midline chest or posterior thoracic pain Sudden onset, may last hours	Blunt trauma, hypertension, inflammatory or degenerative diseases	May have lower blood pressure in legs or one arm, paralysis, murmur of aortic insufficiency, paradoxical pulse, hypertension, shock, death
Tracheobronchitis	Substernal burning discomfort May be referred to anterior chest	Acute viral infections, prolonged cigarette smoking	Cough may or may not be productive May have fever with infection
Other causes	Substernal, retrosternal, epigastric pain or burning Vague tightness to severe crushing	Referred abdominal pain: hiatal hernia, peptic ulcer, gallbladder, acute pancreatitis Hyperventilation syndrome	Symptoms vary with disease Respiratory distress, tachypnea, diaphoresis, numbness of fingers and around mouth Respiratory alkalosis

airways from infection, chronic cough, and excessive nasal drainage, the patient may also experience difficulty swallowing (*dysphagia*).

Interference with the recurrent laryngeal nerve that controls the vocal cords can result in vocal cord paralysis. Damage to the nerve can be caused by tumors of the lung or esophagus, aortic aneurysms, and, rarely, following thoracic (chest) surgery. If bilateral paralysis occurs, severe dyspnea can result secondary to airway obstruction.

Dizziness and Fainting (Syncope)

Syncope is a temporary loss of consciousness caused by reduced blood flow and therefore a reduced supply of oxygen and nutrients to the brain. Reduced cerebral blood flow may be localized (as in cerebral thrombosis, embolism, or atherosclerotic obstruction) or generalized as occurs with obstruction to blood flow from the heart, cardiac arrythmias, and hypovolemia (decreased available blood volume). Pulmonary causes of syncope include pulmonary embolism or hypertension (obstruction of blood flow from the right heart), prolonged bouts of coughing (tussive syncope), or holding one's breath following a deep inspiration (Valsalva maneuver), which results in high intrathoracic pressure and decreased venous return to the heart. Causes of syncope are listed in Table 2–9. While some of these causes of syncope are not associated with poor long-term outcomes, others can be warning signs of sudden death. Patients with cardiac causes of syncope have a 1-year mortality rate of 20% or greater.

Vasovagal or "common dizziness and fainting" is the most usual type of syncope and results from a loss of peripheral venous tone. It can occur with all forms of physical and emotional stress including (but not limited to) pain; venipuncture; prolonged standing, especially in hot weather; and anxiety. Special attention must be given to careful review of all parts of the history and to the physical examination to rule out the organic causes of syncope.

Cough (tussive) syncope[27,28] is the transient loss of consciousness following cough. It occurs most commonly in middle-aged men with underlying COPD who are outgoing and moderately obese and have a great appetite for food, alcohol, and smoking. It rarely occurs in women. The cough may be chronic and is usually dry and unproductive. Typically there is a "tickle" in the patient's throat precipitating a coughing paroxysm; then the patient's face becomes red, vision dims, the eyes become fixed, and the patient suddenly loses consciousness. The attacks usually last only a few seconds, but the patient may fall or slump in a chair since the muscles relax completely. Some patients have reported more than 20 episodes a day. Cough syncope is usually a benign symptom and patients return to their previous activity with little recall of the episode. How-

Table 2–9 Causes of Syncope*
Circulatory control abnormalities
Drugs (very common)
Vasovagal syncope ("common faint")
Orthostatic hypotension
Hypovolemia
Carotid sinus hypersensitivity
Autonomic failure
Cardiopulmonary abnormalities
Valvular and myocardial disease
Prosthetic valve dysfunction
Aortic stenosis
Mitral valve prolapse
Pulmonary stenosis
Pulmonary embolism
Hypertrophic obstructive cardiomyopathy
Acute myocardial ischemia/infarction
Inadequate cardiac filling
Coughing, Valsalva maneuver
Atrial myxoma
Cardiac arrhythmias
Sick sinus syndrome
Atrioventricular (AV) block
Superventricular tachycardia
Ventricular tachycardia
Wolff-Parkinson-White syndrome
Long Q-T syndrome
Metabolic conditions
Hypoxia
Hypocapnia
Hypoglycemia
Intoxication
Neurologic conditions
Neurovascular disease
Convulsive disorders
Generalized seizures
Transient ischemic attack (TIA)
Psychologic conditions
Hysterical fainting
Panic attacks

*Data from references 25, 26.

ever, deaths and serious injury have been reported when the syncope occurred while driving.

A precise description of the syncopal event should include a description of the preceding events as well as coexisting symptoms, including dyspnea, nausea, neurologic events, angina (chest pain), and palpitations or irregular heartbeat. A careful interview of witnesses (if available) and ambulance personnel can be extremely helpful. Additionally, a detailed review of medications and medical history, including known neurologic or heart disease, arrhythmia, pacemaker placement, or known sudden death of a family member, will provide clues to the cause of the syncope.

Swelling of the Ankles (Dependent Edema)

Edema is soft-tissue swelling resulting from an abnormal accumulation of fluid. It may be generalized (*anasarca*), may appear only in dependent body areas (feet and ankles in ambulatory patients, sacral area in patients on bed rest), or may be limited to a single extremity or organ (such as pulmonary edema). Edema is associated with kidney disease, liver disease, cardiac and pulmonary disease, and obstruction of venous or lymphatic drainage of an extremity.

Peripheral (dependent) edema caused by pulmonary disease occurs when the disease process causes narrowing of the capillaries in the lung requiring the right ventricle to generate higher and higher pressures to move blood through the lungs. Gradually the overworked right ventricle becomes enlarged and unable to pump all its blood through the lungs, which results in a damming effect that causes the venous system to become engorged with blood. Because of the high pressure in the veins, fluid is pushed out into the tissues. At first, the edema is only seen in the feet and ankles when the patient has been standing or sitting, and is relieved by rest and elevation of the legs. Later, as the right heart failure worsens, peripheral edema is no longer relieved by rest, and congestion occurs in the abdominal organs as well as the extremities and dependent areas of the body. As the liver becomes congested (*hepatomegaly*), the patient may also complain of pain just below the ribs on the right side (*right upper quadrant pain*). Edema of the bowel and *ascites* (collection of fluid in the abdomen) cause complaints of anorexia, nausea, and sometimes vomiting. Patients may also complain of slowed healing and even skin breakdown in the edematous areas.

Peripheral edema is a sign and a symptom. The examiner may find edematous ankles the patient had not noticed. The presence of edema is such an important factor that the history of the edema should be traced. Precipitating and alleviating factors and associated symptoms should be documented with the history of present illness.

Long Bone, Joint, and Muscle Pain

Patients with chronic pulmonary disease may complain of swelling and pain in the long bones and joints and swelling particularly in the hands, wrists, and jaw. The pathogenesis of the disease process is not understood, but the combination of symptoms occurs frequently enough in patients with pulmonary disorders that the name *pulmonary osteoarthropathy* is used even when the cause is hepatic cirrhosis or congenital heart disease. Additionally, patients with primary lung disease (i.e., viral pneumonia and primary lung cancer) and systemic diseases that affect the lungs (e.g., poliomyelitis) may experience weakness and muscle pain (*myalgia*). The pain may be present at rest or with movement and may affect many muscles or be limited to specific muscle groups.

Fever, Chills, and Night Sweats

Normal body temperature (*euthermia*) varies between 97° and 99.5° F (36° and 37.5° C) orally and is 1° to 2° F (0.5°–1° C) higher in the late afternoon than in the early morning. This normal change of temperature during the day is known as the *diurnal variation*. Body temperature is also affected by age (higher in infants), exercise (increases to as high as 100° F during exertion and returns to normal within 30 minutes), excitement, sudden changes in environmental temperature, digestion, technique and route of measurement (about 1° F higher rectally and about 1° F lower axillary), and use of medications containing antipyretics (drugs that decrease temperature).[29]

Fever (*hyperthermia, pyrexia*) is an elevation of body temperature above the normal range. Fever may be described as *sustained* (continuously elevated, varying little more than 1° F during a 24-hour period), *remittent* (continuously elevated with wide, usually diurnal variations), *intermittent* (daily elevation with a return to normal or subnormal between spikes), or *relapsing* (recurring in bouts of several days interspersed with periods of normal temperature).

Fever is a nonspecific symptom and may be caused by multiple factors including a hot environment; dehydration (inadequate fluid volume in the body); reactions to chemical substances, drugs, or protein breakdown; damage to the heat-regulating center in the hypothalamus; infection; malignant neoplasms; connective tissue disease; and a variety of diseases. In some patients a cause for *fever of unknown origin* (FUO) is never found.

Fever is usually accompanied by many other constitutional symptoms such as vague aching, malaise (vague discomfort, uneasiness), irritability, increased heart rate (9–10 beats per minute for each 1° F of elevation), and if high enough, confusion, delirium, or convulsions. A rapidly increasing fever may be accompanied by chills and shivering or even *rigors* (bone-shaking, teeth-rattling chills) as peripheral vasoconstriction occurs to conserve heat.

Normally humans increase sweat production about threefold with their diurnal drop in temperature at night. However, when the temperature falls abruptly, as occurs with intermittent fever, sweat production may increase fivefold to eightfold, resulting in *diaphoresis*. When this profuse sweating occurs at night soaking the bed clothes, it is clinically significant and is termed *night sweats*.

Since fever is the most common manifestation of infection, it is usually assumed to be caused by an infectious process until proved otherwise. Pulmonary infections, including lung abscess, empyema (infection within the pleural space), tuberculosis, and pneumonia are all accompanied by fever. Acute bacterial infections are usually accompanied by shaking chills, although the occurrence of a single rigor followed by sustained fever suggests pneumococcal pneumonia. Remittent fever is seen with mycoplasmal pneumonia, legionnaires' disease, and acute viral respiratory infections. An immobile or postoperative patient with fever who is *guarding the chest* (not taking deep breaths or coughing because of pain), tachypneic (respiratory rate 26–30/min), and tachycardiac (heart rate greater than 100 beats per minute) may have atelectasis (collapse of a lung segment or lobe). However, it cannot be assumed that the patient does not have an infection because there is no fever. Patients vary greatly in the degree of fever accompanying a disease process. Patients taking high doses of steroids and other drugs that can be used as immunosuppressants may have no fever in the presence of a massive infection.

Fever, like swelling and wheezing, can be a sign or a symptom. Once the temperature is taken during the physical examination, it is clearly evident when fever is present. However, many patients report fever or chills and fever but have never taken their temperature. It is important to clarify why patients think they have a fever and, if the temperature was taken, to document the route and the patient's technique. The patient should be asked to present any temperature charts that have been made and to describe the pattern of the fever and the accompanying symptoms.

When a cause for fever is not readily apparent, careful attention should also be given to the history of travel, recreation, occupation, and exposure to toxins or carriers of infectious diseases. All drugs used, including OTC medications, vitamins, and illicit drugs, should be listed, since many drugs, including antibiotics and blood products, can cause drug-related fever.

Headache, Altered Mental Status, and Personality Changes

Some patients with pulmonary disease complain of headache. When patients cannot get adequate oxygen into their blood, as happens with lung disorders, anemia, or when the amount of oxygen in the inspired air is low (as at high altitude), the amount of oxygen available to the brain is decreased (*cerebral hypoxia*) and headache can occur. As the carbon dioxide level in the blood increases, the cerebral arterial vessels dilate causing vascular headaches with throbbing pain over the entire head.[30] Because hypercapnea worsens during sleep in patients with pulmonary disorders, early-morning headaches may be the first indication that the patient is retaining abnormally high amounts of carbon dioxide. If the hypercapnea persists, headaches may be present throughout the day.

As cerebral hypoxia and hypercapnea increase, progressive changes occur in the patient's mental status. Thought processes and memory deteriorate, the mind wanders, and the patient is easily distracted. Headaches, tremors, uncontrolled movements, hallucinations, and nightmares may occur. If the hypercapnea continues, alertness is affected, progressing to drowsiness, disorientation, stupor, then coma.[31]

Personality changes are not uncommon with advanced pulmonary disorders.[32-37] The patient may complain of forgetfulness or inability to concentrate. On the other hand, the family may report the patient as depressed, anxious, demanding, or denying the disease process and refusing to follow the treatment regimen. As chronic pulmonary disease progresses, life-style options are decreased for the patient and family. Choices of work, play, and even places to live become more limited, and dependency on others increases. Patients must use more and more of their limited energy to breathe and perform the basic tasks of everyday living. Fear of acute respiratory failure, coughing up blood, another hospitalization, and the possibility of death are always present. As a result, it is not uncommon for patients to deny their illness and refuse to cooperate with treatment, use the illness to demand attention, or channel all of their concerns to the illness and use it as a threat to control others.

However, sudden personality changes or alterations in mental status are indicative of an acute problem. Although such changes are nonspecific and may be seen with neurologic or cardiac disease or intoxication, they also result from decreased levels of oxygen and increased levels of carbon dioxide in the blood. A patient with chronic pulmonary disease who experiences an additional insult such as trauma, surgery, unusual stress or exertion, pneumothorax, or inhalation of pollutants may be stressed beyond the ability to adequately oxygenate and remove carbon dioxide from the blood. The patient may have a total change of personality and then deteriorate in a matter of hours. A patient who has been resting quietly and becomes restless deserves the same thorough investigation that would be carried out for the patient who becomes less responsive.

Summary

The history is the foundation of assessment. Ideally, it is obtained from the patient in a professional, conversational, and empathic manner that establishes trust and rapport with the patient. Properly taken, the history provides the interviewer and those reading the history later with an organized, unbiased, detailed, and chronologic description of the development of the problems that caused the patient to seek health care. From the information gained during the history, the examiner determines the emphasis of the physical examination and laboratory studies, and changes in therapy.

The information obtained from the history is termed *subjective* data because it is a description of what the patient experienced or is perceiving that cannot be observed by the interviewer. Subjective manifestations of health problems are termed *symp-*

toms. The chief complaint and history of present illness are the sections of the history that record the development of symptoms that caused the patient to seek health care. The patient's description of how therapy (treatment) modifies the symptoms is recorded as subjective data in the daily progress notes.

The symptoms most commonly reported by patients with respiratory problems include coughing, shortness of breath (dyspnea), sputum production, coughing up blood (hemoptysis), chest pain, and noisy breathing. Voice changes, dizziness and fainting (syncope), swelling of feet and ankles (edema), long bone and joint pain (pulmonary osteoarthropathy), fever, chills, night sweats, headache, altered mental status, and personality changes are also reported. The description of each symptom should include the date, time, and type of onset; the setting and quality of the symptom; the body location and radiation; the severity or quantity; the frequency, duration, and course of each event; the aggravating and alleviating factors: and the associated symptoms.

REVIEW QUESTIONS

1. T   F   *Nonverbal communication is often more valuable in determining the progress of an interview than verbal communication.*

2. T   F   *Proper diagnosis and treatment is determined to a great extent by the accuracy and detail of the patient's history.*

3. *Which of the following would be examples of techniques used in conversational interviewing?*
   a. *using questions such as "What happened next?"*
   b. *saying things like "You feel better now, don't you?"*
   c. *asking for clarification of a symptom*
   d. *a and c*

4. *Proper introduction of yourself to the patient prior to the interview is useful for all the following except:*
   a. *establishing your role*
   b. *asking permission to be involved*
   c. *conveying your sincere interest in the patient*
   d. *identifying diagnostic information*

5. *In what section of the patient history can a detailed description of the patient's current symptoms be found?*
   a. *chief complaints*
   b. *history of present illness*
   c. *past medical history*
   d. *occupational history*

6. *What is the most common symptom in pulmonary disease?*
   a. *wheezing*
   b. *sputum production*
   c. *cough*
   d. *chest pain*

7. *A cough that is described as being persistent for more than 3 weeks would be called which of the following?*
   a. *acute*
   b. *paroxysmal*
   c. *chronic*
   d. *nocturnal*

8. *A patient's complaint of breathlessness or air hunger would be defined as which of the following?*
   a. *hemoptysis*
   b. *wheezing*
   c. *dyspnea*
   d. *cyanosis*

9. T   F   *Chest pain associated with inspiration is termed pleuritic.*

10. *Which of the following problems is associated with hemoptysis?*
    a. *tuberculosis*
    b. *lung carcinoma*
    c. *pneumonia*
    d. *all of the above*

11. *Which of the following is(are) true regarding dependent edema caused by lung disease?*
    a. *it is caused by pulmonary vasodilation*
    b. *accompanying hepatomegaly may be present*
    c. *caused by acute systemic hypertension*
    d. *all of the above*

12. *What term is used to describe shortness of breath in the upright position?*
    a. *orthopnea*
    b. *platypnea*
    c. *eupnea*
    d. *apnea*

REFERENCES

1. Delp MH and Manning RT: *Major's physical diagnosis,* ed 9, Philadelphia, 1981, WB Saunders.
2. Grimes J and Iannopollo E: *Health assessment in nursing practice,* ed 3, Monterey, Calif. 1992, Wadsworth Health Sciences Division.
3. Judge RD, Zuidema GD, and Fitzgerald FT: *Clinical diagnosis: a physiologic approach,* ed 5, Boston, 1989, Little, Brown.

4. Malasanos L, Barkauskas V, and Stoltenberg-Allen, K: *Health assessment,* ed 4, St Louis, 1990, Mosby.
5. Lane W: Patient interview and history taking. In Spittel JA, editor, *Practice of medicine,* vol 1, New York, 1972, Harper & Row.
6. Greenberger NJ and Hinthorn DR: *History taking and physical examination: essentials and clinical correlates,* St Louis, 1993, Mosby.
7. *Nursing 82 Books, Assessment,* Springhouse, Pa, 1982, Intermed Communications.
8. Morton PG: *Nurse's clinical guide to health assessment,* Springhouse, Pa, 1990, Springhouse.
9. Brooks SM: The occupational history and approach to the diagnosis of an occupational pulmonary disorder. In Bone RC and others, editors: *Pulmonary and critical care medicine,* St Louis, 1993, Mosby.
10. Gee JBL: Occupational lung disease. In Simmons DH and Tierney DF, editors: *Current pulmonology,* vol 13, St Louis, 1992, Mosby.
11. George RB, editor: Occupational and environmental diseases. In Bone RC and others, editors: *Pulmonary and critical care medicine,* St Louis, 1993, Mosby.
12. Epler GR, editor: Occupational lung diseases, *Clin Chest Med* 13:1992.
13. Ziskind MM: Occupational pulmonary disease, *Clin Symp* 30:2, 1978.
14. Gold DR: Indoor air pollution, *Clin Chest Med* 13:215, 1992.
15. Alberts WM and Brooks SM: Advances in occupational asthma, *Clin Chest Med* 13:281, 1992.
16. Berstein DI: Occupational asthma, *Med Clin North Am* 76:917, 1992.
17. Burge PS: New developments in occupational asthma, *Br Med Bull* 48:221, 1992.
18. Lopez M and Salvaggio JE: Occupational asthma. In Bone RC and others, editors: *Pulmonary and critical care medicine,* St Louis, 1993, Mosby.
19. American Thoracic Society Medical Section of the American Lung Association: Standards of nursing care for adult patients with pulmonary dysfunction, *Am Rev Respir Dis,* 144:231, 1991.
20. Irwin RS, Rosen MI, and Braman SS: Chronic persistent cough in the adult: the spectrum and frequency of causes and successful outcome of specific therapy, *Am Rev Respir Dis* 123:413, 1981.
21. Smyrnios NA and Irwin RS: Chronic cough. In Tierney DF, editor: *Current pulmonology,* vol 14, St Louis, 1993, Mosby.
22. Seller RH: *Differential diagnosis of common complaints,* ed 2, Philadelphia, 1993, WB Saunders.
23. Irwin RS and Hoolingsworth HM: The upper respiratory tract. In Bone RC and others, editors: *Pulmonary and critical care medicine,* vol 1, St Louis, 1993, Mosby.
24. Holt GA and Kelsen SG: Dyspnea. In Tierney DF, editor: *Current pulmonology,* vol 14, St Louis, 1993, Mosby.
25. Hopson JR and Kienzle MG: Evaluation of patients with syncope: separating the "wheat" from the "chaff," *Postgrad Med* 91:321, 1992.
26. Kapoor WN: Evaluation and management of the patient with syncope, *JAMA* 268:2553, 1992.
27. Bonekat HW, Miles RM, and Staats BA: Cough syncope, *Respir Manage* 18:34, 1988.
28. Linzer M and others: Critical carotid and vertebral arterial occlusive disease and cough syncope, *Stroke* 23:1017, 1992.
29. Mackowiak PA, editor: *Fever: basic mechanisms and management,* New York, 1991, Raven Press.
30. Ryan RE Sr and Ryan RE Jr: *Headache and head pain: diagnosis and treatment,* St Louis, 1978, Mosby.
31. Feinson T: Altered mental status, headache and coma. In Glauser EL, editor: *Signs and symptoms in pulmonary medicine,* Philadelphia, 1983, JB Lippincott.
32. Kent DC and Smith JK: Psychological implications of pulmonary disease, *Clin Notes Respir Dis* 16:3, 1977.
33. Kinzel T: Managing lung disease in late life: a new approach, *Geriatrics* 46:54, 1991.
34. Shusterman DJ and Dager SR: Prevention of psychological disability after occupational respiratory exposures, *Occup Med* 6:11, 1991.
35. Moran MG: Psychological factors effecting pulmonary and rheumatologic diseases: a review, *Psychosomatics* 32:14, 1991.
36. Morgan MD: Experience of using the CRQ (Chronic Respiratory Questionnaire), *Respir Med* 85 (Suppl B):23, 1991.
37. Jones PW, Quirk FH, and Baveystock CM: The St George's Respiratory Questionnaire: *Respir Med* 85 (Suppl B):25, 1991.

BIBLIOGRAPHY

Banner AS: Cough. In Simmons DH, editor: *Current pulmonology,* vol 9, St Louis, 1988, Mosby.
Berstein L, Berstein RS, and Dana RH: *Interviewing: a guide for health professionals,* East Norwalk, Conn, 1974, Appleton-Century-Crofts.
Blacklow RS and others, editors: *MacBrydes' signs and symptoms: applied pathologic physiology and clinical interpretation,* ed 6, Philadelphia, 1983, JB Lippincott.
Block GJ, Nolan JW, and Dempsey, MK: *Health assessment for professional nursing,* New York, 1981, Appleton-Century-Crofts.
Braman SS, editor: Pulmonary signs and symptoms, *Clin Chest Med* 8 (2), June 1987.
Brannin PK: Physical assessment of acute respiratory failure, *Crit Care* 1:27, 1979.
Branwald E: Approach to the patient with disease of the respiratory system. In Isselbacher KJ and others, editors: *Harrison's principles of internal medicine,* ed 11, New York, 1987, McGraw-Hill.
Burnside JW and McGlynn TJ: *Physical diagnosis,* ed 17, Baltimore, 1987, Williams & Wilkins.
Burton GG: Patient assessment procedures. In Barnes TA and Lisbon A, editors: *Respiratory care,* St Louis, 1988, Mosby.
Charan NB and Carvalho P: Cardinal symptoms and signs in respiratory care. In Pierson DJ and Kacmarek RM: *Foundations of respiratory care,* New York, 1992, Churchill Livingston.
Cherniack RM: *Current therapy of respiratory disease 1984–1985,* St Louis, 1984, Mosby.
Cherniack RM and Cherniack L: *Respiration in health and disease,* ed 3, Philadelphia, 1983, WB Saunders.
Cole RB and Mackay AD: *Essentials of respiratory disease,* New York, 1990, Churchill Livingston.
Conn RB Jr, editor: *Current diagnosis,* ed 8, Philadelphia, 1991, WB Saunders.
Drage CW, editor: *Respiratory medicine for primary care,* San Diego, 1982, Academic Press.
Epstein J and Gaines J: *Clinical respiratory care of the adult patient,* Bowie, Md, 1983, Robert J Brady.
Fishman AP: *Pulmonary diseases and disorders,* 3 vols, ed 2, New York, 1988, McGraw-Hill.
Glauser FL, editor: *Signs and symptoms in pulmonary medicine,* Philadelphia, 1983, JB Lippincott.
Guenter C and Welch M: *Pulmonary medicine,* Philadelphia, 1977, JB Lippincott.
Guyton AC: *Textbook of medical physiology,* ed 8, Philadelphia, 1990, WB Saunders.
Horowitz LD and Groves BM, editors: *Signs and symptoms in cardiology,* Philadelphia, 1985, JB Lippincott.
Knowles RD: Building rapport through neuro-linguistic programming, *Am J Nurs* 83:1010, 1983.
Margulis DM and Thaler MS: *The physician's book of lists,* New York, 1983, Churchill Livingstone.
Mengel A: Getting the most from patient interviews, *Nursing '82* 12:46, 1982.
Mennies JH: Smoking: the physiologic effects, *Am J Nurs* 83:1143, 1983.
Mitchel RS and Petty RL, editors: *Synopsis of clinical pulmonary disease,* ed 4, St Louis, 1989, Mosby.

Prior JA and Silberstein JS: *Physical diagnosis: the history and examination of the patient,* ed 6, St Louis, 1981, Mosby.

Rukosky JS: Assessment of the individual with altered respiratory function, *Nurs Clin North Am* 16:195, 1981.

Schroeder SA and others: *Current medical diagnosis and treatment,* Los Altos, Calif, 1992, Lange.

Seller RH: *Differential diagnosis of common complaints,* ed 2, Philadelphia, WB Saunders.

Sexton DL: *Chronic obstructive pulmonary disease: care of the child and adult,* St Louis, 1981, Mosby.

Taylor MS: *Difficult diagnosis,* Philadelphia, 1985, WB Saunders.

Tockman MS: Environmental and occupational lung disease. In Green GM and others, editors: *Yearbook of pulmonary disease,* St Louis, 1987, Mosby.

Wade JF: *Respiratory nursing care: physiology and technique,* ed 3, St Louis, 1982, Mosby.

Walker JK, Wall WD, and Hurst JW, editors: *Clinical methods: the history, physical and laboratory examinations,* ed 3, Boston, 1988, Butterworth.

Williams MH Jr: *Essentials of pulmonary medicine,* Philadelphia, 1982, WB Saunders.

Chapter 3

Vital Signs

Susan Jones Krider

LEARNING OBJECTIVES

Upon completion of this chapter, the reader should be able to accomplish the following:

1. *Recognize the four classic vital signs and the value of monitoring their trends.*

2. *Identify the clinical significance of abnormal sensorium.*

3. *Recognize what the Glasgow coma scale is useful for assessing and its predictive value in terms of patient outcome.*

4. *Recognize the normal values of the following vital signs and common causes of deviation from normal in the adult:*
   a. *pulse*
   b. *respiratory rate*
   c. *blood pressure*
   d. *temperature*

5. *Recognize the following issues related to body temperature measurement:*
   a. *types of devices commonly used*
   b. *factors affecting the accuracy of devices*
   c. *common sites and temperature ranges of those sites for measurement*
   d. *proper method in neonates*

6. *Describe how fever affects the following:*
   a. *oxygen consumption and carbon dioxide production*
   b. *respiratory rate*
   c. *pulse*

7. *Define the following terms:*
   a. *fever*
   b. *tachycardia*
   c. *bradycardia*
   d. *pulsus paradoxus*
   e. *pulsus alternans*
   f. *tachypnea*
   g. *bradypnea*
   h. *systolic blood pressure*
   i. *diastolic blood pressure*
   j. *hypertension*
   k. *hypotension*

LEARNING OBJECTIVES — cont'd

     l. pulse pressure
     m. posture hypotension

  8. *Recognize or list the technique, common sites for palpation, and characteristics to evaluate for the pulse.*

  9. *Describe the technique for determining respiratory rate and blood pressure.*

  10. *Recognize how hypotension affects perfusion and tissue oxygen delivery.*

  11. *Recognize the factors which cause erroneously elevated blood pressure measurements.*

  12. *Identify the mechanism by which pulsus paradoxus is produced.*

Chapter Outline

Obtaining Vital Signs and Clinical Impression
Frequency of Vital Signs Measurement
Trends in the Vital Signs
Comparing Vital Signs Information
Height and Weight
General Clinical Presentation
Questions to Ask Yourself about Clinical Presentation
Level of Consciousness (Sensorium)
Glasgow Coma Scale
Questions to Ask Yourself about Level of
   Consciousness

Body Temperature
Fever
Hypothermia
Measurement of Body Temperature
Questions to Ask Yourself about Temperature

Pulse Rate
Measurement of Pulse Rate
Questions to Ask Yourself about Pulse

Respiratory Rate
Measurement of Respiratory Rate
Questions to Ask Yourself about Respiratory Rate

Blood Pressure
Measurement of Blood Pressure
Effects of the Respiratory Cycle on Blood Pressure
Questions to Ask Yourself about Blood Pressure

Chapter Overview

The first two chapters of this text discussed how to approach and interview the patient to obtain information about what the patient experiences, and what the patient perceives as important. This *subjective* information includes what patients believe about the effectiveness of their treatment, as well as their feeling about how their disease is affecting their quality of life. Patients with chronic disease develop their own practi-

cal knowledge about their symptoms and disease. They are frequently able to determine when their medications and treatment programs need to be changed, and when they are in danger and need emergency care.[1] This practical knowledge is similar to that of an expert clinician though it is based on body sensations and perceptions rather than on *objective* data which can be observed or measured by an examiner or caregiver. This experience-based practical knowledge, as well as the patient's feelings of fear or panic, must be considered as *vital* assessment information and never passed off as simply emotions. In fact, this information is frequently what determines that it is time to obtain *objective assessment information:* vital signs, physical examination, blood gases, and other laboratory and radiologic information.

    This chapter focuses on *vital signs*—the most frequently measured objective data for monitoring vital body functions and often the first and most important indicator that the patient's condition is changing. Vital signs are used to establish a *baseline* (a record of an initial measurement against which future recordings are compared), to observe for trends, to monitor response to therapy, and to identify physiologic problems or improvements.

Obtaining Vital Signs and Clinical Impression

The four classic vital sign measurements are *temperature, pulse, respiration* and *blood pressure*. Though not always listed as vital signs, the patient's *height, weight,* and *level of consciousness* and *responsiveness (sensorium)*, as well as the caregiver's *general clinical impression* are also important observations to be included with the vital signs assessment. Pulse oximetry with heart rate monitoring as well as bedside electrocardiographic (ECG) monitoring are becoming part of the standard vital signs package in some areas. These forms of continuous noninvasive vital signs monitoring are discussed in Chapters 9, 11, and 12. Patients who have intravenous (IV) catheters or are receiving IV

Table 3-1	Signs of Hypoxemia Assessed During Vital Signs Measurement
Vital Signs Measurement	**Sign**
General clinical presentation	Impaired coordination or cooperation
	Difficulty breathing, use of accessory muscles
	Diaphoresis (profuse sweating)
Sensorium (level of consciousness)	Decreased mental function
	Impaired judgment, confusion
	Loss of consciousness
	Decreased pain perception
Respiration	Increased rate and depth of breathing
Heart rate	Tachycardia
	Dysrhythmias [2–7] (irregular heart rate), especially during sleep[8,9]
Blood pressure	Increased blood pressure initially
	Decreased blood pressure
	Cool extremities* (can be felt while taking the heart rate and blood pressure)

* Temperature of the extremities, as well as diaphoresis, can be felt at the time the heart rate and blood pressure are obtained.

fluids or who have undergone vascular or surgical procedures will have wounds, catheter insertion sites, and extremity checks performed and recorded as part of "routine vitals."

Frequency of Vital Signs Measurement

The frequency of vital signs measurement is dependent on the condition of the patient, the nature and severity of the disorder, and the procedures, surgery, or treatments being performed. A baseline measurement should be taken on admission, at the beginning of each shift, prior to any treatment or procedure, and anytime the patient's condition changes. Routine vitals on nonintensive care hospitalized patients are most commonly recorded every 4 to 6 hours (beginning and midshift). Vital signs associated with respiratory care treatments are usually recorded before and after the treatment and occasionally at a midpoint during the treatment to evaluate possible side effects as well as effectiveness of the treatment. Following surgery or certain procedures, vital signs are measured more frequently to ensure the patient's safety; usually every 15 minutes for 2 hours, then every 30 minutes for 1 to 2 hours, then hourly until the patient is stable. The physician's order in the chart is frequently written as: "Vitals q15m × 8, q30m × 4, qh until stable, then routine." Of course, vital signs should always be monitored and recorded as often as necessary for the safety of the patient. If the patient's condition changes unexpectedly or the patient suddenly comments about "not feeling well," vital signs should be measured immediately by the person closest to the patient. Patient safety is in everyone's job description.

Trends in the Vital Signs

A single vital sign measurement gives information about the patient at that moment in time. Each measurement may be evaluated to see if it is high or low compared to the normal value for the patient's age; however, an isolated measurement does not give you much information about what is normal for the individual patient or how the patient is changing or responding to therapy over time. To evaluate whether an individual patient has "normal" vital signs, one must understand what is "normal" for the patient's age and disease. Sometimes the disease or treatment modality causes expected alterations in heart rate, respiratory rate, blood pressure, or temperature which change what is "normal" for an individual patient. If you doubt a finding, repeat the measurement and be sure the patient's position and your technique are correct for the parameter you are measuring. If you still doubt the measurement or if you think the patient may be getting into trouble, get help.

A series of vital sign measurements over time establishes a *trend* and is far more important clinically than any single measurement. Each time vital signs are measured, they should be compared with several previous measurements. Sometimes the patient's condition may be changing slowly and comparison with one or two previous measurements will not indicate the trend, whereas comparison over an entire shift or 24 hours of vital signs may indicate clearly that the patient is slowly deteriorating. Because the trend of vital signs is so important, many physicians insist that vital signs on hospitalized patients be recorded on a multiple-day graph.

Comparing Vital Signs Information

Information can be obtained about the probability that a patient is experiencing or may be developing a particular problem by comparing simultaneous changes in several different vital signs measurements over time. As an example, specific changes in the general appearance of the patient, the level of consciousness, heart and respiratory rate, and blood pressure occur in the patient developing *hypoxemia,* defined as partial pressure of arterial oxygen (Pa_{O_2}) less than 60 mm Hg. Table 3–1 lists the signs of hypoxemia. In the field of medicine, this comparison of multiple signs and symptoms to arrive at the patient's diagnosis is called *differ-*

ential diagnosis. Of course it takes time for the beginning student to learn all these relationships, but remember, the difference between the novice and expert clinician is not just knowledge, it is also the ability to assess and compare multiple types of subjective and objective data over time and to identify patterns and relationships in an individual patient. The key to expert assessment of vital signs at the bedside is to be constantly aware and to look for change:

- *Look* at the patient: Watch facial expressions, body movements, coordination, position, color, skin, effort to breathe or move.
- *Listen* to the patient: Hear words, tones, sounds, rhythms, patterns, silence, feelings, fears.
- *Touch*: Feel moisture, temperature, change in temperature, muscle and skin tone, resistance, quality of pulses.
- *Reassess and analyze*: Collect information in a timely manner, compare it to normal values for the patient and the disease process, mentally update this information whenever you are around the patient. Validate its accuracy. Does the information make sense? Is something wrong with the picture?
- *Trend, trend, trend*: What has changed about the patient? How has the patient changed? Why has he or she changed? What has not changed? Why? What does it mean? Does the change indicate a need for immediate action?

Height and Weight

Height and weight are routinely measured as part of the physical examination and usually as part of every outpatient appointment. For hospitalized patients, the admitting height and weight is either obtained and recorded when the patient goes to preadmitting testing service (PATS) or by the admitting nurse; thereafter, weight is usually measured every day or two. If there is a question of either dehydration or fluid overload, *fluid intake* and *output* and weight may be recorded each shift until the patient's fluid balance is stable. Because weight is often used to calculate medication doses, the weight may be recorded in kilograms (1 kg = 2.2 lb) on the patient's medication record rather than on the vital signs record. Scales and measurement standards should be selected in sizes and styles appropriate for the age of the patient and should be calibrated regularly to ensure their accuracy.

General Clinical Presentation

General observation begins the moment you first see the patient and continues throughout the examination and care. The patient's general appearance gives clues to the level of distress and severity of illness as well as information about the patient's personality, hygiene, culture, and reaction to illness. This first step may dictate the order of care or physical examination. If the patient is in distress, the priority is to evaluate the problem in the most efficient and rapid way possible and intervene or locate someone who can assist the patient. A more complete examination can be completed when the patient is more stable. Some visual signs of distress are included in the following:

Cardiopulmonary distress is suggested by labored, rapid, irregular, or shallow breathing which may be accompanied by coughing, choking, wheezing, dyspnea, anxiety, chest pain, and even a bluish color (cyanosis) of the oral mucosa, lips, and fingers. *Anxiety* is recognized by restlessness, fidgeting, tense looks, difficulty communicating normally and may be accompanied by cool hands and sweaty palms. Patients in *pain* usually present with drawn features, guarding, and shallow breathing: they do not want to move, deep-breathe, or cough, and may be moaning or writhing. Of course, *bleeding* and *loss of consciousness* are other signs of extreme distress that require immediate intervention.

When a patient is not in acute distress, this initial observation provides an opportunity to see the patient as a whole person. Using all your senses—hearing, smell, seeing, touch, and perception—during this head-to-toe inspection will give information about the patient's apparent age, state of health, body structure, nutritional status, posture, motor activity, physical and sensory limitations, and mental acuity. It will help you to assess the reliability of the patient as an historian. It will help you know what type of assistance and teaching the patient may need.

A written description of these initial observations helps others involved in the patient's care know how to plan care and relate to the patient's needs. Usually these descriptive statements are written in language everyone can understand, e.g., "JC is a cooperative, alert, well-nourished, 43-year-old man who appears younger than his stated age and exhibits no indication of distress. He shows no signs of acute or chronic illness and is admitted for ..." You may occasionally find that more specific terms for body types have been used in the written physical examination report. Table 3–2 lists and defines some of those terms.

Questions To Ask Yourself About The Clinical Impression

Questions to ask yourself while doing this portion of the examination include:

- What is the general appearance and attitude of the patient?
- Is the patient in distress?
- How is the patient responding?
- Are there abnormalities in the patient's face or movements?
- Does the patient have any motor or sensory limitations?

Table 3-2   Terms Used to Describe Body Types

Body Type	General Characteristics
Ectomorphic	Slight development, body linear and delicate with sparse muscular development
Endomorphic	Soft, roundness throughout the body, large trunk and thighs with tapering extremities
Mesomorphic	Preponderance of muscle bone and connective tissue, with heavy hard physique of rectangular outline (between endomorphic and ectomorphic)
Sthenic	Average height, well-developed musculature, wide shoulders, flat abdomen, oval-shaped face
Hypersthenic	Short, stocky, may be obese; shorter, broader chest; thicker abdominal wall; rectangular-shaped face
Hyposthenic	Tall, willowy, musculature poorly developed; long, flat chest; abdomen may sag; long neck, triangular-shaped face
Asthenic	Exaggeration of hyposthenic body type
Cachectic	Profound and marked malnutrition, wasting, ill health.
Debilitated	Weak, feeble, lack of strength (with weakness and loss of energy)
Failure to thrive	Physical and developmental delay or retardation in infants and children seen in children with illness but more often in children with psychosocial or maternal deprivation.

Data from references 10–12.

Table 3-3   Glasgow Coma Scale—Record of Patient Recovering from Coma*

	Score		Day 1	Day 2	Day 3	Day 4	Day 5
Eye-opening response	Spontaneous opening	4					X
	To verbal stimuli	3				X	
	To pain	2	X	X	X		
	None	1					
Most appropriate verbal response	Oriented	5					X
	Confused	4					
	Inappropriate words	3				X	
	Incoherent	2		X	X		
	None	1	X				
Most integrated motor response (arm)	Obeys commands	5				X	X
	Localizes pain	4		X	X		
	Flexion to pain	3					
	Extension to pain	2	X				
	None	1					
TOTAL SCORE			5	8	8	11	14

* From Malasanos L, Barkauskas V, and Stoltenberg-Allen K: *Health assessment*, ed 4, St Louis, 1990, Mosby–Year Book.

- Will this patient require assistance, safety precautions, or teaching?

Level of Consciousness (Sensorium)

Evaluation of the patient's level of consciousness is a simple but important task. Adequate cerebral oxygenation must be present for the patient to be conscious, alert, and well oriented. The conscious patient also should be evaluated for orientation as to time, place, and person. This is referred to as evaluating the patient's *sensorium* or mental status. The alert and well-oriented patient, whose orientation as to time, place, and person is accurate, is said to be "oriented × 3," and the sensorium is considered normal.

An abnormal sensorium and a loss of consciousness may occur when cerebral perfusion is inadequate or when poorly oxygenated blood is delivered to the brain. As cerebral oxygenation deteriorates, the patient initially is restless, confused, and disoriented. If tissue hypoxia continues to deteriorate, the patient eventually becomes comatose. An abnormal sensorium also may occur as a side effect of certain medications and in drug overdose cases. Deterioration of the patient's sensorium often indicates the need for mechanical ventilation in the presence of acute respiratory dysfunction.

Evaluation of the patient's sensorium not only helps determine the status of tissue oxygenation but also the ability of the patient to cooperate and participate in treatment. Patients who are alert and oriented can take an active role in their care, whereas those who are disoriented or comatose cannot. The treatment plan is often adjusted according to the evaluation of sensorium.

Glasgow Coma Scale

Many systems for evaluating the patient's level of consciousness have been developed. One assessment tool that allows for objective evaluation based on behavioral response of the patient is the Glasgow coma scale (Table 3-3). This scale can be used to monitor trends in the patient's neurologic condition over several days. A person with normal consciousness would obtain a score of 14.

Although the Glasgow coma scale has been the gold standard for assessing the neurologic function of patients that have been sedated, received anesthesia, suffered head trauma, or near coma, it has limited ability to predict patient outcome. As health care shifts its attention to predicting outcomes, new and more precise prognostic scales and outcome indicators will be developed. A new coma–near-coma scale which uses eight patient responses (auditory, olfactory, tactile, pain, vocalization, threat, visual, and command) has been proposed for use in predicting the potential for rehabilitation in patients that have been categorized as near-vegetative.[13] Variations on the Glasgow coma scale and other prognostic indicator tools are expected to be introduced in the next few years.

Questions to Ask Yourself About Level of Consciousness

Asking yourself questions like the ones below while obtaining vital signs will help you assess the patient's sensorium:

- Is the patient conscious? If medicated, can the patient be aroused easily?
- Is the patient responding and is the response appropriate for the stimulus?
- Is the patient alert?
- Is the patient oriented to person, place, and time?
- Can the patient see, hear, and sense touch?
- Is the patient restless, fidgety, easily distracted?
- Has the patient's responsiveness or behavior changed?

Body Temperature

Normal body temperature for most people is approximately 98.6° F (37° C) with a normal range from 97.0° to 99.5° F and daily variations of 1° to 2° F (see Table 3–4). The body temperature usually is lowest in the early morning and highest in the late afternoon. Most metabolic functions occur optimally when body temperature is within the normal range. Temperature elevation to between 99° and 100° F occurs normally during exercise and takes about 15 minutes to return to normal following exercise. In women, normal temperature increases about 1°F during ovulation and during the first 4 months of pregnancy.

Body temperature is maintained in the normal range by balancing heat production with heat loss. If the body had no ability to rid itself of the heat generated by metabolism, the body temperature would rise approximately 2°F/hr.[14] The hypothalamus plays an important role in regulating heat loss and can initiate peripheral vasodilation and sweating in an effort to dissipate body heat. The respiratory system also helps in the removal of excess heat through ventilation. When the inhaled gas is cooler than the body temperature, the airways warm the gas to body temperature. This warming and subsequent exhalation of the gas now at body temperature aids in removing excess body heat. When the inhaled gas is heated to near body temperature before inhalation, this heat loss mechanism is not functional.

Fever

An elevation of body temperature above normal (*hyperthermia*) can result from disease or from normal activities such as exercise. When the temperature is elevated from disease, this elevation is called *fever,* and the patient is said to be *febrile.* Fever often occurs as a result of microorganisms invading the body and producing an *infection.* Causes and patterns of fever are described in Chapter 2.

A fever results in an increase in the metabolic rate of the body functions and produces an increase in oxygen consumption and carbon dioxide production by the body tissues. For every 1° C elevation of body temperature, oxygen consumption and carbon dioxide production increase approximately 10%. The demand for an increase in the oxygen supply to the tissues and removal of carbon dioxide must be met by an increase in circulation and ventilation. Examination of the febrile patient often reveals increased heart rates and breathing rates. For the patient with significant cardiac or pulmonary disease, the increased demand on these systems may represent an intolerable stress.

Hypothermia

When the body temperature is below normal, *hypothermia* exists. Hypothermia is not common but can occur in persons with severe head injuries that damage the hypothalamus and in persons suffering from exposure to cold environmental temperatures. When the body temperature is below normal, the hypothalamus initiates shivering in an effort to generate energy and vasoconstriction to conserve body heat.

Because hypothermia reduces oxygen consumption and carbon dioxide production by the body tissues, the patient with hypothermia usually has slow and shallow breathing and a reduced pulse rate. Mechanical ventilators in the control mode may need significant adjustments in the depth and rate of delivered tidal volumes as the body temperature of the patient varies above and below normal.

Measurement of Body Temperature

Body temperature is most often measured at one of four sites: the mouth, ear, axilla, or rectum. Rectal temperatures most accurately reflect actual body core temperature. Oral temperature registration is the most acceptable for awake, adult patients, but this method should not be used with infants, comatose patients, or

Table 3–4 Temperature Normals by Site and Time Requirements For Accuracy When Using a Glass Thermometer

| Site | Normal Temperature Ranges | | Time Required |
	Fahrenheit	Centigrade	
Oral	97.0°–99.5°	36.5°–37.5°	3–5 min*
Axillary	96.7°–98.5°	35.9°–36.9°	9–11 min
Rectal	98.7°–100.5°	37.1°–38.1°	2–4 min
Ear	Expected to be very close to rectal		2–3 sec

* Wait 15 minutes after eating or drinking.

orally intubated patients. After the patient has ingested hot or cold liquid or has been smoking, a 10- to 15-minute waiting period is required before an accurate oral temperature can be obtained. For infants and small children who do not tolerate rectal thermometers, axillary temperatures may be taken safely. Axillary temperature is measured for neonates because it approximates their core temperature and avoids injury to the rectal tissues. Feeling the skin temperature to determine elevation of temperature is not reliable because skin temperature varies depending on the body's need to store or release heat, the ambient temperature, and the adequacy of blood circulation to the area.

Temperature normals vary with the site and method of temperature measurement. Additionally, when glass thermometers are used, accuracy is dependent on the length of time the thermometer is allowed to register. See Table 3–4.

The oral temperature is not affected significantly by oxygen administration via nasal cannula, simple mask, or Venti-Mask.[15,16] Therefore it is not necessary to remove the oxygen or take rectal temperatures of patients receiving oxygen via cannula or mask to obtain accurate oral temperature readings.

Oral temperature may not be measured as reliably in patients breathing heated or cooled aerosol via face masks. There is a tendency for oral temperatures to increase slightly with the application of heated aerosol and decrease slightly with cooled aerosol.[17] However, the range of fluctuation is probably too small to influence clinical decisions.

EAR TEMPERATURE. Tympanic thermometry uses a handheld probe placed in the ear canal to detect infrared emissions from the surfaces of the tympanic membrane and ear canal. No direct contact is made with the tympanic membrane. The temperature is digitized by a computer processor and displayed on a liquid crystal screen in less than 3 seconds. The first ear thermometer was introduced to the U.S. market in 1986,[18] after two decades of use in the aerospace industry. This new method has the advantage of being fast, clean, and noninvasive, and avoids the embarrassment and time delays associated with the classic forms of temperature measurement. It is already commonly used in pediatric outpatient offices around the country.

There are, however, concerns about its accuracy and use in the hospital setting.

Multiple studies[19–25] have been performed in different populations and age groups to evaluate correlations with other types of temperature measurement. The effects of examiner technique,[26] ambient temperature changes,[27] middle ear infection, and the influence of wax and exudate in the ear have also been evaluated: results have been mixed. It is clear that there is not 100% equivalence between the temperatures in the ear canal and those in other body sites; however, there is a significant correlation between ear and rectal, oral, and core temperatures.[28] One study[29] found no significant difference between left tympanic and axillary temperature in neonates but a significant difference between right tympanic and axillary temperature. At this writing, axillary temperature is still the route of choice in the neonate.

Questions to Ask Yourself About Temperature

To assure the accuracy of the temperature measurement, ask yourself the following questions:

- What type of thermometer was used?
- What site was used: oral, axillary, rectal, tympanic?
- Was an appropriate amount of time used to obtain the temperature for the method of measurement?
- Had the patient just had a treatment, food, liquid, medication, or other event that could alter the accuracy of the measurement?
- Was the patient observed during temperature measurement? Is there any reason to believe that an elevated temperature was "facticious fever"?
- What is the time of day? Is the temperature highest in the late afternoon and lowest in the early morning, as expected?

Pulse Rate

The pulse rate should be evaluated for rate, rhythm, and strength. Normal pulse rate varies with the age and

Table 3-5	Pulse and Respiratory Rates Referred to Age	
Age	Pulse (beats/min)	Respiratory Rate (breaths/min)
Newborn	90-170	35-45-70 with excitement
1 yr	80-160	25-35
Preschool	80-120	20-25
10 yr	70-110	15-20
Adult	60-100	12-20

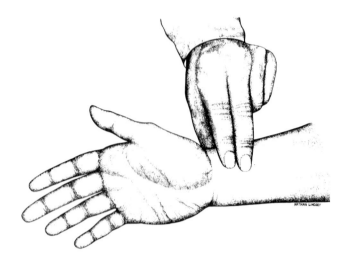

Fig. 3-1. *Technique for assessment of radial pulse.*

status of the patient. As shown in Table 3–5, the younger the patient, the faster the pulse rate. The normal pulse rate for adults is 60 to 100 beats per minute and is regular in rhythm. A pulse rate exceeding 100 beats per minute in an adult is termed *tachycardia.* Common causes of tachycardia include anxiety, fear, exercise, fever, high ambient temperature, low blood pressure, anemia, reduced arterial blood oxygen levels, and certain medications. A pulse rate below 60 beats per minute is termed *bradycardia.* This is less common but can occur when the heart is diseased, as a side effect of certain medications, or in well-conditioned athletes who typically have resting pulse rates in the fifties. Irregularity of the pulse suggests *arrhythmias* (*dysrhythmias*) which are discussed in Chapter 9; *sinus arrhythmia* (acceleration with inspiration), however, is normal in children.

The amount of oxygen delivered to the tissues is dependent on the ability of the heart to pump oxygenated blood. The amount of blood pumped through the circulatory system (cardiac output) is a function of heart rate and stroke volume (volume of blood ejected with each contraction of the ventricle). When the oxygen content of the arterial blood falls below normal, usually from lung disease, the heart tries to compensate by increasing cardiac output to maintain adequate oxygen delivery to the tissues. An increase in cardiac output is accomplished by an increase in heart rate in most persons. For this reason the heart rate is important to monitor in patients with lung disease. These concepts are discussed in more detail in Chapters 11, 13, and 14.

Measurement of Pulse Rate

The most common site for evaluation of the pulse is the radial artery. The examiner's second and third finger pads are used in assessment of the radial pulse (Fig. 3–1). The pulse rate should be counted for 1 minute to evaluate the rate, rhythm, and strength. If the patient's wrist is held above the level of his heart, the pulse may be difficult to obtain. Other common sites available for assessment of the pulse include the brachial artery, the femoral artery, and the carotid artery. When the blood pressure is abnormally low, the more centrally located pulses, such as the carotid pulse in the neck and femoral pulses in the groin, can be identified more easily than the peripheral pulse.

The fullness or volume of the pulse is evaluated. Pulse volume is usually characterized using a 0 to 4 scale: 0 = absent; 1+ = markedly reduced, weak, thready; 2+ = slightly reduced; 3+ = normal; 4+ = bounding. The fullness of the pulse can be reduced for many reasons, including an arterial blood clot, atherosclerosis, diabetes mellitus, dehydration, or any other condition that would cause the blood flow through the artery to decrease.

Spontaneous ventilation may influence the strength of the pulse. When the patient's pulse strength decreases with spontaneous inhalation, it is referred to as *pulsus paradoxus. Pulsus alternans* is an alternating succession of strong and weak pulses and usually is not related to respiratory disease. These concepts are described in more detail in the discussion of blood pressure.

Questions to Ask Yourself About Pulse

To assure the accuracy of the pulse rate, ask yourself the following questions:
- What is the pulse rate? Rhythm? Quality?
- Has the patient been doing something that might raise the pulse temporarily? Is the patient usually anxious at this time?
- Should I take the pulse again later when the patient is resting?
- If the pulse is irregular, did I count it for a full minute?
- Does the pulse vary with respirations?

Respiratory Rate

Respiratory rates vary by age and condition of the patient. Table 3–5 gives reference ranges for patients of various ages. A respiratory rate of 40 breaths per minute is unusual and greater than 60/min is definitely

Table 3-6   *Normal Blood Pressure and Sphygmomanometer Cuff Sizes by Age**

Age	Average blood pressure (mm Hg)	95th percentile (mm Hg)	Cuff Width† (in. [cm])	Cuff Length (in. [cm])
<1 mo	84/	104/	1 [3]	2 [5]
3–6 yr	94/52	110/70	2 [5]	3 [8]
6–10 yr	98/62	114/70	3 [8]	5 [13]
11–13 yr	106/66	124/84	4 [11]	6–7 [17]
14–19 yr	108/64 (girls)	126/82 (girls)	5 [13]	10 [24]
	116/68 (boys)	136/85 (boys)		
20+ yr	90/60–150/90		5 [17]	13 [32]
Obese or thigh measurements			8 [20]	16–17 [42]

* Data from references 31, 32.
† The width of the bladder should be 125% to 155% of the arm diameter and 40% to 50% of the arm circumference.[33]

abnormal at any age. If carefully measured, respiratory rate is a sensitive and reasonably specific marker of acute respiratory disease.[30] *Tachypnea* is the term used to describe respiratory rates above normal. Rapid respiratory rates may occur as the result of exercise, atelectasis, fever, reduced arterial blood oxygen content, metabolic acidosis, anxiety, and pain. A slow respiratory rate, referred to as *bradypnea,* is uncommon but may occur in patients with head injuries or hypothermia, as a side effect of certain medications such as narcotics, and in patients with drug overdose. Along with the rate, the pattern of breathing should be assessed. Evaluation of respiratory patterns is described in Chapter 4.

Measurement of Respiratory Rate

The respiratory rate is counted by watching the abdomen or chest wall move in and out with breathing. With practice, even the subtle breathing movements of the healthy person at rest can be identified easily. In some patients the examiner may need to place his or her hand on the patient's abdomen to identify the breathing rate.

The respiratory rate must be counted when the patient is not aware, as the rate may be altered voluntarily by the patient. One successful method requires counting the respiratory rate immediately after evaluating the pulse, while maintaining your fingers on the patient's radial artery.

Questions to Ask Yourself About Respiratory Rate

To assure the accuracy of the respiratory rate, ask yourself the following questions:
- What is the respiratory rate? Regularity? Pattern?
- What is the depth of respiration?
- Are accessory muscles used for respiration?
- Did patient awareness that respirations were being counted alter the rate or pattern of respiration?
- Did I count the rate for a full minute if the rate was unusually fast, slow, or irregular?

Blood Pressure

Arterial blood pressure is the force exerted against the walls of the arteries as the blood moves through the arterial vessels. Arterial *systolic blood pressure* is the peak force exerted during contraction of the left ventricle. *Diastolic pressure* is the force occurring when the heart is relaxed. *Pulse pressure* is the difference between systolic and diastolic pressures. Normal pulse pressure is 35 to 40 mm Hg. When pulse pressure is less than 30 mm Hg, the peripheral pulse is difficult to detect.

Arterial blood pressure is determined by the force of left ventricular contraction, the peripheral vascular resistance, and the blood volume. The normal values for blood pressure change with age, as shown in Table 3–6. The normal range for systolic pressure in adults is 90 to 150 mm Hg with 120 mm Hg the average. Normal diastolic pressure ranges from 60 to 90 mm Hg with 80 mm Hg the average. Blood pressure is recorded with systolic listed over diastolic, for example, 120/80 mm Hg.

A blood pressure persistently above 140/90 mm Hg is termed *hypertension.* Hypertension may result from an increase in the force of ventricular contraction or when peripheral vascular resistance is elevated.

Hypotension is defined as blood pressure less than 90/60 mm Hg in adults. It may occur as the result of peripheral vasodilation, left ventricular failure, or low blood volume. Perfusion of vital body organs may be significantly reduced with hypotension. Without adequate circulation, oxygen delivery to the tissues is impaired, and tissue hypoxia occurs. For this reason prolonged hypotension must be guarded against.

Changes in posture may produce abrupt changes in the arterial blood pressure in the hypovolemic patient. Normally, when the patient moves from the supine to the sitting position, blood pressure changes very little. When hypovolemia is present, the blood pressure may decrease significantly when the patient rapidly sits up; this is referred to as *postural hypotension.*

Measurement of Blood Pressure

The most common techniques for measuring arterial blood pressure utilize a blood pressure cuff called a *sphygmomanometer.* When the cuff is applied to the extremity, usually the upper arm, and pressurized to exceed systolic blood pressure, the blood flow in the artery is stopped. As the pressure in the cuff is released slowly, blood will pass through the compressed artery when the cuff pressure is just below systolic pressure. The pulsations can be felt by palpation of the artery or sensed by a flow probe or oscillometric sensor and can be used to determine the systolic blood pressure. These techniques are discussed in Chapters 10 and 11. The partial obstruction of the arterial blood flow creates distention of the artery and turbulence that produce sounds called *Korotkoff sounds.* The auscultatory technique for blood pressure measurement utilizes a stethoscope placed over the artery to hear these Korotkoff sounds.

AUSCULTATORY BLOOD PRESSURE MEASUREMENT. To measure the blood pressure a deflated cuff is wrapped snugly around the upper arm with the lower edge of the cuff 1 inch above the antecubital fossa. The brachial pulse is palpated, and the cuff is inflated to a pressure 30 mm Hg higher than the point at which the pulse was obliterated. The bell of the stethoscope is placed over the site of the brachial artery. Then the cuff is deflated at a rate of 2 to 3 mm Hg/sec while observing the manometer.

The systolic blood pressure is recorded from the point at which the initial Korotkoff sounds are heard. The point at which the sounds become muffled is recorded as the diastolic pressure. This muffling sound is the final change in the Korotkoff sounds just before they disappear. At this point the cuff pressure is equal to the diastolic pressure, and no turbulent sounds are created. The examiner must be careful and perform the procedure efficiently, since the pressurized cuff is impairing circulation to the forearm and hand. Since cuff pressures are only estimates of pressure based on blood flow through an artery, anything that alters flow in the artery may result in erroneous blood pressure measurements.

ERRORS IN BLOOD PRESSURE MEASUREMENT. Causes of arterial blood congestion above the cuff that result in erroneously high cuff pressure measurements include the following:

1. Too narrow a cuff. (Cuff and bladder width should be at least the diameter of the arm[33]; see Table 3–6.)
2. Cuff applied too tightly.
3. Cuff applied too loosely. (When the loose bladder is inflated, the edges rise so the por-

tion pressing on the artery has a tourniquet effect.)
4. Excessive pressure placed in the cuff during measurement.
5. Inflation pressure held in the cuff.
6. Incomplete deflation of cuff between measurements.

A low pressure reading is obtained if the cuff is too wide; however, this produces errors in the range of 3 to 5 mm Hg rather than the 40 mm Hg error often obtained when using too narrow a cuff.

Erroneous diastolic pressures occur when pressure is maintained on the artery so that laminar flow is not reestablished. Since turbulent flow can be heard, muffling or disappearance of sound may not occur. Causes include applying the cuff too tightly and pressing the stethoscope too tightly over the artery. When both muffling and disappearance of the sound occur, both pressures are recorded (120/80/60).

Static electricity, ventilators, extraneous room sounds, and presence of an auscultatory gap may also cause erroneous cuff measurements. An auscultatory gap is a drop of 20 to 40 mm Hg with no sound between the first systolic sound and the continuous pulse sound. Inflating the cuff until the palpated radial pulse can no longer be felt prevents missing the "opening snap." When an auscultatory gap is heard, both the opening snap pressure and the pressure where continuous pulses were heard should be recorded (160/140/80).

Effects of the Respiratory Cycle on Blood Pressure

Systolic blood pressure usually decreases slightly with normal inhalation. This decrease in systolic blood pressure is more significant during a forced maximal inhalation. When the systolic pressure drops more than 6 to 8 mm Hg during inhalation at rest, a definite abnormality exists; this is termed *paradoxical pulse.* Paradoxical pulse, also called pulsus paradoxus, is a nonspecific phenomenon that occurs in various circulatory and respiratory conditions such as asthma and cardiac tamponade.[34] The most probable mechanism responsible for this fluctuation in blood pressure centers around the negative intrathoracic pressure created by the respiratory muscles during inhalation. The negative intrathoracic pressure encourages venous blood to return to the right ventricle and discourages arterial blood flow out of the left ventricle. Additionally, the increased venous return to the right ventricle increases the right ventricular filling pressures, which causes the interventricular septum to distend toward the left ventricle. This results in reduced left ventricular filling, reduced stroke volume, and decreased systolic blood pressure simultaneous with inhalation.[35]

The fluctuation in systolic blood pressure with ventilation can be identified most accurately with a sphygmomanometer; however, if the pulse can be felt to wane with inspiration in several accessible arteries, paradoxical pulse is present. To confirm and quantify the presence of paradoxical pulse, a blood pressure cuff is used. The cuff is inflated until no sounds are heard with the stethoscope bell over the brachial artery, and then it is gradually deflated until sounds are heard on exhalation only. The cuff pressure then is reduced slowly until sounds are heard throughout the respiratory cycle. The difference between these two pressure readings indicates the degree of paradoxical pulse. A reading in excess of 6 to 8 mm Hg is significant. The presence of paradoxical pulse may also occur with any disorder causing acute airway obstruction.[36]

Questions to Ask Yourself About Blood Pressure

To assure the accuracy of the blood pressure, ask yourself the following questions:
- Is the correct cuff size being used? Is the cuff applied correctly?
- Is the arm in the standard position when the blood pressure is measured?
- Is the same arm used as was used in previous measurements? Which arm has higher blood pressure?
- If using a mercury column or gauge, is it at eye level?
- Has the patient been in the same position long enough to obtain a stable reading?
- Does the blood pressure change when the patient changes position from supine or sitting to standing?
- Does the patient complain of symptoms such as dizziness when changing position?
- Are things occurring in the environment that would artificially alter the patient's blood pressure?
- If the blood pressure is high, does it decrease if measured again in a few minutes?

Summary

The four classic vital sign measurements are *temperature, pulse, respiration,* and *blood pressure.* Observation of the patient while these vital signs are measured allows the caregiver or examiner to assess the patient's *level of consciousness* (*sensorium*) and develop a *general clinical impression* about the patient's level of distress, severity of illness, ability to cooperate, and need for assistance and education. The frequency of vital sign measurement is dependent on the reason for obtaining the information and the patient's condition. Obtaining one set of vital signs gives information about the patient at that moment in time. Evaluating vital signs over time and comparing the *trends* with information obtained from the history, physical examination, and radiologic and laboratory studies allows for an accurate assessment and appropriate intervention. Careful attention to technique ensures that the measurements are accurate.

REVIEW QUESTIONS

1. T   F   *Abnormal sensorium can be caused by reduced blood flow and/or oxygenation to the brain.*

2. *Which of the following is not included in the measurement of vital signs?*
    a. *pulse*
    b. *respiratory rate*
    c. *urinary output*
    d. *blood pressure*

3. *What is the normal value of the resting pulse rate in the adult?*
    a. *30-60 beats/min.*
    b. *60-100 beats/min.*
    c. *80-120 beats/min.*
    d. *100-150 beats/min.*

4. T   F   *The normal value for the resting respiratory rate in an adult is 6-10 breaths/min.*

5. T   F   *Resting pulse and respiratory rates for neonates and children are normally higher than adults.*

6. *Which of the following changes would be consistent with a fever?*
    a. *decreased respiratory rate*
    b. *increased pulse rate*
    c. *decreased oxygen consumption*
    d. *all of the above*

7. T   F   *Fever is defined as an increase in body temperature above normal due to disease.*

8. *Which of the following methods of temperature measurement is recommended for neonates?*
    a. *oral*
    b. *axillary*
    c. *rectal*
    d. *ear*

9. *Which of the following affects the accuracy of temperature measurement?*
    a. *type of thermometer*
    b. *length of time used for measurement*
    c. *recent ingestion of oral materials*
    d. *all of the above*

10. *"A decrease in the intensity of the palpated pulse during inhalation" is a definition of which of the following?*
    a. *abdominal paradox*
    b. *pulse pressure*
    c. *pulsus paradoxus*
    d. *pulsus alternans*

11. *Which of the following would cause tachycardia in the adult?*
    a. *hypothermia*
    b. *hypoxemia*
    c. *hypertension*
    d. *polycythemia*

12. *Which of the following arterial sites is the most common for evaluating the pulse in the adult patient?*
    a. *pedal*
    b. *temporal*
    c. *radial*
    d. *femoral*

13. *Which of the following would cause tachypnea in the adult?*
    a. *hypothermia*
    b. *narcotic overdose*
    c. *metabolic acidosis*
    d. *hyperoxia*

14. *Which of the following would cause an erroneously high blood pressure measurement?*
    a. *inflation pressure held in the cuff between measurements*
    b. *use of blood pressure cuff that is too wide*
    c. *not enough pressure used in the cuff during measurement*
    d. *a and b*

15. T   F   *Hypotension reduces perfusion and tissue oxygen delivery.*

REFERENCES

1. Jason-Bjerklie S, and others: Clinical markers of asthma severity and risk: importance of subjective as well as objective factors, *Heart Lung* 21:265, 1992.
2. Kleiger RE, and Seinior RM: Long term electrocardiographic monitoring of ambulatory patients with chronic airway obstruction, *Chest* 65:483, 1074.
3. Icalzi RA, and others: Cardiac arrhythmias and left ventricular function in respiratory failure from chronic obstructive pulmonary disease, *Chest,* 97:1092, 1990.
4. Holford FD, and others: Cardiac arrhythmias in hospitalized patients with chronic obstructive pulmonary disease, *Am Rev Respir Dis* 108:879, 1973.
5. Schactman MS, and Greene J: Rhythm disturbances in the patient with pulmonary disease, *Crit Care Nurse* 13:40, 1993.
6. Shih HT, and others: Frequency and significance of cardiac arrhythmias in chronic obstructive lung disease, *Chest* 94:44 1988.
7. Ayres S, and Grace WJ: Inappropriate ventilation and hypoxemia as causes of cardiac arrhythmias, *Am J Med* 4:495, 1969.
8. Flick MR, and Block AJ: Nocturnal versus diurnal cardiac arrhythmias in patients with COPD, *Chest* 75:28, 1979.
9. Tirlapur VG, and Mar MA: Nocturnal hypoxemia and associated electrocardiographic changes in patients with chronic obstructive airway disease, *N Engl J Med* 306:125, 1982.
10. Draper G, and others: Human constitution in clinical medicine, New York, 1944, Hoeber.
11. Malasanos L, Barkauskas V, and Stoltenberg-Allen K: *Health assessment,* ed 4, St Louis, 1990, Mosby–Year Book.
12. O'Toole, M, editor: *Miller-Keane encyclopedia and dictionary of medicine, nursing and allied health,* ed. 5, Philadelphia, 1992, WB Saunders.
13. Caine RL: New coma scale targets patients in low level states, *Headlines* January/February 1993, p. 22.
14. Daily EK, and Schroeder JP: *Techniques in bedside hemodynamic monitoring,* ed 4, St Louis, 1989, Mosby–Year Book.
15. Hasler ME, and Cohen JA: The effect of oxygen administration on oral temperature assessment, *Nurs Res* 31:2665, 1982.
16. Lim-Levy F: The effect of oxygen inhalation on oral temperature, *Nurs Res* 31:151, 1982.
17. Yonkman CA: Cool and heated aerosol and the measurement of oral temperature, *Nurs Res* 31:354, 1982.
18. O'Hara GJ, and Phillips DB: Method and apparatus for measuring internal body temperature utilizing infrared emission. US Patent 4602642, (1986), and 4790324, (1988).
19. Nobel JJ: Infrared ear thermometry, *Pediatr Emerg Care* 8:54–58, 1992.
20. Davis K: The accuracy of tympanic temperature measurement in children, *Pediatr Nurse* 19:267–272, J1993.
21. Erickson RS, and Yount ST: Comparison of tympanic and oral temperatures in surgical patients, *Nurs Res* 40:90–93, 1991.
22. Milewski A, Ferguson KL, and Terndrup TE: Comparison of pulmonary artery, rectal, and tympanic membrane temperatures in adult intensive care unit patients, *Clin Pediatr (Phila)* (Suppl):13, 1991.
23. Terndrup TE, and Milewski A: The performance of two tympanic thermometers in a pediatric emergency department, *Clin Pediatr (Phila)* (Suppl):18, 1991.
24. Chamberlain JM, and others: Comparison of a tympanic thermometer to rectal and oral thermometers in a pediatric emergency department, *Clin Pediatr (Phila)* (Suppl):24, 1991.
25. Talo H, Macknin ML, and Medendorp SV: Tympanic membrane temperatures compared to rectal and oral temperatures, *Clin Pediatr (Phila)* (Suppl):30, 1991.
26. Pransky SM: The impact of technique and conditions of the tympanic membrane upon infrared tympanic thermometry, *Clin Pediatr (Phila)* (Suppl):50, 1991.
27. Zehner WJ, and Terndrup TE: The impact of moderate ambient temperature variance on the relationship between oral, rectal, and tympanic membrane temperatures, *Clin Pediatr (Phila)* (Suppl):61, 1991.
28. Fraden J: The development of thermoscan (R) instant thermometer, *Clin Pediatr (Phila)* (Suppl):11, 1991.
29. Weiss ME: Tympanic infrared thermometry for fullterm and preterm neonates, *Clin Pediatr (Phila)* (Suppl):42, 1991.
30. Gravelyn TR, and Weg JG: Respiratory rate as an indicator of acute respiratory dysfunction, *JAMA* 244:1123, 1980.
31. NIH Taskforce: The second task force on blood pressure control in children—1987, *Pediatrics* 79:1, 1987.
32. Kirkendall WM, and others: AHA Committee Report: recommendations for human blood pressure determinations by sphygmomanometers (abstract), *Circulation* 62:1146A, 1980.
33. Park MK: *Pediatric cardiology for practitioners,* ed 2, St Louis, 1988, Mosby–Year Book.
34. Henkind SJ, Benis AM, and Teichholz LE: The paradox of pulsus paradoxus, *Am Heart J* 114:1966, 1987.
35. Branwald E, editor: *Heart diseases: a textbook of cardiovascular medicine,* ed 2, Philadelphia, 1984, WB Saunders.
36. Rebuck AS, and Pengelly LD: Development of pulses paradoxus in the presence of airway obstruction, *N Engl J Med* 288:66, 1973.

Chapter 4

Physical Examination of the Patient with Cardiopulmonary Disease

Robert L. Wilkins

LEARNING OBJECTIVES

Upon completion of this chapter, the reader should be able to accomplish the following:

1. Recognize the four components of physical examination.

2. Recognize the importance of reviewing the history of present illness prior to performing a physical exam.

3. Recognize the significance of the following during examination of the head and neck:
   a. nasal flaring
   b. cyanosis
   c. pursed-lip breathing
   d. changes in pupillary size in response to light
   e. jugular venous distention
   f. deviated tracheal position

4. Describe the correct method for measuring JVP and expected normal findings.

5. Define the following terminology used to classify thoracic configuration during inspection of the chest:
   a. pectus carinatum
   b. pectus excavatum
   c. kyphosis
   d. scoliosis
   e. kyphoscoliosis
   f. barrel chest
   g. flail chest

6. Recognize the topographic position of the following:
   a. thoracic cage landmarks (suprasternal notch, sternal angle [angle of Louis], vertebral spinous processes [C7 and T1])
   b. lung fissures (oblique [major] and horizontal [minor])
   c. tracheal bifurcation anteriorly and posteriorly
   d. right and left diaphragm anteriorly and posteriorly
   e. lung borders

LEARNING OBJECTIVES — cont'd

7. Define the following terms used to describe breathing pattern during inpsection of the chest:
   a. apnea
   b. Biot's
   c. Cheyne-Stokes
   d. Kussmaul's
   e. apneustic
   f. paradoxical
   g. asthmatic

8. Identify the breathing patterns associated with restrictive and obstructive lung disease.

9. Recognize the clinical significance of accessory muscle usage and retractions/bulging.

10. Recognize the significance of a "clavicular lift" greater than 5 mm during inspiration in patients with COPD.

11. Define the following terms and recognize their significance:
    a. abdominal paradox
    b. respiratory alternans
    c. peripheral cyanosis
    d. central cyanosis

12. Identify causes for increased and decreased tactile fremitus.

13. Identify causes for decreased thoracic expansion as assessed during chest palpation.

14. Recognize a description of subcutaneous emphysema and its clinical significance.

15. Identify causes of increased and decreased resonance during percussion of the lung.

16. Describe the four basic parts of a stethoscope and their uses.

17. Recognize the proper technique for auscultation of the lungs.

18. Recognize the four characteristics of breath sounds that should be evaluated by the examiner during auscultation.

19. Recognize a definition of the following terminology used to describe lung sounds and the mechanisms responsible for producing the sounds:
    a. bronchial or tracheal
    b. bronchovesicular
    c. vesicular (normal)
    d. diminished or reduced
    e. harsh

20. Recognize a definition of the following terminology used to describe abnormal (adventitious) lung sounds and the mechanisms responsible for producing the sounds:
    a. crackles (rales)
    b. wheezes
    c. stridor
    d. pleural friction rub

21. Recognize qualifying adjectives that can be used to describe lung sounds and the importance of using these qualifying adjectives.

22. Recognize the significance of the following auscultatory findings:
    a. monophonic wheeze
    b. polyphonic wheeze
    c. late-inspiratory crackles
    d. inspiratory and expiratory crackles
    e. pleural friction rub
    f. stridor

LEARNING OBJECTIVES — cont'd

23. *Recognize a definition of egophony and bronchophony and the causes for each condition.*

24. *Recognize the topographic location of the apex and base of the heart during examination of the precordium.*

25. *Recognize a definition of point of maximal impulse (PMI), its normal location, and the factors which may cause a shift of the PMI to the right or left.*

26. *Recognize the best location for auscultating sounds produced by the aortic, pulmonic, mitral, and tricuspid valves.*

27. *Recognize what produces the first (S_1), second (S_2), third (S_3), and fourth (S_4) heart sounds.*

28. *Describe what is meant by a "gallop rhythm" and what it signifies.*

29. *Recognize factors that increase or decrease the intensity of the heart sounds.*

30. *Recognize a definition of S_2 "splitting" and a loud P_2 heart sound and what they signify.*

31. *Describe the factors that cause systolic and diastolic heart murmurs.*

32. *Recognize a definition and the significance of hepatomegaly in the cardiopulmonary patient.*

33. *Recognize a definition and the significance of the following during examination of the extremities:*
    a. *digital clubbing*
    b. *cyanosis*
    c. *pedal edema*
    d. *capillary refill*
    e. *peripheral skin temperature*

34. *Recognize the general physical signs of the following abnormal pulmonary pathologies:*
    a. *acute airway obstruction*
    b. *chronic airway obstruction*
    c. *consolidation*
    d. *pneumothorax*
    e. *pleural effusion*
    f. *local bronchial obstruction*
    g. *diffuse interstitial fibrosis*
    h. *acute upper airway obstruction*

Chapter Overview

Physical examination is the process of examining the patient for the physical signs of disease. It is an inexpensive way of obtaining immediate and pertinent information about the patient's health status. The four basic components of the physical examination are *inspection, palpation, percussion,* and *auscultation.*

The patient initially is examined to help determine the correct diagnosis. Once a tentative diagnosis is made, subsequent examinations are valuable to monitor the patient's hospital course and to evaluate the results of treatment. Each examination should be modified according to the patient's history and the purpose of the examination. Through experience, the examiner learns which of the techniques described in this chapter should be used in any situation. Each examination should be performed in a quiet, well-lighted room, and

the examiner should avoid exposing the patient to any unnecessary discomfort.

The skills described in this chapter are not difficult to learn; however, proficiency is attained only with practice. The beginner first should practice the skills on normal persons to improve technique and, more importantly, to obtain an appreciation for normal variations. Abnormalities can be detected only by examiners who have developed an appreciation of normal body functions for comparison.

This chapter emphasizes the techniques of examination used in assessment of the patient with respiratory disease. Because respiratory disease may indirectly alter other body systems, examination of the entire patient is important. The techniques used in examination of the thorax and other body systems for the abnormalities often associated with respiratory disease are reviewed. The typical order in which the initial physical examination is performed and recorded is presented in the box below. See Chapter 3 for a complete discussion of the initial impression and assessment of the vital signs.

A review of the patient's history of present illness and past medical history before examination is helpful, especially if the examiner was not involved in acquiring the patient's medical history. This gives the examiner insight into the physical examination findings to be expected and suggests the techniques to emphasize.

Examination of the Head and Neck

Head

An examination of the head should first identify the patient's facial expression. This may help determine if the patient is in acute distress or suffering from physical pain. The facial expression can also help to evaluate alertness, mood, general character, and mental capacity. Abnormalities produced by respiratory disease include nasal flaring, cyanosis, and pursed lips breathing. Nasal flaring is identified by observing the external nares flare outward during inhalation. This occurs especially in neonates with respiratory distress and indicates an increase in the work of breathing.

When respiratory disease results in reduced oxygenation of the arterial blood, cyanosis may be detected, especially around the lips and oral mucosa. *Cyanosis* is a bluish cast to the skin that clinically may be difficult to detect, especially in a poorly lighted room. The presence of cyanosis is strong evidence that tissue oxygenation may be less than optimal; further investigation is indicated. The absence of cyanosis, however, does not indicate that tissue oxygenation is adequate, because a sufficient hemoglobin concentration must exist before cyanosis can be identified (see Inspection for Cyanosis, below).

Patients with chronic obstructive pulmonary disease (COPD) may use pursed lips breathing during exhalation. This technique is often taught to patients and may even be used by patients who have not had instruction on its benefits. Some patients naturally begin to pucker their lips during exhalation to provide a slight resistance to the exhaled breath. This resistance theoreti-

TYPICAL FORMAT FOR RECORDING THE PHYSICAL EXAMINATION

Initial impression
Age, height, weight, and general appearance

Vital signs
Pulse rate, respiratory rate, temperature, and blood pressure

HEENT (head, ears, eyes, nose, and throat)
Inspection findings

Neck
Inspection and palpation findings

Thorax
Lungs—inspection, palpation, percussion, and auscultation

Heart—inspection, palpation, and auscultation findings

Abdomen
Inspection, palpation, percussion, and auscultation findings

Extremities
Inspection and palpation findings

---

cally provides a slight backpressure in the airways during exhalation and prevents their premature collapse.

Eyes

The pupillary reflexes are evaluated as part of the neurologic examination. Cranial nerves II and III must be intact for normal pupillary reflexes to be present. If the pupils are equal in size, round, and reactive to light and accommodation, the physician may simply write PERRLA (*P*upils *E*qual, *R*ound, *R*eactive to *L*ight and *A*ccommodation) in the patient's chart when reporting examination results. Head trauma, tumors, central nervous system disease, and certain medications can cause abnormal findings. Brain death, catecholamines, and atropine can cause the pupils to become dilated and fixed (*mydriasis*). Parasympathetic stimulants and opiates can cause pinpoint pupils (*miosis*).

Examination of the eyelids is useful when the examiner suspects disease of the cranial nerves. Drooping of the upper lid (*ptosis*) may be an early sign of disease involving the third cranial nerve. Congenital defects, cranial tumors, and neuromuscular diseases such as myasthenia gravis may cause ptosis. Ptosis may represent an early warning sign of respiratory failure when a descending neuromuscular disease such as

myasthenia gravis is occurring. Neuromuscular diseases affecting the cranial nerves may also result in blurred or double vision (*diplopia*), and involuntary, cyclical movement of the eyeballs known as *nystagmus*.

Neck

Inspection and palpation of the neck are of value in determining the tracheal position, in estimating the jugular venous pressure (JVP), and in identifying whether the patient's accessory muscles are in use. Normally, the trachea is located centrally in the neck when the patient is facing forward. The midline of the neck can be identified by palpation of the suprasternal notch at the base of the anterior neck. The midline of the trachea should be directly below the center of the suprasternal notch.

The trachea may be shifted from midline with unilateral upper lobe collapse, pneumothorax, pleural effusion, or lung tumors. The trachea shifts toward the collapsed lung but away from the pneumothorax, pleural effusion, or lung tumor. Abnormalities in the lower lung fields may not shift the trachea unless the defect is severe.

The JVP is estimated by examining the level of the column of blood in the jugular veins. JVP reflects the volume and pressure of the venous blood in the right side of the heart. Both the internal and external jugular veins can be assessed, although the internal jugular is most reliable. Persons with obese necks may not have visible neck veins, even with distention.

In the supine position the neck veins of a healthy person are full. When the head of the bed is elevated gradually to a 45-degree angle from horizontal, the level of the column of blood descends to a point no more than a few centimeters above the clavicle with normal venous pressure. With elevated venous pressure, the neck veins may be distended as high as the angle of the jaw, even when the patient is sitting upright (Fig. 4–1). The degree of venous distention can be estimated by measuring the distance the veins are distended above the sternal angle. The sternal angle has been chosen universally because its distance above the right atrium remains relatively constant (about 5 cm) in all positions. With the head of the bed elevated to a 45-degree angle, venous distention greater than 3 to 4 cm above the sternal angle is abnormal (Fig. 4–2).

Exact quantification of the jugular pressure in terms of centimeters above the sternal angle is difficult and probably exceeds the accuracy needed for most observers. A simple grading scale of normal, increased, and markedly increased is acceptable.

The level of jugular venous distention may vary with breathing. During inhalation the level of the column of blood may descend toward the thorax and return to the previous position with exhalation. For this reason JVP should always be estimated at the end of exhalation.

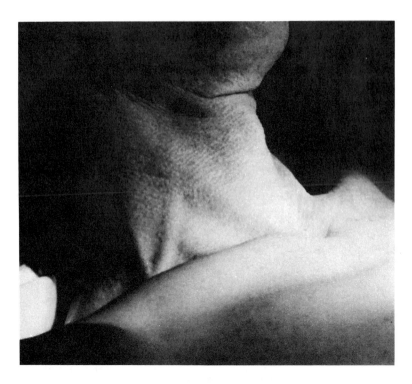

Fig. 4-1 *Photograph of jugular venous distention. (Reproduced by permission from Daily EK, and Schroeder JP:* Techniques in bedside hemodynamic monitoring, *ed 4, St Louis, 1981, Mosby-Year Book.)*

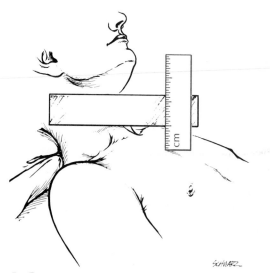

Fig. 4-2 *Estimation of jugular venous pressure. (From Malasanos, Barkauskas V, and Stoltenberg-Allen K:* Health assessment, *ed 4, St Louis, 1990, Mosby-Year Book.)*

The most common cause of jugular venous distention is right heart failure. Right heart failure may occur secondary to left heart failure or chronic hypoxemia. Hypoxemia initiates pulmonary vasoconstriction and increases the resistance to blood flow through the pulmonary vasculature, increasing the workload of the right ventricle. Persistent lung disease with hypoxemia may result in right heart failure and jugular venous distention. Jugular venous distention also may occur with hypervolemia and when the venous return to the right atrium is obstructed by tumors in the mediastinum.

Contraction of the sternomastoid muscle in the neck is an indication that the patient's work of breathing is increased. It is a common finding in patients with airway obstruction. This is discussed in the section on chest inspection.

Lung Topography

The examiner must understand how the lungs are situated within the chest to perform an accurate physical assessment of the respiratory system. Topographic (surface) landmarks of the chest are helpful in identifying the location of underlying structures and in describing the location of abnormalities.

Imaginary Lines

On the anterior chest the midsternal line divides the chest into two equal halves. The left and right midclavicular lines parallel the midsternal line and are drawn through the midpoints of the left and right clavicles respectively (Fig. 4-3).

The midaxillary line divides the lateral chest into two equal halves. The anterior axillary line parallels the midaxillary line and is situated along the anterolateral

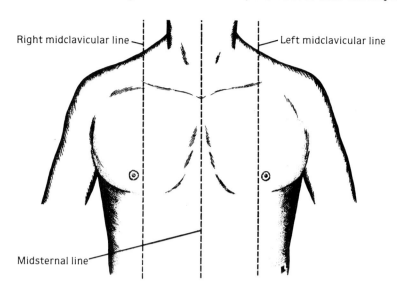

Right midclavicular line

Left midclavicular line

Midsternal line

Fig. 4-3 *Imaginary lines on anterior chest wall.*

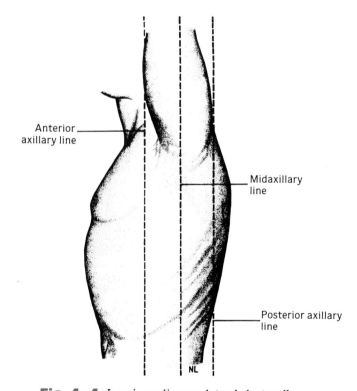

Anterior axillary line

Midaxillary line

Posterior axillary line

Fig. 4-4 *Imaginary lines on lateral chest wall.*

chest. The posterior axillary line is also parallel to the midaxillary line and is located in the posterolateral chest (Fig. 4-4).

Three imaginary vertical lines are drawn on the posterior chest. The midspinal line divides the posterior chest into two equal halves. The left and right midscapular lines parallel the midspinal line and pass through the inferior angles of the scapulae in the relaxed upright patient (Fig. 4-5).

Thoracic Cage Landmarks

On the anterior chest the suprasternal notch is located at the top of the manubrium and can be located by palpation of the depression at the base of the neck. Directly below this notch is the sternal angle, which is also referred to as the *angle of Louis*. The sternal angle can be identified by palpating down from the suprasternal notch until the ridge between the gladiolus and the

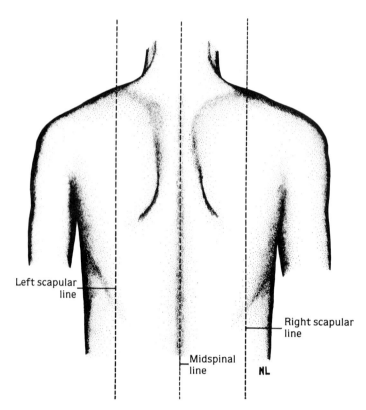

Fig. 4-5 *Imaginary lines on posterior chest wall.*

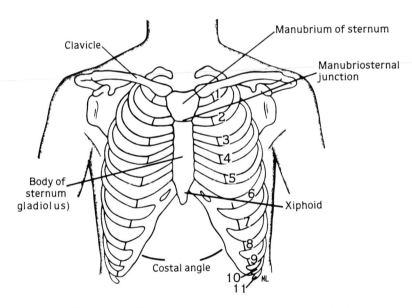

Fig. 4-6 *Thoracic cage landmarks on anterior chest.*

manubrium is identified. This important landmark is visible in most persons. The second rib articulates with the top of the gladiolus at this point (Fig. 4–6). Rib identification on the anterior chest can now be accomplished with this as a reference point. It is recommended that ribs be counted to the side of the sternum, since individual costal cartilages that attach the ribs to the sternum are not identified as easily near the sternum.

On the posterior chest the spinous processes of the vertebrae are useful landmarks (Fig. 4–7). The spinous process of the seventh cervical vertebra (C7) usually can be identified by having the patient extend the head and neck forward and slightly down. At the base of the neck the most prominent spinous process that can be visualized and palpated is C7. The spinous process just below C7 belongs to the first thoracic vertebra (T1). The scapular borders also can be useful

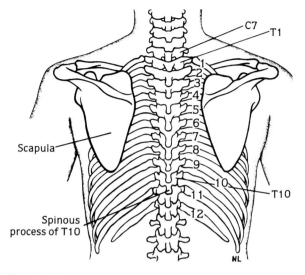

Fig. 4-7 *Thoracic cage landmarks on posterior chest.*

landmarks on the posterior chest. With the patient's arms raised above the head, the inferior border of the scapula approximately overlies the oblique fissure that separates the upper from the lower lobes on the posterior chest.

Lung Fissures

Between the lobes of the lungs are the interlobar fissures. Both lungs have an oblique fissure that begins on the anterior chest at approximately the sixth rib at the midclavicular line. This fissure extends laterally and upward until it crosses the fifth rib on the lateral chest in the midaxillary line and continues on the posterior chest to approximately T3 (Figs. 4–8 and 4–9).

The right lung also has a horizontal fissure that separates the right upper lobe from the right middle lobe. The horizontal fissure extends from the fourth rib at the sternal border around to the fifth rib at the

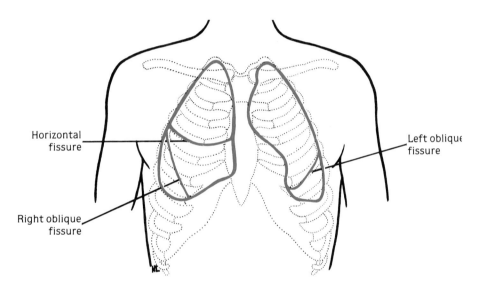

Fig 4-8 *Topographic position of lung fissures on anterior chest.*

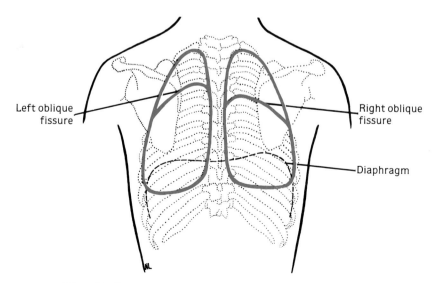

Fig. 4-9 *Topographic position of lung fissures on posterior chest.*

midaxillary line. The left lung rarely has a horizontal fissure.

Tracheal Bifurcation

On the anterior chest the carina is located approximately beneath the sternal angle and on the posterior chest at about T4 (Fig. 4–10).

Diaphragm

The diaphragm is a dome-shaped muscle that lies between the thoracic and abdominal cavities and moves up and down during normal ventilation. At the end of a tidal expiration the right dome of the diaphragm is located at the level of T9 posteriorly and the fifth rib anteriorly. On the left the diaphragm comes to rest at the end of expiration at T10 posteriorly and the sixth rib anteriorly. The right hemidiaphragm is usually a little higher anatomically than the left hemidiaphragm because of the placement of the liver.

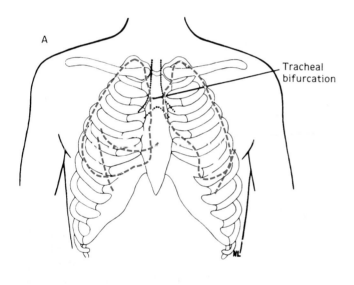

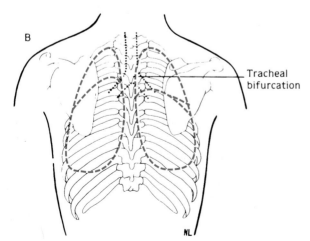

Fig. 4–10 *Topographic position of tracheal bifurcation and lung borders on* **A,** *anterior chest and* **B,** *posterior chest.*

Lung Borders

Superiorly on the anterior chest the lungs extend 2 to 4 cm above the medial third of the clavicles. The inferior borders on the anterior chest extend to approximately the sixth rib at the midclavicular line and to the eighth rib on the lateral chest wall. On the posterior chest the superior border extends to T1, and the inferior border varies with ventilation between approximately T9 and T12 (see Fig. 4–9).

Examination of the Thorax

Inspection

Visual examination of the chest is of value in assessing the thoracic configuration and the pattern and effort of breathing. For adequate inspection the room must be well lighted and the patient should be sitting upright. When the patient is too ill to sit up, the examiner needs to roll the patient carefully onto one side to examine the posterior chest. Male patients should be stripped to the waist. Female patients should be given some type of drape to prevent embarrassing exposure of the breasts.

THORACIC CONFIGURATION. The normal adult thorax has an anteroposterior diameter less than the transverse diameter. The anteroposterior diameter normally increases gradually with age and prematurely increases in patients with COPD. This abnormal increase in anteroposterior diameter is called *barrel chest.* When the anteroposterior diameter increases, the ribs lose their normal 45-degree angle of slope in relation to the spine and become horizontal (Fig. 4–11). Other abnormalities of the thoracic configuration include the following:

Pectus carinatum	Sternal protrusion anteriorly
Pectus excavatum	Depression of part or all of the sternum, which can produce a restrictive lung defect
Kyphosis	Spinal deformity in which the spine has an abnormal anteroposterior curvature
Scoliosis	Spinal deformity in which the spine has a lateral curvature
Kyphoscoliosis	Combination of kyphosis and scoliosis; may produce a severe restrictive lung defect as a result of poor lung expansion

Severe trauma to the chest cage can result in fractures of the ribs and sternum. Abnormal configuration of the thoracic cage may result, especially if multiple ribs are broken. A section of the rib cage may move paradoxically with breathing when multiple ribs are fractured at more than one site. The paradoxical

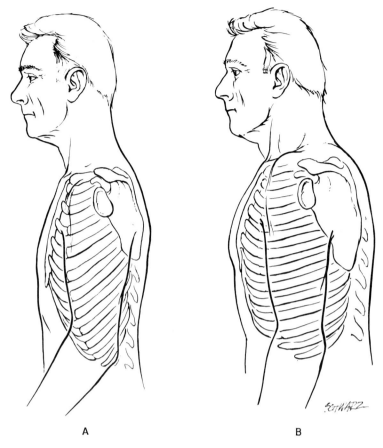

Fig. 4-11 A, *Patient with normal thoracic configuration.* **B,** *Patient with increased anteroposterior diameter. Note contrasts in angle or slope of ribs and development of accessory muscles. (From Malasanos L, Barkauskas V, and Stoltenberg-Allen K:* Health assessment, *ed 4, St Louis, 1990, Mosby-Year Book.)*

motion is seen as a sinking inward of the affected region with each spontaneous inspiratory effort and an outward movement with subsequent exhalation. This paradoxical motion of the affected rib cage is called *flail chest.*

BREATHING PATTERN AND EFFORT. The normal adult at rest has a consistent rate and rhythm of ventilation. The effort of breathing is minimal on inhalation and passive on exhalation. Men typically breathe with their diaphragm, causing the stomach to move slightly outward during inhalation. Women tend to use a combination of intercostal muscles and the diaphragm, producing more chest wall movement than men. Table 4-1 describes the abnormal patterns of breathing.

Changes in the patient's pattern of breathing can provide important clues to the type of respiratory problem present. Patients with restrictive lung disease typically breathe with a rapid and shallow pattern. Acute obstruction of intrathoracic airways, as occurs with asthma, results in a prolonged exhalation time. The approximate inspiratory-to-expiratory (I/E) ratio can be determined by timing the two phases of breathing. With more severe cases of airway obstruction, the

I/E ratio may be 1:3 or 1:4. Acute upper airway obstruction, as occurs with croup or epiglottitis, often results in a prolonged inspiratory time.

Any respiratory abnormalities that increase the work of breathing may cause the accessory muscles of breathing (scalene and sternomastoid) to become active during breathing at rest. This is common in acute and chronic diffuse airway obstruction, acute upper airway obstruction, and disorders that reduce lung compliance.

Significant increases in the effort of breathing cause large swings in pleural pressure. As a result, the skin overlying the chest cage may sink inward during inspiration and bulge outward during exhalation when the work of breathing is increased. Inward depression of the skin during inspiration is known as *retraction.* The opposite movement of the skin during exhalation is known as *bulging.* Obesity and muscular chest walls prevent retractions and bulging from occurring unless the abnormality is severe.

The diaphragm may be nonfunctional in patients with spinal injuries or neuromuscular disease and severely limited in patients with COPD. When this occurs, the accessory muscles of breathing become ac-

Table 4–1 Abnormal Breathing Patterns

Pattern	Characteristics	Causes
Apnea	No breathing	Cardiac arrest
Biot's	Irregular breathing with long periods of apnea	Increased intracranial pressure
Cheyne-Stokes	Irregular type of breathing; breaths increase and decrease in depth and rate with periods of apnea	Diseases of central nervous system, congestive heart failure
Kussmaul's	Deep and fast	Metabolic acidosis
Apneustic	Prolonged inhalation	Brain damage
Paradoxical	Portion or all of chest wall moves in with inhalation and out with exhalation	Chest trauma, diaphragm paralysis
Asthmatic	Prolonged exhalation	Obstruction to airflow out of lungs

tive, even at rest. The respiratory accessory muscles may also become active during acute airway obstruction. In fact retraction of the sternomastoid muscle is an indication of severe obstruction.[1] Its absence, however, does *not* rule out the possibility that severe airway obstruction is present.

In patients with emphysema the lungs lose their elastic recoil and become hyperinflated. This results in the diaphragm being "pushed down" into a less functional position. The accessory muscles then must assist ventilation by raising the anterior chest in an effort to increase thoracic volume. When the accessory muscles are producing a "clavicular lift" of more than 5 mm in this situation, lung function tests have demonstrated consistently the presence of severe obstructive lung disease.[2]

Normally the abdomen moves gently outward with inspiration and inward with exhalation. When the diaphragm becomes fatigued, the accessory muscles of breathing attempt to maintain ventilation by becoming more active. As the accessory muscles contract in an effort to cause gas to flow into the lung, negative intrathoracic pressure causes the diaphragm to be pulled upward and the abdomen to sink inward during inspiration. This is known as *abdominal paradox*. It is an important finding that occurs with paralysis or fatigue of the diaphragm. Diaphragm fatigue is common in COPD patients, especially during weaning from mechanical ventilation.[3] Abdominal paradox may be accompanied by *respiratory alternans*. Respiratory alternans consists of periods of breathing using only the chest wall muscles alternating with periods of breathing entirely by the diaphragm. It is not as common as abdominal paradox but also is an indication that the diaphragm is fatigued. Not all patients with diaphragm dysfunction will develop abdominal paradox[4] or respiratory alternans, but when these clinical signs are present they indicate significant inspiratory muscle fatigue.

INSPECTION FOR CYANOSIS. *Cyanosis* is a bluish discoloration of the skin caused by a relative decrease in the oxygen saturation of the cutaneous capillary blood. Cyanosis may be present only in the extremities (hands and feet), tip of the nose, ear lobes, and lips, in which case it is called *peripheral cyanosis* or

acrocyanosis. Peripheral cyanosis is most often caused by a significant reduction in systemic blood flow (cardiac failure). Slow blood flow results in more substantial desaturation of the capillary blood, since more oxygen is extracted to compensate for the reduction in cardiac output. Peripheral cyanosis results because the blood in the extremities is darker in color owing to its desaturated condition.

Central cyanosis is present when the patient's trunk or more central regions such as the oral mucosa are cyanotic. This occurs when the lungs are not oxygenating the blood adequately or when congenital heart disease causes venous blood to be shunted into the arterial system without passing through the lungs. In summary, central cyanosis is associated with arterial oxygen desaturation and peripheral cyanosis is often related to inadequate circulation.

Palpation

Palpation is the art of touching the chest wall in an effort to evaluate underlying lung structure and function. Palpation is performed to (1) evaluate vocal fremitus, (2) estimate thoracic expansion, and (3) assess the skin and subcutaneous tissues of the chest. Palpation is used in selective patients to confirm or rule out suspected problems suggested by the history and initial physical examination.

VOCAL FREMITUS. The term *vocal fremitus* refers to the vibrations created by the vocal cords during phonation. These vibrations are transmitted down the tracheobronchial tree and through the alveoli to the chest wall. When these vibrations are felt on the chest wall, they are called *tactile fremitus.*

During the assessment of tactile fremitus, the patient is directed to repeat the word *ninety-nine* while the examiner systematically palpates the thorax. The examiner can use the palmar aspect of the fingers or the ulnar aspect of the hand as illustrated in Fig. 4–12. If one hand is used, it should be moved from one side of the chest to the corresponding area on the other side. The anterior, lateral, and posterior chest wall should be evaluated.

The vibrations of tactile fremitus may be increased, decreased, or absent. Increased fremitus re-

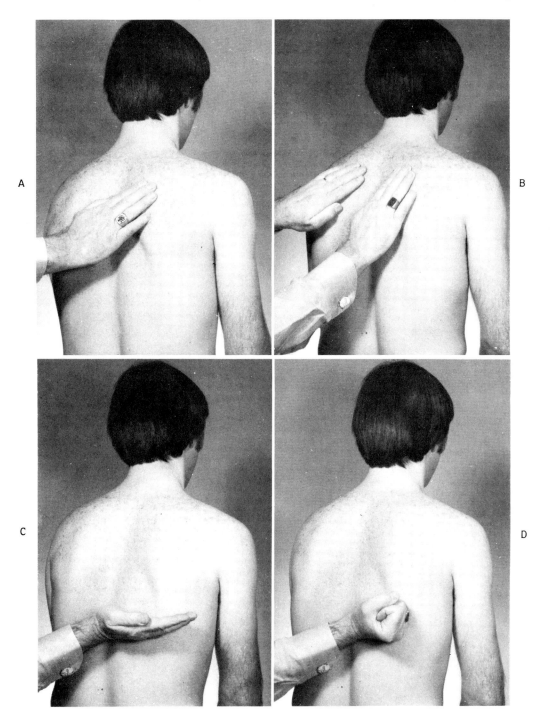

Fig. 4–12 *Palpation for assessment of vocal fremitus.* **A,** *Use of palmar surface of fingertips.* **B,** *Simultaneous application of fingertips of both hands.* **C,** *Use of ulnar aspect of hand.* **D,** *Use of ulnar aspect of closed fist. (From Prior JA, and Silberstein JS:* Physical diagnosis: the history and examination of the patient, *ed 6, St Louis, 1982, Mosby-Year Book.)*

sults from the transmission of the vibration through a more solid medium. The normal lung structure is a combination of solid and air-filled tissue. Any condition that tends to increase the density of the lung, such as the consolidation of pneumonia, results in an increased intensity of fremitus. If the area of consolidation is not in connection with a patent bronchus, fremitus will not be increased but will be absent or decreased.

A reduced tactile fremitus is often present in patients who are obese or overly muscular. Also, when the pleural space lining the lung becomes filled with air (pneumothorax) or fluid (pleural effusion), the vocal fremitus is reduced significantly or is absent.

In patients with emphysema the lungs become hyperinflated with a significant reduction in the density of lung tissue. In this situation the vibrations transmit poorly through the lung tissue, resulting in a bilateral reduction in tactile fremitus. The bilateral reduction in tactile fremitus is more difficult to detect than the unilateral increase in fremitus associated with lobar consolidation. The causes of abnormal tactile fremitus are summarized as follows:

Increased
 Pneumonia
 Lung tumor or mass
 Atelectasis
Decreased
 Unilateral
  Bronchial obstruction with mucus plug or
   foreign object
  Pneumothorax
  Pleural effusion
 Diffuse
  COPD
  Muscular or obese chest wall

The passage of air through airway(s) contaminated with thick secretions may produce palpable vibrations referred to as *rhonchial fremitus.* Rhonchial fremitus often is identified during inhalation and exhalation and may clear if the patient produces an effective cough. It frequently is associated with a coarse, low-pitched sound that is audible without a stethoscope.

THORACIC EXPANSION. The normal chest wall expands symmetrically during deep inhalation. This expansion can be evaluated on the anterior and posterior chest. Anteriorly, the examiner's hands are placed over the anterolateral chest with the thumbs extended along the costal margin toward the xiphoid process. On the posterior chest the hands are positioned over the posterolateral chest with the thumbs meeting at approximately T8 (Fig. 4–13). The patient is instructed to exhale slowly and completely while the examiner's hands are positioned as described. When the patient has exhaled maximally, the examiner gently secures the tips of his or her fingers against the sides of the chest and extends the thumbs toward the midline until the tip of each thumb meets at the midline. The patient is then instructed to take a full, deep breath. The examiner should make note of the distance each thumb moves from the midline. Normally, each thumb moves an equal distance of approximately 3 to 5 cm.

Diseases that affect expansion of both lungs cause a bilateral reduction in chest expansion. This is seen commonly with neuromuscular diseases and COPD. A unilateral (one-sided) reduction in chest expansion occurs with respiratory diseases that reduce the expansion of one lung or a major part of one lung. This may occur with lobar consolidation, atelectasis, pleural effusion, and pneumothorax.

SKIN AND SUBCUTANEOUS TISSUES. The chest wall can be palpated to determine the general temperature and condition of the skin. When air leaks from the lung into subcutaneous tissues, fine beads of air produce a crackling sound and sensation when palpated. This is referred to as *subcutaneous emphysema.*

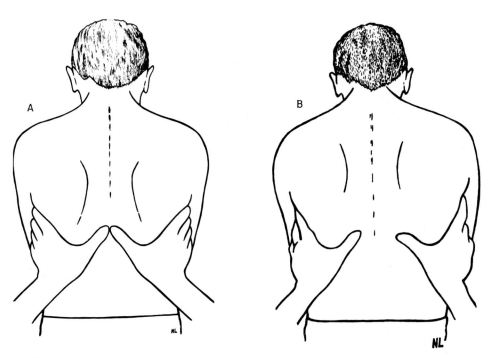

Fig. 4–13 *Estimation of thoracic expansion.* **A,** *Exhalation.* **B,** *Maximal inhalation.*

Percussion of the Chest to Assess Resonance

Percussion is the art of tapping on a surface in an effort to evaluate the underlying structure. Percussion of the chest wall produces a sound and a palpable vibration useful in the evaluation of the underlying lung tissue. The vibration created by percussion penetrates and thus evaluates the lung to a depth of 5 to 7 cm below the chest wall.

The technique most often used in percussion of the chest wall is termed *mediate* or *indirect percussion*. The examiner places the middle finger of the left hand (if the examiner is right-handed) firmly against the chest wall parallel to the ribs with the palm and other fingers held off the chest. The tip of the middle finger on the right hand or the lateral aspect of the right thumb strikes the finger against the chest near the base of the terminal phalanx with a quick, sharp blow. Movement of the hand striking the chest should be generated at the wrist and not the elbow or shoulder (Fig. 4–14).

The percussion note is clearest if the examiner remembers to keep the finger on the chest firmly against the chest wall and to strike this finger and immediately withdraw. The two fingers should be in contact only for an instant. As one gains experience in percussion of the chest, the feel of the vibration created becomes as important as the sound in the evaluation of lung structures.

PERCUSSION OVER LUNG FIELDS. Percussion of the lung fields should be done systematically, testing comparable areas on both sides of the chest consecutively. Percussion over the bony structures and

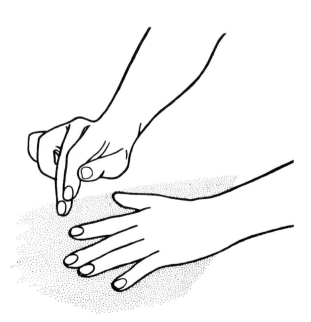

Fig. 4–14 *Technique for indirect chest percussion.*

breasts of the female is not of value and should be avoided. If the patient is asked to raise the arms above the shoulders, this will help move the scapulae laterally and minimize their interference with percussion on the posterior chest wall.

The sounds generated during percussion of the chest are evaluated for intensity (loudness) and pitch. Percussion over normal lung fields produces a sound moderately low in pitch that can be heard easily. This sound is best described as *normal resonance*. When the percussion note is louder and lower in pitch than normal, the resonance is said to be *increased*. Percussion may produce a sound with characteristics just the opposite of resonance, referred to as *dull* or *flat*. This sound is high-pitched, short in duration, and not loud.

CLINICAL IMPLICATIONS. By itself, percussion of the chest is of little value in making a diagnosis. When the percussion note is considered along with the history and other physical findings, it may contribute significantly.

Any abnormality that tends to increase the density of the lung tissue, such as the consolidation of pneumonia, lung tumors, or alveolar collapse (atelectasis), results in a loss of resonance and a dull percussion note over the affected area. Percussion over pleural spaces filled with fluid, such as blood or water, also results in a dull or flat percussion note.

An increase in resonance is detected in patients with hyperinflated lungs. Hyperinflation can occur as a result of acute bronchial obstruction (asthma) and chronic bronchial obstruction (emphysema). When the pleural space contains large amounts of air (pneumothorax), the percussion note increases in resonance over the affected side.

Unilateral abnormalities are easier to detect than bilateral abnormalities because the normal side provides an immediate comparison. The dullness heard from percussion over consolidation is a distinct sound that is easier to detect than the subtle increase in resonance associated with hyperinflation or pneumothorax.

Percussion of the chest has limitations that are often clinically important. Abnormalities of the lungs are difficult to detect if the patient's chest wall is obese or overly muscular. Abnormalities that are small or more than 5 cm below the surface are not likely to be detected during percussion of the chest. Percussion to assess lung resonance is not routinely done on most patients. It is useful, however, in the acutely ill patient suspected of having tension pneumothorax.

DIAPHRAGMATIC EXCURSION. The range of diaphragm movement may be estimated by percussion and is done best on the posterior chest wall (Fig. 4–15). To estimate diaphragm movement, the patient first is instructed to take a deep, full inspiration and hold it. The examiner then determines the lowest

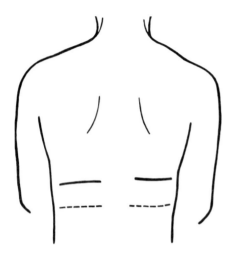

Fig. 4–15 *Assessment of diaphragmatic excursion by percussion. Horizontal lines indicate position of diaphragm at maximal inhalation and exhalation.*

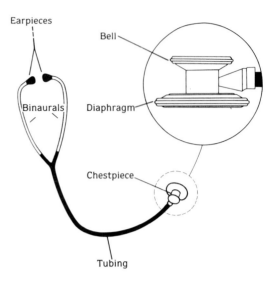

Fig. 4–16 *Acoustic stethoscope.*

margin of resonance by percussing over the lower lung field and moving downward in small increments until a definite change in the percussion note is detected. The patient then is instructed to exhale maximally, holding this position while the percussion procedure is repeated. The examiner should work rapidly to prevent the patient from becoming short of breath. The normal diaphragmatic excursion during a deep breath is about 5 to 7 cm. The range of diaphragm movement is less than normal in certain neuromuscular diseases and in patients with severe pulmonary hyperinflation.

The exact range of movement and position of the diaphragm is difficult to determine by percussion.[5] This probably is because the diaphragm is a dome-shaped muscle with the center of the dome 15 cm beneath the surface of the posterior chest. Percussion can only approximate the position and degree of movement and is not frequently performed.

Auscultation of the Lungs

Auscultation is the process of listening for sounds produced in the body. Auscultation over the thorax is performed to identify normal or abnormal lung sounds. Careful assessment of the patient's lung sounds is useful in making the initial diagnosis and to evaluate the effects of treatment. A stethoscope is used during auscultation for better transmission of sounds to the examiner. Whenever auscultation is performed, the room must be as quiet as possible.

STETHOSCOPE. The stethoscope possesses four basic parts: a bell, a diaphragm, tubing, and earpieces (Fig. 4–16). The bell detects a broad spectrum of sounds and is of particular value when listening to low-pitched heart sounds. It is also valuable in auscultation of the lungs in certain situations, as in the emaciated patient where rib protrusion restricts placement of the diaphragm flat against the chest. The bell

piece should be pressed lightly against the chest when attempting to auscultate low-frequency sounds. If the bell is pressed too firmly against the chest wall, the skin will be stretched under the bell and may act as a diaphragm, filtering out certain low-frequency sounds.

The diaphragm piece is used most often in auscultation of the lungs, since most lung sounds are high frequency. It is also useful in listening to high-frequency heart sounds. The diaphragm piece should be pressed firmly against the chest so that external sounds are not heard.

The ideal tubing should be thick enough to exclude external noises and should be approximately 25 to 35 cm (11–16 in.) in length. Longer tubing may compromise transmission of lung sounds, and shorter tubing is often inconvenient in reaching the patient's chest.

The stethoscope should be examined regularly for cracks in the diaphragm, wax or dirt in the earpieces, and other defects that may interfere with the transmission of sound. It should be wiped off with alcohol on a regular basis to prevent a buildup of microorganisms.

TECHNIQUE. When possible, the patient should be sitting upright in a relaxed position. The patient should be instructed to breathe a little deeper than normal with the mouth open. Inhalation should be an active process and exhalation passive. The bell or diaphragm must be placed directly against the chest wall, since clothing may alter lung sounds or produce distorted sounds. The tubing should not be rubbing against any objects, since this may produce extraneous sounds. Auscultation of the lungs should be systematic, including all lobes on the anterior, lateral, and posterior chest. It is recommended that the examiner begin at the bases, compare side with side, and work toward the lung apices. The examiner should begin at the lung bases because certain abnormal lung sounds (described later) that occur primarily in the dependent lung zones may be altered by several deep breaths. At least one full ventilatory cycle should be evaluated at each stethoscope position. The common errors of auscultation can be summarized as follows:

Errors	Correct technique
Listening to breath sounds through the patient's gown	Place bell or diaphragm directly against the chest wall
Allowing tubing to rub against bed rails or patient's gown	Keep tubing free from contact with any objects during auscultation
Attempting to auscultate in a noisy room	Turn television or radio off
Interpreting chest hair sounds as adventitious lung sounds	Wet chest hair, if thick, before auscultation
Auscultating only the "convenient" areas	Ask alert patient to sit up; roll comatose patient onto side to auscultate posterior lobes

Four characteristics of breath sounds should be specifically listened for by the examiner. First, the pitch (vibration frequency) should be identified. Second, the amplitude or intensity (loudness) is noted. Third, the distinctive characteristics are listened for and noted. Fourth, the duration of inspiratory sound is compared to that of expiration. The acoustic characteristics of breath sounds can be illustrated in breath sound diagrams (Fig. 4–17). Examiners must have a clear understanding of the characteristics of the normal breath sounds described in Table 4–2 to identify subtle changes that may signify respiratory disease.

TERMINOLOGY. In normal persons the sound heard over the trachea has a loud, tubular quality referred to as a *bronchial* or *tracheal* breath sound. Bronchial breath sounds are high-pitched sounds with an expiratory component equal to or slightly longer than the inspiratory component.

A slight variation to the bronchial breath sound is heard around the upper half of the sternum on the anterior chest and between the scapulae on the posterior chest (Fig. 4–18). This is not as loud as the bronchial breath sound, is slightly lower in pitch, and has equal inspiratory and expiratory components. It is referred to as a *bronchovesicular* breath sound.

Auscultating over the lung parenchyma of a normal person yields a soft, muffled sound. This is referred to as a *vesicular* or *normal* breath sound and is lower in pitch and intensity (loudness) than the bronchial breath

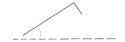

Fig. 4–17 *Diagrammatic representation of normal breath sound. Upstroke represents inhalation and downstroke represents exhalation; length of upstroke represents duration; thickness of stroke represents intensity; angle between upstroke and horizontal line represents pitch.*

sound. The vesicular sound is quite difficult to hear and is heard primarily during inhalation with only a minimal exhalation component (see Table 4–2).

Respiratory disease may alter the intensity of normal breath sounds heard over the lung fields. A slight variation in intensity is difficult to detect even for experienced clinicians. Breath sounds are described as *diminished* when the intensity decreases and *absent* in extreme cases. Breath sounds are described as *harsh* when the intensity increases. Harsh breath sounds may have an expiratory component equal to the inspiratory component and are described as *bronchial* breath sounds in such cases.

Abnormal sounds or vibrations produced by the movement of air in the lungs are termed *adventitious* sounds. Most adventitious lung sounds can be classified as either continuous or discontinuous sounds. Continuous lung sounds are defined as having a duration longer than 25 msc. (This definition is derived from recording and spectral analysis of lung sounds. Examiners are not expected to time the lung sounds.) Discontinuous lung sounds are characteristically intermittent, crackling, or bubbling sounds of short duration, usually less than 20 msc.[6]

The terminology used to describe abnormal lung sounds has had a confusing history. As a result, there has been a lack of standardization among clinicians.[7] Fortunately, the American Thoracic Society (ATS) and the American College of Chest Physicians (ACCP) formed a committee to address the issue of pulmonary nomenclature. Their work was first published in 1975 and suggested that the term *rales* be used to describe discontinuous types of abnormal lung sounds and the term *rhonchi* for continuous types of sounds.[8]

The committee published updated reports in 1977 and 1981 that advocated the term *crackles* for discontinuous types of lung sounds instead of the more popular term *rales*.[9,10] *Rales* had been used in the past to document both continuous and discontinuous types

Table 4-2	Characteristics of Normal Breath Sounds				
Breath Sound	**Pitch**	**Intensity**	**Location**	**Diagram of Sound**
Vesicular or normal	Low	Soft	Peripheral lung areas	
Bronchovesicular	Moderate	Moderate	Around upper part of sternum, between scapulae	
Bronchial	High	Loud	Over trachea	

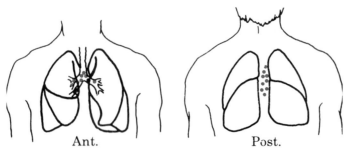

Bronchovesicular Breath Sounds

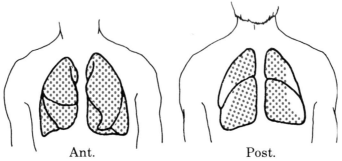

Vesicular Breath Sounds

Fig. 4-18 *Location on chest wall where normal bronchovesicular and vesicular breath sounds are heard. (From Wilkins RL, Hodgkin JE, and Lopez B:* Lung sounds: a practical guide, *St Louis, 1988, Mosby-Year Book.)*

of abnormal lung sounds, and the committee perceived that the more descriptive term *crackles* may be better suited for describing discontinuous types of abnormal lung sounds. Although use of the term *rales* has declined since the committee's recommendations, it remains a popular term among many clinicians.[11] The updates also suggested that high-pitched continuous types of abnormal lung sounds be described as *wheezes* and that *rhonchi* be used specifically for low-pitched, continuous sounds. There is evidence that the term *rhonchi* has been and is being used for both continuous and discontinuous abnormal lung sounds.[12] Consequently, there may be an advantage to abandoning use of the term *rhonchi* and limiting the description of abnormal lung sounds to the terms *crackles* and *wheezes*. For the remainder of this text, to be consistent with these recommendations, the term *crackles* is used for discontinuous lung sounds and *wheezes* for continuous lung sounds.

The reader should be aware that since there is a lack of standardization of lung sound terminology among clinicians, authors of other publications may use different terms to describe abnormal lung sounds. Table 4-3 provides a list of alternative terms that may be used by others.

Another continuous sound, heard primarily over the larynx and trachea during inhalation when upper airway obstruction is present, is known as *stridor*. This is a loud, high-pitched sound that frequently may be

Table 4-3	**Recommended Terminology for Lung Sounds and Other Terms Used**	
Recommended Term	**Classification**	**Other Terms Used**
Crackles	Discontinuous	Rales
		Crepitations
Wheezes	High-pitched, continuous	Sibilant rales
		Musical rales
		Sibilant rhonchus
	Low-pitched, continuous	Sonorous rales
		Rhonchi

heard without the aid of a stethoscope. Stridor is readily recognized by most clinicians.[12]

When abnormal lung sounds are identified, their location and specific characteristics should be noted. Abnormal lung sounds may be high- or low-pitched, loud or faint, scanty or profuse, and inspiratory or expiratory (or both). The timing during the respiratory cycle should be noted also, e.g., late inspiratory. The examiner must pay close attention to these characteristics of abnormal lung sounds because they help determine the functional status of the lungs. Many clinicians do not describe adventitious lung sounds with a qualifying adjective.[13] The importance of using appropriate qualifying adjectives to describe abnormal lung sounds is further emphasized in the following paragraphs.

MECHANISMS AND SIGNIFICANCE OF LUNG SOUNDS. The exact mechanisms responsible for the production of normal and abnormal lung sounds are not understood in detail. There is enough agreement among investigators, however, to allow a general description. This knowledge should give examiners a better understanding of the lung sounds frequently heard through a stethoscope.

Normal Breath Sounds. Lung sounds heard over the chest of the normal person are generated primarily by turbulent flow in the larger airways.[14,15] Turbulent flow creates audible vibrations in the airways, producing sounds that are transmitted through the lung and the chest wall. As the sound travels to the lung periphery and the chest wall, it is altered by the filtering properties of normal lung tissue. Normal lung tissue is known to act as a low-pass filter, which means it preferentially passes low-frequency sounds. This filtering effect can be demonstrated easily by listening over the periphery of the lung while a subject speaks. The muffled voice sounds are difficult to understand because of the filtering properties of the lung.

This filtering phenomenon accounts for the characteristic differences between bronchial breath sounds heard directly over larger airways and vesicular sounds heard over the periphery of the lung. Normal vesicular lung sounds essentially are filtered bronchial breath sounds.

The identification of normal breath sounds over all areas of the chest is helpful in ruling out pneumonia and other chest diseases. In one study the identification of normal breath sounds ruled out pneumonia with greater than 95% certainty in asthmatic patients who arrived in the emergency room complaining of dyspnea. This helped eliminate the need for chest radiographs.[16]

Abnormal Bronchial Breath Sounds. Bronchial breath sounds may replace the normal vesicular sound when the lung tissue increases in density, as occurs in atelectasis and pneumonia. When the normal air-filled lung tissue becomes consolidated, the filtering effect is lost, and similar sounds are heard over large upper airways and the consolidated lung.[17]

Diminished Breath Sounds. Diminished breath sounds occur when the sound intensity at the site of generation (larger airways) is reduced or when the transmission properties of the lung or chest wall are reduced. The intensity of sound created by turbulent flow through the bronchi is reduced with shallow or slow breathing patterns. Obstructed airways (e.g., mucus plugs) and hyperinflated lung tissue inhibit normal transmission of sounds through the lungs. Air or fluid in the pleural space and obesity reduce the transmission of breath sounds through the chest wall.

In patients with chronic airflow obstruction, the intensity of vesicular breath sounds is often reduced markedly throughout all lung fields. This is primarily the result of poor sound transmission through hyperinflated lung tissue, as occurs with emphysema. Shallow breathing patterns also may contribute to reduced breath sound intensity in patients with COPD. Studies have been done correlating the intensity of vesicular lung sounds with pulmonary function tests, and these studies have provided some useful conclusions. A definite, diffuse reduction in breath sound intensity is strong evidence that obstructive pulmonary disease is present and that a significant reduction in expiratory flow rates exists. Normal breath sound intensity heard throughout the lung fields nearly excludes the possibility that significant chronic obstructive abnormalities are present. Mild reductions in breath sound intensity are less predictive.[18–20]

Wheezes. Wheezes are generated by the vibration of the wall of a narrowed or compressed airway as air passes through at high velocity.[14,15] The diameter of an airway may be reduced by bronchospasm, mucosal edema, or foreign objects. The pitch of the wheeze is independent of the length of the airway but is related directly to the degree of airway compression. The tighter the compression, the higher the pitch. Low-pitched continuous sounds are often associated with the presence of excessive sputum in the airways. A sputum flap vibrating in the airstream may produce low-pitched wheezes that clear after the patient coughs.

The significance of expiratory wheezing during unforced breathing has been studied, and several useful conclusions have been reached. Patients with chronic airflow obstruction who do not wheeze are not likely to have significant improvement of expiratory flow rates (measured by spirometry) after bronchodilator therapy. Patients with chronic airflow obstruction who wheeze are more likely to have significant improvement in their expiratory flow rates after bronchodilator therapy. When unforced expiratory wheezing is intense, spirometry consistently demonstrates moderate to severe airway obstruction. Less intense wheezing is associated with a wide range of obstructive defects.[21] Wheezing heard during a forceful expiratory maneuver is identified commonly in persons with obstructed and unobstructed airways and is of no predictive value.

When wheezes are identified, certain characteristics should be noted. Examiners should identify the pitch and intensity and the portion of the respiratory cycle occupied by the wheezing.[22,23] Improvement in the patient's airway caliber with bronchodilator therapy often results in a decrease in pitch and intensity of the wheezing and in a reduction in the portion of the respiratory cycle occupied by wheezing. For example, before treatment the patient may have loud, high-pitched wheezing that is heard during inspiration and expiration. Following bronchodilator therapy the wheezing may decrease in pitch and intensity and be heard only during the later part of exhalation. Since the intensity of wheezing is related to the flow, loud wheezing does indicate that air movement is occurring, whereas soft wheezing may occur with fatigue and the onset of respiratory failure. Clinicians must never rely solely on changes in the intensity of wheezing in assessing the patient's response to therapy.

Wheezing may be polyphonic (having several different musical notes) or monophonic (having a single note). Polyphonic wheezing is limited to exhalation, and its many different musical notes begin and end simultaneously. They indicate that multiple airways are obstructed, as in asthma. Monophonic wheezes may be single or multiple, with each one indicating obstruction of a bronchus. When multiple monophonic wheezes are present, the different notes often begin and end at different times and so overlap. The illusion of widespread airway obstruction is due to the transmission of a few loud notes to most areas of the chest wall. A single monophonic wheeze indicates obstruction of a single airway. This may be present in the patient with an airway tumor that is partially obstructing a major airway.

Crackles. Crackles are often produced by the movement of excessive secretions or fluid in the airways as air passes through. In this situation crackles are usually coarse and heard during inspiration and expiration. They often clear if the patient coughs and may be associated with rhonchial fremitus.

Crackles also occur in patients without excess secretions when collapsed airways pop open during inspiration.[14,24-27] The crackling sound in this situation is caused by the explosive-type equalization of pressure between the collapsed airways and the patent airways above. Airway closure may occur in peripheral bronchioles or in more proximal bronchi. The source of the crackles in this situation may be suggested by certain characteristics described in the following paragraphs.

Larger, more proximal bronchi may close during expiration when there is an abnormal increase in bronchial compliance or if the retractive pressures around the bronchi are low. In this situation crackles usually occur early in the inspiratory phase and are referred to as *early inspiratory crackles* (Fig. 4–19). Early inspiratory crackles are usually scanty (few in number) but may be loud or faint. They are often transmitted to the mouth and are not silenced by a cough or change in position. They most often occur in patients with COPD, as in chronic bronchitis, emphysema, and asthma, and may indicate that a more severe airway obstruction is present.[25]

Peripheral alveoli and airways may close during exhalation when the surrounding intrathoracic pressure increases. Crackles produced by the sudden opening of peripheral airways usually occur late in the inspiratory phase and are referred to as *late inspiratory crackles.* They are more common in the dependent regions of the lungs where the gravitational stress

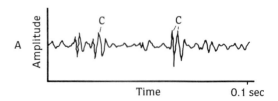

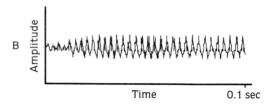

Fig. 4–19 *Time-expanded waveforms demonstrating* **A,** *inspiratory crackles and* **B,** *expiratory polyphonic wheezes. (From Wilkins RL, and others:* Lung-sound terminology used by respiratory care practitioners, *Respir Care 34:36, 1989.)*

predisposes the peripheral airways to collapse during exhalation. They are often identified in several consecutive respiratory cycles, producing a recurrent rhythm. They may clear with changes in posture or if the patient performs several deep inspiratory maneuvers. Coughing or maximal exhalation by the patient may produce the reappearance of late inspiratory crackles. Patients with respiratory disorders such as atelectasis, pneumonia, pulmonary edema, and fibrosis that cause a reduction in lung volume (restrictive disorders) are most likely to have the late inspiratory type of crackles[25] (Table 4–4).

The presence of inspiratory crackles generally is considered an abnormal physical finding, but may occur in normal persons in certain situations.[28,29] Fine inspiratory crackles can be identified in healthy subjects during inhalation from low lung volumes (after maximal exhalation). In addition, an end-expiratory cough may result in the identification of late inspiratory crackles that were not present after a normal expiratory effort. Since crackles can be elicited from normal subjects during inspiration from low lung volumes, they are not necessarily abnormal lung sounds. Perhaps fine, late inspiratory crackles should be considered abnormal only when they occur during inhalation from a resting lung volume.

Pleural Friction Rub. A *pleural friction rub* is a creaking or grating type of sound that occurs when the pleural surfaces become inflamed and the roughened edges rub together during breathing. It may be heard only during inhalation but is often identified during both phases of breathing. Pleural rubs often sound similar to coarse crackles but are not affected by coughing. Pleural rubs are not commonly encountered in the clinical setting and for this reason are often not

Table 4-4 Application of Adventitious Lung Sounds

Lung Sounds	Possible Mechanism	Characteristics	Causes
Wheezes	Rapid airflow through obstructed airways caused by bronchospasm, mucosal edema	High-pitched; most often occur during exhalation	Asthma, congestive heart failure, bronchitis
Stridor	Rapid airflow through obstructed airway caused by inflammation	High-pitched; often occurs during inhalation	Croup, epiglottitis, postextubation
Crackles			
Inspiratory and expiratory	Excess airway secretions moving with airflow	Coarse and often clear with cough	Bronchitis, respiratory infections
Early inspiratory	Sudden opening of proximal bronchi	Scanty, transmitted to mouth; not affected by cough	Bronchitis, emphysema, asthma
Late inspiratory	Sudden opening of peripheral airways	Diffuse, fine; occur initially in the dependent regions	Atelectasis, pneumonia, pulmonary edema, fibrosis

correctly identified when present.[13] The intensity of pleural rubs may increase with deep breathing.

VOICE SOUNDS. If inspection, palpation, percussion, or auscultation of the patient's chest suggests any respiratory abnormality, vocal resonance may be useful. Vocal resonance is produced by the same mechanism as vocal fremitus, described earlier. The vibrations created by the vocal cords during phonation travel down the tracheobronchial tree and through the peripheral lung units to the chest wall. The patient is instructed to repeat the words *one, two, three,* or *ninety-nine* while the examiner listens over the chest wall with the aid of a stethoscope, comparing side with side. The normal, air-filled lung tissue filters the voice sounds, resulting in a significant reduction in intensity and clarity. Pathologic abnormalities in lung tissue alter the transmission of voice sounds, resulting in either increased or decreased vocal resonance.

An increase in intensity and clarity of vocal resonance is referred to as *bronchophony.* Bronchophony occurs as a result of an increase in lung tissue density, as in the consolidation of pneumonia, and is the result of the better transmission of vocal vibrations through consolidation. Bronchophony is easier to detect when it is unilateral and is often associated with bronchial breath sounds, dull percussion note, and increased vocal fremitus.

Vocal resonance is reduced in similar lung abnormalities that result in reduced breath sounds and decreased tactile fremitus. Hyperinflation of lung parenchyma, pneumothorax, bronchial obstruction, and pleural effusion reduce the transmission of vocal vibrations through the lung or chest wall, producing decreased vocal resonance.

When the spoken voice increases in intensity and takes on a nasal or bleating quality, it is referred to as *egophony.* Egophony may be identified over areas of the chest where bronchophony is present. The exact reason for this change in voice-sound character is unknown. It is identified most easily by having the patient say *e-e-e.* If egophony is present, the *e-e-e* will be heard with the stethoscope over the peripheral chest wall as *a-a-a.* Egophony is usually identified only over an area of compressed lung above a pleural effusion.

Whispering Pectoriloquy. Whispering pectoriloquy may be a helpful physical finding, especially in patients with small or patchy areas of lung consolidation. The patient is instructed to whisper the words *one, two, three* while the examiner listens over the lung periphery with a stethoscope, comparing side with side. Whispering creates high-frequency vibrations that are filtered out selectively by normal lung tissue and normally heard as muffled, low-pitched sounds. However, when consolidation is present the lung loses its selective transmitter quality and the characteristic high-pitched sounds are transmitted to the chest wall with clarity over the affected region.

Auscultatory Percussion of the Chest

A technique that uses the combination of auscultation and percussion is known as *auscultatory percussion.* The procedure is simple to perform and requires only the use of a stethoscope. The examiner percusses on the manubrium of the patient with the index finger of one hand while auscultating over the posterior lung fields, comparing side with side.

The advantage of auscultatory percussion over conventional percussion proposed by Guarino[30] in his study of 30 patients with unilateral lung disease is the increased sensitivity to lung abnormalities. Of the 30 patients studied, 28 had abnormal chest x-ray films with normal or uncertain findings during conventional percussion. In the majority of cases, the auscultatory percussion technique readily detected the abnormalities. Before this method can be accepted widely, however, confirmation by other studies needs to be completed.

Examination of the Precordium

As mentioned previously, chronic diseases of the lungs may and frequently do cause abnormalities in other body systems. Recognition of these abnormalities is helpful in identifying respiratory disease and in quantifying its severity. Because of the close working relationship between the heart and lungs, the heart is especially at risk for developing problems secondary to lung disease. The techniques for physical examination of the chest wall overlying the heart (*precordium*) include inspection, palpation, and auscultation. Percussion is of little or no value in the examination and is omitted. For the sake of convenience most clinicians perform the examination of the precordium simultaneously with the examination of the lungs.

Review of Heart Topography

The heart lies between the lungs within the mediastinum and is situated so that the right ventricle is more anterior than the left ventricle. The upper portion of the heart consists of both atria and is referred to commonly as the *base of the heart*. The base lies directly beneath the upper-middle portion of the gladiolus (sternum). The lower portion of the heart, which consists of the ventricles, is referred to as the *apex*. The apex points downward and to the left, extending to a point near the midclavicular line, and usually lies directly beneath the lower left portion of the gladiolus and near the costal cartilage of the fifth rib (Fig. 4–20).

Inspection and Palpation

The purpose of inspecting and palpating the precordium is to identify any normal or abnormal pulsations. Pulsations on the precordium are affected by the thickness of the chest wall and the quality of the tissue through which the vibrations must travel. The normal apical impulse is produced by the thrust of the contracting left ventricle and usually is identified near the midclavicular line in the fifth intercostal space. This systolic thrust may be felt and visualized in many

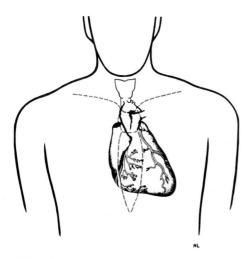

Fig. 4–20 *Topographic position of heart.*

healthy persons; it may be referred to as the *point of maximal impulse (PMI).*

Right ventricular hypertrophy, a common manifestation of chronic lung disease, often produces a systolic thrust (heave) that is felt and may be visualized near the lower left sternal border. The palmar aspect of the examiner's right hand is placed over the lower left sternal border for identification. Right ventricular hypertrophy may be the result of chronic hypoxemia, pulmonary valve disease, or pulmonary hypertension.

In patients with chronic pulmonary hyperinflation (emphysema), identification of the apical impulse is more difficult. The increase in anteroposterior diameter and the alteration in lung tissue contribute to poor transmission of the vibrations of systole to the surface of the chest. Therefore in patients with pulmonary emphysema the intensity of the PMI is often reduced or not identifiable.

The PMI may shift to the left or right with shifts in the mediastinum. Pneumothorax or lobar collapse often shifts the mediastinum, resulting in a shift of the PMI toward the lobar collapse but usually away from the pneumothorax. Patients with emphysema and low, flat diaphragms may have the PMI located in the epigastric area.

The second left intercostal space near the sternal border is referred to as the *pulmonic area* and is palpated in an effort to identify accentuated pulmonary valve closure. Strong vibrations may be felt in this area with pulmonary hypertension (Fig. 4–21).

Auscultation of Heart Sounds

Normal heart sounds are created primarily by the closure of the heart valves. The first heart sound (S_1) is produced by the sudden closure of the mitral and tricuspid valves (atrioventricular) during contraction of the ventricles. When systole ends, the ventricles relax and the pulmonic and aortic valves (semilunar) close, creating the second heart sound (S_2). Because the left side of the heart has a significantly higher pressure created during systole, closure of the mitral valve is louder and contributes more than the closure of the tricuspid valve to S_1 in the healthy person. For the same reason closure of the aortic valve is usually more significant in producing S_2. Whenever the atrioventricular or semilunar valves do not close simultaneously, a split heart sound is heard. A slight splitting of S_2 is normal and often occurs as the result of normal spontaneous ventilation. The normal splitting of S_2 is increased during inhalation because of the decrease in intrathoracic pressure, which improves venous return to the right side of the heart and further delays pulmonic valve closure.

A third heart sound (S_3) may be identified during diastole. S_3 is thought to be produced by rapid ventricular filling immediately after systole. The rapid disten-

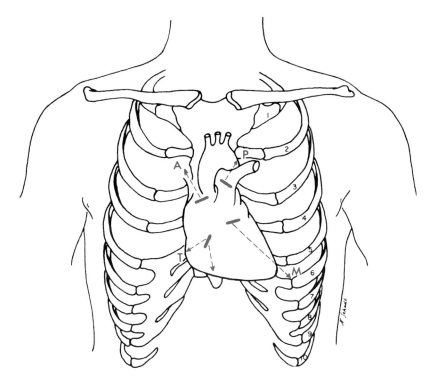

Fig. 4-21 *Anatomic and auscultatory valve area. Location of anatomic valve sites is represented by solid bars. Arrows designate transmission of valve sounds to their respective auscultatory valve areas. M, mitral valve; T, tricuspid valve; A, aortic valve; P, pulmonic valve. (From Prior JA, and Silberstein JS:* Physical examination: the history and examination of the patient, *ed 6, St Louis, 1982, Mosby-Year Book.)*

tion of the ventricles causes the walls of the ventricles to vibrate and produce a sound of low intensity and pitch. It is best heard over the apex. It is normal in young healthy children and is referred to as physiologic S_3 in this situation. In other situations, however, an S_3 is abnormal. For example, in an older patient with a history of heart disease, an S_3 is a definite abnormality and may signify myocardial infarction.

A fourth heart sound (S_4) also may be identified during diastole. S_4 occurs late in diastole just before S_1. S_4 is produced by active filling of the ventricles from atrial contraction just prior to systole. It may occur in healthy persons or be considered a sign of heart disease.

A *gallop rhythm* refers to an abnormal condition in which a third or fourth heart sound, or both, are present. The spacing of the heart sounds results in a unique sequence of sounds that resemble the gallop of a horse. A gallop rhythm suggests that the left or right ventricle, or both, are being overdistended during diastole. This may occur with a diseased ventricle, as in postmyocardial infarction, left-to-right shunts, or ventricular failure from any cause.

Auscultation of the heart sounds may identify alterations in the loudness of S_1 or S_2. A reduction in the intensity of the heart sounds may be the result of cardiac or extracardiac abnormalities. Extracardiac factors include alteration in the tissue between the heart

and the surface of the chest. Pulmonary hyperinflation, pneumothorax, and obesity make identification of both S_1 and S_2 difficult. S_1 and S_2 intensity may also be reduced when the force of ventricular contraction is poor, as in heart failure, or when valvular abnormalities exist.

Pulmonary hypertension produces an increased intensity of S_2 as a result of more forceful closure of the pulmonic valve; this is referred to as an increased P_2. A loud P_2 is a common finding in cor pulmonale. A lack of S_2 splitting with inhalation may also be the result of pulmonary hypertension. An increased P_2 is identified best over the pulmonic area of the chest.

Cardiac murmurs are identified whenever the heart valves are incompetent or stenotic. Murmurs are usually classified as either systolic or diastolic. Systolic murmurs are produced by an incompetent atrioventricular valve or a stenotic semilunar valve. An incompetent atrioventricular valve allows a backflow of blood into the atrium, usually producing a high-pitched whooshing noise simultaneously with S_1. A stenotic semilunar valve produces a similar sound, created by an obstruction of blood flow out of the ventricle during systole.

Diastolic murmurs are created by an incompetent semilunar valve or a stenotic atrioventricular valve. An incompetent semilunar valve allows a backflow of blood into the ventricle simultaneously with or immediately after S_2. A stenotic atrioventricular valve obstructs blood flow from the atrium into the ventricles during diastole and creates a turbulent murmur.

A murmur may also be created by rapid blood flow across normal valves. In summary, the murmurs are created by (1) a backflow of blood through an incompetent valve, (2) a forward flow through a stenotic valve, and (3) a rapid flow through a normal valve.

Auscultation of heart sounds is usually done at the same time the lung sounds are identified. The bell and diaphragm pieces of the stethoscope are used. The diaphragm is most useful for higher frequency sounds such as S_1, S_2, and systolic murmurs. The bell is best used for low-frequency sounds such as gallops and diastolic murmurs. The heart sounds may be easier to identify if the patient leans forward or lies on the left side, since anatomically this moves the heart closer to the chest wall. When the peripheral pulses are difficult to identify, auscultation over the precordium may be an easier method of identifying the heart rate.

Examination of the Abdomen

An in-depth discussion of examining the abdomen is beyond the scope of this text; however, the abnormalities associated with respiratory disease are reviewed.

The abdomen should be inspected and palpated for evidence of distention and tenderness. Abdominal distention may cause impairment of the diaphragm and contribute to respiratory failure. It may also inhibit the patient from coughing and deep breathing, both of which are extremely important in preventing respiratory complications in the postoperative patient.

Palpation and percussion are used on the right upper quadrant (Fig. 4–22) of the abdomen in an effort to estimate the size of the liver. An enlarged liver may be found when chronic right heart failure has occurred as a consequence of chronic respiratory disease. Any respiratory disease that results in a reduction of the oxygen level in the blood causes pulmonary vasoconstriction. If this occurs over a period of months or years, the right ventricle becomes enlarged and fails to pump blood effectively. The venous blood flow returning to the right ventricle is reduced, and engorgement of major veins and organs may occur. The hepatic vein that empties into the inferior vena cava may become engorged in this situation, and the liver may increase in size. This is referred to as *hepatomegaly*.

To identify hepatomegaly, the superior and inferior borders of the liver are located by percussion. Normally, the liver spans about 10 cm at the midclavicular line. If the liver extends more than 10 cm, it is considered enlarged.

Hepatomegaly may be accompanied by the collection of serous fluid in the peritoneal cavity known as

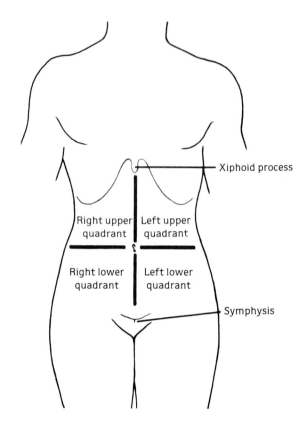

Fig. 4–22 *Division of abdomen into quadrants. (From Prior JA, and Silberstein JS:* Physical examination: the history and examination of the patient, *ed 6, St Louis, 1982, Mosby-Year Book.)*

ascites. Ascites most often results from interference with venous return to the right side of the heart, as occurs in heart failure. Cirrhosis of the liver, depletion of plasma proteins, and sodium retention are common contributing factors. Severe ascites may restrict diaphragm movement, as mentioned above, and contribute to the onset of respiratory failure.

Examination of the Extremities

Respiratory disease may result in numerous abnormalities, identified during inspection of the extremities. These abnormalities include digital clubbing, cyanosis, and pedal edema. Each is discussed briefly.

Clubbing

Clubbing of the digits is a significant manifestation of cardiopulmonary disease. The mechanism responsible for clubbing is not known, but it is often associated with a chronic cardiopulmonary disease. It is identified most commonly in patients with bronchogenic carcinoma, COPD, cystic fibrosis, and chronic cardiovascular disease.

Clubbing is characterized by a painless enlargement of the terminal phalanges of the fingers and toes. It requires years to develop. As the process of clubbing advances, the angle of the fingernail to the nail base advances past 209 degrees and the base of the nail feels "spongy." The profile view of the digits allows easier recognition of clubbing (Fig. 4–23).

Cyanosis

Examination of the digits should identify the presence or absence of cyanosis in any patient suspected of having cardiopulmonary disease. The transparency of the fingernails and skin covering the digits allows cyanosis to be detected initially in this area. Cyanosis occurs whenever 1.5 volumes percent of reduced hemoglobin exist; thus the intensity of cyanosis increases with the amount of hemoglobin in the blood. Patients with a high hemoglobin concentration (polycythemia) develop cyanosis at a lesser degree of tissue hypoxia, whereas patients with low hemoglobin concentrations (anemia) have severe hypoxia before cyanosis occurs. The presence of cyanosis in the digits indicates that the blood flow is not optimal. Tissue oxygenation may not be adequate when cardiac output falls below normal.

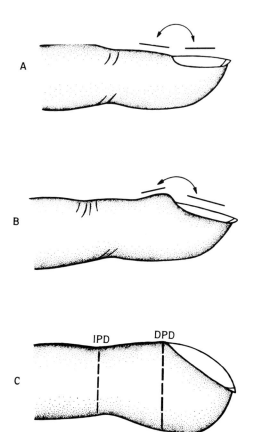

Fig. 4–23 A, *Normal digit configuration.* **B,** *Mild digital clubbing with increased hyponychial angle.* **C,** *Severe digital clubbing; depth of finger at base of nail (DPD) is greater than depth of interpharyngeal joint (IPD) with clubbing.*

Pedal Edema

Pedal edema may be a manifestation of chronic lung disease. Since hypoxemia produces pulmonary vasoconstriction, the right ventricle must work harder than normal whenever significant hypoxemia exists. This chronic workload on the right ventricle may result in right ventricular hypertrophy and poor venous blood flow return to the heart. When the venous return to the right side of the heart is reduced, the peripheral blood vessels engorge, resulting in an accumulation of fluid in the subcutaneous tissues of the ankles, referred to as *pedal edema.* The ankles most often are affected, since they naturally are maintained in a gravity-dependent position throughout the day. The edematous tissues pit (indent) when pressed firmly with the fingertips. Pitting edema should be evaluated for the level of occurrence above the ankle in an effort to quantify the degree of right heart failure. For example, pitting edema occurring at a level well above the knee is much more significant than pitting edema around the ankles only.

Capillary Refill

Capillary refill is assessed by pressing firmly for a brief period on the fingernail and identifying the speed at which the blood flow returns. When cardiac output is reduced and digital perfusion is poor, capillary refill is slow, taking several seconds to appear. In normal persons with good cardiac output and digital perfusion, capillary refill should take less than 3 seconds.

Peripheral Skin Temperature

When the heart does not circulate the blood at a sufficient rate, compensatory vasoconstriction occurs in the extremities to shunt blood toward the vital organs. The reduction in peripheral perfusion results in a loss of warmth in the extremities. Palpation of the patient's feet and hands may provide general information about perfusion. Cool extremities usually indicate inadequate perfusion.

Actual extremity temperature can be compared to room temperature. The extremity should be at least 2°C warmer than room temperature (unless room temperature is equal to or greater than body temperature). When there is less than 2°C difference, perfusion is reduced; a 0.5°C difference indicates that the patient has serious perfusion problems. (See Chapter 11 for a more detailed discussion.)

Physical Signs of Respiratory Disease

The techniques of physical examination provide an inexpensive and rapid way to identify important clinical abnormalities of the cardiopulmonary system. The initial evaluation of the patient with acute disease, needing rapid assessment and treatment, should identify the adequacy of tissue oxygenation and pulmonary function with regard to ventilation and oxygenation.

Tissue oxygen availability is a function of cardiac output and the content of oxygen in the arterial blood. The most accurate assessment of arterial oxygenation is done through analysis of an arterial blood gas sample (see Chapter 6), but in certain situations when time is of the essence or when blood gases are not available, clinical results must be relied on. Clinical signs of acute hypoxemia include tachycardia, hypertension, tachypnea, cyanosis, restlessness, and confusion. Clinical signs of reduced cardiac output and poor tissue perfusion include hypotension, cool extremities with weak or absent pulses, poor capillary refill, semiconsciousness or coma, reduced urine output, and tachycardia. The clinical factors that reflect perfusion are described in more detail in Chapter 11.

Chronic hypoxemia may result in right ventricular hypertrophy and failure. It is referred to as *cor pulmonale,* and is clinically manifested by pedal edema, loud pulmonic valve closure, jugular venous distention, hepatomegaly, and a systolic heave at the lower left sternal border.

By itself, the physical examination usually cannot identify a specific diagnosis, but it can suggest certain pathologic abnormalities of the lungs. When the physical findings are considered along with the history and other diagnostic procedures to be discussed in subsequent chapters, a more specific diagnosis can be suggested. The pathologic abnormalities of the lung that

occur because of specific diseases usually result in characteristic abnormal physical findings. These are summarized in the following paragraphs. Specific respiratory diseases are not emphasized (Table 4–5).

Acute Airway Obstruction

Respiratory distress is usually apparent from observation of tachypnea, tachycardia, intercostal retraction on inspiration, and the use of accessory muscles. The expiratory phase is significantly prolonged. Paradoxical pulse may be present and indicates severe airway obstruction. Expiratory wheezes may be present but may diminish as bronchial obstruction improves or worsens. The lungs are hyperinflated diffusely, resulting in bilateral reduction in tactile and vocal fremitus, reduced vesicular-type breath sounds, and a mild to moderate increase in resonance with percussion. As bronchial obstruction resolves, the physical findings return to normal. Asthma, acute exacerbation of bronchitis, bronchiolitis, or foreign body aspiration may produce this clinical picture.

Chronic Airway Obstruction

At rest the patient may not appear to be in respiratory distress. The respiratory pattern may be normal in rate, but prolongation of the expiratory phase with pursed lips breathing is often noted. The anteroposterior diameter is increased significantly and referred to as *barrel-chested.* Large supraclavicular fossae may be present. The intercostal spaces retract with inspiration, and accessory muscles are used in an effort to lift the anterior chest wall during inspiration, resulting in a

Table 4–5 *Physical Signs of Pulmonary Abnormalities*

Abnormality	Initial impression	Inspection	Palpation	Percussion	Auscultation	Possible Causes
Acute airway obstruction	Appears acutely ill	Use of accessory muscles	Reduced expansion	Increased resonance	Expiratory wheezing	Asthma, bronchitis
Chronic airway obstruction	Appears chronically ill	Increased anteroposterior diameter, use of accessory muscles	Reduced expansion	Increased resonance	Diffuse reduction in breath sounds; early inspiratory crackles	Chronic bronchitis, emphysema
Consolidation	May appear acutely ill	Inspiratory lag	Increased fremitus	Dull note	Bronchial breath sounds; crackles	Pneumonia, tumor
Pneumothorax	May appear acutely ill	Unilateral expansion	Decreased fremitus	Increased resonance	Absent breath sounds	Rib fracture, open wound
Pleural effusion	May appear acutely ill	Unilateral expansion	Absent fremitus	Dull note	Absent breath sounds	Congestive heart failure
Local bronchial obstruction	Appears acutely ill	Unilateral expansion	Absent fremitus	Dull note	Absent breath sounds	Mucous plug
Diffuse interstitial fibrosis	Often normal	Rapid shallow breathing	Often normal; increased fremitus	Slight decrease in resonance	Late inspiratory crackles	Chronic exposure to inorganic dust
Acute upper airway obstruction	Appears acutely ill	Labored breathing	Often normal	Often normal	Inspiratory/ expiratory stridor	Epiglottitis, croup, foreign body aspiration

clavicular lift during inhalation. Breath sounds are often reduced markedly bilaterally and are absent in more severe cases. Adventitious lung sounds that may be identified include early inspiratory crackles and expiratory wheezes. Tactile and vocal fremitus are reduced, and resonance with percussion is increased. The diaphragm is low, flat, and immobile (Fig. 4–24). Bilateral chest expansion is reduced significantly with quiet and deep breathing. In contrast to acute bronchial obstruction, the abnormalities do not resolve. Emphysema and chronic bronchitis may produce this type of clinical picture.

Consolidation

Consolidation of the lung parenchyma (Fig. 4–25) occurs when the alveoli fill with fluid and exudate as a result of a bacterial or viral pneumonia or if a parenchymal tumor develops. The patient usually appears

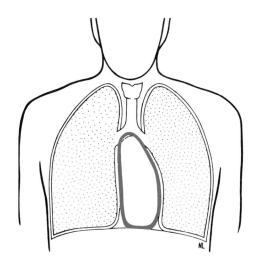

Fig. 4–24 *Chronic pulmonary hyperinflation with low, flat diaphragm and small narrow heart.*

acutely ill, febrile, and breathing is more rapid than normal.

Examination of the chest may identify increased tactile and vocal fremitus, bronchial breath sounds, and a dull percussion note over the area(s) of consolidation. Bronchophony, egophony, and whispering pectoriloquy may be present. Inspiratory crackles may be identified, especially later in the progression of pneumonia as the consolidation resolves. Expansion of the affected side may be reduced. Cyanosis may be present in more severe cases.

Pneumothorax

Air in the pleural space may result in significant abnormalities, depending on the extent of the pneumothorax and underlying lung dysfunction. A small pneumothorax may go unnoticed; however, when lung compression is significant (Fig. 4–26), the patient appears acutely short of breath. Over the pneumothorax, chest expansion is reduced, the percussion note is increased in resonance, breath sounds are absent, and tactile fremitus is absent. The trachea and mediastinal contents shift away from the affected side with tension in the pleural space, as may occur in positive pressure breathing. If the pneumothorax is severe enough to disrupt cardiac function, blood pressure will decrease.

Pleural Effusion

The patient with fluid in the pleural space may or may not appear ill, depending on the cause and size of the effusion. The trachea may be shifted toward the opposite side with larger pleural effusions (Fig. 4–27). The percussion note is dull or flat, tactile fremitus is absent, and breath sounds are reduced or absent over the effusion. Near the upper limit of the effusion, bronchial breath sounds, egophony, and whispering pectoriloquy may be heard; these are caused by compression of the

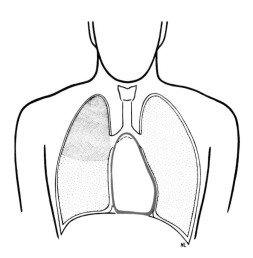

Fig. 4–25 *Right upper lobe consolidation.*

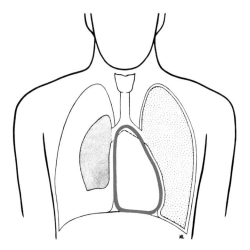

Fig. 4–26 *Large pneumothorax.*

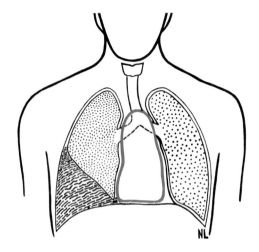

Fig. 4-27 *Large pleural effusion.*

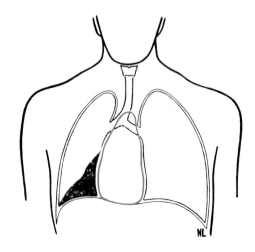

Fig. 4-28 *Atelectasis of right lower lobe.*

underlying lung. Tachypnea is usually present when a significant effusion is present, resulting in atelectasis.

Acute Local Bronchial Obstruction

A sudden complete obstruction of a major bronchus may occur as the result of a mucus plug, bronchogenic carcinoma, or an aspirated foreign body. Distal to the obstructed bronchus, lung parenchyma collapses, resulting in a sudden loss of volume on the affected side. Consequently, the trachea and mediastinal contents shift toward the affected side (Fig. 4-28). The shift may increase during inspiration and decrease with expiration. Over the affected area, chest expansion is reduced, the percussion note is dull or flat, tactile fremitus is reduced or absent, and breath sounds are reduced or absent.

Diffuse Interstitial Fibrosis

The patient is usually in no acute distress at rest but has significant dyspnea on exertion. The respiratory pattern is usually rapid and shallow. Fine late inspiratory crackles are a common finding with auscultation; they are not influenced by body position or coughing. The percussion note is reduced slightly throughout all lung fields, although this finding is difficult to detect. In more severe chronic cases the signs of cor pulmonale develop.

Acute Upper Airway Obstruction

The patient with an acute upper airway obstruction appears in acute distress with labored and often noisy breathing. The accessory muscles are commonly used during inhalation. Inspiratory time may be prolonged with supraglottic obstruction, whereas expiratory time is more often prolonged with subglottic obstruction. Inspiratory stridor may be heard without the aid of a stethoscope. Breath sounds are often clear, but the

sounds of upper airway obstruction may be transmitted to the peripheral chest, making it difficult to identify vesicular or other adventitious breath sounds. The lungs are usually normal to percussion and palpation. Since ventilation is at risk, the patient should not be left alone, and the assessment must be quick and accurate to allow proper treatment. Epiglottitis, foreign body aspiration, laryngospasm, or croup may produce these types of findings.

REVIEW QUESTIONS

1. T F The presence of nasal flaring indicates an increase in pulmonary compliance and decrease in work of breathing.

2. Which of the following may cause an increased jugular venous distention?
    a. chronic hypoxemia
    b. left heart failure
    c. right heart failure
    d. all of the above

3. T F Atelectasis, if large enough, may cause tracheal deviation away from the affected side.

4. T F JVP is measured vertically from the sternal angle with the head of the bed at a 45-degree angle.

5. The JVP is considered elevated if greater than which of the following values?
    a. 0 cm
    b. 1-2 cm
    c. 2-3 cm
    d. 3-4 cm

6. *"An inward depression of the sternum" describes which of the following thoracic configurations?*
    a. *kyphosis*
    b. *pectus excavatum*
    c. *flail chest*
    d. *barrel chest*

7. T   F   *Scoliosis is an s-shaped (lateral) curvature of the spine.*

8. *What spinous process is most prominent with the patient sitting and with their head bent forward?*
    a. *T1*
    b. *C1*
    c. *C7*
    d. *S3*

9. *At which of the following topographic locations is the bifurcation of the trachea located on the anterior chest?*
    a. *over the upper part of the manubrium*
    b. *at the sternal angle*
    c. *rib 4 at the sternum*
    d. *under the xyphoid process*

10. *The minor (horizontal) fissure begins at which of the following locations on the anterior chest?*
    a. *rib 2 at the sternal border*
    b. *rib 4 at the sternal border*
    c. *rib 6 at the sternal border*
    d. *none of the above*

11. *Which of the following best describes an apneustic breathing pattern?*
    a. *prolonged exhalation*
    b. *prolonged inhalation*
    c. *deep and fast*
    d. *lack of breathing*

12. T   F   *Restrictive lung disease is typified by rapid and shallow breathing pattern.*

13. T   F   *Intercostal retractions are indicative of decreased work of breathing.*

14. *A clavicular lift greater than _____ mm indicates severe obstructive airway disease.*
    a. *2*
    b. *3*
    c. *4*
    d. *5*

15. *Which of the following indicate(s) diaphragmatic fatigue?*
    a. *increased JVP*
    b. *abdominal paradox*

    c. *respiratory alternans*
    d. *b and c*

16. *Which of the following would cause an increased tactile fremitus?*
    a. *pneumonia*
    b. *pneumothorax*
    c. *chronic obstructive pulmonary disease*
    d. *obesity*

17. *Which of the following would cause a bilateral decrease in chest expansion?*
    a. *lobar consolidation*
    b. *pneumothorax*
    c. *chronic obstructive pulmonary disease*
    d. *pleural effusion*

18. *Which of the following would cause an increased resonance to percussion of the chest?*
    a. *lobar consolidation*
    b. *pneumothorax*
    c. *pleural effusion*
    d. *atelectasis*

19. T   F   *The diaphragm portion of a stethoscope is used to listen to high frequency sounds such as those over the lungs.*

20. *Normal bronchial breath sounds are produced by which of the following mechanisms?*
    a. *turbulent air flow through large airways*
    b. *filtered sounds through lung tissue*
    c. *passage of air through secretions*
    d. *passage of air through narrowed airways*

21. *Which of the following terms, previously used synonymously with crackle, does the American Thoracic Society suggest be discontinued?*
    a. *wheeze*
    b. *rale*
    c. *rhonchi*
    d. *stridor*

22. *The finding of late inspiratory crackles on auscultation of a patient might indicate which of the following?*
    a. *atelectasis*
    b. *pleural effusion*
    c. *bronchospasm*
    d. *mucosal edema*

23. T   F   *Polyphonic wheezes arise from varying degrees of obstruction of a single bronchus.*

24. *Which of the following is the normal topographic location of the PMI?*
    a. *third intercostal space at the anterior axillary line*
    b. *fourth intercostal space at the anterior axillary line*
    c. *fifth intercostal space at the midclavicular line*
    d. *sixth intercostal space at the midsternal line*

25. *Which of the following locations is best for auscultating the mitral valve?*
    a. *third intercostal space at the anterior axillary line*
    b. *fourth intercostal space at the anterior axillary line*
    c. *fifth intercostal space at the midclavicular line*
    d. *sixth intercostal space at the midsternal line*

26. *T   F   The first (S_1) heart sound is produced as a result of aortic and mitral valve closure.*

27. *T   F   A gallop rhythm is present when the third and/or fourth heart sounds are heard on auscultation and indicates ventricular distention during diastole.*

28. *Which of the following may cause an increased P_2 component of the second heart sound?*
    a. *pulmonary hypertension*
    b. *pulmonary embolism*
    c. *cor pulmonale*
    d. *all of the above*

29. *T   F   Clubbing of the digits may be seen with significant pulmonary or cardiac disease.*

30. *T   F   Reduced capillary refill and cool peripheral skin temperature indicate adequate tissue perfusion status.*

31. *Which of the following signs would be consistent for a patient with pleural effusion?*
    a. *unilateral chest expansion*
    b. *increased resonance to percussion*
    c. *reduced or absent breath sounds*
    d. *a and c*

32. *Which of the following would be consistent for a patient with acute upper airway obstruction?*
    a. *labored breathing*
    b. *normal palpation*
    c. *inspiratory stridor*
    d. *all of the above*

REFERENCES

1. McFadden ER Jr, Kiser R, and de Groot WJ: Acute bronchial asthma: relations between clinical and physiologic manifestations, *N Engl J Med* 288:221, 1973.
2. Anderson CL, Shankar PS, and Scott JH: Physiological significance of sternomastoid muscle contraction in chronic obstructive pulmonary disease, *Respir Care* 25:937, 1980.
3. Cohen CA, and others: Clinical manifestations of inspiratory muscle fatigue, *Am J Med* 73:308, 1982.
4. Mier-Jedrzejowicz A, and others: Assessment of diaphragm weakness, *Am Rev Respir Dis* 137:877, 1988.
5. Williams TJ, Ahmand D, and Morgan WK: A clinical and roentgenographic correlation of diaphragmatic movement, *Arch Intern Med* 141:878, 1981.
6. Murphy RLH, Holford E, and Knowler W: Visual lung sound characterization by time-expanded waveform analysis, *N Engl J Med* 296:968, 1977.
7. Andrews JL, and Badger TL: Lung sounds through the ages, *JAMA* 241:2625, 1979.
8. Report of the ACCP-ATS joint committee on pulmonary nomenclature, *Chest* 67:583, 1975.
9. Report of the ATS-ACCP ad hoc subcommittee on pulmonary nomenclature, *ATS News*, 3:5, 1977.
10. Report of the ATS-ACCP ad hoc subcommittee on pulmonary nomenclature, *ATS News*, 2:8, 1981.
11. Wilkins RL, Dexter JR, and Smith JR: Survey of adventitious sound terminology in case reports, *Chest* 85:523, 1984.
12. Wilkins RL, and Dexter JR: Comparing RCPs to physicians for the description of lung sounds. Are we accurate and can we communicate? *Respir Care* 35:969, 1990.
13. Wilkins RL, and others: Lung sound nomenclature survey, *Chest* 98:886, 1990.
14. Forgacs P: The functional basis of pulmonary sounds, *Chest* 73:399, 1978.
15. Murphy RLH, and Holford SK: Lung sounds, *Basics of RD* (March) 8:3, 1980.
16. Heckerling PS: The need for chest roentgenograms in adults with acute respiratory illness, *Arch Intern Med* 146:1321, 1986.
17. Donnerberg RL, and others: Sounds transfer function of the congested canine lung, *Br J Dis Chest* 74:23, 1980.
18. Bohadana AB, Peslin R, and Uffholtz H: Breath sounds in the clinical assessment of airflow obstruction, *Thorax* 33:345, 1978.
19. Pardee NE, and others: Combinations of four physical signs as indicators of ventilator abnormality in obstructive pulmonary syndromes, *Chest* 77:354, 1980.
20. Pardee NE, Martin CJ, and Morgan EH: A test of the practical value of estimating breath sound intensity, *Chest* 70:341, 1976.
21. Marini JJ, and others: The significance of wheezing in chronic airflow obstruction, *Am Rev Respir Dis* 120:1069, 1979.
22. Baughman RP, and Loudon RG: Quantification of wheezing in acute asthma, *Chest* 86:718, 1984.
23. Baughman RP and Loudon RG: Lung sound analysis for continuous evaluation of airflow obstruction in asthma, *Chest* 88:364, 1985.
24. Forgacs P: Crackles and wheezes, *Lancet* 2:203, 1967.
25. Nath AR, and Capel LH: Inspiratory crackles, early and late, *Thorax* 29:223, 1974.
26. Nath AR, and Capel LH: Inspiratory crackles and mechanical events of breathing, *Thorax* 29:695, 1974.
27. Forgacs P: Lung sounds, *Br J Dis Chest* 63:1, 1969.
28. Thacker RE, and Kraman SS: The prevalence of auscultatory crackles in subjects without lung disease, *Chest* 81:672, 1982.
29. Workum P, and others: The prevalence and character of crackles (rales) in young women without significant lung disease, *Am Rev Respir Dis* 126:921, 1982.
30. Guarino JR: Auscultatory percussion of the chest, *Lancet* 2:1332, 1980.

BIBLIOGRAPHY

Bates B, and Hoeckelman RA: *A guide to physical examination and history taking,* ed 4, Philadelphia, 1987, JB Lippincott.

Cherniak RM, and Cherniack L: *Respiration in health and disease,* ed 3, Philadelphia, 1983, WB Saunders.

Forgacs P: *Lung sounds,* London, 1978, Balliere Tindall.

Judge RD, and Zuidema GD: *Clinical diagnosis: a physiological approach,* ed 5, Boston, 1988, Little, Brown.

Malasanos L, Barkauskas V, and Stoltenberg-Allen K: *Health assessment,* ed 4, St Louis, 1990, Mosby–Year Book.

Prior JA, and Silberstein JS: *Physical diagnosis: the history and examination of the patient,* ed 6, St Louis, 1982, Mosby–Year Book.

Seidel HM, and others: *Mosby's guide to physical examination,* ed 2, St Louis, 1990, Mosby–Year Book.

Wilkins RL, Hodgkin JE, and Lopez B: *Lung sounds: a practical guide,* St Louis, 1988, Mosby–Year Book.

Chapter 5

Clinical Laboratory Studies

Linda W. Chu and Robert L. Wilkins

LEARNING OBJECTIVES

Upon completion of this chapter, the reader should be able to accomplish the following:

1. *Identify the components that make up the formed elements and plasma of the blood.*

2. *Define blood serum and describe how it is obtained.*

3. *Recognize the normal values, and significance of the following hematology lab tests:*
   a. *red blood cells (RBC)*
   b. *hematocrit*
   c. *hemoglobin*
   d. *erythrocyte indices (MCV, MCH, MCHC)*
   e. *white blood cells (WBC)*
   f. *white cell differential*
   g. *reticulocyte count*
   h. *sedimentation rate*
   i. *platelet count*
   j. *coagulation studies (bleeding time, activated partial thromboplastin time [APTT], prothrombin time [PT])*

4. *Define anemia and the most common cause of anemia.*

5. *Identify the potential effect anemia has on oxygen carrying capacity and tissue oxygenation.*

6. *Define left shift in terms of the white blood cell differential and its clinical significance.*

7. *Define primary, secondary, and relative polycythemia and identify how polycythemia affects blood oxygen transport and myocardial work.*

8. *Define leukocytosis and leukopenia.*

9. *Recognize the causes for the following white cell abnormalities:*
   a. *neutrophilia*
   b. *eosinophilia*
   c. *lymphocytosis*
   d. *lymphocytopenia*
   e. *monocytosis*

10. *Identify the effect that AIDS and AIDS-related complex has on the ratio of T helper to T suppresser cells.*

11. *Define leukemia and myeloproliferative disorders.*

12. Recognize the normal values, and significance of the following chemistry lab tests:
    a. electrolytes
    b. anion gap
    c. sweat electrolyte concentration
    d. blood urea nitrogen (BUN) and creatinine
    e. enzymes (aspartate aminotransferase (AST), alanine aminotransferase (ALT), alkaline phosphatase (ALP), acid phosphatase (ACP), lactic dehydrogenase (LDH), creatine kinase (CK), amylase, lipase)
    f. glucose
    g. protein (immunoglobulins, albumin)
    h. lipids (triglycerides, cholesterol, HDL, LDL)
    i. tumor markers
    j. drug monitoring

13. Identify the therapeutic level for theophylline and factors which affect its metabolism and clearance.

14. Recognize a definition of the following medical microbiology terms:
    a. normal flora
    b. gram stain
    c. culture
    d. sensitivity

15. Recognize the type of organism a Ziehl-Neelsen stain is used to identify.

16. Recognize the methods for obtaining a fresh and uncontaminated sputum sample.

17. Identify the factors involved in the macroscopic (gross) sputum examination.

18. Identify the characteristic appearance of the sputum from a patient with bronchiectasis.

19. Identify the microscopic criteria used to determine whether a sputum sample is reliable.

20. Recognize the significance of sputum eosinophilia.

21. Recognize some of the organisms responsible for producing pneumonia and the most common cause of bacterial pneumonia.

22. Identify the indications and method of obtaining a bronchoalveolar lavage (BAL).

23. Identify the significance of the following during pleural fluid examination:
    a. increased pleural fluid amount
    b. "milky" pleural fluid
    c. hemorrhagic pleural fluid
    d. low protein content (< 3 g/dL)
    e. high protein content (> 3 d/dL)

24. Identify the significance of the following tests performed during a urinalysis:
    a. specific gravity
    b. pH
    c. protein content
    d. glucose concentration
    e. ketones
    f. bilirubin
    g. blood
    h. urobilinogen
    i. nitrates
    j. sedimentary constituents

25. Describe or identify the purpose of histologic and cytologic examinations.

26. Identify the malignant tumors responsible for producing the majority of primary lung cancer.

27. Recognize the types of pulmonary samples that can be examined cytologically.

Chapter Outline

Hematology
Complete Blood Count
Red Blood Cell Abnormalities
White Blood Cell Abnormalities
Leukemias and Myeloproliferative Disorders
Reticulocyte Count
Sedimentation Rate
Platelet Count
Coagulation Studies

Chemistry
Electrolyte Concentrations
Blood Urea Nitrogen and Creatinine
Enzymes
Glucose
Protein
Lipids
Tumor Markers
Drug Monitoring

Microbiology
Examination of Pulmonary Secretions

Bronchoalveolar Lavage

Pleural Fluid Examination

Urinalysis

Histology and Cytology

Skin Testing

Chapter Overview

The modern clinical laboratory consists of a formidable array of equipment, and offers a vast number of studies. Most hospitalized patients with respiratory disease have many laboratory tests, and it is important for clinicians to have a basic understanding of at least the commonly ordered tests. This chapter attempts to provide that understanding. Although the emphasis is on interpreting laboratory data in patients with respiratory disease, most of the concepts described are applicable to any patient.

The majority of laboratory tests are performed using peripheral venous blood from the patient. Many other types of body fluids or secretions including sputum, pleural fluid, cerebrospinal fluid, urine, feces, and sweat are also used for various tests.

The blood consists of two major components: the formed elements and the plasma. The formed elements are composed of three types of cells: red blood cells *(erythrocytes)*, white blood cells *(leukocytes)*, and platelets *(thrombocytes)*. These formed elements are made in the bone marrow from stem cells. The stem cells are acted on by cytokines which are proteins of low molecular mass (Fig. 5–1). The cytokines regulate all important biological processes such as cell growth, cell activation, and tissue repair. The plasma contains a myriad of substances including electrolytes, clotting factors, immunologic factors, various proteins, lipids, and hormones; almost every substance the cells in the body use must be transported via the plasma. Plasma from which the clotting factors have been removed (by allowing the blood sample to clot, by centrifuging, and by removing the supernatant) is known as *serum*.

Evaluating laboratory test results requires an understanding of a few basic principles relating to statistical analysis. Normal values are usually expressed as ranges constructed to include 95% of the normal population (two standard deviations). Each laboratory must determine its own normal values using its particular equipment, methods, etc. Therefore the normal values mentioned in this chapter are typical of many laboratories but not absolute for any specific laboratory.

It is possible to obtain a normal test result for a patient with the disease that a laboratory test is designed to detect. Similarly, it is possible for normal patients to have abnormal test results. Therefore laboratory tests must always be evaluated in light of other clinical findings and should be regarded as supplemental information. A diagnosis is seldom, if ever, made from the results of a laboratory test alone. Correlation of clinical findings with laboratory test results leads to more appropriate diagnosis and treatment.

Most clinical laboratories are divided into sections, with all of the tests relating to a particular area being performed in one section. This chapter is subdivided according to the common sections found in most laboratories: hematology, chemistry, microbiology, and urinalysis. Surgical pathology (histology) and cytology are also described, because they relate to the evaluation of pulmonary specimens.

Hematology

Hematology laboratory tests are divided into two main categories. There are tests that evaluate the cellular

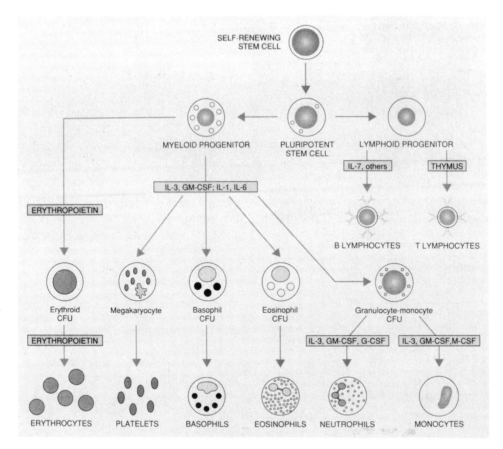

Fig. 5–1 *Maturation of blood cells: the hematopoietic "tree." The maturation of different blood cells is regulated by various cytokines (see text). Note that the names of the various cytokines depicted in this figure are abbreviated: CFU, colony-forming unit; IL, interleukin; GM-CSF, granulocyte-macrophage colony-stimulating factor. (From Abbas, A.K.: Cellular and molecular immunology, Philadelphia, 1991, W.B. Saunders. Used by permission.)*

elements of the blood. These include the complete blood count (CBC), platelet count, and reticulocyte count. There are also tests that evaluate the proteins in the plasma involved in forming blood clots; these tests fall into the general category of coagulation and include the prothrombin time (PT), activated partial thromboplastin time (APTT), and bleeding time. Platelets are also involved in the general function of coagulation.

Complete Blood Count

The CBC includes counting the number of red blood cells (RBCs) and white blood cells (WBCs), evaluating certain RBC factors relating to size and hemoglobin content, and counting the different kinds of WBCs. The counting of RBCs and WBCs is usually done electronically by a machine, whereas the determination of the different types of WBCs, known as the *differential,* is performed either visually (manually) by a technologist or, in larger laboratories, by automated cell counters. Typical normal values are listed in Table 5–1.

RED BLOOD CELLS. Red blood cells are produced in the bone marrow by maturation of nucleated cells known as *normoblasts.* Under normal circum-

stances, as the normoblasts mature, the nuclei become smaller and darker and the cytoplasm acquires a red color as a result of the development of hemoglobin. Before the red cell is released from the bone marrow to circulate in the peripheral blood, the nucleus is lost. RBCs typically have a life span of approximately 120 days.

Normal RBCs assume the shape of a biconcave disk as they circulate to facilitate their primary function of carrying oxygen (Fig. 5–2). Mature RBCs are made up largely of hemoglobin, which imparts to blood its normal red color when oxygen mixes with the hemoglobin in the lung. The RBC count is reported in number of cells per cubic millimeter or per liter (see Table 5–1 for normal values). Without a normal RBC count, the ability of the blood to transport oxygen would be reduced significantly. A normal RBC count, however, does not guarantee a normal hemoglobin level or oxygen-carrying capacity.

HEMATOCRIT (PACKED CELL VOLUME). Hematocrit is the ratio of red cell volume to that of whole blood. It can be determined by centrifuging whole blood so that the blood cells settle and then determining the percent or fraction of the total blood

Table 5-1 Normal Values for the Complete Blood Count Tests

Test	Normal Values
Red blood cell count (RBC)	
Men	$4.6–6.2 \times 10^6/mm^3$
Women	$4.2–5.4 \times 10^6/mm^3$
Hemoglobin (Hb)	
Men	13.5–16.5 g/dL
Women	12.0–15.0 g/dL
Hematocrit (Hct)	
Men	40%–54%
Women	38%–47%
Erythrocyte index	
Mean cell volume (MCV)	80–96 μm^3
Mean cell hemoglobin (MCH)	27–31 pg
Mean cell hemoglobin concentration (MCHC)	32%–36%
White blood cell count (WBC)	4500–11,500/mm³
Differential of white blood cells	
Segmented neutrophils	40%–75%
Bands	0%–6%
Eosinophils	0%–6%
Basophils	0%–1%
Lymphocytes	20%–45%
Monocytes	2%–10%
Platelet count	150,000–400,000/mm³

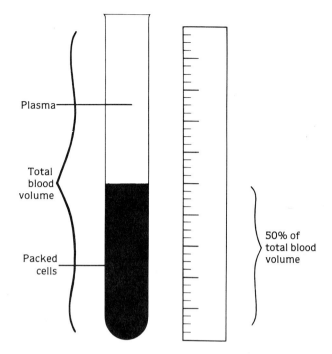

Fig. 5–3 *Determination of hematocrit from centrifuging blood sample. Packed cell volume is half total blood volume; therefore hematocrit is 50% in this example.*

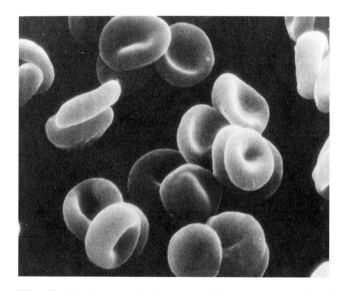

Fig. 5–2 *Normal red blood cells. (Courtesy of Brian Bull, M.D.)*

volume occupied by the RBCs (Fig. 5–3). It is calculated electronically in most laboratories.

HEMOGLOBIN. Hemoglobin (Hb) is the protein that carries oxygen to the tissues; it is the major component of RBCs. Hemoglobin is also important in maintaining acid-base balance by acting as a buffer and by carrying carbon dioxide from the tissues to the lungs. The hemoglobin molecule consists of two portions: the heme group, of which iron is a vital constituent, and the protein, or globin, chains. Each RBC contains between 200 and 300 million hemoglobin molecules.

INDICES. Three erythrocyte indices are either measured or calculated. They indicate the cell size, hemoglobin content, and hemoglobin concentration and are known respectively as mean cell volume (MCV), mean cell hemoglobin (MCH), and mean cell hemoglobin concentration (MCHC). The values are useful in the evaluation and classification of anemias (disorders with decreased RBCs). Interpretation of the RBC indices is described later in this chapter.

WHITE BLOOD CELLS. The WBCs are the circulating blood cells normally nucleated. The cell counting machines measure WBCs similarly to RBCs by lysing the cells and counting the nucleated cells that remain. WBCs normally represent several populations of cells that function as part of the body's immune system in fighting infection. Leukocyte counts are especially helpful in evaluating acute respiratory infections.

DIFFERENTIAL. This portion of the CBC is traditionally performed by examination of a blood smear by a technologist, and it is extremely important. A drop of whole blood is smeared in a thin layer on a glass slide, stained, most commonly by a stain known as Wright's stain, and then examined under the microscope. WBCs (100) are counted and classified as to exact cell type. WBCs normally seen in the peripheral blood are neutrophils (segmented and band forms), eosinophils, basophils, lymphocytes, and monocytes. Neutrophils, eosinophils, and basophils are included in the general category of granulocytes. The differential count defines the percentage of the total WBCs made of

Table 5-2	Normal Absolute and Relative Values for Differential of WBCs	
Cell Type	Relative Value (%)	Absolute Value*
Neutrophils	40–75	1800–7500
Eosinophils	0–6	0–600
Basophils	0–1	0–100
Lymphocytes	20–45	900–4500
Monocytes	2–10	90–1000

*Based on a normal WBC range of 4500 to 10,000 and using the equation: Absolute value = relative value × total WBC.

each cell type. An increase or decrease in the number of a particular cell type may be either absolute or relative. For example, if the total WBC count is elevated and the neutrophils are increased, the lymphocytes may make up a smaller than usual percentage of the WBCs. However, the total absolute number of lymphocytes may be normal. This would represent a relative decrease in lymphocytes associated with an absolute increase in neutrophils. To determine the absolute cell count, the total WBC count is multiplied by the differential count or percentage for the particular cell type of interest (Table 5-2).

Neutrophils are also known as polymorphonuclear neutrophilic leukocytes and segmented neutrophilic granulocytes. Neutrophils usually constitute 40% to 75% of the blood's WBCs. A band is a less mature neutrophil in which the nucleus has not yet segmented. Bands normally make up 0% to 6% of the WBCs. In various abnormal conditions, the more immature cells may be seen: the metamyelocyte, myelocyte, promyelocyte, and myeloblast. (For the normal sequence of granulocyte maturation occurring in the bone marrow, see Fig. 5-4.) Neutrophils contain enzymes that destroy bacteria and other invaders. They also are capable of phagocytosis (engulfment of bacteria and other foreign material). The interpretation of WBC count and differential is described later in this chapter.

Eosinophils are a type of granulocyte having large granules that stain bright red, whereas basophils have large granules that strongly take up the basic stain (dark blue to purple). The function of both cell types is not completely understood; however, they appear to have complementary interactions in allergic reactions. Eosinophils also help defend the body against parasitic infestations. Eosinophils normally constitute 0% to 6% of WBCs, whereas basophils are less plentiful at 0% to 1%.

Lymphocytes are complex cells extremely important in the body's defense against various infections. Two major types of lymphocytes exist: T cells involved in cell-mediated immunity and B cells involved in antibody production (see Fig. 5-1). The types appear similar on a blood smear. Lymphocytes normally make up 20% to 45% of circulating WBCs, with most of the circulating peripheral lymphocytes being T cells.

The separation and counting of T cells and B cells can be done only with special studies. The studies identify the type of cell present by using monoclonal antibodies which react with the surface antigen unique to the T or B cells. This usually is done with a special instrument, known as a flow cytometer, which detects and counts the cells that react with various monoclonal antibodies. T lymphocytes also can be separated into subcategories known as helper and suppressor cells. The helper or inducer cells provide help in antibody production and other immune responses and are identified by a unique surface antigen known as CD4. They are sometimes referred to as T4 cells. The suppressor cells play a role in suppressing or dampening immune responses. These cells have the unique antigen CD8, and are referred to as T8 cells. Studying these lymphocyte subsets is important in the diagnosis and follow-up of patients with acquired immunodeficiency syndrome (AIDS).

Monocytes are the largest WBC normally seen and constitute 2% to 10% of leukocytes in the peripheral blood. In tissue the monocyte is known as a *macrophage*. The primary function of the monocyte is phagocytosis of organisms and other foreign material invading the body.

While performing the differential cell count, the technologist also looks at the RBCs for size and shape and the platelets for size and number. In an increasing number of laboratories, the differential is being performed on automated cell counters which differentiate the types of WBCs based on their differing cytoplasmic chemicals. The blood smear is examined manually, however, whenever any abnormality is found in the automated differential.

Red Blood Cell Abnormalities

Anemia is a decrease in the RBC count, hemoglobin, and hematocrit. When anemia is present, and if the MCV, MCH, and MCHC are abnormally low, the anemia is known as a *microcytic, hypochromic* anemia; that is, the red cells are smaller than normal and contain a lower than normal concentration of hemoglobin. If the anemia is *normocytic, normochromic,* the indices are normal. If the MCV is high, the anemia is known as *macrocytic,* and the RBCs are larger than normal. The MCHC is never high, since it is impossible for RBCs to contain a higher hemoglobin concentration than normal. Anemias may be caused by blood loss, increased destruction of RBCs, or decreased production of RBCs. Anemias may be seen in chronic respiratory infections and malignancies. Severe anemia significantly reduces the oxygen-carrying capacity of the blood and may result in dyspnea and tissue hypoxia.

Probably the most common type of anemia is the result of iron deficiency. This typically occurs when

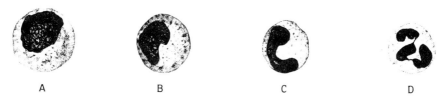

Fig. 5-4 *Granulocyte maturation states:* **A,** myelocyte; **B,** metamyelocyte; **C,** band; **D,** polymorphonuclear leukocyte (segmented form).

there is chronic blood loss and the iron contained in the RBCs leaves the body instead of being recycled as is done normally. Iron deficiency anemia is usually microcytic and hypochromic. Other microcytic, hypochromic anemias include those caused by porphyria (an inherited disease), thalassemia (also an inherited disorder in which there is abnormal hemoglobin synthesis), and the "anemia of chronic disease," occurring in patients who have longstanding inflammatory diseases. This latter type of anemia also may be normocytic, normochromic.

Macrocytic anemia is usually a "megaloblastic" anemia caused by either folate or vitamin B_{12} deficiency. The term *megaloblastic* refers to the typical large, nucleated developing RBC seen in the bone marrow in these cases.

Normochromic, normocytic anemias include anemias caused by many conditions such as acute blood loss, immune hemolytic anemia (antibodies destroying RBCs), and sickle cell disease; other examples include various inherited disorders in which the RBCs are abnormal, and those anemias in which the bone marrow is failing to produce RBCs because of intrinsic bone marrow disease such as tumor infiltration or simply bone marrow failure (aplasia or hypoplasia).

Anemia from any cause reduces the oxygen-carrying capacity of the blood. As a result, tissue oxygenation may suffer, especially if cardiovascular compensatory mechanisms are compromised. The combination of anemia and hypoxemia represents a serious threat to tissue oxygenation.

Polycythemia is an increase in the RBC count, hemoglobin, and hematocrit, and may be either primary or secondary. Secondary polycythemia is most common and is seen in patients who have chronic stimulation of the bone marrow to produce more RBCs secondary to some other disorder. This is commonly seen in patients with congenital heart disease, in those who live at high altitudes, and in patients who have chronic hypoxemia as a result of various pulmonary disorders such as chronic bronchitis or pulmonary fibrosis. Chronic hypoxemia stimulates the bone marrow to produce and release more RBCs, which carry oxygen to the body cells in an attempt to help compensate for the oxygen deficit. Patients with chronic hypoxemic lung disease often have an increased MCV and a reduction in the MCHC.

Chronic cigarette smoking can produce significant elevations of blood carboxyhemoglobin levels. The carboxyhemoglobin levels result from inhalation of carbon monoxide which is produced by burning cigarettes. The carbon monoxide binds tightly with hemoglobin and ties up a portion of the binding sites. As a result, oxygen is blocked from binding with the portion of the hemoglobin bound with carbon monoxide. A significant blood carboxyhemoglobin level can occur in heavy smokers and results in a "functional" anemia. A "smoker's polycythemia" often occurs in such cases in an effort to compensate for the functional anemia.

The degree of secondary polycythemia in patients with chronic hypoxemic lung disease is variable and is probably related to many factors. In some patients a reduced erythrocyte response (e.g., minimal or no polycythemia) may occur when chronic infection is present, when the erythrocytes have a reduced survival time, or when compensatory cardiovascular mechanisms are sufficient.

Primary polycythemia is caused by an uncontrolled proliferation of hematopoietic cells within the bone marrow and is known as *polycythemia vera* (one of the myeloproliferative disorders). Rarely, tumors (especially of the kidneys) produce a substance (erythropoietin) that stimulates the bone marrow to make more RBCs.

Both primary and secondary polycythemia involve a real or absolute increase in the total RBC mass. Sometimes "relative" polycythemia occurs because of a decrease in the plasma volume. This is seen in patients who are dehydrated for various reasons and in a condition known as *spurious* or *stress polycythemia*. This latter condition usually occurs in men who smoke, have hypertension, and are obese.

Although polycythemia is helpful in increasing the oxygen-carrying capabilities of the blood, it may be detrimental to the heart and circulation. Substantially more RBCs increase the viscosity of the blood, causing an increased workload for the heart.

Nucleated RBCs do not normally circulate in the peripheral blood. Their presence may indicate extreme stress being placed on the marrow to produce RBCs, thereby releasing cells at a younger stage. Nucleated RBCs also occur in the peripheral blood in some of the myeloproliferative disorders caused by an uncontrolled or malignant proliferation of bone marrow cells, including the erythroid elements. Nucleated RBCs are also seen commonly in premature infants.

White Blood Cell Abnormalities

An increase in the total WBC count is known as *leukocytosis,* whereas a decrease is known as *leukopenia.* The abnormal count can be defined more specifically by referring to the exact cell type that is either increased or decreased using similar terminology. For example, an increase in neutrophils is referred to as either *neutrophilia* or a *neutrophilic leukocytosis,* and a decrease is *neutropenia.* Increases in the cell counts may be primary (a result of uncontrolled proliferation of cells in the bone marrow) or secondary (a result of stimulation of the bone marrow secondary to other diseases or disorders). Similarly, decreases in cell counts may be caused by either primary bone marrow failure or increased destruction and use of the cells peripherally. Bone marrow failure can occur as a side effect of various drugs and disorders (secondary) or as a result of unknown causes (primary or idiopathic).

Neutrophilia is a common response to various kinds of stress placed on the body. It is typically one of the body's first responses to infection and inflammation. Neutrophilia is a common finding in patients with bacterial pneumonia. It is also seen when there is tissue destruction and in metabolic toxic states. Certain drugs and chemicals (e.g., epinephrine or steroids) also increase neutrophils. When various kinds of stress stimulate the bone marrow to release these cells, the cells are released at an earlier stage than usual. Therefore increased numbers of the young cells, usually bands, appear in the peripheral blood. This is referred to as a *left shift.* When the stimulus is severe, even younger cells may be seen. The degree of the left shift and the severity of the neutrophilia usually correlate with the severity of the initiating cause (e.g., infection). The capability of the bone marrow to respond to stress such as infection is, however, influenced by the state of the immune system, which in turn is affected by general health, age, and many other complex factors. Neutropenia may occur with overwhelming infection when the bone marrow cannot produce cells as fast as they are used.

Eosinophilia or eosinophilic leukocytosis is most characteristic of allergic states and parasitic infestations. Patients with extrinsic types of asthma often have eosinophilia, which is also seen in certain skin and gastrointestinal disorders. Basophilia is primarily associated with certain myeloproliferative disorders. It is rarely seen in hypersensitivity reactions.

Lymphocytosis is typically seen in viral infections, especially infectious mononucleosis. In addition, the lymphocytes in these disorders are often enlarged and have a characteristic appearance referred to as *atypical.* Lymphocytopenia is seen in trauma and acute infection.

Table 5-3 Types of Leukocytosis

Cell Type	Causes For Increase	Appropriate Term
Neutrophil	Bacterial infection, inflammation	Neutrophilia
Eosinophil	Allergic reaction, parasitic infection	Eosinophilia
Lymphocyte	Viral infection	Lymphocytosis
Monocyte	Chronic infections, malignancies	Monocytosis
Basophil	Myeloproliferative disorders	Basophilia

Lymphocytopenia is an important feature of human immunodeficiency virus (HIV) infection, the agent of AIDS. Furthermore, there is alteration of the ratio of T helper (CD4) to T suppressor (CD8) cells in patients with active disease or AIDS-related complex. Normally the helper cells predominate, with the normal ratio being 2:1 to 3:1. This ratio is reduced in AIDS patients and the severity of the reduction is progressive, correlating with the progression of disease.

Monocytosis is characteristic of certain chronic infections, including tuberculosis, syphilis, typhoid fever, brucellosis, and various fungal infections. Monocytosis is also seen in "preleukemia" and other malignancies (Table 5-3).

Leukopenias may involve one specific cell type or commonly all of the WBCs. Probably the most common causes today are chemotherapy and radiation used to treat various malignant tumors. Both radiation and chemotherapy are effective in killing rapidly dividing tumor cells. Hematopoietic cells are among the most rapidly dividing normal cells in the human body and are particularly susceptible to these forms of therapy. Usually the tolerance of the bone marrow determines the maximum dose given when using radiation and chemotherapy. Many other types of drugs may cause various leukopenias, either because of a hypersensitivity or because of a toxic effect on the bone marrow with a decreased production of cells. Sometimes a viral infection causes a generalized decrease in the WBC count. In addition, any time there is significant replacement of the bone marrow by abnormal cells, either myeloproliferative disorders (intrinsic or primary bone marrow malignancies) or metastatic (extrinsic) malignancies, leukopenia may result.

Leukemias and Myeloproliferative Disorders

Leukemias and myeloproliferative disorders are primary malignancies (uncontrolled proliferations) involving bone marrow cells. Leukemia implies a proliferation of a specific type of WBC (usually either lymphocytic or granulocytic) and may be either acute or chronic. Myeloproliferative disorders encompass a spectrum of diseases resulting from an abnormality of the *stem cell* (the precursor of all bone marrow cells), and are often associated with a proliferation of more than one type of cell. Myeloproliferative disorders may terminate as an acute leukemia.

In acute leukemia there is a tremendous proliferation of young cells known as *blasts*. These blasts quickly replace all other cells in the bone marrow and the peripheral blood. WBC counts may be high with a differential showing predominately blasts. The RBCs and platelets are usually decreased. Without treatment the patient would die rapidly. Acute lymphocytic leukemia usually occurs in young children, whereas acute granulocytic or myelogenous leukemia often occurs in young adults. Pure monocytic leukemia is rare and usually occurs in adults. However, many cases of acute myelogenous leukemia prove to be myelomonocytic (the cells have features of both myeloid and monocytic cells) on special testing. This is not surprising since both myeloid and monocytic cells arise from a common precursor cell (see Fig. 5–1).

Chronic leukemias result from a slower proliferation of more mature cells, and even without treatment the patient may live for years. Chronic lymphocytic leukemia is the most common type of leukemia and usually occurs in elderly people. The WBC count again may be quite high, but the differential will show a preponderance of mature lymphocytes. Only late in the disease are other cells decreased. Chronic granulocytic leukemia (CGL) often occurs in middle-aged adults. There is a high WBC count caused mainly by granulocytes in various stages of maturation. Platelets are often increased, and there is progressive anemia. CGL often terminates in acute leukemia, known as *blast crisis,* and is included among the myeloproliferative disorders.

Other myeloproliferative disorders include polycythemia vera, myelofibrosis with myeloid metaplasia, Di Guglielmo syndrome, and essential thrombocythemia. (Polycythemia was previously discussed.) Myelofibrosis begins with a proliferation of granulocytes and megakaryocytes (the cells that make platelets) in the marrow, but fibrous tissue eventually replaces the marrow cells. The patient may have high or low WBC counts depending on the stage of the disease. Di Guglielmo syndrome (sometimes referred to as erythroleukemia) is a rare disorder, more like an acute leukemia involving both WBC and especially RBC precursors. Essential thrombocythemia primarily involves megakaryocytes with increased platelets in the peripheral blood.

Reticulocyte Count

Young RBCs, recently released from the bone marrow, are known as *reticulocytes*. These cells are slightly larger and have an increased amount of RNA in the cytoplasm. Supravital dyes, such as methylene blue or cresyl blue, stain the RNA material to identify these cells. A reticulocyte count is performed by obtaining the percentage of reticulocytes within the RBCs. The reticulocyte count is reported as a percentage or as an absolute number determined by multiplying the percentage times the red cell count. The average reticulocyte count is about 1.5% or $60,000/mm^3$.

The reticulocyte count is a helpful measurement in evaluating anemias. If the absolute reticulocyte count is high, it indicates the marrow is producing increased numbers of RBCs, and the anemia is probably a result of peripheral blood loss or destruction. However, if the reticulocyte count is low, then the anemia is probably the result of decreased bone marrow production.

Sedimentation Rate

If blood is placed in a vertical tube, the RBCs will tend to fall or "sediment" toward the bottom. A measurement of the speed at which they fall (distance per unit of time) is known as the *sedimentation rate.* The most commonly used methods are known as the *Wintrobe* and *Westergren,* which differ mainly by the use of different tube sizes. The sedimentation rate is a nonspecific test that is increased in a multitude of disorders, especially in inflammatory diseases. This is largely because of an increase in various plasma proteins. The proteins surround the RBCs and decrease the normal repelling effect between the cells caused by external negative charges on the cell surface. Anemia also increases the sedimentation rate as a result of the lesser concentration of erythrocytes.

Platelet Count

Platelets are the smallest formed elements in the blood. They have an important function in blood coagulation through formation of blood clots. Platelets are usually counted electronically, with normal platelet counts in the range of 140 to $440 \times 10^9/L$. As with the other blood cells, platelets may be decreased as a result of either increased destruction or use or decreased bone marrow production.

When the platelet count is decreased significantly ($< 50 \times 10^9/L$), patients are likely to have bleeding problems, especially with trauma such as surgery or arterial punctures. The bleeding that results from decreased platelets usually manifests itself as small skin hemorrhages (petechiae and ecchymoses) or oozing from mucosal surfaces. However, when the platelet count becomes extremely low ($< 10–20 \times 10^9/L$), the patient is at risk for serious spontaneous internal hemorrhage (e.g., brain hemorrhage). The disorders most likely to result in decreased platelets are side effects of certain drugs, various bone marrow diseases, and idiopathic thrombocytopenia purpura (ITP), an autoimmune disorder in which antibodies are produced that destroy the person's own platelets.

An increase in platelets may be simply a nonspecific reaction to stress placed on the body or may be caused by bone marrow disease (usually one of the myeloproliferative disorders). If the platelet count is extremely high, there may be an increased tendency to form blood clots *(thromboses)*.

Coagulation Studies

The evaluation of hemostasis (ability to prevent hemorrhage, form a blood clot) can be quite complex, and many tests are available. However, four basic screening tests are generally used: the bleeding time, platelet count (already discussed), APTT, and PT.

The bleeding time measures the ability of the small skin vessels to constrict and evaluates the function of platelets. It is performed by making standardized puncture wounds in the skin and timing how long it takes for the bleeding to stop. Various methods are used, but normal values are usually up to 6 minutes. The bleeding time and platelet count measure the first two steps in the body's defense for preventing hemorrhage, vascular integrity (ability of vessels to constrict) and formation of a platelet plug (requiring adequate numbers of platelets and their normal function).

The final step is the formation of a fibrin clot which results from the interaction of multiple proteins in the plasma. These proteins are labeled with roman numerals, factors I to XIII. There is an intrinsic pathway activated by damaged vascular endothelium and an extrinsic pathway used whenever tissue gains access to circulating blood. The APTT assesses predominantly the intrinsic system by measuring the length of time required for plasma to form a fibrin clot once the intrinsic pathway is activated. Normal values range from 24 to 32 seconds. The PT is performed similarly, using activation of the extrinsic system as a beginning point. Normal values generally range from 12 to 15 seconds. These tests are abnormal if one or more of the involved clotting factors are decreased significantly. Usually, further studies are required to delineate the specific factor(s) implicated. Factor deficiencies may be either congenital (e.g., hemophilia, which is a congenital absence of factor VIII) or acquired (e.g., liver disease with a decrease in factors II, VII, IX, and X). The APTT is also used for monitoring heparin therapy, whereas PT is used for monitoring warfarin (Coumadin) therapy.

Chemistry

Electrolyte Concentrations

Electrolytes are the free ions in body fluids. The normal functioning of all cells depends on proper concentrations of these elements, demanding that the body maintain close control of these substances. Monitoring of electrolyte concentrations of the plasma is extremely

Table 5-4 Normal Values in Chemistry

Test	Normal Value
Sodium	137–147 mEq/L
Potassium	3.5–4.8 mEq/L
Chloride	98–105 mEq/L
Carbon dioxide	25–33 mEq/L
Blood urea nitrogen	7–20 mg/dL
Creatinine	0.7–1.3 mg/dL
Total protein	6.3–7.9 g/dL
Albumin	3.5–5.0 g/dL
Cholesterol	150–220 mg/dL
Glucose	70–105 mg/dL

important in patients whose body fluids are being endogenously or exogenously manipulated (e.g., intravenous therapy, renal disease, or diarrhea).

The four electrolyte concentrations commonly measured are sodium (Na^+), potassium (K^+), chloride (Cl^-), and bicarbonate (HCO_3^-). Most commonly, the HCO_3^- is approximated by measuring the total CO_2. Ninety percent of the total CO_2 is made up of HCO_3^-. Normal values for the electrolyte concentrations and other common chemistry tests are listed in Table 5–4.

Sodium is the major cation (an ion having a positive charge) of extracellular fluid. The kidney, influenced by hormones secreted by the adrenal gland (aldosterone) and hypothalamus (antidiuretic hormone [ADH]), regulates the concentration of sodium in the serum very closely. Normal values are 137 to 147 mEq/L.

Sodium affects many vital functions and is mainly responsible for the osmotic pressure of the extracellular fluid. Increased serum Na^+ *(hypernatremia)* is seen when the body loses water without salt (e.g., profuse sweating, diarrhea, renal diseases, or prolonged hyperpnea), if there is lack of sufficient water intake, and when there are hormonal abnormalities known as *Cushing's disease* and *hyperaldosteronism*. These last two diseases have increased levels of hormones that cause the kidney to retain sodium. Patients with hypernatremia will typically complain of excessive thirst and a dry, sticky mouth. Decreased sodium concentration *(hyponatremia)* occurs when there is excess sodium loss compared to the degree of water loss, including diarrhea, nephrosis, and diuretic therapy. It also occurs with certain hormonal disorders known as *Addison's disease* and with syndrome of inappropriate secretion of ADH (SIADH). Addison's disease results from adrenal destruction and loss of aldosterone which impairs sodium reabsorption. SIADH occurs in a variety of central nervous system diseases and lung diseases and malignancies and causes the kidney to retain excessive H_2O. Complicating disorders such as lung tumors and pulmonary infections may produce hyponatremia by SIADH. Most often, however, hyponatremia occurs as a result of salt and water retention.

Patients with severe hyponatremia ($<$ 115 mEq/L) usually show confusion, abnormal sensorium, muscle twitching, and sometimes even seizures. At the same time, with true hyponatremia the clinical signs of hypovolemia (tachycardia, hypotension, oliguria) may be present.

Potassium is the chief cation occurring within cells. Extracellularly the concentration is low, with the usual serum concentration in the range of 3.5 to 4.8 mEq/L. *Hypokalemia,* or decreased serum K^+, occurs when K^+-containing fluid is lost (e.g., with vomiting, diarrhea, kidney diseases, diuretic therapy, and metabolic alkalosis [see Chapter 6]). The hormones that cause retention of sodium cause loss of potassium; therefore patients with Cushing's disease and hyperaldosteronism have hypokalemia. Hypokalemia usually disturbs the cardiac, skeletal muscle, and gastrointestinal systems. As a result, the patient may have a weak and rapid pulse that is irregular. Muscular weakness and abdominal distention are also common. *Hyperkalemia,* an elevated K^+, is seen primarily in various types of kidney diseases, metabolic acidosis, and extensive tissue damage, causing release of intracellular K^+ into the plasma. Hyperkalemia causes the patient to feel weak, tired, and nauseated and may lead to muscle paralysis.

Interpretation of the K^+ concentration must take into account the acid-base status of the patient. Changes in extracellular pH have an effect on the equilibrium between plasma and intracellular K^+ concentration. Hydrogen (H^+) and K^+ ions are transported and exchanged across the cell membrane to help maintain a more normal pH in the extracellular fluid. Therefore if acidosis exists, a normal serum K^+ indicates K^+ depletion, and a low serum K^+ indicates severe depletion. When alkalosis is present, a reduced serum K^+ exists in the presence of normal intracellular K^+ stores. The serum K^+ level can be considered to reflect the intracellular or total body potassium status only if no acid-base abnormalities are present.

Abnormalities in K^+ level are particularly important in patients recovering from respiratory failure. Optimal effectiveness of the respiratory muscles is needed when the patient is being weaned from mechanical ventilation. Hypokalemia and severe hyperkalemia may prevent effective contraction of the diaphragm and accessory breathing muscles. As a result, clinicians should optimize serum K^+ levels prior to attempting weaning.

Chloride is the chief anion (an ion having a negative charge) in the extracellular fluid. Normal concentration is 98 to 105 mEq/L. Decreased serum Cl^- *(hypochloremia)* occurs when there is prolonged vomiting (loss of HCl), metabolic acidosis, chronic respiratory acidosis, addisonian crisis, and certain kidney diseases. Increased serum Cl^- *(hyperchloremia)* is seen with prolonged diarrhea (loss of HCO_3^-), certain kidney diseases, and sometimes hyperparathyroidism.

Also, patients with cystic fibrosis have increased synthesis of Cl^- in their sweat, which can be measured (see discussion below).

HCO_3^- is the second most plentiful anion in the serum and is extremely important in acid-base balance within the body. An increase in serum HCO_3^- occurs with metabolic alkalosis or as compensation for respiratory acidosis, whereas a decrease occurs with metabolic acidosis or as compensation for respiratory alkalosis. The H_2CO_3 (carbonic acid)–HCO_3^- buffer system, however, interacts with many other blood components in an attempt to compensate for various mechanisms that may upset the delicate acid-base balance of the body.

Other electrolyte concentrations that are sometimes measured include calcium (Ca^{2+}), phosphorus (PO_4^-), and magnesium (Mg^{2+}). The Ca^{2+} level is controlled closely by parathyroid hormone (PTH) and vitamin D. Patients with increased PTH have increased calcium (hypercalcemia). Since bone contains a large amount of calcium, certain bone diseases result in hypercalcemia. Hypocalcemia occurs in vitamin D deficiency (rickets) and in various other hormonal aberrations. PO_4^- metabolism is closely linked to that of Ca^{2+}. Abnormalities of Mg^{2+} concentrations are uncommon but can be seen in a variety of diseases. Hypomagnesemia and hypocalcemia have been associated with respiratory muscle weakness.

ANION GAP. Evaluation of the electrolyte concentrations provides information regarding the balance between cations and anions in the extracellular fluid. This is accomplished by calculation of the *anion gap.* The anion gap is derived from the difference between the commonly measured cations and anions. The measurable electrolyte concentrations contributing to the anion-cation relationship are Na^+, Cl^-, and HCO_3^-. K^+ contributes minimally to the extracellular ions and is usually not considered. To calculate the anion gap, the serum Cl^- and HCO_3^- are subtracted from the serum sodium $[Na^+ - (Cl^- + HCO_3^-)]$. With normal electrolyte concentrations the anion gap falls between 8 and 16 mEq/L. If the K^+ concentration is included in the cations, the normal value for the anion gap is between 12 and 20 mEq/L. Calculation of the anion gap helps identify the occurrence and clarify the cause of metabolic acidosis (see Chapter 6). An elevated anion gap ($>$ 16 mEq/L) usually occurs when fixed acids are produced (as in lactic acidosis) or added to the blood (as in poisoning), resulting in metabolic acidosis *(anion gap acidosis).*

ELECTROLYTE CONCENTRATION OF SWEAT. The electrolyte concentration of the patient's sweat may be analyzed to assist in the diagnosis of cystic fibrosis. The sweat glands of patients with cystic fibrosis have a diminished ability to reabsorb Na^+ and Cl^-. As a result, a high concentration of Na^+ and Cl^- ($>$ 60–80 mEq/L) is present in the sweat. Although analysis of the electrolyte concentration of sweat is an important diagnostic test for cystic fibrosis, some patients with cystic fibrosis may have minimally elevated or normal sweat Cl⁻ levels.

Blood Urea Nitrogen and Creatinine

The most common screening tests in assessing renal function are the blood urea nitrogen (BUN) and creatinine (Cr). Urea is a waste product synthesized in the liver from ammonia, which is the end product of protein (amino acid) breakdown. Therefore urea is constantly being formed and is excreted by the kidneys. Normally the serum level is maintained in the range of 7 to 20 mg/dL. Many kidney diseases result in decreased filtration and thereby increased retention of urea, leading to an elevated serum level. Other conditions such as shock and heart failure, in which there is decreased renal perfusion and thereby decreased filtration, also cause an elevated urea level. Diet (protein intake), the state of hydration, and various hormones that affect protein metabolism also influence the BUN.

Creatinine is another waste product constantly formed within muscle tissue and filtered out by the kidneys. The serum concentration of creatinine (0.7–1.3 mg/dL) is usually quite constant and reflects the balance between production of creatinine (proportional to the body's muscle mass) and its filtration by the renal glomerulus. The creatinine level rises in kidney diseases in which 50% or more of the renal nephrons are destroyed. Creatinine is also elevated in muscle diseases. Neither the BUN nor the creatinine level is sensitive to early renal disease.

When the BUN and creatinine are elevated as a result of renal failure, metabolic acidosis is often present, since the renal function for acid-base balance is impaired (see Chapter 6). Metabolic acidosis stimulates the respiratory system to increase ventilation and reduce the arterial carbon dioxide tension ($Paco_2$) as a compensatory mechanism. Therefore, patients with renal failure often have increased respiratory rates and may appear to be short of breath. If the patient with renal failure also has respiratory disease, the onset of metabolic acidosis can add intolerable stress and result in respiratory failure.

Enzymes

Enzymes are found in all of the body's cells. These substances are responsible for most chemical reactions. When there is destruction of tissue cells, enzymes are released into the blood. Many enzymes occur widely throughout the body, but certain enzymes are associated with specific organs. Therefore, sometimes elevation of a particular enzyme is a clue to a diseased organ. Most enzymes are measured by assessing their activity in catalyzing chemical reactions. The results are usually expressed in units that reflect the rate of the reaction.

Since many enzymes occur in multiple organs, *isoenzymes* (slightly different chemical forms of the same enzyme) that may be more specific for a particular site or disease have been identified in some cases. Most isoenzymes are identified by electrophoresis.

New terminology has recently been adopted for naming many of the enzymes. Most enzymes are commonly referred to by a series of capital letters that are abbreviations for the chemical names. In the following discussion, eight enzymes commonly tested in most hospitals are discussed. Both the old and new names are given, with the newer name listed first. In some cases, the older name is still used and understood more widely.

Aspartate aminotransferase (AST), formerly known as serum glutamic-oxaloacetic transaminase (SGOT) occurs in many tissues throughout the body. The highest concentrations are in heart and liver tissue, and the highest serum concentrations are seen in diseases involving those two types of tissue. The highest levels occur with acute hepatitis. Elevated AST levels occur on the second day following myocardial infarction. Although elevated AST levels occur in many diseases, the enzyme is used primarily in assessing liver disease and possible myocardial infarction.

Alanine aminotransferase (ALT), formerly known as serum glutamic-pyruvic transaminase (SGPT), is a liver enzyme that is elevated in hepatic disease similarly to AST. However, ALT is elevated minimally or not at all in myocardial infarction or other heart diseases unless there is secondary severe liver congestion with destruction of some liver tissue. Therefore ALT is helpful in deciding whether an AST elevation is the result of disease in the liver or in some other organ, especially the heart, since AST occurs in many organs, whereas ALT occurs in high concentrations mainly in the liver.

Alkaline phosphatase (ALP) is another enzyme useful in evaluating liver disease. Liver ALP is elevated in many liver diseases, but the highest values occur in liver disease caused by extrahepatic obstruction of the bile duct. ALP also occurs in bone, placenta, spleen, kidney, and intestine. The enzyme occurring in each of these organs has minor chemical differences specific for the type of tissue. These subtypes are referred to as isoenzymes and can be separated somewhat by certain chemical reactions and electrophoresis. Apart from liver disease, the other main category for which ALP determinations are useful clinically is that of bone diseases. In any type of bone disease in which there is increased new bone formation, a significantly elevated ALP is the result. Usually it can be determined by clinical features and other liver enzyme studies, without performing isoenzyme determinations, whether an ALP elevation is the result of hepatic or bone disease.

Acid phosphatase (ACP) occurs in high concentrations in the prostate gland. Lesser levels of a chemically different acid phosphatase occur in RBCs and platelets. Significantly elevated levels of ACP are seen almost exclusively in prostatic carcinoma that has metastasized (spread) outside of the prostate gland. Prostate specific antigen (PSA) is another substance specific for prostate origin that can be identified and quantified in the blood. It is being used increasingly to screen for prostate cancer.

Lactate dehydrogenase (LDH) is an enzyme that occurs in high concentrations in heart, liver, skeletal muscle, brain, kidney, and RBCs. Therefore elevated LDH levels occur in a wide variety of diseases. It is possible by electrophoresis to separate LDH into five isoenzymes, with each source of the enzyme having typical concentrations of these different isoenzymes. However, there is considerable overlap in the patterns from different organs. Myocardial and red blood cell LDH are similar to each other but distinctly different from liver and skeletal muscle LDH, which are also similar to each other. The highest LDH elevations occur in patients with megaloblastic anemia, widespread carcinoma, and severe shock. Moderate elevations occur with acute myocardial infarction, beginning at 24 hours after infarction and lasting up to 2 weeks. In addition, with myocardial infarction there is a distinct isoenzyme pattern (LDH_1 greater than LDH_2), referred to as a *flipped* pattern. Moderate LDH elevations also occur in pulmonary infarction, usually within 24 hours of the onset of pain. LDH elevations are also seen in muscular diseases, leukemia, hemolytic anemia, infectious mononucleosis, liver disease, renal disease, and hypothyroidism.

Creatine kinase (CK), also known as creatine phosphokinase (CPK), occurs in significant amounts in skeletal muscle, myocardium, and brain tissue. Isoenzyme patterns characteristic for the source of the enzyme can be determined by electrophoresis. CK values are elevated primarily in myocardial infarction and various skeletal muscle diseases. CK originating in the brain does not cross the blood-brain barrier and therefore does not appear in serum. In acute myocardial infarction the CK elevation can be detected within the first 8 hours after infarction and persists for several days. Although high CK values generally occur because of myocardial or skeletal muscle disease, for uncertain reasons high levels have occurred with pulmonary infarction and pulmonary edema. The CK enzyme is made up of two subunits, which may be either identical or different. The CK isoenzyme that occurs in the brain is made up of two similar subunits and is referred to as CK-BB. The isoenzyme occurring in skeletal muscle is also made up of two identical subunits and is called CK-MM. The CK present in the myocardium has one component similar to that found in brain and one similar to that found in muscle and is known as CK-MB. The CK normally present in the blood is all from the skeletal muscle or CK-MM type. The presence of a CK-MB band on electrophoresis is characteristic of myocardial infarction.

Amylase and lipase are enzymes used primarily in assessing pancreatitis. Amylase in the blood and urine is predominantly from the pancreas and salivary glands. Elevated serum levels occur within a few hours after the onset of pancreatitis. There is also markedly increased excretion of amylase in the urine, and determination of urinary amylase is more sensitive than serum amylase. Serum amylase may also be elevated in pancreatic carcinoma (usually late in the disease); diabetic ketoacidosis; and diseases of the gallbladder, stomach, and small intestine. Serum lipase levels are also elevated in acute pancreatitis, but those elevated levels appear later, rising more slowly. Their presence may help confirm the diagnosis of pancreatitis.

Glucose

Glucose is the major substance produced from the digestion of dietary carbohydrates. Glucose is absorbed into the blood and carried to various cells throughout the body, where it is metabolized for energy production. Insulin is necessary in order for cells to use glucose circulating in the blood. Patients with diabetes have decreased insulin levels or at least a cellular resistance to insulin, which is manifested by a decreased use of blood glucose and increased levels of glucose in blood or plasma, a condition known as *hyperglycemia*. Therefore determination of blood glucose levels is essential to the diagnosis of diabetes. Hyperglycemia is also seen in Cushing's disease and in patients being treated with steroids. Many other hormones also affect the level of blood glucose, and hyperglycemia may occur in various hormonal disorders. When significant elevation of blood glucose is present the patient's acid-base status should be evaluated. If metabolic acidosis is occurring, uncontrolled diabetes with ketoacidosis is probably the cause, and this represents a potentially dangerous situation. *Hypoglycemia* (low blood glucose) is a syndrome associated with such signs as sweating, shaking, weakness, headaches, and lethargy and can be the result of various hormonal, drug-induced, or digestive diseases. Evaluation of blood glucose levels is also important in patients receiving parenteral solutions containing glucose.

It is important in evaluating glucose levels to know when the patient last ate in relation to when the blood was drawn. The "fasting" plasma glucose level (blood drawn after an overnight fast) is normally in the range of 70 to 105 mg/dL. After ingestion of carbohydrate, the glucose level normally rises in the first 60 to 90 minutes and then returns to the normal fasting level within 2 hours. The single most sensitive test in screening for diabetes is the "2-hour postprandial" glucose level, that is, a glucose level drawn 2 hours after a meal or glucose challenge.

Classically, the most sensitive test in diagnosing diabetes mellitus is the "3-hour glucose tolerance test."

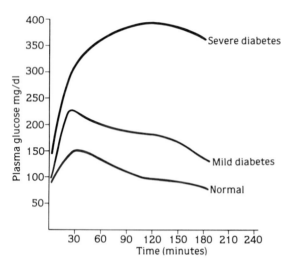

Fig. 5–5 *Typical blood glucose response to glucose tolerance test in normal persons and those with diabetes.*

In this test a standard glucose load is given, and plasma levels of glucose are determined at 30 minutes, 1 hour, 2 hours, and 3 hours after the glucose is ingested. The normal pattern and two typical diabetic patterns are shown in Fig. 5–5.

Significant hypoglycemia is thought to be present if the plasma glucose falls below 45 mg/dL, especially if clinical symptoms are present concurrently. Hypoglycemia occurring after a meal is known as *reactive hypoglycemia*. An extended glucose tolerance test, carried on for 5 hours with plasma levels tested every 30 minutes, is sometimes useful in evaluating patients with possible hypoglycemia. Probably the most common cause of reactive hypoglycemia is early, mild, or prediabetes.

Protein

The plasma contains a wide variety of proteins that are essential not only for normal metabolic functioning but also as the body's chief building substance. The enzymes and coagulation factors discussed earlier are proteins. Immunoglobulins and hormones are also proteins. The major serum protein is albumin, which functions as a transport and storage substance for many hormones, drugs, and electrolytes. Albumin is also important in maintaining the osmotic pressure of blood. It is maintenance of the osmotic pressure that keeps the water component of plasma in vascular spaces and helps promote "dryness" of tissues such as lung tissues. Albumin also plays a primary role in lipid metabolism. The two most commonly ordered tests assessing protein are the total protein and albumin analyses.

Total protein analysis is a rough screening test used to detect gross abnormalities in overall protein synthesis. A decreased total protein would be seen in severe liver disease (many proteins are secreted in the liver) and in severe malnutrition. The total protein level has many limitations and does not reveal which of the

many serum proteins may be causing an abnormality. If abnormalities are suspected, often a serum protein electrophoresis (SPEP) is performed. This test involves using an electric current to separate the serum proteins into specific groups. It generally does not identify specific proteins but patterns characteristic of certain disorders (e.g., liver disease and renal disease). In addition, the detection of *monoclonal gammopathy* (secretion of abnormal immunoglobulin by lymphocytes or plasma cells) is most successful with serum protein electrophoresis. Normally the plasma cells (immunoglobulin secreting cells) secrete a wide variety of different immunoglobulins, which form a broad band with electrophoresis. However, in multiple myeloma (malignant proliferation of plasma cells), each plasma cell secretes the same immunoglobulin, resulting in a high concentration of one immunoglobulin and forming a narrow band or "spike" pattern on electrophoresis. This pattern is also occasionally seen in certain types of malignant lymphoma, in some infections, and in elderly people without disease.

Albumin is secreted by liver cells and makes up more than 60% of the total serum protein. Decreased albumin levels *(hypoalbuminemia)* are seen in various forms of protein malnutrition and in severe liver disease with a decrease in functioning liver tissue. Chronic inflammation, severe acute disease, and kidney disease (with loss of albumin) can also result in hypoalbuminemia. Significant hypoalbuminemia leads to loss of fluid from vascular spaces and causes edema in various tissues throughout the body (e.g., pulmonary edema).

Lipids

The lipids include a wide variety of complex substances used throughout the body as fuel storage and as building blocks for the secretion of a wide variety of substances such as hormones and cell walls. The two lipids most commonly measured in routine screening tests are triglycerides and cholesterol.

Triglycerides represent the main storage lipid in humans, and fatty tissue is made up chiefly of these substances. Cholesterol is the widely publicized substance in eggs and other dietary animal proteins and is also synthesized by the body. Cholesterol is extremely important in the synthesis of various hormones. Most of the attention focused on the serum levels of various lipids results from the correlation of increased lipid levels with a greater incidence of atherosclerotic disease. Many more sophisticated tests analyzing various lipids by centrifugation or electrophoresis are available but are beyond the scope of this book. Lipids should usually be assessed in fasting patients, since dietary intake does affect the serum level, especially of triglycerides. The cholesterol level normally increases with age, with average values for adults being around 160 mg/dL at 20 years, 200 mg/dL at 40 years, and 215 mg/dL at 60 years. There is probably a difference between the average value and the ideal value. The ideal value, or the value that would be desirable for optimal health, is probably considerably lower. The triglyceride level in adults after 35 years of age averages about 140 to 150 mg/dL.

More recently, the emphasis has been on assessment of the lipoproteins. These are usually studied by means of ultracentrifugation or electrophoresis, allowing separation of the three main categories: VLDL (very low-density lipoproteins), LDL (low-density lipoproteins), and HDL (high-density lipoproteins). The amount of cholesterol occurring within these separate categories gives more useful information than a simple total cholesterol level, especially when the cholesterol level is elevated. Although increased total cholesterol is a risk factor for cardiovascular disease, *decreased* HDL cholesterol level is also a risk factor. Therefore, if the elevated cholesterol is primarily HDL, there may not be an increased risk of cardiovascular disease.

Tumor Markers

Owing to the prevalence of cancer in our society, there has been tremendous interest in identifying substances in the blood that can be easily detected and that indicate the presence of cancer in the body. Various hormones, enzymes, proteins, and oncofetal antigens have been found to be associated with various types of tumors.

Tumors derived from organs that normally secrete hormones may retain the property of hormonal secretion. In addition, nonendocrine tumors may produce "ectopic hormones," and the evaluation of serum levels of those hormones may be useful in the diagnosis and follow-up of the tumors. Lung carcinoma, especially the small-cell or oat cell type, is one of the most common tumors with ectopic hormone production. Hormones sometimes produced by lung tumors include ACTH (adrenocorticotropic hormone), PTH, ADH, GH (growth hormone), and TSH (thyroid-stimulating hormone).

An oncofetal antigen is an antigen that is normally expressed by the cell only in fetal life. However, with the aberrations that take place in the development of cancer, the cancer cells may again express these fetal antigens. The most commonly tested oncofetal antigen is carcinoembryonic antigen (CEA). CEA is present in abundance in fetal life in the developing intestine and lung. Adult patients with gastrointestinal, lung, and various other types of cancer may have elevated levels of CEA in their blood. However, CEA is not specific for any type of malignancy and can be elevated in many benign conditions including hypothyroidism and inflammation and in cigarette smokers. CEA is most useful in following patients with known colorectal cancer. An elevated CEA level occurring more than 6 weeks after resection of a colon cancer indicates recurrent disease. CEA levels can also be used in assessing tumor response to chemotherapy in lung cancer. Alpha-fetoprotein (AFP) is another oncofetal antigen used in the assessment of liver cell carcinoma (hepatoma) and testicular tumors. CA 125 is an oncofetal antigen sometimes identified in ovarian cancer.

Other tumor markers include prostatic acid phosphatase (PAP) and PSA for prostatic carcinoma. Also, T and B cell typing, as discussed under lymphocytes, is used for marking lymphomas and leukemias.

Drug Monitoring

Determining the level of various drugs within a patient's plasma can be of great benefit to the physician prescribing the drug. This is important with drugs that can be harmful in higher-than-therapeutic ranges and especially with those drugs for which the toxic level is only slightly above the therapeutic range. It also is important in assuring that a therapeutic concentration is attained (e.g., in antibiotics in which a certain level is necessary to kill the organisms). Because of individual variation in the rate of absorption, metabolism, and excretion of drugs, there can be large variances in the blood levels of different patients taking the same drugs on the same dosage schedule. Drugs that may be tested include cardiac drugs (digoxin, digitoxin, lidocaine); anticonvulsants (phenytoin, barbiturates); tranquilizers (diazepam, chlordiazepoxide, phenothiazines); salicylates; theophylline; and various antibiotics (gentamicin). Most of these substances are identified and quantitated by some form of chromatography (gas chromatography or high-performance liquid chromatography) or radioimmunoassay (RIA). RIA is also used for quantitative analysis of many hormones and involves identifying the substance by an antibody specific for that substance, which is labeled by a radioactive material. The radioactive label allows quantifying of the substance by counting the radioactivity. A similar method known as enzyme immunoassay (EIA) is gaining widespread use. EIA uses an enzyme to mark and quantify the substance being identified by the antibody. This method has the advantage of avoiding radioactive materials.

Theophylline is discussed because of its importance and widespread use in various pulmonary disorders. It is usually measured by chromatographic methods, and the normal therapeutic range is 10 to 20 μg/mL. The level should be obtained after there has been time to reach the plateau or maximal level and just before the next dose. Side effects such as nausea, vomiting, loss of appetite, and abdominal pain usually occur when the level is greater than 20 μg/mL, but some patients begin to experience these side effects at levels in the range of 15 to 20 μg/mL. More severe symptoms such as cardiac arrhythmias, seizures, and

Table 5-5	Factors Affecting Theophylline Clearance
Increased Clearance	**Decreased Clearance**
Young children	Liver disease
Smokers	Congestive heart failure
	Cimetidine
	Cor pulmonale
	Severe exacerbation of chronic obstructive pulmonary disease

cardiac and respiratory arrest occur in the range of 30 to 60 µg/mL. Serum theophylline levels are determined by the dosage given and the ability of the liver to metabolize the drug. Factors that affect theophylline metabolism by the liver are listed in Table 5–5.

Microbiology

Medical microbiology, sometimes referred to as *bacteriology,* involves the isolation and identification of microorganisms from body tissues and fluids. A detailed discussion of the many organisms that may be isolated is beyond the scope of this book, but a few general comments and a discussion relating to sputum examination follow.

The microbiology laboratory receives a wide variety of specimens. The handling of each specimen is determined by the site of origin of the sample and the specific organisms suspected by the patient's physician. An optimal amount of information is gained from the specimen when the laboratory is provided with the proper clinical information. Many body sites are normally sterile, and the isolation of any organisms from these sites may be significant. Blood, pleural fluid, ascitic fluid, and tissue samples do not contain microorganisms in a state of health, and if collected in a sterile manner, will not grow any type of organisms when cultured. Other samples such as stool, urine, and sputum regularly contain or are routinely contaminated with large numbers of microorganisms known as *normal flora.* With these specimens, the number and type of organisms isolated must be evaluated to determine whether they represent pathogenic organisms or normal flora. Although bacteria are the most common organisms isolated, laboratories also may identify fungi, protozoa, helminths (worms), rickettsiae, and viruses. These different types of organisms require different procedures for proper identification. Viruses are often identified only in referral laboratories.

The initial step involved in the examination of most specimens is the immediate preparation and examination of a direct smear of the specimen. The smear may be stained by various methods, depending on the type of organism suspected. A gram stain is used most commonly for bacterial organisms. Bacteria present are usually seen well after staining and may be classified as either gram-positive or gram-negative, depending on their staining reactions. In addition, the shape of the organism can be determined, allowing further classification of bacteria as cocci (spherical) or rods (elongate). Another rapid bacterial stain often used for sputum and other specimens is the acid-fast stain (e.g., the Ziehl-Neelsen stain), which allows presumptive identification of the tuberculous and related organisms. The information derived from the gram stain in combination with clinical information often allows the physician to suspect the proper diagnosis. Treatment may then be initiated on the basis of the preliminary diagnosis.

The definitive identification of microorganisms is made by culturing the specimen on various types of media promoting the growth of organisms. Culture results are usually available anywhere from 24 hours to many weeks later. Most bacteria grow in 24 to 48 hours, but some bacteria (e.g., the tubercle bacillus) and fungi may require 6 weeks or more to grow. After an organism grows, additional time may be required for tests to permit full identification. Procedures allowing more rapid culture and identification of organisms are currently being introduced into many laboratories. Rapid identification methods often involve immunologic reactions for specific organisms.

Along with the culture, a sensitivity test is often performed. The bacteria are cultured in the presence of various antibiotics, thereby permitting the determination of whether an organism is "sensitive" to a particular antibiotic, that is, whether the antibiotic in appropriate concentration prevents the growth of organisms. This kind of information is of great clinical importance in selecting the proper antibiotic therapy in the hospital setting.

Examination of Pulmonary Secretions

SPUTUM COLLECTION. The goal of sputum collection is to obtain fresh, uncontaminated secretions from the tracheobronchial tree. This goal is achieved more readily when the alert patient is carefully instructed on the importance of the procedure and how the sample must come from the "windpipe." The patient should be instructed to rinse the mouth out with water and even brush the teeth prior to expectorating a specimen. This will help reduce contamination of the specimen with oral microbes. Most patients with respiratory infections have little problem producing secretions for analysis with an effective cough. However, occasionally the respiratory secretions may be minimal and sputum induction is necessary to obtain an acceptable sample. Sputum is induced from the patient's tracheobronchial tree by application of mists capable of increasing the flow of bronchial secretions (bronchorrhea) and stimulating a cough. The resulting mild bronchorrhea and cough should assist in transporting pathologic specimens to the oropharynx for expectoration. Most often sputum induction is accomplished through application of heated or ultrasonic aerosol with hypertonic solutions.

In certain situations in which the patient has an unproductive cough and sputum induction is unsuccessful, sputum sampling may be achieved through bronchoscopic lavage (see below). Transtracheal aspiration may also be helpful in obtaining a specimen from the patient in a coma with a respiratory infection.

SPUTUM EXAMINATION. At the bedside the sample should be grossly examined to determine its origin. Legitimate sputum samples from the tracheobronchial tree typically are more viscous and purulent in nature than saliva. The specimen obviously containing mostly saliva should be discarded. Macroscopic examination of the sputum also identifies such characteristics as color, presence of blood, general viscosity, and odor. Yellow or green sputum frequently occurs when secretions are retained and may be seen in response to an allergic or infectious process. Stringy, mucoid sputum may be a sign of bronchial asthma. Certain respiratory infections may produce "classic" sputum samples. For example, respiratory infections with *Pseudomonas aeruginosa* typically produce thick, green sputum with a unique musty odor. Bronchiectasis typically produces a three-layered sputum sample that is foul-smelling. Thick secretions may indicate the patient's need for effective hydration or aerosol treatment.

The first step in sputum examination is the preparation of a gram-stained smear. The gram stain is used to determine if the sputum is a reliable sample. A commonly used criterion for an acceptable sample is the presence of more than 25 leukocytes (neutrophils) per low-power field. In addition, epithelial cells (from the mouth) should not be too numerous. These criteria help assure that the specimen to be cultured is truly sputum originating from the source of infection. Otherwise, only saliva from the mouth may be obtained, and culture results may be misleading. Saliva contains a large number of bacteria, but they are probably not the organisms responsible for the respiratory infection. Exceptions do occur; for example, an immunocompromised patient may not have large numbers of leukocytes in the sputum, even in the presence of infection.

Once it has been determined that the sputum sample is reliable, the results of the gram stain may lead to a presumptive diagnosis of bacterial pneumonia if large numbers of similar bacteria are found. In addition, the gram stain reaction (positive or negative) and the shape of the bacteria may indicate the type of organism responsible for the infection. Such results are always presumptive, and a definitive diagnosis is made only by isolation of the organism from cultures. Identification of numerous eosinophils in the sputum indi-

may occur with chylous effusions in leakage of the thoracic duct fluid content) into the pleural space. He fluid is most often due to malign trauma, infections, pulmonar disorders. It is importan (from needle insertio pleural fluid.

The level of also be determ is charact caused fluid ist

Bronchoalveolar Lavage

In certain situations, bronchoalveolar lavage (BAL) is performed during bronchoscopy by injecting a large volume of sterile fluid into the patient's lung. This fluid mixes with the respiratory secretions within the airways and alveoli and is subsequently withdrawn for analysis in the laboratory. BAL has two main functions: (1) to evaluate the need for therapy in patients with interstitial lung disease by analysis of the cells obtained in the lavage solution; (2) to serve as a diagnostic tool in diseases such as *Pneumocystis carinii* pneumonia and asbestosis. BAL is contraindicated in patients with significantly reduced pulmonary function, reduced blood oxygen levels (hypoxemia), significant cardiovascular disease, or serious electrolyte disturbances.

Once the lavage solution is recovered from the patient, the sample is sent to the laboratory for microscopic analysis. Lavage solution obtained from healthy nonsmokers is 91% to 95% machrophages, 6% to 8% lymphocytes, and 1% granulocytes (neutrophils and eosinophils). The cellular composition of this fluid shows characteristic alterations in various diseases such as pulmonary sarcoidosis.

Pleural Fluid Examination

Normal pleural fluid is clear and pale yellow in color. Usually only small amounts of fluid are present (< 20 mL). Increased pleural fluid occurs most commonly with heart failure but also with liver disease, infections, and tumors. Opaque or turbid fluid is characteristic of infections in which there are large numbers of WBCs in the fluid. Actual cell counts may be performed on the fluid. The type of WBC present may be useful in determining the type of infection present. Milky fluid

which there is
with its high lipid
morrhagic or bloody
ancy but can occur with
infarct, and various other
to rule out a traumatic tap
n) as the source of blood in

protein occurring in pleural fluid may
ined. A protein level of less than 3 g/dL
ristic of a transudate. Transudates are
by mechanical factors with simple effusion of
across undamaged lining cells, and are character-
c of disorders such as heart failure and cirrhosis.
Exudates result from effusion of fluid and cells across
damaged lining cells, have a protein content of 3 g/dL
or greater, and are characteristic of infections, trauma,
infarct, rheumatoid disease, and tumors. Culture of the
fluid for microbiologic organisms and cytologic examination for malignant cells are other tests commonly
performed on pleural fluid and are described elsewhere
in this chapter.

Urinalysis

Urinalysis is one of the most commonly performed
tests in the clinical laboratory. It is helpful as a crude
screening test for kidney disease and reflects the metabolic status of the patient. The examination of urine
may also indicate the likelihood of urinary tract infection before culture results. The following features are
usually noted in routine urinalysis: appearance, specific
gravity, pH, protein, glucose, ketones, blood, bilirubin,
urobilinogen, nitrite, and microscopic examination of
urinary sediment.

The appearance simply denotes the color and
whether the urine appears clear or cloudy. The specific
gravity indicates the concentration of the urine. More
concentrated urine is normally seen in dehydration,
whereas more dilute urine is present with high fluid
intake and in some kidney diseases in which the
kidney is unable to concentrate urine normally. The pH
of the urine reflects the acid-base status of the patient.
The presence of protein in the urine, known as
proteinuria, is usually indicative of renal disease.
Glucose appears in the urine *(glucosuria)* most commonly in diabetes but is sometimes caused by renal
disease. Ketones occur with starvation and in diabetes
mellitus. *Hematuria,* or blood in the urine, may
originate in either the kidney or the bladder from a
wide variety of causes. Bilirubin occurs in the urine in
the conjugated form and is seen in the urine when
there is an obstruction to the outflow of bile from the
liver. Urobilinogen appears in some liver diseases and
hemolytic states. Nitrates may indicate that significant
numbers of bacteria are present. Most of the substances just mentioned are tested for by reagent strips

and are quantitated only roughly. The degree of
quantitation is on a scale of 1^+ to 4^+ and sometimes
includes trace amounts of less than 1^+.

The urine may then be centrifuged, and the
sediment examined microscopically. The presence and
numbers of any blood cells (RBCs, WBCs), casts, and
crystals are noted. Large numbers of WBCs may indicate the presence of infection. Various types of casts
may occur and generally indicate renal disease.

Histology and Cytology

A small biopsy of lung tissue may be obtained either
through a bronchoscope (bronchoscopic biopsy) or at
the time of thoracotomy (open lung biopsy). The tissue
samples obtained are sent to the histology or surgical
pathology laboratory. The tissue is processed in such a
way that it can be cut very thin, placed on a slide, and
stained so that the cells are visible when examined by a
pathologist with a microscope. This can yield valuable
information concerning infectious processes, chronic
lung diseases, and benign and malignant tumors. An
acid-fast (Ziehl-Neelsen) stain can be done on tissue to
identify mycobacteria. Gomori's methenamine silver
(GMS) and periodic acid–Schiff (PAS) stains may be
done to identify fungal organisms. GMS stains also
identify the *Pneumocystis* organisms causing increasing
numbers of infections, such as pneumonia, in immunocompromised patients. Tissue gram stains may also be
done.

Sometimes a specific lung lobe or an entire lung is
surgically removed. These tissues are examined thoroughly to determine presence of tumor, size of tumor,
surgical margins, and presence of regional lymph node
metastasis. If any information regarding the pathology
is needed by the surgeon during surgery, a frozen
section may be made. Freezing the tissue permits
immediate sectioning (slicing) of the tissue and preparation of a slide, whereas normal processing of tissue is
an overnight procedure. With a frozen section, the
pathologist can examine the tissue and relay the necessary information to the surgeon while the operation is
in progress.

Tumors of the lung may be either benign or
malignant. A classification of malignant lung tumors is
shown in the accompanying box. Benign lung tumors
are less common than malignant tumors, with hamar-
toma (a benign proliferation of elements normally occurring in the lung) being seen most often. The first
four tumors listed in the box (squamous cell carcinoma,
small-cell carcinoma, adenocarcinoma, and large-cell
carcinoma) represent the majority of primary lung
tumors and are often referred to as *bronchogenic carcinoma.* These tumors are usually related to smoking
(with the possible exception of adenocarcinoma) and
are highly malignant. Secondary or metastatic tumors
to the lung are also very common. Carcinoid tumors

**MODIFIED WORLD HEALTH
ORGANIZATION HISTOLOGIC TYPING
OF MALIGNANT TUMORS***

1. Squamous cell carcinoma
2. Small-cell carcinoma
    Oat cell carcinoma
    Intermediate cell type
3. Adenocarcinoma
    Bronchioloalveolar carcinoma
4. Large-cell carcinoma
    Giant cell carcinoma
5. Carcinoid tumor
6. Bronchial gland carcinoma
    Adenoid cystic carcinoma
    Mucoepidermoid carcimona

Indented categories represent common subtypes.

and bronchial gland carcinomas are much less common and are usually less aggressive. They are sometimes referred to as low-grade carcinomas (they were previously called bronchial adenomas). Tumors consisting of a mixture of cell types and other rare types of tumor may occur.

Cytology is the study of fluids, secretions, or other body samples that contain cellular material but not actual fragments of intact tissue as in biopsies. The cells are smeared on a glass slide, (Papanicolaou smear), stained, and examined by a pathologist. Often the presence of malignancy and even the type of malignancy can be determined in this manner. Pulmonary samples that can be examined cytologically include sputum, bronchial washings, bronchial brushings, and pleural fluid. A newer, growing field in cytology is fine needle aspiration (FNA). In FNA a relatively small needle (usually 22 gauge) is inserted into a mass and some of the cellular material is aspirated into the needle and then expressed and smeared onto a slide. The slide is then stained and examined, often yielding very accurate information about the nature of the mass. FNA of lung masses is performed under radiologic guidance. For many years this procedure has been widely used in this country to evaluate lung masses and has proved to be a safe, relatively simple, and effective way to diagnose malignant tumors and other processes prior to surgery. Sometimes surgery can be avoided by using the FNA procedure.

Skin Testing

Over the years skin testing has proved to be a useful means of diagnosing disease entities that involve the entire body as well as the lungs. The diseases include tuberculosis (TB), coccidioidomycosis, histoplasmosis, sarcoidosis, blastomycosis, and allergic disorders.

The procedure requires a small amount of the protein "essence" of the organism or substance involved in causing the disease to be injected under the skin. The accuracy of the test depends on the material being placed precisely in the subcutaneous layer of the skin. Great care must be exercised to be sure this occurs.

Many patients develop a condition, referred to as *anergy,* in which their immune system does not react to skin testing. Unfortunately, some of the diseases diagnosed by skin testing render the patient anergic. Conditions that may cause a person to become anergic are aging, cancer, starvation or debilitation, and sarcoidosis. To evaluate the patient's reactions, a "marker" skin test is employed along with the material being used to test for a specific disease. If the marker test does not produce a reaction, the absence of a reaction to the skin test for disease is meaningless. The examiner should not accept this negative skin reaction as evidence that the patient does not have the suspected disease. The markers used are extracts of material everyone has encountered and has an immunity against but to which no disease has developed. Some of the common markers used are protein derivatives of mumps, the fungus *Trichophyton,* and streptokinase-streptodornase (SKSD).

The most commonly used skin test is the test for TB. The test requires that 0.1 mL of a material called *purified protein derivative (PPD)* be injected into the subcutaneous layer of skin. The test is evaluated 48 to 72 hours later. Two distinct skin reactions are necessary for the test to be considered positive: an induration (raised welt) and an area of erythema (redness). The area of erythema is sometimes mistakenly interpreted as a positive result. The indurated area must also be present and be at least 10 mm in diameter for the reaction to be considered positive.

There are times when it is unwise or nonproductive to use the tuberculin test. Many people born and raised outside of the United States are vaccinated with a vaccine called *BCG* (bacille Calmette-Guérin). These people, along with those who have already had tuberculosis, should not be skin-tested for TB, since they have a positive response in the absence of active tuberculosis.

Case Study 1

B.K. is a 22-year-old white woman who was brought to the emergency room by her mother with chief complaints of cough, fever, and chills for the past 3 days. B.K. has a history of Down syndrome and lives at home with her parents. Initial examination reveals tachycardia, tachyp-

nea, fever, and normal blood pressure. Chest auscultation identifies bronchial breath sounds and inspiratory and expiratory coarse crackles of the right lower lobe. The admitting physician orders a sputum gram stain and culture, CBC count, and a chest film. The initial laboratory results are:

CBC:	Results	Normals
WBC ($\times 10^9$/L)	19.5	4.5–11.5
RBC ($\times 10^{12}$/L)	4.2	4.2–5.4
Hb (g/dL)	10.6	11.5–15.5
Hct	34.9%	38%–47%
MCV (μm^3)	77.0	80–96
MCHC	30.4%	32%–36%
White blood cell differential:		
Segmented neutrophils	82%	40%–75%
Lymphocytes	8%	20%–45%
Monocytes	4%	2%–10%
Eosinophils	1%	0%–6%
Basophils	0	0%–1%
Band neutrophils	7%	0%–6%

Gram stain: 2+ gram-positive cocci; 1+ pus cells with many epithelial cells

Interpretation: *Leukocytosis is present and appears to be due to an increase in the neutrophils consistent with a bacterial infection. The slight increase in immature neutrophils (bands) represents a left shift indicating stress on the bone marrow to release more neutrophils to fight the infection. The relative decrease in the percentage of lymphocytes is due to the absolute increase in the number of neutrophils and is not an abnormality.*

The RBC count is within normal limits; however, the decrease in hemoglobin, hematocrit, MCV, and MCHC are consistent with a microcytic, hypochromic anemia. This needs further investigation to identify the cause, but iron deficiency anemia is a likely reason.

The gram stain of the sputum sample indicates that it was heavily contaminated with secretions from the mouth since many epithelial cells were present. The sample should be discarded and another sputum sample obtained.

Case Study 2

C.J. is a 65-year-old woman who was brought to the emergency room by her husband. C.J. is complaining of severe shortness of breath, weakness, and cough. C.J. has a long history of chronic obstructive pulmonary disease (COPD) with a 90-pack-year smoking history. She currently admits to smoking one pack per day. In the emergency room C.J. appears acutely and chronically ill and is found to be using her accessory muscles to breathe. She is cyanotic and has decreased breath sounds bilaterally. C.J. is started on oxygen by nasal cannula and the attending physician orders a CBC, electrolyte determination, and other appropriate tests. The results:

Test	Results	Normals
WBC ($\times 10^9$/L)	19.9	4.5–11.5
RBC ($\times 10^{12}$/L)	5.1	4.2–5.0
Hb (g/dL)	15.3	12–15 g/dL
Hct	47.5%	34%–46%
MCV (μm^3)	98.2	82–98
MCHC	31.6%	33%–35%
Segmented neutrophils	76%	40%–75%
Lymphocytes	12%	20%–45%
Monocytes	5%	2%–10%
Eosinophils	4%	0%–6%
Basophils	2%	0%–1%
Electrolytes (mEq/L):		
Na^+	137	137–147
K^+	4.8	3.5–4.8
Cl^-	87	98–105
Co_2	41	23–33

Interpretation: *The increase in WBCs suggests leukocytosis and appears to be due to an increase in the number of circulating neutrophils. This may be in response to a bacterial infection or acute stress. The RBC count, hemoglobin, and hematocrit are slightly increased consistent with polycythemia. These RBC differential findings are consistent with secondary polycythemia typical for patients with a chronic lung disease in which the arterial blood oxygen levels are persistently low.*

The electrolyte values reveal a decreased serum Cl^- and an increased serum CO_2. This is most likely related to the patient's long-term history of COPD. Some COPD patients chronically retain CO_2 owing to poor pulmonary function. To compensate for the elevated CO_2 the kidneys retain increased levels of serum HCO_3^- in an effort to maintain a near-normal serum pH. The resulting metabolic buildup of serum HCO_3^- is reflected as an increased CO_2 in the venous blood sample. The increase in serum CO_2 (HCO_3^-) causes the kidneys to excrete more than the usual amount of Cl^- in an effort to maintain electrical neutrality. As a result, serum Cl^- levels are typically reduced in patients with chronically elevated serum CO_2.

REVIEW QUESTIONS

1. *Which of the following is not a component of the formed elements of the blood?*
   a. *red blood cells*
   b. *lipids*
   c. *white blood cells*
   d. *platelets*

2. T   F   *Blood serum is plasma from which the clotting factors have been removed by liquid chromatography.*

3. T   F   *In the presence of a significantly reduced RBC count, a normal oxygen carrying capacity of the blood can still be maintained.*

4. Which of the following statements is(are) true regarding hemoglobin?
   a. it functions in oxygen transport
   b. it is the main component of RBCs
   c. it functions in carbon dioxide transport
   d. all of the above

5. What is normal range for white blood cells?
   a. $1000-3000/mm^3$
   b. $3000-5000/mm^3$
   c. $4500-10000/mm^3$
   d. $600-14000/mm^3$

6. Which of the following white cell types normally makes up the majority of the differential?
   a. neutrophils
   b. eosinophils
   c. basophils
   d. lymphocytes

7. T   F   A tissue monocyte is called a macrophage.

8. Which of the following is the most common cause of anemia?
   a. drug-induced RBC lysis
   b. acute blood loss
   c. iron deficiency
   d. none of the above

9. Which of the following is not true regarding polycythemia?
   a. it can be caused by chronic hypoxemia
   b. it is defined as an increase in RBC, hemoglobin, and hematocrit
   c. it increases oxygen carrying capacity of the blood
   d. it decreases the workload on the heart

10. A left-shifted white cell differential is evidenced by which of the following findings?
    a. an increase in the number of eosinophils
    b. a decrease in the number of segmented neutrophils
    c. an increase in the number of bands (immature neutrophils)
    d. a decrease in the number of lymphocytes

11. Which of the following is a common finding in patients with bacterial pneumonia?
    a. neutrophilia
    b. leukopenia
    c. lymphocytopenia
    d. eosinophilia

12. Which of the following is a common finding in a patient with an allergic reaction?

    a. neutropenia
    b. leukopenia
    c. eosinophilia
    d. monocytosis

13. Viral infections typically produce which of the following abnormalities?
    a. lymphocytosis
    b. eosinophilia
    c. basophilia
    d. monocytosis

14. T   F   AIDS increases the ration of T helper to T suppressor cells.

15. T   F   Leukemia is defined as an uncontrolled increase in the number of white blood cells.

16. T   F   The sedimentation rate is a nonspecific test used to determine the general presence of disease.

17. Which of the following tests is used to assess the patient's blood clotting ability?
    a. RBC
    b. hemoglobin
    c. hematocrit
    d. prothrombin time

18. Which of the following electrolytes closely affects muscle function?
    a. sodium
    b. potassium
    c. chloride
    d. phosphorus

19. Which of the following electrolytes is mainly responsible for extracellular water balance?
    a. calcium
    b. sodium
    c. magnesium
    d. potassium

20. What is the normal range for the anion gap?
    a. 2-5 mEq/L
    b. 6-10 mEq/L
    c. 12-20 mEq/L
    d. 22-29 mEq/L

21. Anion gap is useful in assessing which of the following situations?
    a. cause of metabolic alkalosis
    b. cause of metabolic acidosis
    c. cause of respiratory acidosis
    d. cause of respiratory alkalosis

22. An increase in the sweat electrolyte concentration is typical of which of the following diseases?
    a. cystic fibrosis
    b. patent ductus arteriosus
    c. bronchiectasis
    d. epiglottitis

23. Which of the following tests is(are) a measure of kidney function?
    a. BUN
    b. creatine kinase
    c. creatinine
    d. a and c

24. Which of the following enzymes would be elevated in a patient who has had a myocardial infarction?
    a. AST
    b. LDH
    c. CPK
    d. all of the above

25. Which of the following is the therapeutic level for theophylline?
    a. 2-5 μg/mL
    b. 5-10 μg/mL
    c. 10-20 μg/mL
    d. 20-30 μg/mL

26. Which of the following would decrease the clearance of theophylline?
    a. cigarette smoking
    b. congestive heart failure
    c. youthful age
    d. all of the above

27. Which of the following bacteriologic tests is used to determine the effectiveness of antibiotics on a particular organism?
    a. gram stain
    b. culture
    c. sensitivity
    d. Acid-fast

28. T   F   Bacteria that are usually present in a healthy person are called normal flora.

29. A Ziehl-Neelsen stain is used to identify which of the following organisms?
    a. S. aureus
    b. P. aeruginosa
    c. S. pneumoniae
    d. M. tuberculosis

30. Which of the following items are evaluated during a macroscopic (gross) sputum examination?
    a. color
    b. consistency
    c. volume
    d. all of the above

31. T   F   A sputum sample with many epithelial cells present would be considered a reliable sample.

32. Which of the following is the most common cause of bacterial pneumonia?
    a. S. pneumoniae
    b. P. aeruginosa
    c. H. influenza
    d. K. pneumoniae

33. Which of the following findings is consistent with pleural infection?
    a. bloody pleural fluid
    b. low pleural fluid protein levels
    c. opaque/turbid pleural fluid
    d. all of the above

34. T   F   Pleural fluid with a high protein content is called a transudate.

35. Which of the following tests performed during urinalysis could be a help in diagnosing diabetes mellitus?
    a. glucose
    b. pH
    c. ketones
    d. all of the above

36. Proteinuria is usually indicative of which of the following?
    a. COPD
    b. kidney disease
    c. cardiovascular disease
    d. spinal meningitis

37. T   F   Adenocarcinoma is responsible for producing primary lung carcinoma.

38. T   F   Cytologic studies are used to examine tissue samples by freezing and sectioning.

39. Which of the following may cause a patient to have a negative reaction to a skin test?
    a. they do not have the disease
    b. they are anergic
    c. the disease has progressed to a point beyond treatment
    d. a and b

40. Which of the following is true regarding a PPD?
    a. it is positive with coccidioidomycosis infection
    b. it is positive if the patient has previously had a BCG vaccine
    c. it is negative if the induration produced is 12 mm in diameter
    d. none of the above

BIBLIOGRAPHY

Donahoe M, and Rogers RM: Laboratory evaluation of the patient with chronic obstructive pulmonary disease; In Cherniack NS: *Chronic obstructive pulmonary disease,* Philadelphia, 1991, WB Saunders.

Finegold M, and Martin J: *Diagnostic microbiology,* ed 7, St Louis, 1986, Mosby–Year Book.

Fraser RG, and Pare JAP: *Diagnosis of diseases of the chest,* ed 3, Philadelphia, 1988, WB Saunders.

Henry J: *Clinical diagnosis and management by laboratory methods,* ed 18, Philadelphia, 1991, WB Saunders.

McDowell EM, and Beals TF: *Biopsy pathology of the bronchi,* Philadelphia, 1987, WB Saunders.

Spencer H: *Pathology of the lung,* ed 4, New York, 1985, Pergamon Press.

Tietz W: *Textbook of clinical chemistry,* Philadelphia, 1976, WB Saunders.

Tilkian SM, Conover MG, and Tilkian AG: *Clinical implications of laboratory tests,* ed 4, St Louis, 1987, Mosby–Year Book.

Williams J, and others: *Hematology,* ed 3, New York, 1983, McGraw-Hill.

Wintrobe MM: *Clinical hematology,* ed 9, Philadelphia, 1993, Lea & Febiger.

Chapter 6

Interpretation of Blood Gases

Robert L. Wilkins

LEARNING OBJECTIVES

Upon completion of this chapter, the reader should be able to accomplish the following:

1. *Recognize why arterial blood is useful in determining respiratory status instead of venous blood.*

2. *Identify the importance of reviewing the laboratory data that reflects clotting ability prior to performing an arterial puncture.*

3. *Identify the common sites for arterial puncture.*

4. *Identify the test used to determine collateral circulation of the radial artery, how to perform this procedure, and how to interpret its results.*

5. *Recognize how the following factors would generally affe*
   a. *air bubbles in the syringe*
   b. *not putting the sample on ice*

6. *Identify the normal duration of arterial puncture si*

7. *Identify the normal values for the following blood*
   a. *pH*
   b. *Pao_2*
   c. *$Paco_2$*
   d. *HCO_3*
   e. *Sao_2*
   f. *$P(A-a)o_2$*
   g. *Cao_2*
   h. *BE*
   i. *$P\bar{v}o_2$*

8. *Recognize the significance and the fac*
   a. *Pao_2*
   b. *$P(A-a)o_2$*
   c. *Sao_2*
   d. *Cao_2*

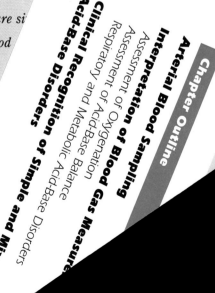

Chapter Outline

Arterial Blood Sampling

Interpretation of Blood Gas Measure
Assessment of Oxygenation
Assessment of Acid-Base Balance
Respiratory and Metabolic Acid-Base Disorders

Clinical Recognition of Acid-Base Disorders
Acid-Base Disorders of Simple and Mixed

LEARNING OBJECTIVES — cont'd

    e. $P\bar{v}o_2$
    f. $C(a\text{-}v)o_2$
    g. $HbCO$

9. Recognize a definition of hypoxia and hypoxemia.

10. Identify the general classifications of hypoxemia.

11. Identify the physiologic causes, mechanisms, and most common physiologic cause of hypoxemia.

12. Describe how the physiologic causes of hypoxemia respond to supplemental oxygen administration.

13. Describe how increases and decreases in $Paco_2$, body temperature, and blood pH affect the oxyhemoglobin dissociation curve and related Sao_2 measurements/oxyhemoglobin affinity.

14. Recognize how shifts in the oxyhemoglobin dissociation curve affect oxygen transport at the tissues and lungs.

15. Identify a definition, the normal value, and the significance of measuring P50.

16. Recognize a definition, the significance, and the factors that affect the following acid-base parameters:
    a. pH
    b. $Paco_2$
    c. Plasma HCO_3^-
    d. standard HCO_3^-
    e. BE

17. Identify the Henderson-Hasselbalch equation and the ratio of HCO_3 to $Paco_2$ needed to maintain a pH of 7.40.

18. Define simple and mixed acid-base abnormalities.

19. For the following simple acid-base disorders identify the basic mechanism of impairment, how the disorder is compensated for, common causes, and the expected values of compensating components:
    a. respiratory acidosis
    b. respiratory alkalosis
    c. metabolic acidosis
    d. metabolic alkalosis

20. For the simple acid-base disorders, identify the degree of compensation present given pH, $Paco_2$, HCO_3^- and BE values.

21. Recognize a definition of mixed acid-base disorders, common causes, and given pH, $Paco_2$, HCO_3^- and BE values, interpret the following mixed acid-base disorders:
    a. metabolic and respiratory alkalosis
    b. metabolic and respiratory acidosis

22. Recognize the relative speed of the respiratory and metabolic compensatory mechanisms.

    Recognize the significance of the 95% confidence-limit bands as used to assess acid-base status.

    the results of an arterial blood gas, interpret the acid-base and oxygenation status of the patient.

ments

Simple Disorders
Limitations of Compensation for Acid-Base Disorders
Mixed Acid-Base Disorders

Summary of Interpreting Blood Gas
Measurements
   id-Base Assessment
   nation Assessment

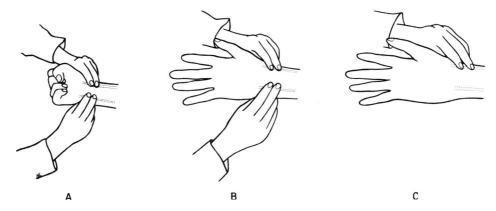

Fig. 6-1 *Assessment of collateral circulation before radial artery sampling.* **A,** *Patient clenches fist while examiner obstructs radial and ulnar arteries.* **B,** *Patient gently opens hand while pressure is maintained over both arteries.* **C,** *Pressure over ulnar artery is released, and changes in color of patient's palm are noted.*

Chapter Overview

Analysis of the arterial blood sample provides precise measurement of acid-base balance and of the lungs' ability to oxygenate the blood and remove excess carbon dioxide. For these reasons, assessment of the patient with respiratory dysfunction is more accurate and complete if arterial blood gas (ABG) measurements are reported. Accurate interpretation of the measurements, however, requires knowledge of the patient's total clinical picture, including any treatment the patient is receiving. This chapter provides insight into interpretation of ABG measurements in the clinical setting.

Arterial blood is used to assess respiratory function because it contains oxygen and carbon dioxide levels primarily determined by the lungs. Venous blood does not reflect respiratory function, since it has been exposed to peripheral vascular beds where gas exchange with the tissues alters the oxygen and carbon dioxide concentrations of the blood (Table 6-1). Mixed venous blood samples from the right atrium or pulmonary artery are useful to evaluate overall tissue oxygenation and are discussed later in this chapter. Peripheral venous blood, instead of arterial blood, may be obtained accidently during the sampling procedure, especially in the patient with hypotension. Analysis of venous blood reflects local metabolic rates and is of little value. An inaccurate assessment will result if the venous sample is analyzed and interpreted as arterial.

Because of the cost and risk to the patient, ABG analysis must be performed only when clinically indicated. If ABG measurements are not obtained when needed, improper assessment and treatment of the patient may result. ABG analysis is indicated if the patient's symptoms, medical history, physical examination, or laboratory data suggest significant abnormalities in respiratory or acid-base status. The analysis is helpful in evaluating the effects of treatment and should also be obtained when significant changes in mechanical ventilation settings are initiated.

Arterial Blood Sampling

The arterial blood sample is obtained by inserting a needle into a major artery (*arteriotomy*). Before arterial puncture, it may be helpful to review the patient's chart for clinical laboratory studies that reflect the patient's blood clotting ability (see Chapter 5). Abnormalities such as low platelet counts or increased bleeding time may indicate that postpuncture bleeding will pose a problem. In such cases the puncture site should be pressurized longer than usual to prevent hemorrhage (see discussion, below).

The arterial blood sample may be obtained from the radial, dorsalis pedis, brachial, or femoral arteries in the adult.[1] The radial artery is the preferred puncture site since it is accessible and easy to stabilize after the puncture.[2] Adequate collateral circulation can be evaluated and is usually available if the radial artery becomes obstructed during the puncture procedure.

The degree of collateral circulation to the hand is evaluated by a modified *Allen test* before puncture of the radial artery. To perform this test the patient is first instructed to make a tight fist. The examiner then compresses both the radial and ulnar arteries (Fig.6-1).

Table 6-1	**Normal Arterial and Venous Blood Gas Measurements**	
	Arterial*	Venous*
pH	7.35–7.45	7.34–7.37
P_{O_2}	80–100 mm Hg	38–42 mm Hg
P_{CO_2}	35–45 mm Hg	44–46 mm Hg
HCO_3^-	22–26 mEq/L	24–30 mEq/L

*Assumes normal respiratory and cardiac function in a patient breathing room air at sea level.

The patient is instructed to open the fist gently to a relaxed position, revealing a blanched palm and fingers. The pressure over the ulnar artery is released while the patient's palm is observed for changes in color. If collateral flow is adequate, the patient's hand will "pink up" within 10 to 15 seconds; this constitutes a positive Allen test. A positive result documents that collateral blood flow is adequate and the radial artery is an acceptable puncture site. If the test is negative (the palm does not pink up rapidly), the radial artery is not an acceptable site for puncture. In such cases the other wrist should be evaluated or the brachial artery used for the puncture site.

Because arteriotomy causes trauma to the puncture site, an indwelling arterial catheter should be used when a need for frequent sampling is anticipated. The catheter must be inserted by well-trained personnel and its use reserved for patients in an intensive care unit under close observation.

Regardless of which artery is chosen, the process of arterial puncture must be well planned and carefully executed by a skilled technician. The sample must be obtained without exposure to the environment. Exposure can occur when large air bubbles are trapped within the syringe. The oxygen and carbon dioxide gas tensions of the bubbles may equilibrate with the blood and result in erroneous measurements.[2] Once the sample is obtained, air bubbles should be removed and the sample stored in an ice water bath to inhibit continued metabolism within the sample.[3] Immediate placement of the sample in ice water is important when the patient's white blood cell count is elevated.[4,5] Attention to the blood sample must not prevent proper care of the puncture site. The wound should be pressurized after the needle is withdrawn for a period of at least 3 to 5 minutes or longer if clotting problems exist.

Once the arterial sample is obtained and the puncture site stabilized, the sample is taken to the laboratory for analysis. The iced sample should be analyzed within 1 hour to obtain the most accurate results.[1] Samples not placed in an ice water bath should be analyzed within 10 minutes.[1] For the results to be reliable, analysis of the blood sample must be performed with properly maintained and calibrated equipment.

Interpretation of Blood Gas Measurements

The measurements obtained from analysis of arterial and mixed venous blood samples are useful in evaluation of the following:
1. Oxygenation status (Pa_{O_2}, Sa_{O_2}, Ca_{O_2}, $P\overline{v}_{O_2}$)
2. Acid-base balance (pH, Pa_{CO_2}, HCO_3^-, base excess)
3. Adequacy of ventilation (Pa_{CO_2})

Abbreviations associated with blood gas interpretation are as follows:

Acid-base

pH	Hydrogen ion concentration in blood
HCO_3^-	Plasma bicarbonate concentration
Pa_{CO_2}	Partial pressure of carbon dioxide in arterial blood
BE	Base excess

Oxygenation

Pa_{O_2}	Partial pressure of oxygen in arterial blood
PA_{O_2}	Partial pressure of oxygen in the alveoli
Sa_{O_2}	Percent saturation of hemoglobin with oxygen in arterial blood
Ca_{O_2}	Content of oxygen in arterial blood (mL/dL)
$P\overline{v}_{O_2}$	Partial pressure of oxygen in mixed venous blood
Fi_{O_2}	Fraction of oxygen in inspired gas (often expressed as a percentage)
$P(A-a)_{O_2}$	Difference in pressure between alveoli and arterial blood of oxygen
Pi_{O_2}	Partial pressure of oxygen in inspired gas

The following discussion describes the use of blood gases to assess oxygenation and acid-base balance in the clinical setting.

Assessment of Oxygenation

The important process of evaluating the oxygenation status of the patient involves two basic steps. First, the measurements provided by blood gas analysis must be evaluated to identify the quantity of oxygen transported in the blood. Second, the patient's tissue oxygenation status must be determined. The following discussion describes the evaluation of measurements available from blood gas analysis that reflect oxygenation. This is followed by a brief description of the basic techniques used in clinical assessment of the patient's overall oxygenation condition. The clinical assessment of tissue oxygenation is also discussed in Chapters 11 and 12.

Oxygen in the blood is primarily transported bound to hemoglobin. A smaller portion is transported as dissolved gas in the blood plasma. Assessment of the basic blood gas measurements reflecting oxygenation involves interpreting data that identify the partial pressure of oxygen in the plasma (Pa_{O_2}), the amount of oxygen bound to hemoglobin (Sa_{O_2}), and the total content of oxygen in the arterial blood (Ca_{O_2}).

PARTIAL PRESSURE OF OXYGEN IN ARTERIAL BLOOD (Pa_{O_2}).

NORMAL VALUE: Approximately 75 to 95 mm Hg on room air

Pa_{O_2} is a measurement of the pressure or tension of oxygen in the plasma of the arterial blood. Pa_{O_2} reflects the ability of the lungs to allow the transfer of oxygen from the environment to the circulating blood.

The normal predicted Pa_{O_2} is dependent on the barometric pressure, the patient's age, and the concentration or fraction of the inspired gas that is oxygen (Fi_{O_2}). Healthy lungs allow oxygen to move from the alveoli to the blood in direct proportion to the alveolar partial pressure of oxygen (PA_{O_2}). At sea level, where the barometric pressure is 760 mm Hg, the PA_{O_2} and

Table 6-2 Relationship Between Age and Normal Predicted Pa_{O_2}*

Age (yrs)	Predicted Pa_{O_2} (mm Hg)
≤10	95–103
20	91–99
30	87–95
40	83–91
50	78–86
60	74–82
70	70–78
80	66–74
90	62–70

Predicted Pa_{O_2} (supine position) = 103.5 – (0.42 × age) ± 4

*Adapted from Burton G and Hodgkin JE: *Respiratory care, a guide to clinical practice*, ed 3, Philadelphia, 1990, JB Lippincott.

predicted Pa_{O_2} are higher than at an elevated altitude where the barometric pressure may be significantly below 760 mm Hg. The predicted normal Pa_{O_2} of a person living in Denver, Colorado (elevation of 5280 ft) is significantly below that of a person of the same age living at sea level.

As age increases, the efficiency of the lungs to oxygenate the blood is reduced; the predicted normal Pa_{O_2} is also reduced (Table 6–2).

PA_{O_2} and therefore Pa_{O_2} are influenced by the $F_{I_{O_2}}$ according to the following equation:

$$PA_{O_2} = F_{I_{O_2}}(P_B - P_{H_2O}) - (Pa_{CO_2} \times 1.25)$$

where

$F_{I_{O_2}}$ = fraction of inhaled gas that is oxygen
P_B = barometric pressure
P_{H_2O} = water vapor pressure in alveoli, assumed to be 47 mm Hg
Pa_{CO_2} = partial pressure of carbon dioxide in the arterial blood, assumed to be equal to the partial pressure of carbon dioxide in the alveoli
1.25 = mathematic factor that takes into account the ratio of carbon dioxide production to oxygen consumption

For example, a patient breathing room air at 760 mm Hg with a Pa_{CO_2} of 40 mm Hg would have a predicted Pa_{O_2} of 100 mm Hg.

$$PA_{O_2} = 0.21 (760 \text{ mm Hg} - 47 \text{ mm Hg}) - (40 \times 1.25)$$
$$= (0.21 \times 713 \text{mm Hg}) - 50 \text{ mm Hg}$$
$$= 150 \text{ mm Hg} - 50 \text{ mm Hg}$$
$$= 100 \text{ mm Hg}$$

When the measured Pa_{O_2} is below the predicted range for a patient breathing room air, regardless of the actual $F_{I_{O_2}}$, it is termed *hypoxemia*. As long as the Pa_{O_2} remains above the minimally acceptable limit, hypoxemia does not exist, regardless of the actual $F_{I_{O_2}}$. *Hypoxia* is a term often associated with hypoxemia and indicates a condition in which tissue oxygenation is inadequate. Hypoxemia may result in hypoxia in patients with limited cardiac performance, but the two

terms are not synonymous. Hypoxemia may be classified as mild, moderate, or severe according to the measured Pa_{O_2}. For patients breathing 21% oxygen (room air) and under the age of 60 years, a Pa_{O_2} of less than 60 to 79 mm Hg is considered mild hypoxemia; a Pa_{O_2} of 40 to 59 mm Hg is considered moderate hypoxemia; and a Pa_{O_2} of less than 40 mm Hg is considered severe hypoxemia. At any age, a Pa_{O_2} of less than 60 to 65 mm Hg is considered hypoxemia and a Pa_{O_2} of less than 40 mm Hg is considered severe hypoxemia.

Hypoxemia is most often the result of lung disease in which the transfer of oxygen from the inhaled gas to the blood is impaired. The physiologic causes of hypoxemia fall into the following general categories.

Ventilation-Perfusion ($\dot{V}/\dot{Q}$) Mismatching. For gas exchange to take place in the lungs, theinhaled gas must come into intimate contact with the blood. This requires close matching of ventilation with the blood perfusing the pulmonary circulation. When the matching of ventilation and perfusion is less than optimal, it is referred to as $\dot{V}/\dot{Q}$ mismatching, and hypoxemia results. $\dot{V}/\dot{Q}$ mismatching is by far the most common cause of hypoxemia in cases of respiratory dysfunction. Extreme degrees of $\dot{V}/\dot{Q}$ mismatching are referred to as wasted or dead space ventilation and shunt (Fig. 6–2). *Dead space ventilation* is defined as ventilation without perfusion. This occurs when perfusion of the lungs is reduced. Perfusion without ventilation is defined as *shunt.*

Shunt. Two types of shunting exist: *anatomic shunting* and *capillary shunting*. Anatomic shunting refers to blood that travels from the right side of the heart to the left side without passing through the pulmonary capillary bed. Normally this is less than 3% of the cardiac output. Congenital heart defects represent one of the most common problems that may cause an increase in the anatomic shunt. Capillary shunting refers to blood that passes through a portion of the pulmonary capillary bed that has reduced or no ventilation. *True shunting* is present when alveolar ventilation is absent in a particular alveolar-capillary (AC) unit and *relative shunting* exists when the ventilation is significantly less than the perfusion in an AC unit. Relative shunting also is referred to as a low $\dot{V}/\dot{Q}$.

The portion of the cardiac output ($\dot{Q}_T$) shunted via anatomic shunt is symbolized as $\dot{Q}_S$. The Q is the symbol for blood flow and s stands for shunted blood. The fraction of the blood flow shunted can also be symbolized as $\dot{Q}_S/\dot{Q}_T$.

The term *physiologic shunt* refers to the combined effect of capillary and anatomic shunting. Clinicians often use this term to describe the total shunt when the exact cause of the shunting is not known. The physiologic shunt is symbolized as *Qsp.*

The amount of AC units affected by the shunting will determine the Pa_{O_2}. Significant shunting (>15% of

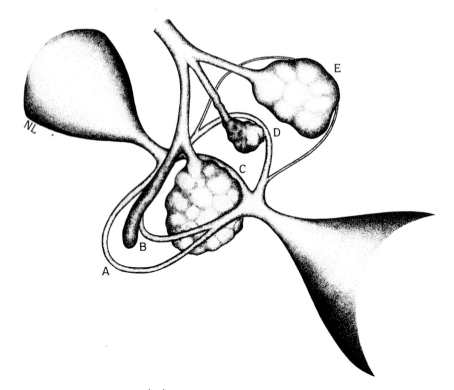

Fig. 6-2 *Spectrum of ventilation-perfusion ($\dot{V}/\dot{Q}$) matching.* **A,** *Blood returning to left ventricle without entering pulmonary vasculature: anatomic shunt.* **B,** *Blood flow through nonventilated areas: capillary shunt.* **C,** *Normal matching of ventilation with perfusion.* **D,** *Perfusion in excess of ventilation: shunt effect.* **E,** *Ventilation in excess of perfusion: dead space or wasted ventilation.*

the cardiac output) results in hypoxemia because the shunted blood fails to pick up oxygen in the lung. Hypoxemia from shunting responds poorly to an increase in F_{IO_2}. Clinicians must suspect shunting as the cause of the hypoxemia any time the patient's Pa_{O_2} does not increase significantly in response to increases in F_{IO_2}. See Chapter 12 for a discussion of shunt measurement.

Diffusion Defect. Abnormalities in the lung structure that slow the diffusion of oxygen from the inhaled gas through the alveolar-capillary membrane result in hypoxemia from diffusion defect. True examples of diffusion defect are not common. Hypoxemia occurring from diffusion defect is typically responsive to oxygen therapy.

Overall Hypoventilation. Elevation of Pa_{CO_2} from hypoventilation reduces the Pa_{O_2}. As Pa_{O_2} falls, Pa_{O_2} decreases also. If the hypoventilation is occurring in a patient with lung disease, the hypoxemia is usually a result of a combination of $\dot{V}/\dot{Q}$ mismatching and hypoventilation. When hypoventilation occurs in patients without lung disease (e.g., drug overdose), the hypoxemia is strictly the result of an elevated Pa_{CO_2}.

Hypoxemia may also occur with low P_{IO_2}. Pa_{O_2} is directly determined by the partial pressure of oxygen in the inhaled gas (P_{IO_2}). At high altitudes the P_{IO_2} is significantly below that at sea level and hypoxemia occurs even if respiratory function is optimal. Patients with a marginal Pa_{O_2} at sea level should avoid traveling to high altitudes without supplemental oxygen.

One other situation in which a reduction in P_{IO_2} may occur is when the patient is attached to breathing circuits. If equipment should fail, the patient may not receive proper F_{IO_2} and hypoxemia will occur. This can take place while the patient is receiving general anesthesia or mechanical ventilation. For this reason, the F_{IO_2} should be closely monitored during mechanical ventilation.

OXYGEN SATURATION (Sa_{O_2}).

NORMAL VALUE: greater than 95%

The Sa_{O_2} is an index of the actual amount of oxygen bound to hemoglobin expressed as a percentage of the total capacity. Some laboratories report only a calculated Sa_{O_2} when equipment is not available for actual measurements. True Sa_{O_2} can be determined only from a co-oximeter and is more reliable. Calculated Sa_{O_2} may be erroneously high, especially with carbon monoxide poisoning. (See discussion of carboxyhemoglobin, later in this chapter.)

The relationship between Pa_{O_2} and Sa_{O_2} is demonstrated by the *oxyhemoglobin dissociation curve* (Fig. 6-3). This curve demonstrates that Pa_{O_2} and Sa_{O_2} do not have a linear relationship. As Pa_{O_2} increases above 80 mm Hg in the flat part of the curve, Sa_{O_2} increases very little, whereas Pa_{O_2} changes below 80 mm Hg in the steep portion of the curve cause significant changes in Sa_{O_2} and thus oxygen content.

The Sa_{O_2} measurement is affected by body temperature, arterial blood pH, Pa_{CO_2}, and other factors (see accompanying box). Alkalosis, hypocapnia, hypo-

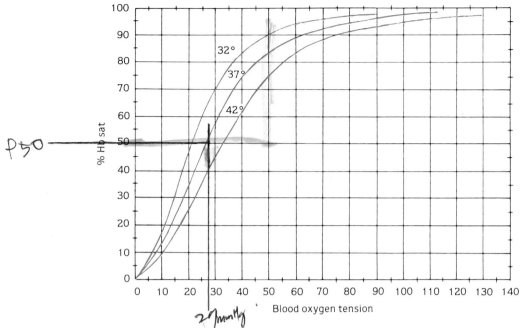

Fig. 6-3 *Oxygen dissociation curve of blood at a pH of 7.40, showing variations at three temperatures. For a given oxygen tension, the lower the blood temperature, the more the hemoglobin holds onto its oxygen, maintaining higher saturation. (From Scanlon LL, Spearman CB, and Sheldon RL:* Egan's fundamentals of respiratory therapy, *ed 5, St Louis, 1990, Mosby-Year Book.)*

FACTORS INFLUENCING THE OXYGEN DISSOCIATION CURVE

Shift to left (increase in hemoglobin-oxygen affinity)

Alkalosis ↓H⁺
Hypocapnia ↓PaCO₂
Reduction in body temperature ↓Temp
Fetal hemoglobin
Carboxyhemoglobin

Shift to right (decrease in hemoglobin-oxygen affinity)

Acidosis ↑H⁺
Hypercapnia
Fever

---

thermia, etc. shift the curve to the left, resulting in higher SaO_2 values at the same PaO_2. Conversely, acidosis, hypercapnia, and fever shift the curve to the right and result in lower SaO_2 values for the same PaO_2. In other words, shifts to the left cause tighter or easier binding of oxygen with hemoglobin and make unloading of oxygen at the tissues more difficult, whereas shifts to the right have the opposite effect, resulting in decreased oxygen affinity for hemoglobin, allowing easier unloading of oxygen at the tissues.

Concept of P-50. When the oxygen dissociation curve is shifted, the middle portion is displaced to a greater degree than the upper or lower ends. Thus the most sensitive indicator of a curve shift is measurement of the PO_2 at 50% hemoglobin saturation. As a result the concept of P-50 was introduced to identify the PO_2 value at which the hemoglobin is 50% saturated under specific conditions of laboratory measurement (37° C, PCO_2 40 mm Hg, and pH 7.40). Normally in healthy arterial blood the P-50 is 27 mm Hg. A P-50 other than 27 mm Hg identifies a shift in the dissociation curve and also the direction and degree of the shift. For example, if the hemoglobin affinity for oxygen is increased for some reason (as in stored blood with reduced 2, 3-diglycerophosphate [DPG] activity), hemoglobin will be 50% saturated at a lower PO_2. Therefore a P-50 of 22 mm Hg indicates that the oxygen affinity has increased, and P-50 values above 27 mm Hg indicate that oxygen affinity has decreased.

It is important to note that changes in pH, PCO_2, and body temperature will shift the oxygen hemoglobin dissociation curve but will not affect the P-50 measurement, since the blood sample is corrected for these parameters when it is determined. As a result, the P-50 measurement indicates the shift in the dissociation curve caused by factors other than changes in pH, PCO_2, and body temperature. The clinical value of P-50 is not clear, and in most cases it is not used at the bedside.

ARTERIAL OXYGEN CONTENT (CaO_2).

NORMAL VALUE: 16 to 20 mL/dL blood

The CaO_2 is a function of the amount of oxygen bound to hemoglobin and dissolved in the plasma. It is one of the most important blood gas measurements since it significantly influences tissue oxygenation. Since most oxygen (99%) is carried in the blood bound to hemoglobin, CaO_2

Table 6–3 Relationship Between Hemoglobin Concentration, Pao₂, Saturation, and Oxygen Content*

Hemoglobin (g/dL)	Pao₂ (mm Hg)	Sao₂ (%)	Cao₂ (vol%)
5.0	50	86	5.9
5.0	100	96	6.7
7.5	50	86	8.8
7.5	100	96	9.9
10.0	50	86	11.7
10.0	100	96	13.2
12.5	50	86	14.6
12.5	100	96	16.4
15.0	50	86	17.4
15.0	100	96	19.6

*Using factor of 1.34 mL of oxygen per gram of hemoglobin.

cannot be normal without adequate circulating red blood cells containing hemoglobin (Hb) (Table 6–3).

Cao_2 is calculated from the following:

$$\frac{\begin{array}{l}1.34^* \text{ mL} \times \text{Hb} \times \text{Sao}_2 = O_2 \text{ combined with Hb} \\ +0.003 \text{ mL} \times \text{Pao}_2 = O_2 \text{ dissolved in plasma}\end{array}}{\text{Total} = \text{Cao}_2(\text{vol\%})}$$

Anemic patients without lung disease may have normal Pao_2 and Sao_2, but Cao_2 is reduced because of the inadequate amount of hemoglobin, and tissue hypoxia may occur without adequate circulatory compensation. Conversely, patients with polycythemia may have mild reductions in Pao_2 and Sao_2 while maintaining Cao_2 values within or near normal limits (see Table 6–3). As with Sao_2, true measurements of Cao_2 can be achieved only from a co-oximeter. Cao_2 measurements from laboratories without a co-oximeter are only calculated values.

A reduced measured Cao_2 can also occur when the hemoglobin is bound to other gases. In such cases a normal level of hemoglobin in the circulating blood is of little value because most of it is not available for transporting oxygen. For example, carbon monoxide poisoning is probably present in the patient who has inhaled a significant amount of smoke from a fire. Carbon monoxide has an increased affinity for hemoglobin and binds tightly with any hemoglobin it contacts. Measured Cao_2 will be very low even though adequate hemoglobin and dissolved oxygen are present in the circulating blood (see discussion of carboxyhemoglobin later in this chapter).

ALVEOLAR-ARTERIAL OXYGEN DIFFERENCE [P(A–a)O₂].

NORMAL VALUE: 10 to 15 mm Hg on room air

The $P(A–a)O_2$ is a measurement of the pressure difference between the alveoli and the arterial blood of oxygen. In normal lungs, oxygen is transferred readily from the alveoli to the blood, and only a small Po_2 difference is present. When the lungs become dis-

eased, oxygen gas exchange is often hindered and a larger $P(A–a)O_2$ develops.

The predicted normal $P(A–a)O_2$ is dependent on the FIO_2 and the age of the patient. When the patient is breathing room air, the normal $P(A–a)O_2$ can be estimated by multiplying 0.4 times the patient's age. The higher the FIO_2 and the older the patient, the larger the predicted normal $P(A–a)O_2$. The $P(A–a)O_2$ is determined by subtracting the Pao_2 (obtained from ABG measurements) from the calculated PAO_2 (obtained from use of the alveolar air equation described earlier in this chapter). Calculation of the PAO_2 requires a known FIO_2 and $Paco_2$. The $P(A–a)O_2$ cannot be determined in patients breathing supplemental oxygen with low-flow devices (nasal cannula) for which the FIO_2 is not known.

An increase in $P(A–a)O_2$ is strictly an indication of respiratory defects in oxygenation ability. Most respiratory dysfunctions that produce hypoxemia are accompanied by an elevated $P(A–a)O_2$.

There are two situations in which hypoxemia may occur with a normal $P(A–a)O_2$: primary hypoventilation and high altitudes. Primary hypoventilation elevates the alveolar and arterial Pco_2 and reduces PAO_2. In this situation, hypoxemia may occur, but $P(A–a)O_2$ remains within normal limits.

At high altitudes PIO_2 is markedly reduced and hypoxemia occurs. The hypoxemia is the result of a decrease in PAO_2 and $P(A–a)O_2$ remains within normal limits. In summary, hypoxemia occurring with a normal $P(A–a)O_2$ is caused by either a decreased PIO_2 or primary hypoventilation.

PARTIAL PRESSURE OF OXYGEN IN MIXED VENOUS BLOOD (P$\overline{v}$O₂).

NORMAL VALUE: 38 to 42 mm Hg

The heart and lungs must work together to provide adequate tissue oxygenation, since oxygen delivery is a function of cardiac output and the Cao_2. Pao_2, Sao_2, and Cao_2 only provide evaluation of the respiratory component, leaving the assessment of tissue oxygenation incomplete.

One dimension capable of providing an indication of the tissue oxygenation status in most cases is the $P\overline{v}O_2$. A true mixed venous sample can be achieved only by sampling the pulmonary artery blood via a pulmonary artery catheter. For this reason, analysis of $P\overline{v}O_2$ is usually reserved for the patient in an intensive care unit where pulmonary artery catheters can be maintained adequately.

Normally only about 25% of the oxygen in the arterial blood is given up at the tissue vascular beds. If oxygen extraction (consumption) remains constant as cardiac output decreases, the venous oxygen level is reduced below normal. The venous oxygen level is also reduced in patients with limited cardiac performance when oxygen consumption increases, as with fever. $P\overline{v}O_2$ is therefore a reflection of the relationship between oxygen delivery to the tissues and the rate at which oxygen is consumed.

*Some authors use 1.39.

A $P\bar{v}_{O_2}$ below 35 mm Hg is strong evidence that tissue oxygenation is less than optimal, and further evaluation is warranted. A normal $P\bar{v}_{O_2}$ may indicate that tissue oxygenation is adequate, but it is not always reliable. In certain situations $P\bar{v}_{O_2}$ may not predict tissue perfusion.[6]

A sudden decrease in $P\bar{v}_{O_2}$ most often occurs when circulation is impaired and oxygen delivery to the tissues is reduced. This may happen with hypovolemia, the addition of positive pressure ventilation, or left heart failure.[7] Rapid assessment of the cause of the decrease in $P\bar{v}_{O_2}$ must be done so that appropriate treatment can be implemented.

ARTERIOVENOUS OXYGEN CONTENT DIFFERENCE C(a–v)$_{O_2}$.

NORMAL VALUE: 3.5 to 5.0 vol%

Measurement of C(a–v)$_{O_2}$ (commonly referred to as the arteriovenous oxygen difference) requires simultaneous sampling of arterial and mixed venous blood. The mixed venous sample must be acquired from a pulmonary artery catheter to be most reliable. The two blood samples are taken to the laboratory for analysis and determination of the Ca$_{O_2}$ and C$\bar{v}_{O_2}$. The difference between the oxygen content of the two samples provides an estimation of the tissue perfusion and oxygenation according to the following equation:

$$\dot{Q}T = \frac{\dot{V}_{O_2}}{C(a-v)_{O_2}}$$

The equation demonstrates that in a patient with a steady oxygen consumption ($\dot{V}_{O_2}$), the cardiac output ($\dot{Q}T$) and C(a–v)$_{O_2}$ are inversely proportional. As $\dot{Q}T$ decreases, C(a–v)$_{O_2}$ increases; as $\dot{Q}T$ increases, C(a–v)$_{O_2}$ decreases. $\dot{V}_{O_2}$ can usually be assumed to be stable in most patients unless the patient is restless or having significant variations in body temperature.

Increases in C(a–v)$_{O_2}$ in a patient with a stable $\dot{V}_{O_2}$ indicate that the perfusion of the body organs is decreasing. Without adequate perfusion, the tissues do not receive adequate oxygenation and tissue hypoxia occurs. When the C(a–v)$_{O_2}$ exceeds 6.0 vol%, cardiovascular decompensation is occurring and tissue oxygenation is inadequate.

A reduction in C(a–v)$_{O_2}$ occurs when perfusion exceeds the normal level with a steady $\dot{V}_{O_2}$ or when $\dot{V}_{O_2}$ is reduced significantly (as with hypothermia) with a normal $\dot{Q}T$. A C(a–v)$_{O_2}$ below 3.5 vol% may also occur when the tissue utilization of oxygen is impaired.

CARBOXYHEMOGLOBIN (HbCO).

NORMAL VALUE: approximately 0.5%

The HbCO is a reflection of the quantity of carbon monoxide (CO) bound to the hemoglobin molecules and can be obtained only from the co-oximeter. Carbon monoxide is a highly diffusible, odorless, and colorless gas that has an affinity for hemoglobin 200 to 250 times that of oxygen. Inhalation of gas containing carbon monoxide

results in a tight bond between the carbon monoxide and the hemoglobin and shifts the oxyhemoglobin dissociation curve to the left. Hemoglobin bonded with carbon monoxide is less capable of carrying oxygen, and Ca$_{O_2}$ decreases accordingly. The resulting shift to the left of the oxyhemoglobin dissociation curve further promotes tissue hypoxia by inhibiting the unloading of oxygen from the hemoglobin to the tissues.

A mild elevation of HbCO (5%–10%) occurs with tobacco or cigarette smoking and exposure to polluted environments.[8] A more significant elevation of HbCO, greater than 10%, occurs from inhalation of large amounts of smoke or automobile exhaust. In such cases Ca$_{O_2}$ (but not necessarily Pa$_{O_2}$) is reduced significantly and tissue oxygenation may be in jeopardy. The patient generally complains of headache, dyspnea, and nausea, and appears hypoxic (tachycardia, tachypnea, etc.), but cyanosis does not occur. At HbCO levels of 40% to 60% visual disturbance, myocardial toxicity, loss of consciousness, and eventually death occur. Laboratories without a co-oximeter do not easily detect the abnormality, since measured Pa$_{O_2}$ and calculated Sa$_{O_2}$ are often normal.

CLINICAL ASSESSMENT OF OXYGENATION.

The ultimate goal of respiratory and cardiovascular function is to provide adequate oxygenation of the body tissues. Therefore assessment of oxygenation should evaluate the ability of the lungs to oxygenate the blood and the ability of the cardiovascular system to distribute the blood. Respiratory function can be evaluated by interpreting the ABG measurements previously reviewed and summarized in the following discussion. ABG analysis, however, cannot assess the adequacy of tissue oxygenation. Tissue perfusion and oxygenation are evaluated better in the nonintensive care unit setting by using the findings of a physical examination as described in Chapters 4 and 11.

Hypoxemia occurs when the respiratory system fails to adequately oxygenate arterial blood. The Pa$_{O_2}$, Sa$_{O_2}$, and usually Ca$_{O_2}$ are reduced. The degree of abnormality can be assessed by looking at the relationship between F$_{IO_2}$ and Pa$_{O_2}$ or at P(A–a)$_{O_2}$. Large P(A–a)$_{O_2}$ values indicate severe respiratory abnormality. Hypoxemia occurring with a normal P(A–a)$_{O_2}$ may be the result of low P$_{IO_2}$ at high altitude or hypoventilation. The P(A–a)$_{O_2}$ cannot be calculated when the F$_{IO_2}$ is not known.

If hypoxemia exists on an F$_{IO_2}$ of 0.21 and the sum of the Pa$_{O_2}$ and Pa$_{CO_2}$ is 110 to 130 mm Hg, the cause of the hypoxemia is hypoventilation. If the sum is less than 110 mm Hg, the cause of the hypoxemia is related to defects in the lungs' ability to oxygenate the blood. If the sum of the Pa$_{O_2}$ and the Pa$_{CO_2}$ is greater than 130 mm Hg, the patient is probably breathing supplemental oxygen, or an error has occurred.

The most important factor indicating the oxygenation status of the arterial blood is the Ca$_{O_2}$. Assessment of the hemoglobin concentration from either the complete blood count (CBC) or co-oximeter measurement is crucial in identifying the potential for Cao_2. A reduction in hemoglobin (anemia) disallows the possibility of a normal Cao_2, regardless of the Pao_2 and Sao_2, since 99% of the Cao_2 is bound to hemoglobin.

Other than hypoxemia and anemia, a reduction in Cao_2 can occur with carbon monoxide poisoning. Carbon monoxide poisoning is usually suggested by the initial history (exposure to smoke or automobile exhaust) and confirmed by co-oximeter measurements. Sao_2 and Cao_2 are reduced markedly, and the Pao_2 is above the predicted value for the Sao_2. Without co-oximeter measurements, carbon monoxide poisoning is difficult to identify, especially if the patient is comatose and the history of present illness is not provided.

The clinical recognition of hypoxemia is often first suggested by the patient complaining of shortness of breath, especially with exertion. Common clinical manifestations of hypoxemia include tachycardia, tachypnea, hypertension, cyanosis, and confusion. Cyanosis is identified when the level of hemoglobin is at or near normal and its saturation with oxygen drops below 85% to 90%. Cyanosis is not recognized in the patient with anemia even if the hypoxemia is severe. As hypoxemia worsens to the extent of tissue hypoxia, metabolic acidosis, bradycardia, and hypotension occur and the patient often becomes comatose. In the intensive care unit, $P\overline{v}o_2$ less than 35 mm Hg and increases in $C(a-v)o_2$ above 5 vol% may indicate tissue hypoxia.

Tissue hypoxia also may occur with normal arterial oxygenation when inadequate perfusion exists. Clinical signs of an inadequate cardiac output include hypotension, cool extremities, weak or absent pulses, reduced urine output, and coma (see Chapter 11).

Assessment of Acid-Base Balance

Normal metabolism produces approximately 12,000 mEq of acid each day. It is the responsibility of the lungs and kidneys to excrete the metabolic acids, maintaining an appropriate acid-base balance in the body. Numerous blood buffers are also available to prevent a buildup of acid in the body. The lungs remove most metabolic acids by removing carbon dioxide from the blood through the process of ventilation. The respiratory system serves as an important regulator of acid-base balance through the control of Pco_2. The kidneys remove a smaller quantity of acid but help restore the buffer capacity of the body fluids by replenishing the HCO_3^- concentration. Respiratory or renal dysfunction may cause a breakdown in the process of maintaining acid-base balance and result in acid-base disorders.

Accurate assessment of the patient's acid-base balance requires interpretation of the measurements provided by blood gas analysis. The measurements that reflect acid-base status are described in the following paragraphs. This is followed by a discussion of the common acid-base disorders and the clinical situations in which they occur.

HYDROGEN ION CONCENTRATION (pH).

NORMAL VALUE: 7.40 with a range of 7.35 to 7.45

The arterial blood pH is a measurement of the hydrogen ion (H^+) concentration in the plasma. Since *acids* are defined as solutions capable of donating H^+ and *bases* as solutions capable of accepting H^+, the pH is a reflection of the acid-base status of the arterial blood.

The actual concentration of H^+ in the arterial blood serum is low (0.00004 mEq/L) and is a cumbersome number with which to work. To solve this problem it has been proposed to convert the H^+ term to pH by taking the negative logarithm (base 10) of the H^+, resulting in more manageable numbers. Because pH is a logarithmic expression of the H^+, changes in pH of 1 unit (e.g., changes from 7.40 to 6.40) represent a tenfold alteration in the H^+ of the blood.

The relationship between pH and H^+ is expressed as follows and demonstrates an important concept: H^+ and pH are inversely related.

pH	[H⁺]*	pH	[H⁺]*
7.80	16	7.20	63
7.70	20	7.10	80
7.60	26	7.00	100
7.50	32	6.90	125
7.40	40	6.80	160
7.30	50		

*Reported in nanomols per liter.

As H^+ increases from the addition of acids, pH decreases. Therefore pH values below 7.35 represent increases in the H^+ concentration, and the blood is *acidotic* or *acidemic*. When the pH increases above 7.45, the H^+ has decreased and the blood is *alkalotic* or *alkalemic*. It is more exact to refer to deviations in plasma pH with the terms *acidemia* and *alkalemia* than with *acidosis* and *alkalosis* since the reported pH is that of the blood plasma and the latter terms do not indicate the compartment that is sampled.

The pH of the arterial blood is important to monitor, since the majority of body functions occur optimally at or near a pH of 7.40. Significant alterations in pH have a profound effect on many systems of the body, especially the central nervous system (CNS).[9] Acidosis results in depression of the CNS. The patient with acidosis initially appears lethargic and disoriented. As the acidosis worsens, the patient eventually becomes comatose. The major effect of alkalosis is overexcitability of the CNS and peripheral nerves. The nerves become so responsive that they automatically and repetitively depolarize, resulting in tetany. Extreme alkalosis may result in muscular spasms of the extremities, face, and body. Respiratory failure may occur if the nerves and muscles of ventilation are involved. Significant alterations in arterial blood pH also may reduce the ability of the heart muscle (myocardium) to contract and effectively pump blood throughout the body.

PARTIAL PRESSURE OF ARTERIAL CARBON DIOXIDE (Pa_{CO_2}).

NORMAL VALUE: 35 to 45 mm Hg

Pa_{CO_2} is a reflection of the respiratory component of acid-base status. It identifies the degree of ventilation in relation to the metabolic rate. Carbon dioxide is a waste product of normal metabolism and must be removed, at least in part, by the lungs exchanging air with the blood. In healthy persons, as the metabolic rate increases (as with fever or exercise), ventilation also increases to maintain a normal Pa_{CO_2}. A normal or increased metabolism without adequate ventilation results in an elevated Pa_{CO_2} and represents a failure of the respiratory system to remove carbon dioxide at an acceptable rate. An elevated Pa_{CO_2}, above 45 mm Hg, referred to as *hypercapnia* or *hypercarbia,* is most often the result of less than adequate alveolar ventilation (*hypoventilation*). A Pa_{CO_2} value of less than 35 mm Hg, referred to as *hypocapnia* or hypocarbia, occurs when alveolar ventilation exceeds normal levels (*hyperventilation*).

Pa_{CO_2} alters pH according to the following equation:

$$CO_2 + H_2 \rightleftharpoons H_2CO_3 \rightleftharpoons HCO_3^- + H^+$$

An increase in Pa_{CO_2} shifts the equilibrium equation to the right, resulting in an increase in H^+; this is referred to as *respiratory acidosis*. A decrease in Pa_{CO_2} shifts the equation to the left and lowers H^+; this is referred to as *respiratory alkalosis*. Respiratory acid-base disorders are compensated for by appropriate adjustments in the plasma HCO_3^- concentration by the kidneys and are discussed later in this chapter.

Pa_{CO_2} is the most reliable measurement for evaluating the effectiveness of ventilation and should be interpreted in light of the patient's minute volume ($\dot{V}_E$). A normal Pa_{CO_2} should be accompanied by a normal $\dot{V}_E$. An increased $\dot{V}_E$ should result in hypocapnia unless metabolism is increased or dead space ventilation is increased. If $\dot{V}_E$ is increased and Pa_{CO_2} is normal or elevated, a definite abnormality exists and the effectiveness of ventilation is reduced. This occurs when the portion of the tidal volume (V_T) that does not come in contact with blood flow is increased; this is referred to as *dead space* or *wasted ventilation*. An increase in dead space ventilation occurs most often when the perfusion of the lungs is reduced.

A reduction in $\dot{V}_E$ below normal usually produces hypercapnia unless metabolism is reduced significantly. If the $\dot{V}_E$ is reduced and Pa_{CO_2} is elevated, the effectiveness of ventilation may be normal but the quantity insufficient. In this case the cause of hypoventilation usually lies outside the lungs and is often the result of neuromuscular disease or response to certain medications such as morphine, that depress the drive to breathe.

ARTERIAL BLOOD BICARBONATE (HCO_3^-).

NORMAL VALUE: 22 to 26 mEq/L

The plasma HCO_3^- is primarily a reflection of the metabolic component of acid-base balance and is regulated by the renal system. When plasma HCO_3^- levels decrease below normal, the pH also decreases, since HCO_3^- is a base; metabolic acidosis results. Metabolic alkalosis occurs when the plasma HCO_3^- increases, resulting in an elevated pH. The HCO_3^- level may also change as a compensatory response to primary changes in Pa_{CO_2} levels; this usually requires 12 to 24 hours to occur.

The plasma HCO_3^- is affected slightly by acute changes in Pa_{CO_2} according to the following equation:

$$CO_2 + H_2O \rightleftharpoons H_2CO_3 \rightleftharpoons H^+ + HCO_3^-$$

Increases in Pa_{CO_2} shift the reaction to the right and result in immediate but small increases in plasma HCO_3^-. Decreases in Pa_{CO_2} shift the equation to the left and result in a reduced HCO_3^- level. For every 10 to 15 mm Hg increase in Pa_{CO_2} above 40 mm Hg, the HCO_3^- increases 1 mEq/L. For every 5 mm Hg decrease in Pa_{CO_2} below normal, the serum HCO_3^- decreases by 1 mEq/L.

Standard Bicarbonate. Since plasma HCO_3^- levels are influenced by acute alterations in Pa_{CO_2}, some laboratories report a standard HCO_3^-. *Standard bicarbonate* is defined as the plasma HCO_3^- concentration that would be present if the Pa_{CO_2} were 40 mm Hg. This theoretically eliminates the "respiratory" influence on plasma HCO_3^- and allows evaluation of the pure metabolic component. The normal standard HCO_3^- is 22 to 26 mEq/L.

BASE EXCESS AND BASE DEFICIT.

NORMAL VALUE: ±2 mEq/L

Base excess is a measurement reflecting the nonrespiratory portion of acid-base balance. It is a standard deviation of the standard HCO_3^- that takes the buffering capabilities of the red blood cells into account. The calculation of base excess is made from the measurements of pH, Pa_{CO_2}, and hematocrit concentration. The hematocrit is considered in the calculation because red blood cells contain significant blood buffers. The total quantity of buffer anions in the blood is 45 to 50 mEq/L or about twice that of HCO_3^-. Thus HCO_3^- accounts for only about half of the total buffering capacity of the blood. Therefore the base excess provides a more complete analysis of the metabolic buffering capabilities.

Base excess is reported as a positive or negative value depending on which direction the buffer base has deviated from normal. The larger the value, the more severe the deviation in the metabolic component. A positive value indicates that either base has been added or acid removed, whereas a negative value (*base deficit*) indicates that acid has been added or base removed.

Measurement of base excess allows analysis of the pure metabolic components of acid-base balance. Changes in plasma HCO_3^- from metabolic components alter base excess, whereas acute changes in plasma HCO_3^- from the respiratory component (P_{CO_2}) do not.

Respiratory and Metabolic Acid-Base Disorders

The previous discussion demonstrates that there are two basic types of acid-base disorders: metabolic and respiratory. Metabolic disorders are recognized by identifying abnormalities in plasma HCO_3^-, whereas respiratory disorders alter Pa_{CO_2}. The effects of Pa_{CO_2} and plasma HCO_3^- on acid-base balance are defined in the following Henderson-Hasselbalch equation:

$$pH = pK + \log \frac{HCO_3 \text{ (renal)}}{Pa_{CO_2} \times 0.03 \text{ (lungs)}}$$

where

$pK = 6.1$ ionization constant
$0.03 =$ solubility factor to convert mm Hg to mEq

Normal example:

$$pH = 6.1 + \log \frac{24}{40 \times 0.03}$$
$$= 6.1 + \log 20$$
$$= 6.1 + 1.30$$
$$= 7.40$$

The equation demonstrates that arterial blood pH is determined by the ratio of HCO_3^- to Pa_{CO_2}. This ratio is normally 20:1. Changes in one component disrupt the 20:1 ratio, resulting in an abnormal pH. Abnormalities in one component can be compensated for by changes in the other component to return the ratio to 20:1. Therefore, pH is not determined by absolute values of Pa_{CO_2} and plasma HCO_3^- but by the ratio of one to the other.

For example, an increase in Pa_{CO_2} from 40 mm Hg to 60 mm Hg changes the ratio from 20:1 to 20:18.8 or 13.3:1. This results in a pH of 7.23 according to the Henderson-Hasselbalch equation:

$$pH = 6.1 + \log \frac{24}{60 \times 0.03}$$
$$pH = 6.1 + \log \frac{24}{1.8}$$
$$pH = 6.1 + \log 13.33$$
$$pH = 6.1 + 1.13$$
$$pH = 7.23$$

Most acid-base abnormalities occur as simple disorders. Simple disorders involve a primary abnormality in one component (either Pa_{CO_2} or HCO_3^-) that may be compensated for by changes in the other component. Therefore a near normal pH does not rule out the possibility of an acid-base disorder but may indicate that compensation has occurred. When a combination of simple disorders occurs, a mixed acid-base disorder exists. The recognition of simple and mixed acid-base disorders in the clinical setting is described in the following section.

Clinical Recognition of Simple and Mixed Acid-Base Disorders

In many situations the most meaningful and accurate interpretation of ABG measurements is obtained by considering the results in relation to other clinical findings. This is especially true in interpreting mixed acid-base disorders. The following discussion focuses first on interpreting simple acid-base disorders. These are important and must be understood before mixed disturbances can be interpreted. The discussion then proceeds to mixed acid-base disorders and the clinical situations in which they may occur.

Simple Disorders

RESPIRATORY ACIDOSIS. Simple respiratory acidosis is an abnormal condition in which there is a primary reduction in alveolar ventilation relative to the rate of carbon dioxide production. It is recognized by identifying an elevated Pa_{CO_2} and indicates that ventilation is inadequate. Respiratory acidosis is present whenever the Pa_{CO_2} is elevated above normal or when it is higher than the expected level of compensation. Respiratory acidosis may occur from a wide variety of respiratory and nonrespiratory abnormalities. They are as follows:

Respiratory
  Acute upper airway obstruction
  Severe diffuse airway obstruction (acute or chronic)
  Massive pulmonary edema
Nonrespiratory
  Drug overdose
  Spinal cord trauma
  Neuromuscular disease
  Head trauma
  Trauma to thoracic cage

Respiratory acidosis is compensated for as the kidneys increase the reabsorption of HCO_3^-. Acute respiratory acidosis is usually uncompensated, since renal changes of plasma HCO_3^- are slow to occur. Uncompensated respiratory acidosis is identified by an elevated Pa_{CO_2}, a decreased pH, and a normal plasma HCO_3^- and base excess. Partial compensation occurs when the plasma HCO_3^- is elevated above the normal range but the pH is not yet within normal limits. If the plasma HCO_3^- is elevated enough to return the pH to within normal range, it is termed *completely compensated respiratory acidosis*. The plasma HCO_3^- does not rise enough to overcorrect the pH above 7.39 because the impetus of the body to compensate diminishes as the pH gets closer to normal.

When respiratory acidosis occurs, identifying the expected change in plasma HCO_3^- is useful to determine if the degree of compensation is appropriate. For acute respiratory acidosis, the plasma HCO_3^- increases

1 mEq/L for each 10 to 15 mm Hg that the Pa_{CO_2} increases. In chronic respiratory acidosis, the plasma HCO_3^- is expected to increase 4 mEq/L for each 10 mm Hg that Pa_{CO_2} increases. If the expected compensation is not occurring, a complicating metabolic disorder may be present.

If the respiratory acidosis is caused by a neuromuscular or airway obstruction disorder, the patient will be short of breath and breathing rapidly. In contrast, if the respiratory center is impaired (e.g., with narcotics), the respiratory rate will be reduced.

The combination of an acutely elevated Pa_{CO_2} and acidosis usually has a significant effect on the clinical findings and produces an anesthetic effect on the CNS. The patient with hypercapnia is often confused, semiconscious, and eventually comatose. Coma may be observed at CO_2 tensions above 70 mm Hg if the onset of hypercapnia is acute. Even higher levels of P_{CO_2} may be well tolerated in patients with chronic respiratory acidosis. As the Pa_{CO_2} acutely increases, the patient may complain of a headache and appear sleepy and lethargic. Since hypercapnia is often associated with hypoxemia in patients breathing room air, the clinical manifestations of hypoxemia are also identified commonly.

Since elevations in Pa_{CO_2} cause systemic vasodilation, cardiovascular manifestations may be seen with hypercapnia. Peripheral vasodilation and an increased cardiac output promote warm flushed skin and a bounding pulse. Arrhythmias are occasionally observed. Cerebral vasodilation also occurs, resulting in elevated intracranial pressures, retinal venous distention, papilledema, and headache. Increases in serum HCO_3^- levels as a result of renal compensation are accompanied by decreased chloride levels.

RESPIRATORY ALKALOSIS. Simple respiratory alkalosis is an abnormal condition in which there is a primary increase in alveolar ventilation relative to the rate of carbon dioxide production. Respiratory alkalosis is identified by a Pa_{CO_2} below the expected level and indicates that ventilation is exceeding the normal level. Hyperventilation is usually the result of an increased stimulus or drive to breathe. This occurs with pain, hypoxemia (Pa_{O_2} <55–60 mm Hg), acidosis, and anxiety.

Respiratory alkalosis is compensated for by the kidneys excreting plasma HCO_3^-. A normal plasma HCO_3^- with a low Pa_{CO_2} and increased pH is referred to as *uncompensated respiratory alkalosis*. Partial compensation occurs when the plasma HCO_3^- falls below normal but the pH is still above 7.45. Full compensation occurs when the plasma HCO_3^- decreases enough to return the pH to within normal range.

The expected compensatory change in plasma HCO_3^- with respiratory alkalosis is dependent on the severity of the hyperventilation and length of time it has been occurring. Acute respiratory alkalosis should result in a decrease in plasma HCO_3^- of 1 mEq/L for

every 5 mm Hg the Pa_{CO_2} decreases. For chronic respiratory alkalosis, the plasma HCO_3^- should decrease 5 mEq/L for every decrease of 10 mm Hg in Pa_{CO_2}. If the expected compensation is not present, a complicating metabolic disorder may be present.

One advantage of a reduction in Pa_{CO_2} is the increase in Pa_{O_2}. According to Dalton's law, a reduction in Pa_{CO_2} allows an increase in Pa_{O_2} and potentially in Pa_{O_2}. Therefore, when hypoxemia and respiratory alkalosis occur together, it is safe to say that the Pa_{O_2} would probably be even lower if the Pa_{CO_2} increased to normal. If Pa_{O_2} is barely adequate and respiratory alkalosis is present, it is likely that hypoxemia would occur if Pa_{CO_2} returned to normal range.

Clinical signs and symptoms associated with respiratory alkalosis include tachypnea, dizziness, sweating, tingling in the fingers and toes, and muscle weakness and spasm.[10] Respiratory alkalosis may be induced accidently in patients receiving intermittent positive pressure breathing treatments when the treatments are administered improperly or with mechanical ventilation when not properly monitored.

METABOLIC ACIDOSIS. Metabolic acidosis is identified when the plasma HCO_3^- or base excess falls below normal. This occurs whenever buffers are not produced in sufficient quantities or when they are lost excessively. In addition, metabolic acidosis can occur when an increased load of H^+ ions is present or when a decreased ability to excrete acids exists.[11] Following is an outline of the causes of metabolic acidosis:

> Loss of HCO_3^-
>> Diarrhea
>> Renal disease
> Increase in metabolic acid production
>> Ketoacidosis
>> Lactic acidosis
>> Ingestion of certain toxins (e.g., methanol)
> Posthypocapnia disorder

When metabolic acidosis occurs as a result of the buildup of organic or inorganic acids in the body, the anion gap is elevated above 16 mEq/L (see Chapter 5 for a discussion of the anion gap).

Normal metabolism requires both oxygen and glucose. When either element is not present in sufficient quantity, an increased amount of nonvolatile acids is produced and accumulates in the blood. A lack of cellular oxygen results in the formation of lactic acid; this is termed *lactic acidosis*. Lactic acidosis is accompanied by signs of tissue hypoxia. The oxygen deficits must be corrected rapidly, usually by improving arterial blood oxygenation and perfusion.

A lack of cellular glucose occurs with diabetes and starvation. Metabolism without sufficient glucose produces ketone bodies from the breakdown of proteins and is termed *ketoacidosis*.

Metabolic acidosis may also be the result of renal failure. The kidneys are responsible for excreting excess

H^+ ions and reabsorbing HCO_3^- ions. Renal disease may disrupt either or both functions and result in metabolic acidosis. In such cases other signs of renal failure are usually present, including increases in blood urea nitrogen and creatinine and decreases in urine output.

Metabolic acidosis is compensated for by a reduction in $Paco_2$ through hyperventilation. Uncompensated metabolic acidosis rarely occurs, since $Paco_2$ is rapidly altered by changes in ventilation. A normal or elevated $Paco_2$ in the presence of metabolic acidosis indicates that a ventilatory defect is also occurring. The predicted compensatory alteration in $Paco_2$ for metabolic acidosis can be estimated by the following equation:

$$Paco_2 = (1.5 \times HCO_3^-) + 8 \pm 2$$

If the $Paco_2$ is not at the expected level, a respiratory abnormality may also be present.

In most cases metabolic acidosis will cause a rapid and significant response by the respiratory system. Slow and deep ventilation, referred to as Kussmaul's respiration, is the most common and obvious sign of metabolic acidosis. This change in the pattern of breathing may not be clinically obvious, especially if the acidosis is not severe. With more severe cases, the patient may complain of dyspnea, headache, nausea, and vomiting. Confusion and stupor may follow. Constriction of the venous blood vessels often occurs with acidosis and may shift the blood flow to the pulmonary system. Pulmonary edema may result. Arrhythmias can occur with severe acidosis when pH or Pao_2 decrease significantly.

METABOLIC ALKALOSIS. Metabolic alkalosis is identified by an elevation of the plasma HCO_3^- above normal. This occurs whenever HCO_3^- ions accumulate in the blood or when an abnormal number of H^+ ions are lost from the plasma. Following is a listing of the most common causes of metabolic alkalosis:

    Hypokalemia or hypochloremia
    Nasogastric suction (loss of stomach acid)
    Persistent vomiting (loss of stomach acid)
    Posthypercapnia disorder
    Diuretic therapy
    Steroid therapy
    Excessive administration of sodium bicarbonate

Certain electrolyte imbalances have the potential for reducing the number of H^+ ions in the plasma or increasing the number of HCO_3^- ions. Hypokalemia (reduced plasma potassium) promotes movement of H^+ ions into the intracellular fluids in exchange for K^+ ions. Hypokalemia also increases the renal excretion of H^+ ions, further increasing the blood base.

Hypochloremia (reduced plasma chloride) results in the loss of anions from the blood plasma, and these must be replaced by another anion, usually HCO_3^-, to maintain electrical balance. Therefore hypochloremia may lead to increases in the plasma HCO_3^- concentration and metabolic alkalosis.

Gastric suction often results in excessive loss of the hydrochloric acid (HCl) of the stomach. The combination of losing H^+ ions and Cl^- ions leads to a proportionate increase in the blood base.

Excess administration of bicarbonate occurs most often during cardiopulmonary resuscitation. Cardiac arrest and tissue hypoxia result in metabolic acidosis, treated by the rapid administration of bicarbonate. If bicarbonate administration is not monitored carefully with ABG measurements, an excessive amount may be administered, resulting in metabolic alkalosis.

Metabolic alkalosis is compensated for by hypoventilation and an elevation of $Paco_2$. Hypoventilation does not occur to a significant degree in the awake, alert patient; metabolic alkalosis tends to remain uncompensated. In the comatose patient, metabolic alkalosis may result in significant hypoventilation and hypercapnia. In such cases the hypercapnia tends to promote hypoxemia unless the Fio_2 is increased above room air levels.

Uncompensated metabolic alkalosis is identified by an elevated plasma HCO_3^-, an increase in pH, and a normal $Paco_2$. Partial compensation occurs when the $Paco_2$ is elevated above 45 mm Hg but the pH is not yet within normal range. Complete compensation is identified when the $Paco_2$ rises enough to return the pH to normal. Predicting the expected compensation for metabolic alkalosis is difficult for the reasons mentioned previously. In situations where the $Paco_2$ is elevated significantly in the presence of metabolic alkalosis, the hypercarbia may actually represent respiratory acidosis.

Limitations of Compensation for Acid-Base Disorders

When severe alterations from the normal range occur with one acid-base component, it is not always possible for the other component to compensate completely. In a patient with a primary metabolic acid-base disorder and a normal respiratory system, compensation by elevated or decreased $Paco_2$ can occur only within the limitations of the respiratory system. Primary respiratory acid-base disorders can be compensated for by changes in plasma HCO_3^- only within the limitations of the renal system.

The likelihood of compensation returning the pH to a normal range is inversely proportional to the degree of the primary disturbance. For example, in chronic respiratory acidosis, at a $Paco_2$ of 50 mm Hg, 75% of the patients may have a pH within a normal range. At a $Paco_2$ of 60 mm Hg, the likelihood decreases to 15%.[12]

The extent of compensation that is possible for any respiratory or metabolic disorder has been determined by human and animal studies. The data accumulated from these studies have been developed into 95% confidence limit bands.[12] The confidence limit bands describe the compensation limits the majority (95%) of patients are able to achieve, and aid in the proper interpretation of acid-base disorders.

For example, a pH of 7.38 and $Paco_2$ of 85 mm Hg with an elevated plasma HCO_3^- traditionally would be interpreted as completely compensated respiratory acidosis. However, the 95% confidence limit bands demonstrate that the majority of patients cannot elevate HCO_3^- enough to fully compensate for a $Paco_2$ of 85 mm Hg.[13] In this example, the correct interpretation would probably be chronic respiratory acidosis with a superimposed metabolic alkalosis. Serial ABG measurements and consideration of other clinical data are usually helpful in the interpretation of ABG measurements, since the exact limitations of compensation cannot be determined for any one patient.

It has been suggested that when major alterations of $Paco_2$ or plasma HCO_3^- occur, the degree of compensation should be classified as *uncompensated, less than maximal,* or *maximal,* regardless of actual pH. For example, a patient with severe metabolic acidosis can hyperventilate the $Paco_2$ down only to about 15 mm Hg, even with normal lungs. If the pH is still below 7.35, the correct assessment would be maximally compensated severe metabolic acidosis, not partially compensated.

Mixed Acid-Base Disorders*

When two of the simple acid-base abnormalities previously reviewed occur simultaneously, a mixed acid-base disorder results. Mixed disorders are less common than simple disorders and can be more difficult to identify. When both components of acid-base balance (HCO_3^- and $Paco_2$) simultaneously deviate from the normal range toward either acidosis or alkalosis, the mixed acid-base disorder can be identified more readily. However, if one component alters toward acidosis or alkalosis and the other component alters toward the opposite acid-base imbalance, the mixed disorder is more difficult to recognize.

Accurate interpretation of mixed disorders requires a complete understanding of the simple disorders and the clinical situations in which they occur. In most situations the first clue to a mixed acid-base disorder comes from the clinical findings of the patient's history, physical examination, and other laboratory tests. Also, each simple disorder alters acid-base balance and electrolyte concentration in a predictable manner. Identification of mixed disorders requires a thorough understanding of the extent of metabolic and respiratory compensation that should occur for each simple disorder. When the degree of compensation for what is thought to be the primary simple disorder is not appropriate, a mixed disorder is usually present (Table 6-4).

*Portions of this section are adapted from Narins RG, and Emmett M: Simple and mixed acid-base disorders: a practical approach, Medicine (Baltimore) 59:161, 1980.

Table 6-4 **Summary of Expected Compensation for Acute and Chronic Acid-Base Disorders**

Primary Disorder	Expected Compensation
Acute respiratory acidosis	For a 15 mm Hg increase in $Paco_2$ the HCO_3^- increases 1mEq/L; significant compensation takes 24-48 hr
Chronic respiratory acidosis	For every 10 mm Hg the $Paco_2$ increases, the HCO_3^- increases 4 mEq/L
Acute respiratory alkalosis	For every 5 mm Hg decrease in $Paco_2$, HCO_3^- decreases 1 mEq; significant compensation requires 24-48 hr
Chronic respiratory alkalosis	HCO_3^- falls 5 mEq/L for every 10 mm Hg fall in $Paco_2$
Metabolic acidosis	$Paco_2$ = last two digits of pH $Paco_2 = (1.5 \times HCO_3^-) + 8 \pm 2$
Metabolic alkalosis	$Paco_2$ change is variable $Paco_2$ usually does not elevate above 50-55 mm Hg For each 1 mEq/L increase in HCO_3^-, $Paco_2$ increases 0.6 mm Hg

A brief review of the criteria and clinical situations associated with the more common mixed acid-base disorders follows. More in-depth discussions of mixed acid-base disorders are available in the literature.[12,14]

RESPIRATORY AND METABOLIC ACIDOSIS. Mixed acid-base disorders such as respiratory and metabolic acidosis are identified easily by an elevated $Paco_2$ and a reduction in plasma HCO_3^-. Hypercapnia and low plasma HCO_3^- act synergistically to reduce pH significantly. Even mild hypercapnia ($Paco_2$ = 50 mm Hg) occurring with a moderate reduction in plasma HCO_3^- (15-17 mEq/L) results in profound acidosis (pH = 7.15). This mixed disorder occurs in a variety of situations, including the following.

Cardiopulmonary Resuscitation. Sudden failure of the heart to pump blood results in apnea and diffuse tissue hypoxia. The combination of tissue hypoxia and hypoventilation, often seen during resuscitation, is manifested as lactic and respiratory acidosis. Adequate ventilation, oxygenation, and perfusion must be reestablished if resuscitation is to be successful.

Chronic Obstructive Pulmonary Disease (COPD) and Hypoxia. Many patients with COPD have chronic elevation of $Paco_2$. Even if hypoxemia is also present, most patients with COPD maintain adequate tissue oxygenation by increasing hematocrit and oxygen extraction. However, metabolic acidosis may occur with significant electrolyte disturbances, sudden hypotension, renal failure, or anemia. Sudden hypotension and anemia result in tissue hypoxia and lactic acidosis. In these situations plasma HCO_3^- may be reduced and $Paco_2$ may remain elevated, resulting in the mixed acid-base disorder.

Poisoning and Drug Overdose. Many cases of poison and drug overdose result in depression of the respiratory center and respiratory acidosis. The poisons and drugs may also be metabolized to strong acids and produce metabolic acidosis. The hypoventilation is usually recognized as a result of shallow and slow breathing. The history of drug overdose or poisoning and the clinical signs of hypoventilation should be enough to prompt initiation of intubation and mechanical ventilation without waiting for ABG results. The metabolic acidosis is identified only by ABG measurements and is treated with infusion of bicarbonate in some cases.

METABOLIC AND RESPIRATORY ALKALOSIS. This mixed acid-base disorder is recognized by identifying an elevated plasma HCO_3^- and a $Paco_2$ below normal. The additive effects of simultaneous respiratory and metabolic alkalosis may result in severe alkalosis. The superimposition of one disorder on the other does not allow any compensation for either primary disorder. The resulting degree of alkalosis depends on the severity of the two primary disorders but is usually significant. Two clinical situations that can result in these mixed disorders are reviewed briefly.

Critical Care Unit. Respiratory alkalosis in the critical care unit may be induced by hypoxemia, hypotension, neurologic damage, excessive mechanical ventilation, anxiety, pain, or any combination of these and other problems. Metabolic alkalosis often results from nasogastric suctioning, vomiting, blood transfusions, or antacid therapy. The prognosis of patients in the critical care unit diminishes as arterial blood pH exceeds 7.55.[15]

Ventilator-Induced Alkalosis. Frequently, ventilator-induced alkalosis occurs when patients with COPD are intubated and mechanically ventilated. These patients often have chronic hypercapnia with compensatory elevated plasma HCO_3^- levels. Acute respiratory failure may occur, requiring the temporary institution of mechanical ventilation. If the mechanical ventilation is excessive and reduces $Paco_2$ to a normal range (35–45 mm Hg) or below, respiratory alkalosis will result. The plasma HCO_3^- remains elevated, yielding the mixed alkalosis. This problem can be avoided if initial respiratory measurements are set to maintain $Paco_2$ at normal values for that patient or if the ventilator is adjusted to lower $Paco_2$ slowly.

METABOLIC ACIDOSIS AND RESPIRATORY ALKALOSIS. Mixed disorders such as metabolic acidosis and respiratory alkalosis may be more difficult to recognize, since either abnormality is usually compensated for by the other. Most often metabolic acidosis occurs as the primary disorder and is compensated for by a predictable degree of hypocapnia. Whenever metabolic acidosis is accompanied by a $Paco_2$ that is lower than the predicted level for the degree of acidosis, a respiratory alkalosis is occurring simultaneously. In this situation the pH may be elevated slightly above 7.40 and give the appearance of a compensated respiratory alkalosis. Conversely, this mixed disorder may be diagnosed in a patient with primary respiratory alkalosis when the degree of reduction in plasma HCO_3^- exceeds the predicted amount. Serial ABG measurements and clinical evaluation of the patient make the assessment of this mixed disorder accurate.

The situations that cause metabolic acidosis or respiratory alkalosis have already been reviewed. Critically ill patients are most likely to have mixed acid-base disorders and have been shown to have a poor prognosis when this mixed acid-base disorder occurs.[14]

METABOLIC ALKALOSIS AND RESPIRATORY ACIDOSIS. When a patient with respiratory acidosis has an inappropriate elevation of plasma HCO_3^- concentration, this mixed disorder may be diagnosed. Conversely, when a patient with a known metabolic alkalosis has an inappropriately elevated $Paco_2$, a complicating respiratory acidosis is occurring. The pH in such situations is determined by the severity of each simple disorder and may be below, above, or within normal range. A pH of 7.40 occurring simultaneously with significant abnormalities in $Paco_2$ and plasma HCO_3^- indicates that a mixed disorder is present, since normal compensation of a single disorder never returns pH to 7.40.

A typical clinical situation in which this mixed disorder may occur is treatment of the patient with COPD who has chronic respiratory acidosis. This type of patient is often treated with diuretics and steroid therapy, which are capable of inducing metabolic alkalosis. The complicating metabolic alkalosis may promote further hypoventilation and worsen the clinical picture. Metabolic alkalosis can make weaning of the patient from mechanical ventilation difficult since it decreases the patient's drive to breathe. Recognition and treatment of the metabolic alkalosis is vital to optimizing the patient's respiratory function and often results in a significant reduction in $Paco_2$.

Summary of Interpreting Blood Gas Measurements

Acid-Base Assessment

STEP 1. Identify the pH measurement. If pH is within normal range, a normal acid-base status, a completely compensated acid-base disorder, or a mixed acid-base disorder is present. A normal acid-base status is obvious by a normal $Paco_2$ (35–45 mm Hg) and plasma HCO_3^- (22–26 mm Hg). If plasma HCO_3^- and $Paco_2$ are both abnormal with a pH within the normal range, either a fully compensated or mixed acid-base disorder is present.

If pH is below 7.35, an acidosis is occurring. Look at plasma HCO_3^- and $Paco_2$ to identify which is contributing to the acidosis. An elevated $Paco_2$ (>45 mm Hg) in-

Table 6-5 Summary of Simple Acid-Base Disorders*			
	pH	Paco$_2$	HCO$_3^-$
Respiratory alkalosis			
Uncompensated	↑	↓	N
Partially compensated	↑	↓	↓
Fully compensated	N	↓	↓
Respiratory acidosis			
Uncompensated	↓	↑	N
Partially compensated	↓	↑	↑
Fully compensated	N	↑	↑
Metabolic acidosis			
Uncompensated	↓	N	↓
Partially compensated	↓	↓	↓
Fully compensated	N	↓	↓
Metabolic alkalosis			
Uncompensated	↑	N	↑
Partially compensated	↑	↑	↑
Fully compensated	N	↑	↑

*N = within normal range; ↑ = increased above normal range; ↓ = decreased below normal range.

dicates respiratory acidosis, whereas a decrease in plasma HCO$_3^-$ (<22 mEq/L) indicates metabolic acidosis.

If pH is greater than 7.45, alkalosis is present. An increase in plasma HCO$_3^-$ (>26 mEq/L) indicates metabolic alkalosis, whereas a decrease in Paco$_2$ (<35 mm Hg) indicates respiratory alkalosis.

STEP 2. Once the acid-base disorder is identified as respiratory or metabolic, look for the degree of compensation occurring. Respiratory acidosis is compensated for by an elevation in plasma HCO$_3^-$, and respiratory alkalosis is compensated for by a decrease in plasma HCO$_3^-$. Metabolic acidosis is compensated for by a decrease in Paco$_2$, and metabolic alkalosis is compensated for by an elevation in Paco$_2$.

Generally, the degree of compensation is classified as *uncompensated* when the compensatory component is within normal range; *partially compensated* when the compensatory component is appropriately abnormal but pH is not yet within normal range; and *fully compensated* when the compensatory component alters enough to return the pH to normal range. Full compensation is not likely if the primary disorder is severe. When fully compensated acid-base disorders are present, the original abnormality can be identified by comparing the pH to the Paco$_2$ and plasma HCO$_3^-$. If the pH is on the acid side of 7.40 (7.35–7.39), the acid-base component that would lend itself to acidosis (either increased Paco$_2$ or decreased plasma HCO$_3^-$) is the one being compensated for. If the pH is on the alkaline side of 7.40 (7.41–7.45), the acid-base component that would lend itself to alkalosis (either decreased Paco$_2$ or increased plasma HCO$_3^-$) is the one being compensated for (Table 6–5).

Compensation for a primary acid-base disturbance often occurs in a predictable manner. This is particularly true for metabolic acidosis, respiratory alkalosis, and respiratory acidosis. A mixed acid-base problem is probably present when the predicted compensation is not present.

Oxygenation Assessment

STEP 1. Identify the Pao$_2$ and determine if it is below or within normal range. The normal predicted Pao$_2$ is dependent on the patient's age, Fio$_2$, and barometric pressure. Generally, a Pao$_2$ below 80 mm Hg in a patient less than 60 years of age is abnormal, and hypoxemia is occurring. A Pao$_2$ of 60 to 79 mm Hg is considered mild hypoxemia; 40 to 59 mm Hg is considered moderate hypoxemia; and less than 40 mm Hg is considered severe hypoxemia. A significant difference between Pao$_2$ and Pao$_2$ [P(A–a)o$_2$] indicates shunt, V̇/Q̇ mismatching, or diffusion defect. Hypoxemia with a normal P(A–a)o$_2$ may occur with an elevated Paco$_2$ and when breathing at high altitude.

STEP 2. Identify the degree of Sao$_2$ on the hemoglobin. Sao$_2$ should be maintained above 90% in the upper flat portion of the oxyhemoglobin dissociation curve in most cases. In the upper portion of the curve, moderate decreases in the Pao$_2$ do not cause significant reductions in Sao$_2$ and oxygen content of the hemoglobin. If the Sao$_2$ is 70% in the steep part of the oxyhemoglobin dissociation curve, small changes in Pao$_2$ will produce significant changes in Sao$_2$. Sao$_2$ may be abnormally decreased with hypoxemia and carbon monoxide poisoning. Actual measurement of Sao$_2$ with a co-oximeter is crucial when carbon monoxide poisoning is suspected.

STEP 3. Identify the hemoglobin concentration and Cao$_2$, if available. Hemoglobin and Cao$_2$ measurements from co-oximeters are reliable. Cao$_2$ measurements from laboratories without co-oximeters are calculated and may not be accurate. A recent hemoglobin measurement from the CBC can provide an estimation of the oxygen-carrying capacity of the blood. A normal Pao$_2$ and Sao$_2$ are of little value without an adequate hemoglobin concentration.

STEP 4. Assess the adequacy of tissue oxygenation using available data. Tissue oxygenation is dependent on adequate oxygenation and circulation of the arterial blood. Evaluation of circulation and tissue oxygenation can be achieved by assessment of the sensorium, blood pressure, extremity temperature and pulses, and mixed venous oxygen (Pv̄o$_2$).

Case Study 1

J.B. is a 52-year-old white man admitted to the hospital following a sudden onset of severe chest pain and shortness of breath. Thirty minutes after admission to the intensive care unit, J.B. suffered a cardiopulmonary arrest. Cardiopulmonary resuscitation was initiated and was successful after approximately 10 minutes.

The initial examination after cardiopulmonary resuscitation revealed that J.B. had hypotension with a spontaneous respiratory rate of 40 breaths per minute and a heart rate of 120 beats per minute. He was comatose, with central cyanosis, cool extremities, inspiratory and expiratory course crackles, and weak pulses. The initial blood gas measurements after resuscitation were as follows:

Results		Normal Range
pH	7.16	7.35–7.45
$Paco_2$	40 mm Hg	35–45 mm Hg
Pao_2	60 mm Hg	74–82 mm Hg
Sao_2	85%	>92%
Cao_2	11 vol%	16–20 vol%
BE	(−14)	±2
HCO_3^-	14 mEq/L	22–26 mEq/L
Fio_2	1.0	—
$P(A–a)o_2$	665 mm Hg	50–70 mm Hg

Interpretation and Discussion. *The pH is well below normal, indicating that acidosis is present. The plasma HCO_3^- is reduced and the $Paco_2$ is normal, indicating metabolic acidosis as the primary problem.*

When primary metabolic acidosis is occurring, the expected compensatory change in $Paco_2$ can be calculated by using the following formula:

$$Paco_2 = (1.5 \times HCO_3^-) + 8 \pm 2$$
$$\text{Expected } Paco_2 = (1.5 \times 14) + 8 = 29 \pm 2$$

Since the measured $Paco_2$ is above this value, a ventilatory disorder also must be occurring. A lack of adequate pulmonary perfusion is probably resulting in an increase in wasted or dead space ventilation. Metabolic and respiratory acidosis are present in this case.

The Pao_2 of 60 mm Hg is considered mild hypoxemia; however, considering that J.B. is breathing 100% oxygen, the Pao_2 is significantly below the predicted value. The $P(A–a)o_2$ is elevated markedly because of shunt, $\dot{V}/\dot{Q}$ mismatching, or diffusion defect, or a combination of these. The Sao_2 and Cao_2 are significantly below normal. Since Cao_2 is reduced proportionately more than Sao_2, the patient must be anemic.

The clinical signs of tissue hypoxia and metabolic acidosis are probably related. The lack of adequate oxygenation and circulation of the arterial blood is resulting in anaerobic metabolism and lactic acidosis. Whenever hypoxemia and the clinical signs of inadequate perfusion occur simultaneously, metabolic acidosis from the production of lactic acid is a definite possibility.

Case Study 2

K.M. is a 12-year-old boy brought to the emergency room with chief complaints of shortness of breath and cough. His past medical history was positive for allergies and atopic disorders (eczema). His family history was also positive for allergies and asthma. Physical examination revealed the following:

Pulse—124 beats/min
Respiratory rate—35/min
Blood pressure—120/76 mm Hg
Temperature—98.9° F

K.M. was restless and used his accessory muscles to breathe. Bilateral expiratory wheezes were heard on auscultation. His chest was clear to percussion but appeared hyperexpanded. His expiratory phase was prolonged. The CBC demonstrated a light increase in white blood cells as a result of eosinophilia. The hemoglobin and hematocrit levels were within normal limits. ABG measurements were as follows:

Results		Normal Range
pH	7.49	7.35–7.45
$Paco_2$	32 mm Hg	35–45 mm Hg
Pao_2	68 mm Hg	95–103 mm Hg
Sao_2	91.5%	>95%
Cao_2	16 vol%	16–20 vol%
HCO_3^-	22 mEq/L	22–26 mEq/L
BE	(−1)	±2
Fio_2	0.21	—
$P(A–a)o_2$	40 mm Hg	<10 mm Hg

Interpretation and Discussion. *The pH is alkalotic and corresponds to the decrease in $Paco_2$. Since plasma HCO_3^- is within normal range, the acid-base status is classified as uncompensated respiratory alkalosis.*

Pao_2 and Sao_2 are reduced mildly and are considered mild hypoxemia. The Cao_2, however, is within the lower limits of normal. Therefore anemia must not be present. The increase in $P(A–a)o_2$ indicates that the respiratory disturbance is causing shunt, $\dot{V}/\dot{Q}$ mismatching, or diffusion defect. The clinical signs of hypoxemia are evident by the tachycardia and tachypnea. The hypoxemia probably would be worse if the patient were not hyperventilating the $Paco_2$ below normal.

The respiratory alkalosis is a result of the tachypnea and "air hunger." The patient has an increase in the work of breathing because of diffuse airways obstruction as evidenced by the expiratory wheezing. It is important to note that although the ABG measurements do not identify any severe abnormalities, the patient's cardiopulmonary system is working hard to maintain these borderline measurements. Without proper treatment, the patient could deteriorate easily.

Case Study 3

C.B. is a 57-year-old white man with a history of chronic cough and sputum production. He was admitted to the hospital for abdominal surgery. On admission C.B. was noted to be using his accessory muscles to breathe, and he appeared mildly short of breath at rest. He had diminished breath sounds bilaterally, increased anteroposterior diameter, and increased resonance to percussion. He has an 80-pack-year smoking history. As part of the preoperative evaluation, blood gases were drawn and revealed the following:

Results		Normal Range
pH	7.41	7.35–7.45
$Paco_2$	61 mm Hg	35–45 mm Hg
Pao_2	66 mm Hg	76–84 mm Hg
Sao_2	91.4%	>93%
Cao_2	12.2 vol%	16–20 vol%
HCO_3^-	37 mEq/L	22–26 mEq/L
BE	+11	±2
Fio_2	2 L/min via nasal cannula	

Interpretation and Discussion. *The pH is within normal range; however, the $Paco_2$ and plasma HCO_3^- are elevated above normal. The initial temptation is to interpret the acid-base status as completely compensated metabolic alkalosis, since the pH is on the alkaline side of 7.40. However, in light of the patient's history and physical examination findings and since patients with normal respiratory systems usually do not hypoventilate significantly to compensate for metabolic alkalosis, the correct interpretation is probably respiratory acidosis and metabolic alkalosis. A mixed acid-base disorder is occurring. A cause for metabolic alkalosis must be sought to optimize respiratory function before surgery.*

Mild hypoxemia is present even though the patient is breathing supplemental oxygen via nasal cannula. The hypoxemia is probably a result of hypoventilation and $\dot{V}/\dot{Q}$ mismatching. The Cao_2 is reduced because of the hypoxemia and anemia.

Case Study 4

V.S. is a 25-year-old woman with no previous history of cardiopulmonary disease. She was admitted to the hospital with a history of frequent urination, excessive thirst, and nausea for the past 3 days. At the time of admission her skin was warm and dry and her breathing was notably deep. She was drowsy but coherent. Blood gas and chemistry results were as follows:

Results		Normal Range
pH	6.96	7.35–7.45
$Paco_2$	17 mm Hg	35–45 mm Hg
Pao_2	110 mm Hg	90–99 mm Hg
Sao_2	99.9%	>95%
Cao_2	19 vol%	16–20 vol%
HCO_3^-	3.5 mEq/L	22–26 mEq/L
BE	−24	±2
Fio_2	0.21	
Na^+	142 mEq/L	137–147 mEq/L
K^+	5.7 mEq/L	3.5–4.8 mEq/L
Cl^-	106 mEq/L	98–105 mEq/L

Interpretation and Discussion. *The pH is well below normal range (acidemia) and corresponds to the decrease in plasma HCO_3^-. The Pco_2 is significantly reduced, indicating that the respiratory system is attempting to compensate for the severe metabolic acidosis.*

The expected compensation for the metabolic acidosis can be calculated:

$$Pco_2 = (1.5 \times 3.5) + 8 \pm 2$$
$$Pco_2 = (5.25) + 8 \pm 2$$
$$Pco_2 = 13.25 \pm 2$$

Since the measured Pco_2 is 17 mm Hg, a slight respiratory problem may be present. This slight increase in the Pco_2 above the expected level is probably explained by the fact that severe decreases in pH (<7.1) do not increase the patient's drive to breathe as much as when the pH is near 7.1.

The anion gap is 32 mEq/L. This result is well above the normal range of 8 to 16 and indicates that an anion gap acidosis is present, consistent with severe diabetic ketoacidosis.

The patient's oxygenation status is normal, with the Pao_2 actually above the predicted normal range. This has occurred because the profound hyperventilation has reduced the $Paco_2$ and simultaneously raised the Pao_2 and Pao_2.

REVIEW QUESTIONS

1. T F *Arterial blood reflects lung function better than venous blood because it is not affected by tissue metabolism.*

2. *Prior to obtaining an arterial blood gas the patient's clotting parameters should be evaluated because:*
   a. *they may affect the patient's Pao_2*
   b. *if reduced they may hinder filling of the syringe with blood during the draw*
   c. *bleeding time may be prolonged if they are elevated*
   d. *all of the above*

3. *Which of the following is a common site for arterial puncture?*
   a. *radial artery*
   b. *aorta*
   c. *temporal artery*
   d. *jugular artery*

4. *Which of the following tests is done to check the collateral circulation of the radial artery prior to puncture?*
   a. *Wilson's test*
   b. *perfusion scan*
   c. *Sack's test*
   d. *Allen's test*

5. *For the above test, "pinking up" of the hand is normal if it occurs within _____ seconds.*
   a. *10-15*
   b. *15-20*
   c. *20-25*
   d. *25-30*

6. T   (F)   *Air bubbles in the blood gas syringe after puncture do not affect the values obtained during the analysis of the blood gas.*

7. *An arterial puncture site should normally be compressed for a minimum of _____ minutes after the puncture.*
    a. 1-2
    b. 3-5
    c. 5-7
    d. 8-10

8. *What is the normal value for arterial pH?*
    a. 7.20-7.30
    b. 7.35-7.45
    c. 7.45-7.50
    d. greater than 7.50

9. *What is the normal value for Pa_{O_2}?*
    a. 50-60 mmHg
    b. 60-70 mmHg
    c. 70-80 mmHg
    d. 80-100 mmHg

10. *What is the normal value for Ca_{O_2}?*
    a. 16-20 vol%
    b. 12-16 vol%
    c. 8-12 vol%
    d. 4-8 vol%

11. *What is the normal value for Pv_{O_2}?*
    a. 25-29 mmHg
    b. 32-35 mmHg
    c. 38-42 mmHg
    d. 45-55 mmHg

12. *Which of the following factors affects the Pa_{O_2}?*
    a. patient age
    b. altitude
    c. inspired oxygen concentration
    d. all of the above

13. *Which of the following is the best indicator of oxygen transport?*
    a. Pa_{O_2}
    b. Sa_{O_2}
    c. Ca_{O_2}
    d. $P(A\text{-}a)_{O_2}$

14. (T)   F   *Pv_{O_2} can be used an indicator of tissue oxygenation.*

15. (T)   F   *A decrease in tissue oxygenation is called hypoxia.*

16. *Which of the following physiologic causes of hypoxemia is the most common?*
    a. hypoventilation
    b. V/Q mismatch
    c. shunt
    d. diffusion defect

17. *Which of the following physiologic causes of hypoxemia is not corrected by supplemental oxygen administration?*
    a. hypoventilation
    b. V/Q mismatch
    c. shunt
    d. diffusion defect

18. *Which of the following shift the oxyhemoglobin dissociation curve to the left?*
    a. increased Pa_{CO_2}
    b. decreased pH
    c. increased body temperature
    d. none of the above

19. T   (F)   *A shift in the oxyhemoglobin dissociation curve to the right results in an increased affinity of hemoglobin for oxygen.*

20. T   F   *A shift in the oxyhemoglobin dissociation curve to the left is an advantage at the tissues.*

21. *Which of the following is true regarding P–50?*
    a. it is normally 27 mmHg
    b. if it is increased it indicates a shift in the oxyhemoglobin curve to the left
    c. it is affected by changes in pH
    d. it is the saturation at a Pa_{O_2} of 50 mmHg

22. *The negative log of the hydrogen ion concentration is defined as which of the following?*
    a. Pa_{CO_2}
    b. BE
    c. standard $H_{CO_3}^-$
    d. pH

23. (T)   F   *An arterial blood pH less than 7.35 is termed acidosis.*

24. T   (F)   *Alkalosis results in depression of the central nervous system and may lead to coma.*

25. *Which of the following parameters is the respiratory component of acid-base status?*
    a. Pa_{CO_2}
    b. $H_{CO_3}^-$
    c. Pa_{O_2}
    d. BE

26. (T)   F   *An increase in Pa_{CO_2} will cause a direct increase in plasma $H_{CO_3}^-$.*

27. *Which of the following is the best indicator of metabolic acid base status?*
    a. plasma HCO_3^-
    b. BE
    c. standard HCO_3^-
    d. T40 HCO_3^-

28. Which of the following ratios of HCO_3^- to $Paco_2$ will result in a pH of 7.40?
    a. 20:1
    b. 10:0.5
    c. 7:0.35
    d. all of the above

29. Which of the following is a correct representation of the Henderson-Hasselbalch equation?
    a. $pK = pH - \log (Paco_2 \times 0.03)/HCO_3^-$
    b. $pK = pH + \log HCO_3^-/(Paco_2 \times 0.03)$
    c. $pH = pK + \log HCO_3^-/(Paco_2 \times 0.03)$
    d. $pH = pH - \log HCO_3^-/(Paco_2 \times 0.03)$

30. T F An example of a simple acid-base disorder would be one in which both the respiratory and metabolic components cause alkalosis.

31. A 32-year-old male presents to the E.R. after a traffic accident with the following data: P -118, RR - 27, BP - 100/68, paradoxical chest movement on left side, breath sounds - decreased on left, ABG (21%): pH 7.32, $Paco_2$ 70, Pao_2 57, HCO_3-23, BE O, Sao_2 86, Cao_2 15.2, Hgb 13.0, P(A-a) o_2 18. Based on the above information the primary cause of the patient's hypoxemia is
    a. overall hypoventilation
    b. V/Q mismatch
    c. diffusion defect
    d. shunt

32. Which of the following are true regarding respiratory alkalosis?
    a. the $Paco_2$ less than 35 mmHg
    b. it is compensated for by an increase in HCO_3^-
    c. would be called "completely compensated" if the pH were 7.52
    d. would be called partially compensated if the pH were in the normal range

33. A patient has the arterial blood gas results below:

pH	7.25
$Paco_2$	32 MMHG
HCO_3^-	16 MEQ/L
BE	-10 MEQ/L

    On the basis of these findings, the patient is suffering from:
    a. compensated metabolic acidosis
    b. uncompensated respiratory acidosis
    c. uncompensated metabolic acidosis
    d. compensated respiratory acidosis

34. A 35-year-old, 54 Kg woman with congestive heart failure enters the E.R. short of breath, arterial blood gas shows the following:

pH	7.50
$Paco_2$	30 mmHg
HCO_3^-	23 mEq/L
BE	+2 mEq/L

    The patient's ABG results indicate:
    a. uncompensated respiratory alkalosis
    b. compensated respiratory acidosis
    c. uncompensated metabolic alkalosis
    d. uncompensated metabolic acidosis

35. Given the following ABG results, interpret the acid-base status:

pH	7.44
$Paco_2$	25 mmHg
HCO_3^-	17 mEq/L
BE	-6 mEq/L

    a. compensated metabolic acidosis
    b. uncompensated respiratory alkalosis
    c. uncompensated respiratory acidosis
    d. compensated respiratory alkalosis

36. A 17-year-old male is brought into the E.R. Vitals are pulse 100/min, respiratory rate 4/min, BP 100/65. The patient was at a party where he was discovered by his friends to be slumped in a chair and unresponsive. ABG results are as follows:

pH	7.29
$Paco_2$	68 mmHg
HCO_3^-	31 mEq/L
BE	+ 1 mEq/L

    The patient's acid-base status would be classified as:
    a. ...ratory acidosis
    ...ratory acidosis

37.

39. T   F   A chronic decrease in $Paco_2$ of 5 mmHg causes a decrease in plasma HCO_3^- by 1 mEq/L.

40. Which of the following could cause a metabolic acidosis?
    a. kidney disease
    b. diabetic ketoacidosis
    c. diarrhea
    d. all of the above

41. Answer the following questions based of the blood gas data listed below:

pH	7.21
$Paco_2$	67
Pao_2	49
Sao_2	76
Hb	10.1
Cao_2	10.4
plasma HCO_3^-	26
BE	-2

Which of the following is true regarding the Pao_2?
    a. it is adequate
    b. it shows mild hypoxemia
    c. it shows moderate hypoxemia
    d. it shows severe hypoxemia

Which of the following is true regarding oxygen carrying capacity?
    a. it is normal
    b. it is increased
    c. it is decreased
    d. unable to determine with the given data

The acid-base status would be classified as which of the following?
    a. an uncompensated metabolic alkalosis
    b. a partially compensated metabolic alkalosis
    c. an uncompensated respiratory acidosis
    d. a partially compensated respiratory acidosis

Which of the following could cause this patient's problem?
    a. anxiety and fear
    acute airway obstruction
    tic acid production
    e above

REFERENCES

1. AARC Clinical practice guideline: sampling for arterial blood gas analysis, *Respir Care* 37:913, 1992.
2. Shapiro BA and others: *Clinical application of blood gases,* ed 4, St Louis, 1989, Mosby–Year Book.
3. Kelman GR and Nunn JF: Nomograms for correction of blood Po_2, Pco_2, pH, and base excess for time and temperature, *J Appl Physiol* 21:1484, 1966.
4. Matchuny JK: Unexplained hypoxemia in a leukemia patient, *Respir Care* 67:742, 1988.
5. Shohat M and others: Determination of blood gases in children with extreme leukocytosis, *Crit Care Med* 16:787, 1988.
6. Vaughn S and Puri VK: Cardiac output changes and continuous mixed venous oxygen saturation measurement in critically ill, *Crit Care Med* 16:495, 1988.
7. Astiz ME and others: Relationship of oxygen delivery and mixed venous oxygenation to lactic acidosis in patients with sepsis and acute myocardial infarction, *Crit Care Med* 16:655, 1988.
8. Shy CM and others: *Health effects of air pollution,* New York, 1978, American Thoracic Society.
9. Guyton AC: *Textbook of medical physiology,* ed 6, Philadelphia, 1981, WB Saunders.
10. Glass LB and Jenkens CA: The ups and downs of serum pH, *Nursing* 13:34, 1983.
11. Neiberger RE: An approach to metabolic acidosis for the respiratory care practitioner, *Respir Care* 37:258, 1992.
12. McCurdy DK: Mixed metabolic and respiratory acid-base disturbances: diagnosis and treatment, *Chest* 62:355, 1972.
13. Burton GG, Hodgkin JE, and Ward JJ: Respiratory care: a guide to clinical practice, ed 3, Philadelphia, 1991, JB Lippincott.
14. Narins RG and Emmett M: Simple and mixed acid-base disorders: a practical approach, *Medicine (Baltimore)* 59:161, 1980.
15. Wilson RF and others: Severe alkalosis in critically ill surgical patients, *Arch Surg* 105:197, 1972.

BIBLIOGRAPHY

Effros RM: Acid-base balance. In Murray JF and Nadel JA, editors: *Textbook of respiratory medicine,* Philadelphia, 1988, WB Saunders.
Flenley DC: Blood gas and acid-base interpretation, *Basics of RD,* 10:1, (Sept) 1981.
Jones NL: *Blood gases and acid-base physiology,* ed 2, New York, 1987, Thieme-Stratton, Inc.
Kacmarek RM: Assessment of gas exchange and acid-base balance. In Pierson DJ and Kacmarek RM, editors: *Foundations of respiratory care,* New York, 1992, Churchill Livingstone.
Kacmarek RM, Mack CW, and Pimas S: *The essentials of respiratory therapy,* ed 2, St Louis, 1985, Mosby–Year Book.
Lane EE and Walker JF: *Clinical arterial blood gas analysis,* St Louis, 1987, Mosby–Year Book.
Malley WJ: *Clinical blood gases,* Philadelphia, 1990, WB Saunders.
Shapiro BA and others: *Clinical application of blood gases,* ed 4, St Louis, 1989, Mosby–Year Book.
Spearman CB, Sheldon RL, and Egan DF: *Egan's fundamentals of respiratory therapy,* ed 5, St Louis, 1990, Mosby–Year Book.

Chapter 7

Pulmonary Function Testing

Richard L. Sheldon

LEARNING OBJECTIVES

Upon completion of this chapter, the reader should be able to accomplish the following:

1. *Recognize the general purpose of performing pulmonary function tests (PFTs).*

2. *Recognize the situations in which PFTs are indicated.*

3. *Identify a definition of the following terms:*
   a. spirometer
   b. spirograph
   c. spirogram

4. *Identify how the following factors affect PFT measurements:*
   a. height and weight
   b. gender
   c. age
   d. patient effort

5. *Identify the standard equipment found in a PFT lab and its basic uses.*

6. *Recognize the primary abnormalities associated with obstructive and restrictive lung disease.*

7. *Given a specific site of airway obstruction, identify the part of the spirogram affected.*

8. *Identify the criteria for establishing a restrictive defect and the diseases that can cause restrictive patterns.*

9. *Identify two diseases that exhibit combined restrictive and obstructive defects.*

10. *Recognize a definition, approximate normal value, factors affecting, and significance of the following spirometric volumes and capacities:*
    a. tidal volume (V_T)
    b. minute volume ($\dot{V}_E$)
    c. total lung capacity (TLC)
    d. vital capacity (VC) and slow vital capacity (SVC)
    e. residual volume (RV)
    f. expiratory reserve volume (ERV)
    g. functional residual capacity (FRC)

LEARNING OBJECTIVES — cont'd

    h. inspiratory reserve volume (IRV)
    i. inspiratory capacity (IC)
    j. maximal voluntary ventilation (MVV)

11. *Identify the theory and methods used to measure RV and FRC using the following techniques:*
    a. body plethysmography
    b. open circuit nitrogen washout
    c. closed circuit helium dilution

12. *Identify a definition, approximate normal value, factors affecting, and significance of the following spirometric flow measurements:*
    a. forced expiratory volume at 1 second (FEV_1) and FEV_1/FVC
    b. forced expiratory volume at 3 seconds (FEV_3) and FEV_3/FVC
    c. forced expiratory flow 25% to 75% ($FEF_{25\%-75\%}$)
    d. peak expiratory flow (PEF)

13. *Given a description of a flow volume loop or a tracing of a flow volume loop identify the respective patterns for obstructive and restrictive disease.*

14. *Identify the following regarding before and after PFT bronchodilator assessment:*
    a. purpose
    b. criteria for improvement
    c. validity in asthma versus other chronic obstructive pulmonary diseases (COPD)

15. *Identify the method of measurement, normal value, factors affecting, and significance of the following specialized pulmonary function studies:*
    a. diffusion capacity (DLCO)
    b. airway resistance (Raw)
    c. compliance (CL) studies
    d. nitrogen washout
    e. closing volume (single breath nitrogen test)
    f. volume of isoflow ($Viso\dot{V}$)
    g. respiratory quotient (RQ)
    h. bronchoprovocation testing
    i. work of breathing (WOB)

16. *Recognize the general applications to respiratory care and pulmonary medicine of the following exercise tests:*
    a. stress electrocardiograph
    b. ventilatory capacity
    c. blood gases before and after exercise
    d. exercise challenge
    e. anaerobic threshold
    f. maximal oxygen uptake ($\dot{V}o_2$ max)

17. *Identify the significance of the following applications of pulmonary function testing:*
    a. smoking cessation
    b. intensive care
    c. surgery
    d. sleep apnea
    e. environmental lung diseases

18. *Given a PFT, interpret the results in terms of obstructive, restrictive, or normal lung function.*

Purpose of Pulmonary Function Testing

There was no easy, noninvasive way to document and track the physiologic effects of disease on the lungs before pulmonary function testing (PFT) became available. First, normal values had to be established for differences in age, sex, and patient size (height) before abnormalities could be recognized. Then came years of data gathering to profile the pulmonary function abnormalities seen with certain lung diseases. The work of data gathering for the purpose of establishing normal values continues. The limits of normalcy usually set within a 95% confidence band may not be as useful in some clinical settings as once thought. For instance, questions have been raised about the effects of culture and altitude on predicted normal values for specific patient populations.[1]

PFT is a way to determine the functional status of the lungs as it relates to how much gas (air) can be moved in and out of the lungs, how fast the gas can be moved, the stiffness of the lung and chest wall, the diffusion characteristics of the alveolar-capillary membrane through which the gas moves, and how well the lung responds to therapy. By using a combination of lung function tests, a nearly complete assessment of the pulmonary system can be made. The purpose of this chapter is to present the fundamentals of interpreting PFT results.

The patient is brought to a laboratory for testing where the necessary equipment is carefully maintained and calibrated by a skilled technician. In most cases, the patient should be stable and not in need of acute treatment before complete PFT is performed. For example, the asthmatic in acute distress is not likely to tolerate much of the PFT that requires significant effort. Presently, PFT is used for the following:

1. Screening for the presence of pulmonary disease (especially useful in determining which patients will be most harmed by smoking[2])
2. Evaluating the patient prior to surgery to determine the ability of the patient to tolerate the surgical procedure
3. Evaluating the patient's condition for weaning from a ventilator (see Chapter 12)
4. Researching pulmonary physiology
5. Documenting the progression of pulmonary disease or the effects of therapy
6. Studying the effects of exercise on the patient's lung function.

The primary instrument used in PFT has been the *spirometer*. It is designed to measure lung volumes and can only measure the lung volume compartments that exchange gas with the atmosphere. Spirometers with electronic signal outputs also measure flow (volume per unit of time). A device may be attached to the spirometer that graphically records the movement of gas in and out of the chest. This attachment is referred to as a *spirograph* and the resulting tracing is a *spirogram*.

Standardization of the methods for performing tests and reporting the results is necessary because of the numerous laboratories and variety of testing equipment available. There is no central regulatory body for pulmonary function laboratories at this time, although several groups might wish to accomplish this: the Joint Commission for Accreditation of Hospitals (JCAH), the U.S. government, industry, or state agencies.

Normal Values

The usefulness of PFT improves with the ability to accurately predict normal ranges. Then, as the measured values deviate from the normal predicted values, a judgment can be made regarding the severity of the disease process or the rate of recovery taking place within the lung. The following basic variables may have an impact of lung function and must be considered.

Height and Weight

Height is the most important factor influencing lung size and predicted values. Generally, the taller the person, the larger the lung size and predicted lung volumes.

As a person gains weight, lung size does not necessarily change unless the lower range of weight gain is considered separately from the higher range of weight gain. If a person gains weight by putting on muscle, a "muscularity" effect is seen by an increase in lung size. As the weight gain continues because of an increase in body fat, there is a reduction in lung size, which, if allowed to continue, results in the obesity effect and reduced lung volumes. This two-phased weight effect makes it difficult to predict normal values in PFT. To account for this change in body habitus, the concept of surface area may be a better scale for predicting normal lung volumes than height and weight.

Gender

Some measurements in lung function are relative to the sex of the individual. When individuals are matched for height and weight, males normally have larger lungs than females.

Age

The vital capacity (VC) (maximal amount of air that can be exhaled after a maximal inspiratory effort) increases in a person until the middle twenties. Lung size begins to decrease as the person ages past the twenties. An average 20-year-old has a predicted VC slightly over 5 L. By age 70, the same person's predicted VC will have fallen to approximately 4 L.

Other Considerations

Other poorly defined predictors of pulmonary function may include race, environmental factors, and altitude.

Presently the data are difficult to obtain and inconclusive when these variables are included as predictors.

In considering patient performance, it should be noted that many of the pulmonary function tests require maneuvers that are effort-dependent, and thus variability occurs in each person on a day-by-day basis. This should be taken into consideration when interpreting and reviewing test results with a patient, especially when comparing current with previous studies.

High-quality pulmonary function data require that attention be paid to the issues that can lead to errors in measurement and interpretation. Routine procedures which can reduce errors include: (1) accurate calibration of all testing equipment; (2) selecting reference equations and lower limits of normal appropriate for both the patients studied and the equipment being used to study them (pediatric vs. adult patients); (3) avoiding the use of too many measurements to generate an interpretation; and (4) taking into consideration the clinical state of the patient when doing the interpretation (as an example, for the patient who has experienced a thoracotomy [surgical removal of one lung] interpretation is unique).[3]

Standard Pulmonary Function Laboratory Equipment

Most equipment is now available with microprocessors to handle computerized evaluation and reporting. The modern pulmonary function laboratory has the following equipment (blood gas equipment is not included here):

1. Spirometer with spirograph (for routine flows and volume)
2. Body plethysmograph (for total lung capacity and airways resistance studies)
3. Diffusion system (for measuring lung diffusion)
4. Gas analysis (carbon dioxide, carbon monoxide, helium, nitrogen, and oxygen)

There are guidelines published by the American Thoracic Society as "Spirometry Update" which include information about testing equipment, quality control, test performance and technician training.[4]

Classification: Obstructive vs. Restrictive Defects

Pulmonary function abnormalities can be grouped into two main categories: (1) obstructive and (2) restrictive defects. This grouping of defects is based on the fact that the routine spirogram, as the centerpiece of PFT, measures two basic components: flow and volume. The abnormality is obstructive if expiratory flow is below normal. If lung volume is reduced, a restrictive disease is probably present.

Obstructive Defects

Obstruction can occur in the upper airways (larynx, trachea, right or left mainstream bronchus), large airways (those greater than 2 mm in diameter), or small airways (less than 2 mm). The anatomic site of obstruction to flow may be suggested by the part of the spirogram that is abnormally altered. Upper airway obstruction will result in reduced flow rates in the initial 25% of a forced expiratory VC maneuver. Obstruction in the smaller airways will cause reduced flow rates in the later portion of the exhaled volume.

Restrictive Defects

A restrictive defect is present when lung volumes are reduced to less than 80% of predicted levels as measured by the routine spirogram or body plethysmograph. This category of disease includes such causes as chest wall dysfunction, neurologic diseases resulting in paralysis of the muscles of inspiration, dysfunction of the diaphragm, absent lung tissue, and scarring of the lungs as with interstitial lung disease. Atelectasis and obesity represent two of the more common causes of a restrictive lung defect.

Combined Defects

Certain diseases can result in both obstructive and restrictive defects. Two examples are sarcoidosis* and emphysema. Sarcoidosis in its final stages severely reduces volume and limits airflow.

A better example of combined defects is severe emphysema, which results in obstruction to airflow out of the lungs. Thus the residual volume gas in the lung slowly increases and eventually restricts the volume of air that can be inspired. The net result is a combined obstructive and restrictive defect.

Anatomy of a Normal Spirogram

Before defining each part of the spirogram, it is worthwhile to note that volumes are single compartments in the lung. Adding two or more volumes together results in what is called a *capacity*.

Volumes and Capacities Routinely Identified are as Follows (Fig. 7-1):

1. Tidal volume (V_T)
2. Minute volume ($\dot{V}_E$)
3. Vital capacity (VC)
4. Total lung capacity (TLC)
5. Residual volume (RV)
6. Expiratory reserve volume (ERV)
7. Functional residual capacity (FRC)
8. Inspiratory reserve volume (IRV)
9. Inspiratory capacity (IC)
10. Maximal voluntary ventilation (MVV)

Tidal Volume

Tidal volume is the volume of air exhaled or inhaled during quiet breathing. The average values for healthy adults show considerable variation but usually fall between 350 and 600 mL. A decreased V_T can occur with both restrictive and obstructive disease. A fall in V_T without an increase in rate may result in hypoventilation and retention of arterial carbon dioxide tension (Pa_{CO_2}). Restrictive lung disease usually causes the patient to breathe with a smaller V_T. The breathing rate of the patient with restrictive lung disease increases in proportion to the loss in lung volume.

Minute Volume

The *minute volume* is the volume of gas expired over 1 minute. $\dot{V}_E$ is determined by adding each measured V_T in 1 minute or, if the patient's V_T is consistently the same size, by multiplying the rate times the average V_T. Normal $\dot{V}_E$ ranges from 4 to 12 L/min at rest, depending on the size of the patient. The $\dot{V}_E$ is the best index of ventilation when used in conjunction with arterial blood gas measurements. The $\dot{V}_E$ should increase in response to exercise, fever, pain, hypoxia, and acidosis, regardless of whether the acidosis is caused by carbon dioxide retention (respiratory acidosis) or lactic acid or ketone body retention (metabolic acidosis).

Vital Capacity

Vital capacity is measured after the person has taken the deepest breath possible. The following exhaled volume should be the maximal amount the patient can exhale and is measured as the VC. If the patient forcefully exhales the volume, it is called the forced

---

*Sarcoidosis is a disease of unknown etiology characterized by the deposition of micronodules, called *noncaseating granulomas*, throughout the body. The granulomas have a predilection for the lungs. They also invade the brain, eyes, heart, liver, skin, and lymph nodes. Sarcoidosis has profound immunologic consequences. Treatment is usually inadequate. Some cases are self-limiting, with an occasional patient showing spontaneous remission of the entire disease process. The usual course is a slow progression of lung fibrosis.

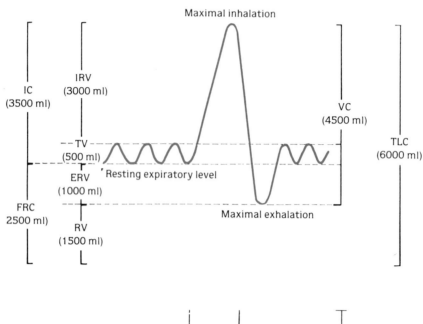

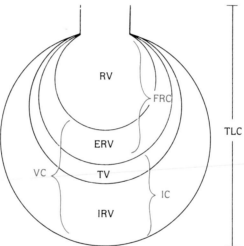

Fig. 7-1 *Lung volumes and capacities. Representation of a normal spirogram and divisions of lung volumes and capacities. Numbers are for average-sized young adults. See text for abbreviations. (From Scanlon CL, Spearman CB, and Sheldon RL,* Egan's fundamentals of respiratory therapy, *ed 5, St Louis, 1990, Mosby–Year Book.)*

vital capacity (FVC) and is the usual way the VC is reported (Fig. 7-2).

VC is not thought of as abnormally increased, only as abnormally decreased. Both restrictive and obstructive diseases can decrease VC. Restrictive lung disorders reduce FVC by shrinking the lung. Obstructive lung dysfunction causes a decrease in the FVC by causing a slow rise in the RV. Since the lung is contained in the thoracic cage, which is a relatively rigid structure, room must be made for this expanding RV. The only space readily available is that used by VC. Therefore, as the RV increases, VC decreases.

VC is also reported as slow vital capacity (SVC). The SVC test is performed by having the patient completely exhale, slowly, following a maximal inspiration. A slow exhalation may allow more air to be exhaled from the lung, since a slow exhalation helps reduce air trapping. In some patients forceful exhalation causes airways to close prematurely because of the high intrathoracic pressures produced. This early closure may spuriously decrease the measured VC volume as gas is trapped distal to the airway closure and cannot be exhaled. The SVC is intended to reduce the likelihood of this happening and allows for all of the VC volume to be exhaled and measured. If measured FVC is significantly smaller than SVC, air trapping is occurring.

VC is an important preoperative assessment factor. Significant reduction in VC (less than 20 mL/kg of ideal body weight) indicates that the patient is at a high risk for postoperative respiratory complications. This is because VC reflects the patient's ability to take a deep breath, to cough, and to clear the airways of excess

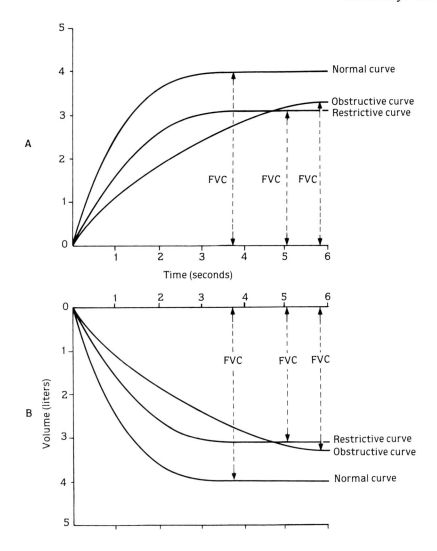

Fig. 7-2 *Forced vital capacity (FVC) curves comparing normal, obstructive, and restrictive disorders.* **A,** *Curves as they appear on commonly available spirometers with tracings beginning at bottom left corner.* **B,** *Same curves as they appear on some spirometers that begin tracings at upper left corner. (From Scanlon CL, Spearman CB, and Sheldon RL: Egan's fundamentals of respiratory therapy, ed 5, St Louis, 1990, Mosby–Year Book.)*

secretions (see Chapter 12). VC is also useful in evaluating the patient's need for mechanical ventilation. A VC of less than 10 to 15 mL/kg indicates that the patient's ventilatory reserve is decreased significantly.

Total Lung Capacity

Total lung capacity is the sum of the VC and the RV (RV is described below). TLC is a function of the person's size, age, and sex. It is increased with most obstructive lung diseases and decreased with restrictive disorders. To measure TLC, the RV must be determined. The RV or FRC is obtained in one of the three ways: (1) body plethysmograph (body box); (2) open circuit nitrogen washout; or (3) closed circuit helium dilution. After the residual volume is obtained, it is added to the VC to determine TLC. More is said about VC and RV and how

the FRC relates to the RV later in this chapter. The following is a brief description of the body plethysmograph, open circuit nitrogen washout method, and closed circuit helium dilution method.

BODY PLETHYSMOGRAPHY (BODY BOX). The body plethysmograph (Fig. 7-3) takes advantage of Boyle's law, which says that the pressure and volume of a gas vary inversely if temperature is constant. The body plethysmograph measures all of the gas within the chest. When the patient is placed in the body box, there are two volumes being considered: the volume of the gas in the lung (the unknown) and the volume of the box itself (known). The formula for identifying the unknown volume is derived from the following:

$$\frac{\text{Unknown lung gas volume } (V_1)}{\text{Known body box gas volume } (V_2)} = \frac{\text{gas pressure of the box } (P_2)}{\text{gas pressure of the lung } (P_1)}$$

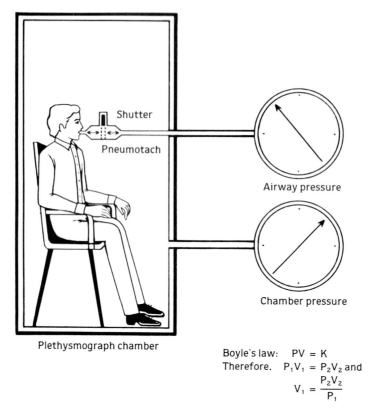

Boyle's law: PV = K

Therefore, $P_1V_1 = P_2V_2$ and

$$V_1 = \frac{P_2V_2}{P_1}$$

Fig. 7-3 *Body plethysmography method for measuring lung volumes. Initial alveolar volume (P₁); initial thoracic gas volume (unknown) (V₁); test of alveolar pressure (shutter closed) (P₂); test of thoracic gas volume (shutter closed) (V₂). (From Spearman CB, Sheldon RL, and Egan DF:* Egan's fundamentals of respiratory therapy, *ed 4, St Louis, 1982. Mosby–Year Book.)*

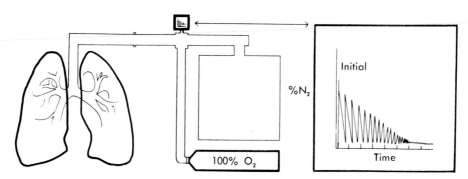

Fig. 7-4 *Indirect spirometric method for determining functional residual capacity and residual volume. Nitrogen washout method. (From Scanlon CL, Spearman CB, and Sheldon RL:* Egan's fundamentals of respiratory therapy, *ed 5, St Louis, 1990, Mosby–Year Book.)*

Thus

$$V_1 = \frac{V_2 \times P_2}{P_1}$$

OPEN CIRCUIT NITROGEN WASHOUT METHOD. The nitrogen washout method is shown in Fig. 7-4. This method requires that the patient breathe 100% oxygen and measures the nitrogen washout down to a low concentration. This test is based on the principle that the gas within the lung is approximately 79% nitrogen. If the amount of nitrogen washed out of the lungs is measured, this measurement represents 79% of the unknown lung volume.

There are several problems with this method: (1) the actual amount of nitrogen "resident" in the lung before washout starts cannot be precisely measured and therefore an estimate is required; (2) there is a significant amount of nitrogen washed out of the tissue with the nitrogen washed out of the lung; (3) if a patient's lungs have significant areas of poor communication with outside air, as in emphysema, this test along with the helium dilution method will underestimate total lung volume.

The test assumes that the nitrogen concentration in the lungs is in equilibrium with the nitrogen in the atmosphere. The patient breathes 100% oxygen for approximately 7 minutes. As the nitrogen washes out of the lung, the volume and nitrogen percentages of the exhaled gas are measured. The test is stopped when the nitrogen concentration plateaus. The following formula is then applied:

$$\text{FRC} \times N_2\% \text{ at start of test} = \text{expired volume} \times N_2\% \text{ at end of test}$$
$$\text{or } V_1 \times N_1 = V_2 \times N_2$$

CLOSED SYSTEM HELIUM DILUTION

METHOD. The closed system helium dilution method is illustrated in Fig. 7–5. It is another way to measure FRC and RV. As with the nitrogen washout method, the RV is added to the VC to determine TLC.

Helium is used because it is an inert gas and is not significantly absorbed from the lungs by the blood. This test is based on the principle that if a known volume and concentration of helium are added to the patient's respiratory system, the helium will be diluted in proportion to the size of the lung volume to which it is added.

Helium is breathed at VT while oxygen is added to replace the oxygen that is consumed by the patient during the test. Since the patient adds carbon dioxide to the closed system, the carbon dioxide must be absorbed out of the closed system to prevent an increase in the dilutional effect on the helium and a falsely enlarged FRC measurement.

If leaks occur with this method, the measured volumes will be overestimated. Other factors influencing the quality of the test include: (1) the blower speed of the device; (2) when the technician stops the test

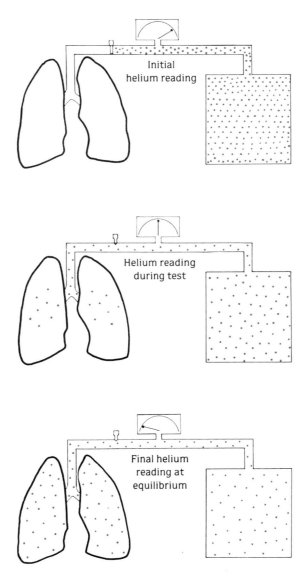

Fig. 7–5 *Indirect spirometric method for measuring functional residual capacity and residual volume. Helium dilution method. (From Scanlon CL, Spearman CB, and Sheldon RL: Egan's fundamentals of respiratory therapy, ed 5, St Louis, 1990, Mosby–Year Book.)*

after equilibration is achieved; and (3) the ventilatory pattern of the patient being tested. As just mentioned, if parts of the lung communicate poorly with the atmosphere, the results will be inaccurate.

The patient breathes in a closed system of a known volume containing a known concentration of helium. The test usually takes about 7 minutes. When the helium meter shows that equilibrium has been reached, the following formula can be used:

$$\text{Volume in spirometer} = \frac{\text{helium added (in milliliters)}}{\text{\% helium at first reading}}$$

The FRC can now be calculated using V for the volume in the spirometer with the following formula:

$$\text{FRC} = \frac{(\text{initial helium} - \text{final helium}) \times V \times \text{BTPS}}{\text{final helium}}$$

where BTPS = values at body temperature and pressure standardized.

Residual Volume

Residual volume measurement cannot be obtained from the routine spirogram. It is obtained from the studies already described under the TLC section. RV can be determined by subtracting the VC from the TLC or by subtracting the ERV from the FRC (see below). RV is the amount of gas left in the lung after exhaling all that is physically possible. RV is reduced in restrictive dysfunction and increased in moderate to severe obstructive dysfunction. RV increases with obstructive disease as air trapping occurs.

Expressed as a ratio to TLC and VC, RV is normally 25% of TLC and 33% of VC. This ratio is a dependable measurement and clinically useful. If RV is greater than 33% of VC, chronic obstructive pulmonary disease (COPD) is probably present. In restrictive dysfunction the ratio is usually normal. There are no clinical states in which RV/TLC or RV/VC is reduced.

Expiratory Reserve Volume

The *expiratory reserve volume* is the volume that can be maximally exhaled following a passive exhalation. This volume is of limited clinical usefulness. It is reduced in obese persons, in those making a poor effort to perform the test, and in those with restrictive disease.

Functional Residual Capacity

When the values representing RV and ERV are added together, the resulting capacity is the *functional reserve capacity*. This is the "resting volume" in the lungs following exhalation of a V_T breath. It represents a balance between the expanding chest wall forces and the contractile-rebound forces of lung tissue.

Any dysfunction that causes a loss of lung tissue (such as emphysema) increases FRC, since the forces that expand the chest wall have a decreasing amount of opposition. Respiratory disorders that cause partial or more complete collapse of the lung (e.g., pneumothorax) reduce FRC.

Inspiratory Reserve Volume and Inspiratory Capacity

Inspiratory reserve volume and *inspiratory capacity* are measured by the routine spirogram but are not used widely in evaluating pulmonary dysfunction. Both of these measurements can be normal in restrictive and obstructive diseases (see Fig. 7–1).

Measurement of Flows

On the expiratory side of the FVC curve, data are found regarding the contractile state of the airways. This part of the curve evaluates the amount of obstruction present in the patient's airways. To better study this curve, the recording device is sped up at the instant the patient starts to exhale. This spreads the recording out and allows for more detailed study of its shape. One of the features that separates an expensive PFT device from a less costly one is the timing device gears and mechanisms that recognize the instant expiration starts and automatically speed up the recorder. Flows routinely identified are the following:

1. Forced expiratory volume at 1 second (FEV_1)
2. Forced expiratory volume at 3 seconds (FEV_3)
3. Forced expiratory flow, midexpiratory phase ($FEV_{25\%-75\%}$)
4. Peak expiratory flow (peak flow, PEF)

FORCED EXPIRATORY VOLUME AT 1 SECOND. The FEV_1 measures the maximal volume of air exhaled during the first second of expiration. It is a forced maneuver, highly significant, and the best indicator of obstructive diseases. It reflects the flow characteristics in the larger airways.

The FEV_1 is reported as a raw number, but it is best expressed as a percentage of the observed FVC (FEV_1/FVC). The normal value varies with age, sex, and height, although most patients should be able to exhale approximately 75% of their VC in 1 second. The FEV_1/FVC is decreased in acute and chronic obstructive pulmonary disease and is usually normal in purely restrictive disorders.

Acute reductions in FEV_1, as occur in asthma, cause ventilation-perfusion mismatching and hypoxemia. The degree of hypoxemia generally depends on the severity of the airway obstruction. The more severe the airway obstruction, as assessed by the reduction in FEV_1, the more significant the hypoxemia.[1] Acute decreases in FEV_1 initially result in respiratory alkalosis in most cases. Only when the reduction in FEV_1 is severe (less than 20% of the predicted value) will hypercapnia and respiratory acidosis occur.

FORCED EXPIRATORY VOLUME AT 3 SECONDS. The FEV_3 looks at the 3-second point of the expired curve and gives an indication of the flow in the smaller airways. It is not as reproducible and sensitive as the FEV_1 but is helpful.

The FEV_3 can also be reported as a percentage of the FVC and tends to decrease normally with age, as does the FEV_1. Normal FEV3/FVC is approximately 95%.

FORCED EXPIRATORY FLOW, MIDEXPIRATORY PHASE. The $FEF_{25\%-75\%}$ is a different way of looking at expiratory flows and is a sensitive test. It is expressed in liters per second and is therefore a real indicator of flow (speed). The first 25% of the exhaled curve is disregarded because of the lungs' initial inertia. The last 25% is also disregarded because of effort dependency. This leaves the middle 50% of the curve's slope to reflect the degree of airway patency. This measurement is sensitive enough to be an early indicator of obstructive dysfunction. $FEF_{25\%-75\%}$ can also be reduced in restrictive dysfunction, but its primary usefulness is in evaluating obstructive disorders. There are other points along the expired curve that are also observed, including the $FEF_{50\%}$ and the $FEF_{75\%}$. These measurements show the 50% and 75% points, respectively, on the expired slope. They are not as useful as the $FEF_{25\%-75\%}$.

PEAK EXPIRATORY FLOW. The PEF is the maximum flow rate achieved by the patient during the FVC maneuver. It may be recorded in liters per second or liters per minute. PEF may be determined by identifying the steepest part of an FVC spirogram or by use of a handheld portable flowmeter. Use of a portable device allows rapid and repeatable assessment of PEF in a variety of clinical settings such as the emergency room or the outpatient setting.[5]

In asthmatics, the PEF correlates well with the FEV_1 and can be used to identify the severity of the airways obstruction.[3,4] If the PEF is less than 100 L/min, severe obstruction is present; 100 to 200 L/min indicates moderate obstruction; and PEF over 200 L/min suggests mild disease.[6] Once therapy is started, PEF is useful in guiding management of the asthmatic patient, providing objective data regarding the patient's response to therapy. Since inexpensive portable devices are available, PEF measurements can be used by the asthmatic patient to self-monitor home care.[6,7]

Maximal Voluntary Ventilation

Maximal voluntary ventilation measurement requires the patient to breathe as rapidly and fully as possible for 12 to 15 seconds. The total volume exhaled is measured to obtain total volume. This volume is then multiplied by the appropriate number (5 if tested for 12 seconds, 4 if tested for 15 seconds) and reported as the volume moved by the lungs in 1 minute. It is realized that this number is probably larger than if the patient actually performed the maneuver for 1 full minute. Because of rapid fatigue of the respiratory muscles or possible syncope from hyperventilation, it is unreasonable to have the patient inhale and exhale rapidly for a full minute. Healthy young adults have a predicted MVV of about 170 L/min.

The MVV reflects the status of the respiratory muscles, compliance of the thorax-lung complex, and airway resistance (Raw). Normal values vary widely. Only large decreases in MVV are clinically significant. The test is popular with surgeons as a quick assessment of the state of the patient's lungs before surgery. A poor performance on this test suggests that the patient may have significant respiratory problems postoperatively. Since this test is very effort-dependent, it is generally not useful.

Flow Volume Curves (Flow Volume Loops)

Flow volume loops are generated by integrating flow with volume on graph paper. This flow volume loop allows a pattern to be seen that is distinctive for certain diseases. Fig. 7–6 shows a typical flow volume loop. The inspiratory loop is shown below the horizontal line and the expiratory loop is shown above the line. This test can be particularly useful in looking for upper airway obstruction and small (less than 0.2 mm in diameter) air-

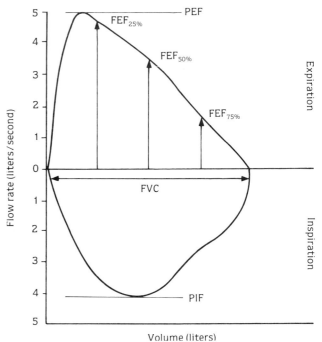

Fig. 7–6 *Flow volume loop. Peak expiratory flow (PEF); peak inspiratory flow (PIF); forced expiratory flow at X% of FVC (FEV%); forced vital capacity (FVC). (From Spearman CB, Sheldon RL, and Egan DF:* Egan's fundamentals of respiratory therapy, *ed 5, St Louis, 1990, Mosby–Year Book.)*

way obstruction. Restrictive disease is shown as a shortened loop in the horizontal volume line (Fig. 7–7).

Pulmonary Function Testing Before and After Aerosol Bronchodilators

In most pulmonary function laboratories, if airway obstruction is identified, bronchodilators are administered to the patient after the routine flow and volume study (spirogram). This is done to assess the reversibility of the airway obstruction seen on the initial spirogram. The type of drug used is a β_2 sympathomimetic, but the specific drug is not standardized from one laboratory to another. The bronchodilator is delivered to the patient as an aerosol via a metered dose inhaler (MDI). It is recommended that two out of three of the measurements FVC, FEV_1, and $FEF_{25\%-75\%}$ improve before response to the inhaled bronchodilator is considered to be present. The amount of improvement needed is as follows:

- FVC: increase greater than 10% to 15%
- FEV_1: increase of 200 mL or 15% over baseline FEV_1
- $FEF_{25\%-75\%}$: 20% to 30% increase

A positive response to a bronchodilator is thought to be most often predictive of subsequent usefulness in asthmatic patients but can be misleading in other COPD patients. This is due to the day-by-day variability seen in the natural course of the disease coincidentally occurring when the PFT is done.

A common question is, If there is no response to bronchodilators, should they be used in treatment?

Bronchodilators are given a trial even when there is no positive response documented by the laboratory. Prolonged exposure to these drugs or a combination of steroids and sympathomimetics may be required before a response is seen clinically. Often the response to bronchodilators in the laboratory setting is a predictor of ease of control in the clinical setting. If there is no response to the bronchodilator in the laboratory, clinical control may be difficult.

Specialized Pulmonary Function Studies

There is a group of studies that go beyond the routine spirogram and that are usually available only at larger medical centers. The special tests that are described below are often used to clarify or quantify the lung abnormalities detected by the simple spirogram. Some of these tests can also be used to detect abnormalities that are present but not detectable by spirograms. These studies include the following:

1. Diffusion capacity (DLCO)
2. Airway resistance (Raw)
3. Compliance studies (static, dynamic, static-effective, and frequency-dependent) (CL)
4. Nitrogen washout
5. Closing volume (CV)
6. Volume of isoflow (VisoV)
7. Respiratory quotient (RQ)
8. Exercise testing

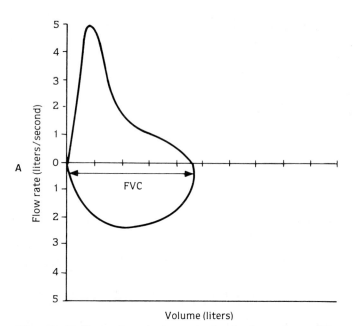
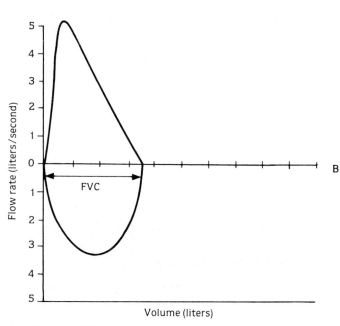

Fig. 7–7 *Flow volume loops comparing* **A,** *obstructive and* **B,** *restrictive disorders. FVC, forced vital capacity. (From Spearman CB, Sheldon RL, and Egan DF:* Egan's fundamentals of respiratory therapy, *ed 5, St Louis, 1990, Mosby–Year Book.)*

9. Bronchoprovocation testing (i.e., methacholine [Provocholine] challenge)
10. Work of breathing (WOB)

Diffusion Capacity

The ability of gas to diffuse across the alveolar-capillary membrane can be measured. The determinants of gas exchange across the membrane include the following:

1. Diffusion coefficient of the gas used in testing
2. Surface area of the membrane
3. Thickness of the membrane
4. Blood volume and flow in the pulmonary capillary tree
5. Distribution of the inspired gas
6. Hematocrit

Diseases that reduce surface area of the membrane, such as emphysema, can reduce DLCO. Emphysema also has a negative impact on the distribution of the inhaled gas. Interstitial diseases such as pulmonary fibrosis, asbestosis, and sarcoidosis alter the integrity of the membrane and cause a reduction in diffusion. The perfusion status of the pulmonary capillaries determines the ability of oxygen in the lung to be absorbed across the alveolar-capillary membrane. Minimal diffusion will occur if the blood volume of the pulmonary capillaries is significantly reduced. The patient's hematocrit also affects DLCO for the same reason. The hemoglobin level of the blood will influence the carrying capacity of the blood since oxygen is carried primarily by the red blood cells.

Diffusion is measured by using carbon monoxide at minute levels (0.4%). Because of carbon monoxide's intensive affinity for hemoglobin (over 200 times greater binding power to hemoglobin than oxygen), the ability of carbon monoxide to diffuse is limited by the membrane and not by capillary blood flow. It is therefore a diffusion-limited gas rather than a perfusion-limited gas.

Using carbon monoxide in a closed system, its rate of removal from this closed system is an indication of the biologic state of the membrane. DLCO is measured in millimeters per minute per millimeter of mercury and reported as both the raw number and percentage of predicted value. Normal DLCO is approximately 25 mL/min/mm Hg.

Other important considerations in measuring diffusion and distribution of inspired gas are alveolar oxygen ($P_{A}O_{2}$) and carbon dioxide tensions ($P_{A}CO_{2}$) and hematocrit and pulmonary capillary blood flow.

Airway Resistance (Raw)

Narrowing of the airways in acute and chronic obstructive pulmonary disease causes airflow resistance to increase. It is sometimes useful to document the precise Raw level as a means of indicating the severity of the disease and effect of therapy. The equipment used to determine Raw is shown in Fig. 7–8. This study uses the same closed, tightly sealed body box (plethysmograph) described earlier for the determination of TLC.

Normally Raw is greater on expiration than on inspiration. It increases with any pathologic process that

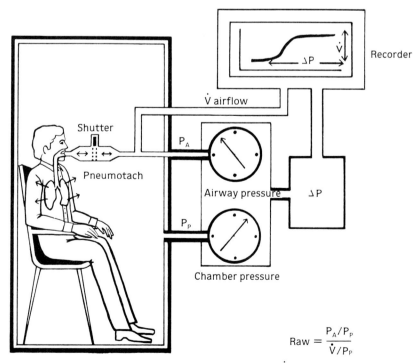

$$Raw = \frac{P_A/P_P}{\dot{V}/P_P}$$

Fig. 7–8 *Measurement of airway resistance* (Raw) *by body plethysmograph.* $\dot{V}$ = *ventilation;* P_A = *airway pressure;* P_P = *chamber pressure. (From Scanlon CL, Spearman CB, and Sheldon RL:* Egan's fundamentals of respiratory therapy, *ed 5, St Louis, 1990, Mosby–Year Book.)*

narrows the airways causing inflammation, edema, or bronchoconstriction. Since the elastic rebound of the lung tends to hold the airways open, loss of elasticity causes the airway to collapse on exhalation and thus increases resistance. This process is seen in emphysema.

The normal resistance is 0.5 to 3.0 cm H_2O/L/sec at a flow rate of 0.5 L/sec. Sometimes resistance is reported as conductance, which is the reciprocal of resistance. Resistance is usually reported as a percentage of normal. A report of 100% ± 20% is considered within normal limits.

Compliance Studies

Compliance is defined as volume change per unit of pressure change. Compliance measurements are useful in identifying the relative stiffness of the lung. Lungs with low compliance require greater pressure changes to expand with a specific volume as compared to more compliant lungs. Esophageal pressure closely approximates intrapleural pressure and can be used to identify changes in thoracic pressures that occur with changes in lung volume. Lung compliance can be determined by having the patient swallow a balloon catheter approximately 10 cm into the esophagus. The proximal end of the catheter is connected to a pressure transducer, and serial pressure measurements are recorded at various lung volumes. For the patient who is intubated, intrathoracic pressure can be determined by using a pressure manometer in line with the breathing circuit, avoiding the need for an esophageal balloon.

Compliance may be measured either at a point of no flow (static compliance) or when gas is flowing into the lung (dynamic compliance). Healthy persons exhibit values for dynamic compliance that are slightly less than values for static compliance. When Raw is elevated, however, dynamic compliance will decrease well below static compliance. Both static and dynamic compliance values will decrease when the lung becomes stiffer, as with atelectasis, pneumonia, and pulmonary fibrosis.

The total compliance of the respiratory system is made up of two distinct compliance units: lung tissue and chest wall. These two compliance units are parallel and not in series; therefore the effect of the sum of the two units would be expressed as the following:

$$\frac{1}{\text{Total CL}} = \frac{1}{\text{CL of the thorax}} + \frac{1}{\text{CL of the lung}}$$

The compliance curve is derived from the following formula:

$$CL = \frac{\text{Change in volume}}{\text{Change in pressure}}$$

The typical compliance curves for various diseases are shown in Fig. 7–9. The flat curve reflects a stiff lung, whereas the curve for emphysema demon-

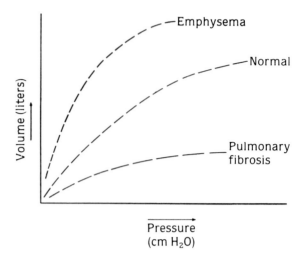

Fig. 7–9 *Pressure-volume curves.*

strates a highly compliant lung that has lost its recoil ability.

Nitrogen Washout

Nitrogen washout is used to determine if there is gross maldistribution of ventilation. As the patient breathes 100% oxygen, the nitrogen analyzer measures a continuously diminishing concentration of nitrogen from the lungs. "Fast ventilatory spaces" may occur and, if so, will empty first. "Slower ventilating spaces" empty slowly and erratically, making the downward slope uneven. This pattern confirms the presence of uneven ventilation as commonly seen in obstructive lung diseases such as emphysema (Fig. 7–10).

Closing Volume (CV)

Closing volume is a special form of nitrogen washout used for early diagnosis of obstruction in the small airways. In the standard nitrogen washout test the patient "washes out" the lung nitrogen by breathing in 100% oxygen for 7 to 10 minutes. In contrast, the CV is determined by having the patient take in a single breath of 100% oxygen and then slowly exhale while the levels of nitrogen in the exhaled breath are monitored. Normally, four phases are seen on the test curve (Fig. 7–11). Phase I is the extreme upper airway (dead space) gas consisting of 100% oxygen; phase II is a mixture of dead space and alveolar gas; phase III is a plateau produced by the exhalation of alveolar gas; phase IV is identified by an abrupt increase in the concentration of nitrogen, which continues until the patient reaches RV. Phase IV occurs when the small airways in the dependent lung zones close, which stops gas flow out of the bases. Gas flow out of the apices now dominates exhalation, and it has a higher concentration of nitrogen than gas from the lower lung zones. This occurs because the lower lung regions receive more of the 100% oxygen inhaled than the upper regions, since

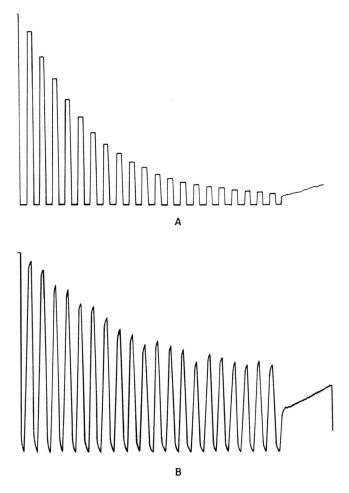

Fig. 7-10 *Nitrogen washout tracing showing* **A,** *normal and* **B,** *abnormal washout curves.*

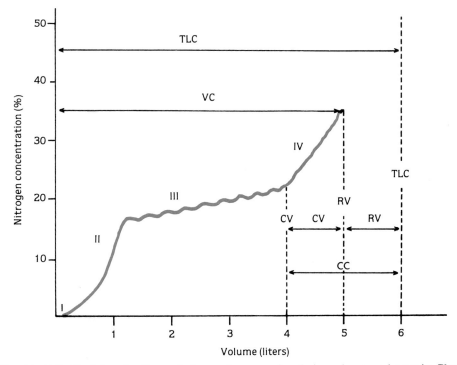

Fig. 7-11 *Single-breath nitrogen test curve for measuring closing volumes and capacity. Phase I: expired dead space gas. Phase II: mixed dead space and alveolar gas. Phase III: alveolar plateau, see text for abbreviations. Phase IV: airway closure. (From Spearman CB, Sheldon RL, and Egan DF:* Egan's fundamentals of respiratory therapy, *ed 5, St. Louis, 1990, Mosby–Year Book.)*

there is proportionately more of the RV gas in the apices after maximum exhalation than in the bases.

There are some difficult technical problems in getting an accurate and useful curve. As a consequence, some laboratories have stopped offering the closing volume as a diagnostic aid. Nevertheless, four varied but valuable test results are available from the closing volume curve:

1. Closing volume: representation of the state of the small airways; early airway narrowing can be detected in this test
2. Delta nitrogen (ΔN_2): index of distribution of ventilation
3. TLC and RV: done by integrating the area under the expired nitrogen curve
4. Fowler method: determination of anatomic airway dead space

Phase IV of the curve is where the CV occurs. CV is often reported as a percentage of the VC and in this situation the term *closing capacity* may be used. Closing capacity is determined by adding the CV to the RV. CV is reported as a percentage of VC and closing capacity is reported as a percentage of TLC. Plus or minus 20% of the predicted value is considered normal. The normal predicted value increases with age. The value increases abnormally in early obstruction of the small airways.

Volume of Isoflow ($V_{iso}\dot{V}$)

This test is done to determine the portion of the VC remaining in the lung at which airflow is independent of gas density. Since helium has a significantly lower density than air, it is used for this test. The patient performs a standard FVC maneuver while breathing air. Next the subject breathes a mixture of 80% helium and 20% oxygen and repeats the FVC test. The two FVC curves are then superimposed to identify the point at which flow becomes identical and therefore independent of gas density. Normally, the $V_{iso}\dot{V}$ occurs when 10% to 20% of the VC remains in the lung. An increase in the $V_{iso}\dot{V}$ is consistent with obstruction of the small airways or loss of elastic recoil.

Respiratory Quotient (RQ)

The ratio of carbon dioxide produced to oxygen consumed is called the *respiratory quotient*. Using appropriate collectors to accurately measure the volume of expired gas and then analyzing the amount of carbon dioxide and oxygen in the expired gas, one can determine carbon dioxide produced and oxygen consumed.

Many metabolic activities affect the RQ. One of the most frequent uses of the RQ is to assess which food group (fats, carbohydrates, or protein) is being metabolized for energy. If the RQ is 0.7, fats are the sole energy source. If the RQ is 1.0, carbohydrates are the main source of energy. Depending on the activity level

and nature of the food being ingested, the RQ can shift. Normally, it is 0.8 to 0.85, showing a mixed metabolism pattern.

There are many clinical applications for this information. One important use is in assessing the patient who is being weaned from a ventilator. Since a patient who is being fed a diet made up exclusively of glucose (carbohydrate) produces more carbon dioxide than usual, the WOB increases to blow off this excess carbon dioxide load. Carbon dioxide is a direct byproduct of carbohydrate metabolism, and the more of this foodstuff eaten, the more carbon dioxide produced. Knowledge of the patient's RQ allows intelligent adjustment of the patient's diet and may speed up the process of weaning the patient from the ventilator (see Chapter 15).

Exercise Testing

A complete review of exercise testing is not feasible here. The information has become so vast that entire books are written on the subject. The following list of possible exercise tests and their uses should serve as an introduction to this fascinating field in pulmonary medicine.

1. *Stress electrocardiography (ECG): used for the noninvasive detection of coronary artery disease.*
2. *Ventilatory capacity: assesses the patient's ability to respond to exercise with the appropriate increase in rate and depth of ventilation.*
3. *Blood gases (arterial oxygen [Pao_2] and carbon dioxide tension [$Paco_2$]), alveolar-arterial oxygen tension difference [$P(A-a)o_2$], pH, base excess, before and after exercise: detects the presence of oxygenation, ventilation, and oxygen usage problems not apparent at rest.*
4. *Exercise challenge: the patient exercises hard, and then the spirogram is used to see if this challenge has incited the development of bronchospasm. Exercise-induced bronchospasm is a variant of asthma and usually responds to specific treatment when correctly identified.*
5. *Anaerobic threshold: when the body is stressed enough during exercise, there is a point at which oxygen need exceeds availability, and a backup mode of metabolism called anaerobic (without oxygen) metabolism is brought into action. Exercise testing is useful to identify this point in persons such as athletes in training and patients with heart disease who may need an individualized exercise program that is safe for them. With proper exercise, the anaerobic threshold can be increased.*
6. *Maximal oxygen uptake ($\dot{V}o_2max$): designed to show the level of exercise that causes the patient to reach maximum oxygen consumption. Obtaining this information requires a well-ordered and well-staffed laboratory with calibrated equipment.*

Bronchoprovocation Testing

The most common cause of undiagnosed cough is "occult" asthma. Frequently the routine spirogram is normal in patients suspected of having nonspecific bronchial hyperresponsiveness, i.e., asthma. This hyperresponsiveness is a constant feature of asthma even though airflow obstruction is often absent at the time of routine testing. Other causes of wheezing exist. Methods of uncovering this hyperresponsive state in a safe controlled setting are necessary to determine which episodes of wheezing are due to asthma and which ones are not.

In these settings bronchoprovocative testing is useful. Several easy and safe techniques are used to document bronchial hyperresponsiveness. Challenging the patient with inhaled histamine or methacholine is most commonly used. These medications have parasympathomimetic properties and therefore may induce bronchospasm. Spirogram studies are done, following the administration of the provoking agent, to determine the response of the airways. Healthy subjects without hyperactive airways tolerate the challenge without significant reduction in pulmonary function values. A 20% decrease in FEV_1 or other reliable measure of expiratory flow, suggests that the patient has hyperactive airways.

The technique may be used safely in an outpatient setting if protocol is carefully followed.[7] Other challenge techniques include cold air and exercise.

Work of Breathing

The healthy person at a resting state uses 2% to 5% of his or her total oxygen consumption each minute to maintain gas exchange. As the lung becomes diseased the oxygen consumed by the respiratory system increases in most cases. In shock, the oxygen cost to breathe may be as high as 50% of all the oxygen brought into the body. This steals oxygen from other oxygen-dependent areas such as white blood cells battling infection, the heart and brain, and the kidneys and liver trying to detoxify harmful byproducts of metabolism.

In the intensive care unit (ICU) setting it is becoming easier to document a high WOB. WOB can be increased with external and internal factors. Breathing circuits and artificial airways represent factors that may impose external increases in the WOB. Internal factors that may increase the WOB include airway obstruction and reduced lung or chest wall compliance. Regardless of the cause, an increase in the WOB must be reduced so available oxygen can be rerouted to areas of great physiologic need. The tests available to determine WOB are the following:

1. Oxygen consumption ($\dot{V}_{O_2}$ in mL/min)
2. Energy expenditure (EE, in kcal/day)
3. $\Delta \dot{V}_{O_2}$
4. Respiratory power input
5. Mouth occlusion pressure (PO.1): respiratory muscle drive
6. Oxygen cost of breathing
7. Tension time index: approximation of energy demand
8. Mechanical work: pressure-volume curves as generated from the ventilator

Several of the tests listed above are considered experimental tools. Currently, ventilator manufacturers are working on making ventilator systems that provide information related to the mechanical work (pressure-volume curves) as part of the feedback loops to the practitioner. Practitioners armed with such information can make adjustments in the ventilator settings to reduce WOB and thus wean the patient faster. Weaning from mechanical ventilation is less likely when more than 15% of the total $\dot{V}_{O_2}$ is used by the respiratory muscles.

Other Applications of Pulmonary Function Testing

Pulmonary function testing is useful in a variety of clinical settings. The following discussion presents some of the additional ways PFT can be valuable.

Smoking Cessation

There has been a significant drop in the consumption of cigarettes in the United States since the Surgeon General's report in the mid-1960s. This report, and many since, detailed the dangers of smoking cigarettes.

PFT can be done on smokers to reinforce the need for smoking cessation, especially if considerable loss of lung function is documented. Smokers may be more motivated to stop smoking if evidence is presented to them that clearly demonstrates the damage cigarettes have imposed on their airways and lung function.

More important, PFT has proved to be the most useful single predictor of who will have cardiopulmonary disease as a result of smoking. Smoking is the main risk factor in the development of coronary artery disease (ahead of hypertension and abnormal cholesterol levels). Early changes in FEV_1 and FVC better predict future problems than does an ECG.[2]

The Intensive Care Unit

In these days of cost containment, the word *expensive* has been substituted for *intensive* in order to make a point about the extreme cost of hospitalizing patients in ICUs. Frequently the speed at which patients can be transferred to step-down units depends on how rapidly they can be weaned from their ventilator.

Specific weaning criteria are frequently published but these criteria are only guides to suggest if a patient is weanable (see Chapter 12). The entire clinical setting of the patient including electrolyte status, blood gases, nutrition, infection, and so forth bears heavily on whether or not weaning will be successful.

As our understanding of the adult respiratory distress syndrome (ARDS) and multiorgan failure (MOF) improves, methodologies initially considered to be useful only as research tools are being reconsidered. These tools include methods to determine lung water and WOB.[9]

Surgery

In patients anticipating surgery who have known pulmonary disease or who have symptoms of dyspnea, cough, etc., PFT is crucial. Regardless of history or symptoms, patients who are to have all or part of a lung removed need to have PFT performed prior to surgery.

If the FEV_1 is less than 2 L, differential perfusion lung scans are recommended to assess the impact on oxygenation and ventilation resulting from the proposed lung resection. It is widely accepted than a postoperative FEV_1 less than 800 mL places a patient at high risk after surgery and may condemn him or her to a life of dyspnea. It should be noted that this number has not been scientifically validated.[10]

Sleep Apnea

Approximately a third of our life is spent asleep, a state of profound physiologic change compared to when we are awake. Only recently have we begun to understand this remarkable phenomenon called sleep (see Chapter 16).

PFT testing can be an important tool in the assessment of patients with sleep-disordered breathing. Sleep apnea can occur as a result of central nervous system problems (central sleep apnea, CSA) or airway obstructive problems (obstructive sleep apnea, OSA). OSA makes up approximately 90% of sleep apnea patients. Of this group, 20% have COPD. PFT needs to be done in this group to better direct daytime treatment of chronic lung disease along with the nighttime treatment of sleep apnea.[11] PFT can be helpful in assessing the patient primarily with CSA.[12] In such patients a mixed obstructive and central apnea is often present and PFT may prove useful in evaluating the degree and severity of upper airway obstruction.

Environmental Lung Diseases

It is recognized that 20% of the general population has some form of lung disease: a restrictive defect, COPD, or lung cancer. The workplace is recognized as a place where lung disease can start or can be made worse. Teams made up of PFT technicians, physicians, and statisticians have worked to lessen the impact of the

work environment on lung disease. Annual changes in the FEV_1 must be carefully interpreted because lung disease has the potential for serious economic impact on both employee and employer.[13]

Clinical Interpretation of Pulmonary Function Testing

Pulmonary function testing is used to identify and evaluate obstructive and restrictive respiratory disorders (Table 7–1). Obstructive defects cause a reduction in the measurements of flow, including FEV_1/FVC, $FEF_{25\%-75\%}$, and PEF. VC is normal in mild obstructive disease but decreases as the obstruction becomes more severe. FRC and TLC are initially normal to mildly increased with acute airway obstruction, but are increased significantly with chronic defects such as emphysema. MVV is reduced in more severe cases.

Clinically, acute decreases in flow rate measurements are associated with dyspnea, hypoxemia, hypocapnia, tachypnea, use of accessory breathing muscles, expiratory wheezing, crackles, and paradoxical pulse. Chronic airflow impairments are associated with an increased anteroposterior diameter of the chest, reduced voice and breath sounds, use of accessory muscles, increased resonance to percussion, and low, flat diaphragms (see Chapter 4).

Restrictive lung disorders are recognized by identifying a reduction in VC, RV, FRC, and TLC. The measurements of flow may be normal or mildly reduced. The FEV_1/FVC is normal in pure restrictive disorders.

Clinically, the patient who has restrictive lung disease may show signs of dyspnea on exertion, cyanosis, rapid shallow breathing, digital clubbing, reduced breath sounds, and late inspiratory crackles. In chronic advanced cases, the signs of chronic right heart failure (cor pulmonale) occur (see Chapter 4).

Case Study 1

M.W. is a 70-year-old man with a chief complaint of dyspnea on exertion. The dyspnea has increased gradually over the last several years. M.W. denies a history of cough, sputum production, smoking, working in a polluted environment, or respiratory disease.

Physical examination reveals tachypnea, tachycardia, jugular venous distention, decreased breath sounds, digital clubbing, and kyphoscoliosis.

Personal data:
Age—70 years
Height—66 in.
Weight—155 lb
Sex—male
Spirometry report:

Table 7-1 Summary of Pulmonary Function Tests*

Measurement	How Determined	Units	Disease Process	Usefulness
TLC	Body box	Liters and % predicted	↑Obstructive: ↓ restrictive	+++
VC	Spirogram	Liters and % predicted	↓Obstructive: ↓ restrictive	++++
ERV	Spirogram	Liters and % predicted	↓ restrictive	+
FRC	Derived: spirogram and body box or nitrogen washout/helium dilution	Liters and % predicted	↑Obstructive: ↓ restrictive	+++
RV	Derived: spirogram and body box or nitrogen washout/helium dilution	Liters and % predicted	↑ Obstructive: ↓ restrictive	+++
V_T	Spirogram	Liters and % predicted	↑/N Obstructive: ↓/N restrictive	++
IRV	Spirogram	Liters and % predicted	↑/N Obstructive: ↓/N restrictive	+
IC	Spirogram	Liters and % predicted	↑/N Obstructive: ↓/N restrictive	+
MVV	Spirogram	L/min	↓ Obstructive: ↓ restrictive	+++
Frequency f	Clock	No./min	↑ Obstructive and restrictive	+++
$\dot{V}_E$	Derived: $f \times V_T$	L/min	↑ Obstructive ↓ restrictive	+++
FEV_1	Spirogram	% Predicted	↑ Obstructive and restrictive	++++
FEV_3	Spirogram	% Predicted	↑ Obstructive and restrictive	+++
$FEF_{25\%-75\%}$	Spirogram	% Predicted	↓ Obstructive	+++
PF	Spirogram	% Predicted	↓ Obstructive	++
FEV_1/FVC	Spirogram	% Predicted	↓ Obstructive	++++
DLCO	Carbon monoxide uptake	% Predicted	↓ Emphysema and restrictive	+++
CV	Nitrogen washout	% Predicted	↑ Obstructive	++
Raw	Body box	% Predicted	↑ Obstructive	+++
Compliance	Esophageal balloon	L/cm H_2O pressure	↑ Obstructive: ↓ restrictive	+++

* = normal; + = least useful; ++++ = most useful.

	Predicted	Observed	Predicted %
FVC (L)	3.78	1.46	39
SVC (L)	3.78	1.42	38
ERV (L)	0.67	0.34	51
IC (L)	3.10	1.07	35
FEV_1 (L)	2.57	1.40	54
FEV_3 (L)	3.59	1.46	41
FEV_1/FVC	70%	96%	—
FEV_3/FVC	95%	100%	—
MVV (L/min)	114	76	67
$FEF_{25\%-75\%}$ (L/min)	2.46	2.01	82
PEF (L/sec)	5–8	6.20	—

Lung volume studies (body box):

	Predicted	Observed	Predicted %
Predicted			
VC (L)	3.78	1.79	47.4
ERV (L)	0.67	0.15	22.0
IC (L)	3.10	1.64	52.9
FRC (L)	2.42	2.01	83.0
RV (L)	1.75	1.86	106
TLC (L)	5.78	3.65	63.2
RV/TLC	30%	51%	

Interpretation and Discussion: *Spirometry reveals a significant reduction in FVC, IC, FEV₁, and FEV₃. However, the measurements of flow are within normal limits. The lung volume studies identify a reduction in VC, IC, and TLC. The findings are consistent with restrictive lung disease. Arterial blood studies are indicated to further evaluate the degree of respiratory impairment.*

The lung function studies are typical for a patient with kyphoscoliosis. Kyphoscoliosis causes a reduction in the size of the thoracic cage and severely compromises lung expansion.

Case Study 2

J.D. is a 38-year-old man with a chronic complaint of dyspnea on exertion. His dyspnea has increased significantly over the past year and now occurs with minimal exertion. J.D. denies cough, chest pain, or sputum production. He has a 40-pack-year smoking history. His family history is positive for COPD. There is no history of exposure to environmental pollutants. Clinical examination is positive for chronic airflow obstruction (see Chapter 4).

Personal data:
Age—38
Height—76 in.

Weight—188 lb
Sex—male
Spirometry report:

	Predicted	Observed	Predicted %
FVC (L)	6.06	3.39	56
SVC (L)	6.06	4.49	74
ERV (L)	1.38	1.99	145
IC (L)	4.69	2.49	53
FEV_1 (L)	4.52	0.95	21
FEV_3 (L)	5.76	1.84	32
FEV_1/FVC	75%	28%	—
FEV_3/FVC	95%	54%	—
MVV (L/min)	189	48	25
$FEF_{25\%-75\%}$ (L/sec)	4.39	0.34	8
PEF (L/sec)	5–8	1.40	—

Lung volume studies (body box):

	Predicted	Observed	Predicted %
Predicted			
VC (L)	6.06	4.88	80.5
ERV (L)	1.38	1.83	133.0
IC (L)	4.69	3.05	65.1
FRC (L)	3.24	9.75	301.2
RV (L)	1.86	7.92	425.7
TLC (L)	7.75	12.80	165.1
RV/TLC	24%	61.90%	257.8

Interpretation and discussion: *Spirometry results demonstrate a reduction in FVC, SVC, IC, FEV$_1$, and FEV$_3$. The measurements of flow FEV$_1$/ observed FVC, and FEF$_{25\%-75\%}$ are also reduced markedly. At first glance this appears to be a combined restrictive and obstructive lung defect. However, the lung volume studies clearly reveal that the reduction in FVC is the result of air trapping, and only an obstructive defect is present.*

The significant difference in FVC and SVC measurements suggests that air trapping is occurring, especially during forced expiratory maneuvers.

Studies done after the use of bronchodilators and arterial blood gases and DLCO measurements would be helpful to further evaluate J.D.'s respiratory status. There should be a high index of suspicion for the presence of alpha$_1$-antitrypsin deficiency in this patient. The DLCO is expected to be markedly reduced if emphysema is the cause of this patient's dyspnea.

REVIEW QUESTIONS

1. T   F   PFTs measure the ability of the lungs to exchange respiratory gases.

2. In which of the following situations is a PFT not *useful?*
    a. documenting the progression of pulmonary disease
    b. evaluating the probability of getting a pulmonary disease
    c. exercise evaluation
    d. weaning from mechanical ventilation

3. The tracing obtained from a PFT is called a
    a. spirograph
    b. spiroagnew
    c. spirogram
    d. spirometer

4. Which of the following factors is the most important in predicting PFT measurements?
    a. weight
    b. age
    c. gender
    d. height

5. T   F   Males generally have larger lung volumes and flows compared to females of similar height and weight.

6. T   F   Most PFTs are independent of patient effort.

7. Which of the following pieces of standard PFT equipment is used to determine total lung capacity and resistance of the airways?
    a. body plethysmography
    b. spirometry
    c. diffusion systems
    d. all of the above

8. Which of the following are consistent with obstructive lung disease?
    a. increased expiratory flows
    b. decreased expiratory flows
    c. decreased lung volumes and flows
    d. increased lung volumes and flows

9. An anatomic obstruction located in the upper airway will affect which part of the spirometric tracing?
    a. initial portion
    b. middle portion
    c. end portion
    d. all of the above

10. Which of the following is true regarding restrictive lung disease?
    a. it is characterized by reduced lung volumes on the PFT
    b. it can be caused by obesity
    c. expiratory flows are generally normal
    d. all of the above

11. T   F   Emphysema can produce both obstructive and restrictive defects in lung function.

12. Which of the following is true regarding tidal volume (V$_T$)?
    a. it is normally 4–5 L
    b. it is normally 50% of TLC
    c. it is defined as the volume inhaled and exhaled during quiet breathing
    d. it is increased in restrictive lung disease

13. Total lung capacity is the sum of which of the following?
    a. tidal volume and vital capacity
    b. inspiratory reserve volume and expiratory reserve volume
    c. residual volume and expiratory reserve volume
    d. vital capacity and residual volume

14. Which of the following tests is useful in determining the need for mechanical ventilation?
    a. FEV_1
    b. FVC
    c. $FEF_{25\%-75\%}$
    d. TLC

15. T F A vital capacity of 12 mL/Kg would suggest a high risk for postoperative pulmonary complications.

16. T F TLC is increased in most obstructive lung diseases.

17. Residual volume is normally which of the following values?
    a. 25% of VC
    b. 25% of V_T
    c. 33% of VC
    d. 33% of TLC

18. Which of the following is/are true regarding FRC?
    a. it is the sum of the RV and ERV
    b. it is increased in obstructive disease
    c. it is reduced in restrictive disease
    d. all of the above

19. Body plethysmography is based on which of the following gas laws?
    a. Boyle's law
    b. Charles' law
    c. Dalton's law
    d. universal gas law

20. Open circuit nitrogen washout can be helpful in measuring which of the following?
    a. RV
    b. TLC
    c. FRC
    d. all of the above

21. Which of the following tests is the best indicator of obstructive lung disease?
    a. FEV_3
    b. $FEF_{25\%-75\%}$
    c. FEV_1
    d. VC

22. Which of the following is the normal value for FEV_1?
    a. 25% of VC
    b. 50% of VC
    c. 60% of VC
    d. 75% of VC

23. T F A large reduction in FEV_1 would result in moderate to severe hypoxemia.

24. T F A PEF of 120 L/min indicates severe airway obstruction.

25. T F A shortened flow volume loop on the horizontal axis indicates obstructive lung disease.

26. Which of the following is/are true regarding pre and post bronchodilator PFTs?
    a. it is used to assess the reversibility of airway obstruction
    b. an increase in FVC by 5% is considered proof of improvement
    c. it is useful in all forms of obstructive lung diseases
    d. all of the above

27. Which of the following is/are true regarding a DLCO?
    a. it will be increased in emphysema
    b. it uses 0.4% CO_2 as a test gas
    c. it will decrease with decreasing lung surface area
    d. it is normally 35 mL/min/mmHg

28. T F A lung with an increased compliance requires less pressure to expand than a lung with reduced compliance.

29. Which of the following is/are true regarding bronchoprovocation testing?
    a. it is used to test for "occult" asthma
    b. methacholine is commonly used as bronchoprovocation agent
    c. histamine is commonly used as bronchoprovocation agent
    d. all of the above

30. Which of the following exercise tests is useful in determining coronary artery disease?
    a. ventilatory capacity
    b. exercise challenge
    c. stress electrocardiograph
    d. anaerobic threshold

31. The results of a PFT are as follows:
    Patient data
    age: 68 years old
    height: 63 inches
    weight: 135 pound
    sex: male

Spirometry	Observed	Predicted	% Predicted
FVC	1.33 L	3.38 L	39
SVC	1.35 L	3.38 L	40
ERV	0.48 L	1.03 L	47
IC	1.01 L	2.35 L	43
FEV_1	1.21 L	2.36 L	51
FEV_3	1.29 L	3.21 L	40
FEV_1/FVC	91%	70%	-
FEV_3/FVC	97%	95%	-
MVV	77 L/min	97.5 L/min	79
$FEF_{25\%-75\%}$	2.0 L/sec	2.41 L/sec	83
PEF	6.1 L/sec	7.66 L/sec	80

Lung Volume Studies	Observed	Predicted	% Predicted
VC	1.44 L	3.38 L	43
ERV	0.27 L	1.03 L	26
IC	1.17 L	2.35 L	50
FRC	2.51 L	3.03 L	83
RV	2.24 L	2.00 L	112
TLC	3.68 L	5.38 L	68
RV/TLC	61%	37%	165

Which of the following is the correct interpretation of this PFT?

    a. restrictive disease

    b. obstructive disease

    c. combined obstructive and restrictive disease

    d. normal PFT

REFERENCES

1. Clausen JL: Prediction of normal values in pulmonary function testing, *Clin Chest Med* 10:135–143, 1989.
2. Petty TL: Spirometry in smoking-related diseases, *IM Intern Med* 12:35–49, 1991.
3. Crapo RO and others: Pulmonary function testing: sources of error in measurement and interpretation, *South Med J* 82-875–879, 1989.
4. McKay RT and others: Pulmonary function testing: guidelines for medical surveillance and epidemiological studies, *Occup Med* 6:43–57, 1991.
5. Mueller GA and others: Pediatric pulmonary function testing in asthma, *Pediatr Clin North Am* 39:1243–1258, 1992.
6. George RB: Monitoring of patients during acute asthma attacks. In Lavietes M and Reichman LB, editors: *Diagnostic aspects and management of asthma,* Norwalk, Conn, 1981, Purdue Frederick.
7. Shim C: Assessment of the response to inhaled pulmonary drugs. In Witek T and Schachter EN, editors: *Problems in respiratory care,* Philadelphia, 1988, JB Lippincott.
8. Rosenthal RR: Approved methodology for methacholine challenge, *Allergy Proc* 10:301–312, 1989.
9. Macnaughton PD and others: Pulmonary function testing in the intensive care unit, *Respir Med* 84:437–443, 1990.
10. Cottrell JJ and others: Preoperative assessment of the thoracic surgical patient, *Clin Chest Med* 13:47–53, 1992.
11. Fletcher EC: Chronic lung disease in the sleep apnea syndrome, *Lung* 168(Suppl): 751–761, 1990.
12. Hanly PJ: Mechanisms and management of central sleep apnea, *Lung* 170:1–17, 1992.
13. Enright PL: Surveillance for lung disease. Quality assurance using computers and a team approach, *Occup Med* 7:209–225, 1992.

BIBLIOGRAPHY

Bates DV, Macklem PT, and Christie RV: *Pulmonary function in disease,* Philadelphia, 1971, WB Saunders.

Clausen JL: *Pulmonary function testing guidelines and controversies,* New York, 1982, Academic Press.

Jones NL and others: *Clinical exercise testing,* Philadelphia, 1975, WB Saunders.

Madama VC: *Pulmonary function testing and cardiopulmonary stress testing,* New York, 1993, Delmar.

Miller WF, Scacci R, and Gast LR: *Laboratory evaluation of pulmonary function,* Philadelphia, 1987, JB Lippincott.

Ruppel G: *Manual of pulmonary function testing,* ed 5, St Louis, 1994, Mosby–Year Book.

Scanlan CS, Spearman CB, and Sheldon RL, editors: *Egan's fundamentals of respiratory therapy,* ed 5, St Louis, 1990, Mosby–Year Book.

Chapter 8

Clinical Application of the Chest Radiograph

Richard L. Sheldon

LEARNING OBJECTIVES – cont'd

9. *Identify the technique, indications, and advantages/disadvantages for tomography and computerized tomography.*

10. *Identify the relative use and indications for magnetic resonance imaging in lung disease.*

11. *Recognize the technique and indications for performing lung scans.*

12. *Identify how the following problems affect lung scans:*
    a. *thromboembolism*
    b. *atelectasis*
    c. *pneumonia*

13. *Recognize the technique and indications for the use of pulmonary angiography.*

14. *Recognize the proper technique for assessing the following during technical evaluation of the chest x-ray:*
    a. *placement on view box*
    b. *adequacy of exposure*
    c. *patient rotation*
    d. *depth of inspiration*

15. *Recognize the proper technique for performing a systematic descriptive evaluation (interpretation) of the chest x-ray.*

16. *Identify the significance of the following special radiographic evaluation signs:*
    a. *silhouette sign*
    b. *air bronchogram*

17. *Recognize the limitations of the chest radiograph.*

18. *Recognize the typical clinical and chest radiographic findings for the following lung diseases:*
    a. *atelectasis*
    b. *pneumothorax*
    c. *hyperinflation*
    d. *interstitial lung disease*
    e. *congestive heart failure*
    f. *pleural effusion*
    g. *consolidation*

Chapter Outline

Production of the Radiograph

Indications for the Chest X-Ray Examination

Radiographic Views
  Standard and Special Views
  Portable Chest Film

Tomography

Computed Tomography
  Lung Tumors
  Chronic Interstitial Lung Disease
  Acquired Immune Deficiency Syndrome
  Occupational Lung Disease
  Pneumonia
  Bronchiectasis
  Chronic Obstructive Pulmonary Disease

Magnetic Resonance Imaging

Lung Scanning

Pulmonary Angiography

Evaluation of the Chest Radiograph
  Review of Clinical Findings
  Placing the Chest X-ray on the View Box
  Interpretation
  Limitations

Clinical and Radiographic Findings in Lung Disease
  Atelectasis
  Pneumothorax
  Hyperinflation
  Interstitial Lung Disease
  Congestive Heart Failure
  Pleural Effusion
  Consolidation

Chapter Overview

The introduction of x-ray technology in the early part of this century gave medical workers a chance to see inside the human body without cutting into it. The result of this advance was revolutionary. It ushered in the era of modern medicine. Finally, the ability to detect disease expanded beyond what the examiners could identify with the history and physical examination.

The ease, accuracy, and reliability of radiographic examination allowed for its use to proliferate at a rapid rate. Within a decade or two radiology became an entire hospital-based department and soon a special discipline within the field of medicine.

The use of x-rays in assessment of the body soon became so pervasive that whenever a patient reported a physical complaint to a physician, the area of the body involved with the complaint received an x-ray examination. Often the area received repeated x-ray examinations. This can result in clinicians depending on the x-ray examination to such a degree that other assessment skills may not be developed fully. The most accurate clinical assessment usually results from a combination of interviewing, physical examination, and radiographic evaluation. This chapter emphasizes the clinical manifestations associated with the pathologic abnormalities of the lung identified by x-ray examination.

A short description is given of the physics related to radiographs and the use of standard and special views in assessment of the patient with pulmonary disease. This is followed by a discussion of techniques for interpreting the chest film. Finally, some of the more common pathologic abnormalities seen on chest x-ray films and their related clinical findings are presented.

Production of the Radiograph

X-rays are electromagnetic waves that radiate from a tube through which an electric current has been passed. The tube is made of a cathode that is attached to a low-voltage electron source (transformer). The end of the cathode wire is inside the vacuum-sealed tube, and as electrons flow through the wire, they are "boiled off," accelerate across a short gap, and strike a positively charged tungsten plate called the *anode*. The electrons coming off the cathode wire are focused to hit a small area on the anode. This area is called the *target*.

On striking the target, the electrons undergo physical changes, which result in the emission of x-rays. These x-rays are emitted in all directions, but because of the construction of the tube, only the few that escape through the window are actually used; the rest are absorbed harmlessly into the wall of the x-ray machine (Fig. 8–1).

X-rays are not reflected back like light rays but penetrate matter. Their ability to penetrate matter is dependent on the density of the matter. Dense objects such as bone absorb more x-rays (allow less penetration) than air-filled objects such as lung tissue. A sheet of film is placed next to the patient's thorax opposite to where the x-ray tube is located to generate a chest film.

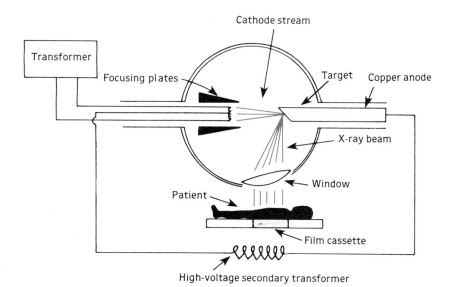

Fig. 8–1 *Electric current is generated by the transformer, passes through focusing plates, and arrives at the cathode. Electrons are "boiled off," making a cathode stream. The cathode stream then strikes the anode target and is transformed into x-rays. X-rays leave the sealed vacuum x-ray tube through a window and strike the patient, pass through the patient, and cast a shadow on the film cassette making an "x-ray picture." (From Scanlon CL, Spearman CB, and Sheldon RL:* Egan's fundamentals of respiratory therapy, *ed 5, St. Louis, 1990, Mosby–Year Book.)*

The x-ray machine emits x-rays which pass through the patient and are absorbed proportional to the density of the tissue through which it is passing. X-rays that pass through low-density (air-filled) objects strike the film full force and turn it black (radiolucent). X-rays that strike bone are partially absorbed; therefore, less darkening of the corresponding area on the x-ray film is seen (radiopaque). Radiopaque areas are seen as white shadows on the film. The four different densities seen on the chest film (also referred to as chest radiograph) are bone, air, water, and fat.

The distance between the source of the x-ray and the patient is an important consideration. The closer the patient is to the source, the greater the magnification and distortion of the objects seen on the chest film. This concept can easily be demonstrated by placing your hand below a lamp and observing the shadow created on the surface below. The shadow becomes smaller and sharper as your hand is moved away from the light source and closer to the surface.

The patient and the film are positioned approximately 6 ft from the x-ray source for the conventional chest x-ray examination. At this distance the images seen on the chest film are in good focus, and the magnification effect is minimized.

Indications for the Chest X-Ray Examination

The ability to "see inside" the body with the use of radiographs has proved to be of great benefit, especially when assessing the contents of the thorax. Production of the chest film has become one of the most popular and important procedures performed in the hospital. It can be used in the following ways:

1. Detecting alterations of the lung caused by pathologic processes
2. Determining the appropriate therapy
3. Evaluating the effectiveness of treatment
4. Determining the position of tubes and catheters
5. Observing the progression of lung disease

Though the chest film provides important information regarding the status of the lungs, obtaining and interpreting the film must never delay fundamental treatment of the patient with obvious signs of hypoxia. In most situations, when the members of the health care team are well trained and work together, a chest film can be obtained without interrupting assessment and treatment.

Radiographic Views

Standard and Special Views

The standard chest radiographs are taken in two directions. First, with the patient standing upright with his back to the x-ray tube, the anterior thorax is pressed against a metal cassette containing the film, and his or her arms are positioned out of the way. The patient is instructed to take a deep breath just before exposure. The x-ray beam leaves the source, strikes the patient's posterior chest, moves through the chest, exits through the front (anterior), and then strikes the film. Since the beam moves from posterior to anterior, this is called a *posteroanterior (PA) view.* Since the heart is in the anterior half of the thorax, there is less cardiac magnification with a PA view. The patient is then turned sideways, and a lateral or side view is obtained. Generally, a left lateral view (left side against the cassette) is preferred. The left lateral view provides less cardiac magnification and a sharper view of the left lower lobe, which is partially obscured on the PA view by the cardiac shadow. However, if right-sided lesions are present, a right lateral view will provide a sharper view of the lesion.

Other views are sometimes obtained when special problems are identified. A lateral decubitus view is taken with the patient lying on the right or left side to see if free fluid (pleural effusion or blood) is present in the chest. As little as 25 to 50 mL of pleural fluid can be detected with the lateral decubitus view. This view is also helpful in the identification of pneumothorax. Since air tends to rise and water tends to fall, patients with a suspected right-sided pneumothorax should be placed on their left side for radiologic examination and patients with suspected right-sided pleural fluid should be placed on their right side. Projections made at approximately a 45-degree tube angulation from below, referred to as *apical lordotic,* are sometimes required for a closer look at the right middle lobe or the top (apical region) of the lung. When the tube is angled upward, the shadows of the clavicles are projected above the thorax.

Oblique views are helpful in delineating a pulmonary or mediastinal lesion from structures that overlie it on the PA and lateral views. Oblique views are often obtained when bilateral lesions are present and help localize the abnormality. In this view the patient is turned 45 degrees to either the right or left with the anterolateral portion of the chest against the film.

Although chest radiographs are usually taken with the patient at full inspiration, an expiratory film can be helpful in certain situations. For example, a small pneumothorax can be difficult or impossible to detect in a routine inspiratory film. As the patient exhales, however, the lung volume is reduced, while the pleural air volume remains the same. The pneumothorax now occupies a greater percentage of the thoracic volume and therefore stands out more. In addition, the lung is more dense in the expiratory position, and the contrast allows for the air density within the pleural space to be more easily visualized.

Portable Chest Film (Anteroposterior View)

Patients in intensive care units are too sick to be transported to the x-ray department for a standard PA chest film. In this instance a portable x-ray machine is brought to the patient's bedside and positioned in front of the patient. The film cassette is placed carefully behind the patient's back. Thus the x-ray beam moves from front to back (anterior to posterior), generating an *anteroposterior (AP)* film, instead of the usual PA film. The distance from the patient to the beam's origin must be consistent so as not to cause a magnification effect.

Interpreting an AP film requires advanced skills. The AP film frequently is not centered, is either over-exposed or underexposed, and/or is not taken when the patient is in full inspiration. There may be many extrathoracic shadows superimposed on the film. These extra shadows include bedding, gowns, electrocardiogram leads, and tubing. The clinician has to be able to read the film accurately despite this artifact.

AP portable films are obtained to evaluate the lung status, gain information on how well lines and tubing are positioned, and see the results of invasive therapeutic maneuvers. Some of the lines and tubes needing evaluation are discussed in the following paragraphs.

ORAL AND NASAL TRACHEAL TUBES. Evaluation of oral and nasal tracheal tubes is necessary to be sure that the inferior tip of the tube comes to rest appropriately 3 to 5 cm above the carina. Accidental placement of the endotracheal tube in the right or left mainstem bronchus or esophagus must be recognized immediately to minimize potential harm to the patient.

CENTRAL VENOUS PRESSURE LINE. Evaluation of the central venous pressure (CVP) line is necessary to be sure that the catheter tip is in proper position. The catheter is placed into either the right or left subclavian or jugular vein and should come to rest in the vena cava or right atrium of the heart. During placement of central catheters, it is possible to enter the lung accidentally by passing through the wall of the vein, entering the pleural space, and thus causing the lung to collapse. If fluids are being delivered (e.g., blood replacement, total parenteral nutrition [TPN]), the fluid will end up in the chest cavity instead of the bloodstream. An AP portable chest film is absolutely required immediately after the line is thought to be in position and before it is sutured in place.

PULMONARY ARTERY CATHETER PLACE-MENT. After the pulmonary artery catheter (Swan-Ganz catheter) is placed, an AP portable x-ray film is important to identify the tip position and the catheter's day-by-day effect on the lung. Catheter placement problems just described relative to CVP lines are equally applicable to pulmonary artery line placement. Fig. 8–2 shows a pulmonary artery catheter in its most common correct position.

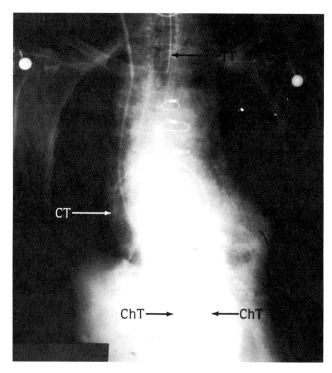

Fig. 8–2 *Pulmonary artery catheter (Swan-Ganz catheter) in its usual position in right lower lung field. This view does not indicate whether the catheter is anterior or posterior within the chest. CT, catheter tip; TT, tracheal tube; ChT, chest tube.*

NASOGASTRIC FEEDING TUBES. Evaluation of nasogastric (NG) feeding tubes is necessary to be sure that they are located appropriately in the stomach and small bowel. Occasionally the NG tube can be accidently inserted into the trachea. An AP portable chest film can identify this complication and avoid further harm to the patient.

CHEST TUBES. Chest tubes placed into the pleural space surrounding the lung have to be evaluated frequently for placement position and therapeutic effect.

PROCEDURES REQUIRING EVALUATION WITH AN AP PORTABLE FILM.

1. *Thoracentesis: temporary placement of a needle into the pleural space to withdraw fluid for analysis (pleural effusion analysis).*
2. *Pericardiocentesis: temporary placement of a needle into the sac surrounding the heart to draw off abnormally accumulated fluid for both treatment and analysis.*
3. *Bronchoscopy: a device used for direct viewing of the larynx, trachea, and large airways can be passed down an oral or nasal tracheal tube. This device, called a bronchoscope, allows for visualization of the trachea and some bronchi. Tissue and secretions can be obtained for analysis, or if a lobe or segment is blocked, the offending blockage can be removed. After this is done, an AP portable x-ray film is obtained to look for any positive or negative effects of the procedure.*

Tomography

Tomograms are a special type of x-ray examination in which the x-ray tube is rotated throughout exposure on an armature above the patient, focusing the rays into a central point or "cut" (Fig. 8–3). In the case of chest tomograms the patient is placed in the supine position on the x-ray table, and the armature holding the x-ray tube is rotated above the patient. Starting at the patient's back as a reference point, consecutive 1-cm cuts are made, moving progressively anteriorly. Tomograms are useful for pinpointing chest lesions, thus detailing their shape and size.

This form of tomography has been replaced almost completely by computed tomography (CT). Other forms of imaging of the body inspired by the concept of tomography have also gained great acceptance. Most noteworthy is magnetic resonance (MR). The clinical use of CT and MR are presented below.

Computed Tomography

Computed tomography (CT scanning) is a high-technology approach to evaluating patients via x-ray examination. The technique requires computed enhancement of x-ray shadows. What results is an amazingly clear look at internal anatomy. CT scanning has revolutionized radiology and is especially useful in pulmonary medicine.

This technique is so widely used in U.S. hospitals that CT scanners are available to scan heads and chests in most hospitals and are used nearly around the clock. Big metropolitan hospitals have these scanners inside emergency rooms for easy evaluation of trauma cases. The technique and equipment has advanced to allow high-resolution CT scanning. This advance has increased the sensitivity of CT scanning to

where lesions can now be detected even before the patient begins to complain of symptoms.

The clarity of the image produced has made CT scanning indispensable in the medical management of pulmonary disease. The only drawback to the use of this technique is its cost, about $800 per procedure. CT scanning is extremely useful in the following areas.

Lung Tumors

Currently the most important use for CT scanning in the lung cancer patient is to determine whether or not a lesion originating outside the chest has metastasized (spread) to the lung. The need for mediastinoscopy has been significantly reduced by the use of CT scanners in this situation. In looking for spread of cancer from extrathoracic sites to the lung, CT scanning is much superior to conventional radiography. High-resolution CT scanning will detect peripheral nodules as small as 2 to 3 mm.

Once a peripheral carcinoma of the lung (coin lesion) has been identified, CT is helpful in placing a biopsy needle into the lesion. Pneumothorax is the main complication and has been reported in from 10% to 60% of cases, with chest tube insertion being required in 5% to 15% of the cases.[1]

Chronic Interstitial Lung Disease

High-resolution CT scanning is superior to conventional films in the evaluation of diffuse, interstitial lung disease (Fig. 8–4). The CT scan will demonstrate considerable changes even when the conventional chest film is read as normal. Well over 100 diseases involve the pulmonary interstitium with 10 of these diseases constituting 80% to 90% of all cases.[2] CT scanning is used selectively because of its high cost. Current research in this area is aimed at identifying the radiographic appearance of each individual interstitial

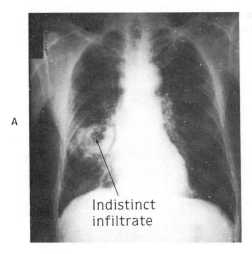
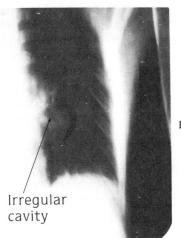

Indistinct infiltrate

Irregular cavity

Fig. 8–3 A, *Lesion in the right lung is indistinct.* **B,** *Single tomographic "cut" taken from a series of cuts done for a tomogram study of the lesion. Every other structure is blurred out except for the lesion in question. Note the irregular cavity highly suggestive of squamous cell carcinoma.*

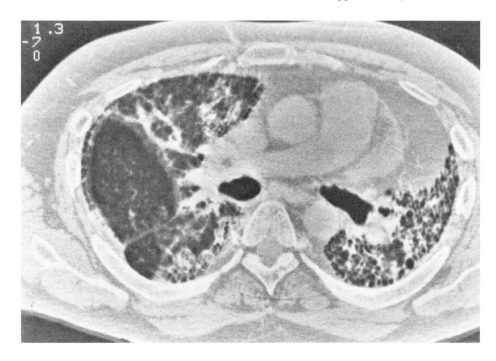

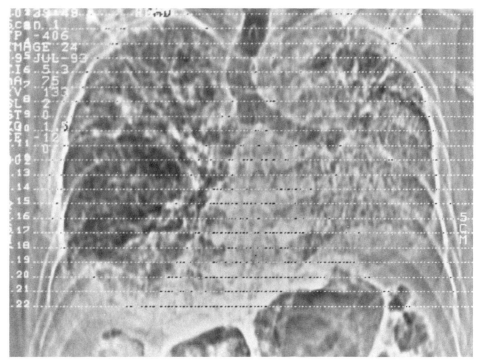

Fig. 8-4 **Top,** *CT scan done for a patient with both bullous emphysema and interstitial lung disease.* **Bottom,** *A scout film with the patient seen on frontal view. The scout film is to reference the cuts as the CT scanning descends down the chest. Detail is poor. Note the tortuous (twisted) trachea, large bullae on the right, and the fibrosis in both lungs, seen on the scout film.* **Top** *shows a cut done below the bifurcation of the trachea. The large bullae in the right chest are now seen in detail. The septa between it and the smaller bullae are seen. Their exact location is now known. Cuts above and below will indicate their size. Throughout both lungs are seen ragged markings indicating severe interstitial fibrosis.*

disease with CT scanning. Eventually this may reduce or eliminate the need for open or closed lung biopsy which is more expensive and dangerous.

Acquired Immune Deficiency Syndrome (AIDS)

Computed tomographic scanning can be useful in the early detection of pneumonias which occur secondary to AIDS. The technique is also useful in detecting abscesses and cavities. The mediastinum can also be evaluated for enlarged lymph nodes secondary to either infection or the lymphoma-like cancers seen in AIDS.[3]

Occupational Lung Disease

The lung diseases resulting from the inhalation of dusts, fumes, irritant gases, organisms, and smoke are called pneumoconioses, or extrinsic alveolitis. Inhaling dusts and fumes can cause numerous respiratory problems such as asthma and pulmonary fibrosis. CT scanning is very helpful in identifying the changes seen in the pleura and the lung parenchyma associated with occupational lung disease. The initial nodules and subsequent fibrosis are clearly seen on CT scan. Pleural plaques seen with asbestosis are readily demonstrated with CT scan.[4]

Pneumonia

The cost of CT has restricted its use in the evaluation of most pneumonias. However, CT scans of the lung are superior to conventional chest films in the visualization of pneumonias and related pathologic changes in the hila and pleura. Opportunistic pneumonias are detected sooner and more precisely by CT as compared to plain films.[5]

Bronchiectasis

In the past, bronchiectasis was visualized best by using the bronchogram. This dangerous and invasive method has now been replaced by the CT scan. The frequency with which unsuspected bronchiectasis is present has surprised many investigators.[6]

Chronic Obstructive Pulmonary Disease

Computed tomographic scans of the emphysematous chest are almost breathtaking in their clarity and detail. The diagnosis of emphysema via conventional radiography is 65% to 80% accurate. With CT scanning, emphysematous changes of even mild to moderate degree are seen with such ease as to make diagnosis consistently in the high 90% range[7] (see Fig. 8-4).

Magnetic Resonance Imaging

The role of MR imaging in the diagnosis of intrathoracic lung disease has been limited. It has been used in conjunction with CT scans but so far MR imaging has added little or no new information to the understanding of lung disease. The one area in which MR imaging may be a little better than CT scanning is in the evaluation of hila. MR imaging is better able to differentiate hilar lymph node enlargement from enlarged hilar blood vessels than is CT.[8] This information is critical in determining to what extent lung cancer has spread. The patient is inoperable if a lung cancer has spread to the hilum and thus enlarged it.

Another area where MR imaging may be superior to the CT scan is in the evaluation of chest wall invasion by lung cancer and in the evaluation of the specific cancer called Pancoasts tumor or superior sulcus tumor (Fig. 8-5). These tumors occur high in the lung and invade the nearby chest wall. The axillary nerves and superior mediastinal blood vessels may also be involved in the tumor spread.[9] MR imaging can determine the precise position of the tumors and the involvement with surrounding structures.

Lung Scanning

Lung scans are obtained by measuring gamma radiation emitted from the chest after radiopharmaceuticals are injected into the bloodstream or inhaled into the lung. This procedure, once thought of as a sophisticated research technique, is now widely available. Lung scanning is useful for studying the distribution of ventilation and perfusion and the effect disease may have on these two important functions. The major clinical application of lung scanning is in the evaluation of patients suspected of having a pulmonary embolism.

To perform perfusion lung scans, particulate radionuclides are injected into a peripheral vein. The venous blood flow then carries the particles to the pulmonary circulation where the radionuclides lodge in the pulmonary capillaries because the particles are larger than the capillaries. The particles remain lodged for a considerable time and can be scanned to identify the distribution of perfusion in the lungs (Fig. 8-6). A reduction in pulmonary blood flow to a part of the lung can be detected because the radioactivity over the affected area is decreased. This reduction in blood flow occurs with pulmonary embolism or any respiratory disease such as atelectasis or pneumonia that causes a localized area of vasoconstriction.

Ventilation lung scans are performed by having the patient breathe a radioactive gas or a nebulized aerosol of a radioactive material. Poorly ventilated regions can be easily detected because the radioactive material will not enter the affected lung regions. The

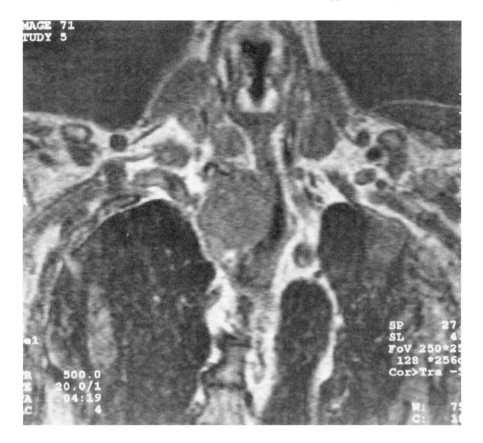

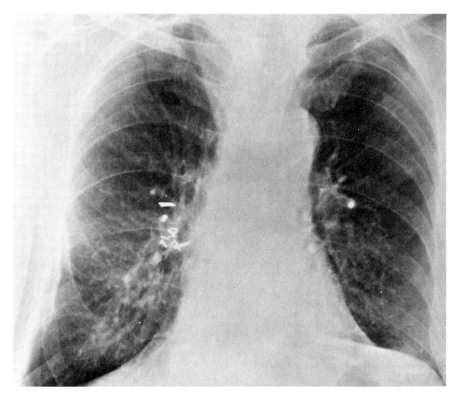

Fig. 8–5 **Top,** *Magnetic resonance (MR) imaging shows an apical tumor in the right lung displacing the trachea to the left.* **Bottom,** *Except for a slight leftward shift of the trachea, the standard x-ray film gives no clue that there is a cancer hidden in the right apex.*

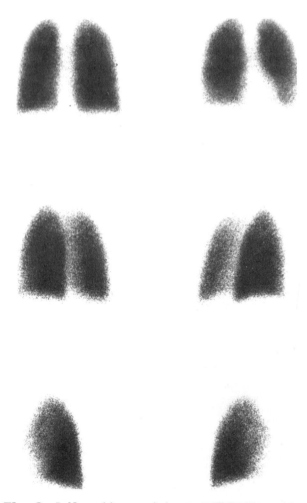

Fig. 8-6 *Normal lung perfusion scan. There is no evidence of perfusion defects in the anterior, posterior, oblique, or lateral views of the lungs.*

ventilation scan is then compared with the perfusion scan to identify the matching of ventilation to perfusion (Fig. 8-7). When a pulmonary embolism is present, the ventilation scan is usually normal, while the perfusion scan shows a defect in the affected region. If the patient has pneumonia or atelectasis, both ventilation and perfusion scans will be abnormal. In some cases of pulmonary embolism, the clot may cause atelectasis in the affected region and therefore lead to abnormal ventilation and perfusion. In such cases the lung scan results are not diagnostic for pulmonary thromboembolic disease.

The diagnosis of pulmonary embolism is frequently difficult. The current approach is to obtain a ventilation-perfusion scan as the first step. The current radiology wording for reporting the results of a ventilation-perfusion scan is "high probability," "indeterminant," or "low probability." "High probability" suggests that the scan is positive for pulmonary embolism but not 100% conclusive since lung scans are not diagnostic. "Indeterminant" indicates that the lung scan has an abnormality but the defect may or may not be consistent with a pulmonary embolism. "Low probabil-

ity" suggests that the lung scan is not demonstrating an abnormality typical of pulmonary embolism.

A recently reported large multicenter study has confirmed the concerns of clinicians having to diagnose patients with pulmonary embolism using Ventilation-perfusion scans and this reporting system. "High probability" scans are false-positive 12% to 14% of the time and "low probability" scans miss 16% to 40% of patients that have pulmonary embolism. This means that 12% to 14% of patients can potentially come under prolonged therapy with dangerous blood thinners (heparin and coumarin for at least 2–4 months) or that 16% to 40% of patients may not be treated for a condition that is life-threatening.[10] The solution to the problems lies in the use of the more invasive pulmonary angiogram.

Pulmonary Angiography

Angiography of the pulmonary circulation is most often done to evaluate thromboembolic disease of the lungs. It is generally done only after lung scanning and when results of the ventilation-perfusion scan are uncertain. To perform pulmonary angiography a contrast medium is injected into the pulmonary artery or into one of its branches. Angiographic proof of pulmonary embolism is considered to be identification of one or more filling defects (Fig. 8-8). The decision to use it must be made carefully since this procedure is invasive and costly.

Evaluation Of The Chest Radiograph

This section is intended to introduce the basic principles involved with evaluation of the chest radiograph. It cannot teach the reader to interpret chest films any more than a book on surgery can teach the reader to operate. Interpreting chest films is a skill obtained only through hours of dedicated practice. The beginner is encouraged to view chest films initially with the help of qualified experts.

Familiarity with the anatomic landmarks seen on normal chest films is extremely helpful in learning to recognize abnormalities. Fig. 8-9 identifies the more important landmarks on a normal PA chest radiograph.

Review of Clinical Findings

The clinician will benefit from reviewing the patient's history and physical examination findings before viewing the chest film. This information can provide insight into the abnormalities to be looked for on the chest film.

Placing the Chest Film on the View Box

The chest film must be placed on the view box as if the patient were facing the clinician (i.e., the right side of

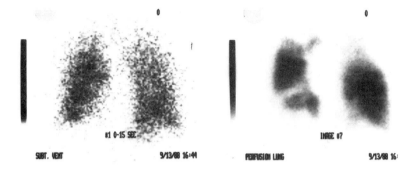

Fig. 8-7 *Abnormal ventilation-perfusion scan. The ventilation study (left scan) demonstrates bilateral lung filling without gross defects; however, the perfusion scan (right scan) shows multiple subsegmental perfusion defects of both lungs. These findings are highly suggestive of pulmonary emboli.*

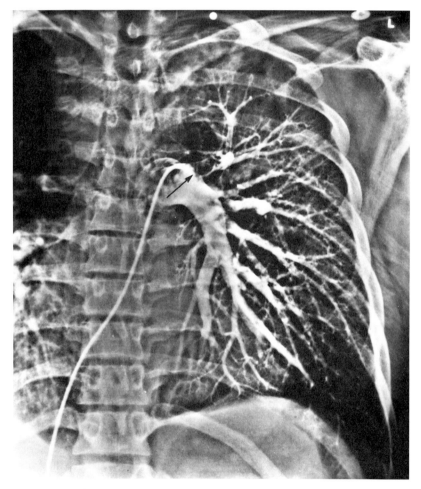

Fig. 8-8 *Abnormal pulmonary angiogram. The radiograph demonstrates a large clot in the pulmonary vascular tree. A small amount of dye was able to slip around the clot and outline the embolus (arrow).*

the patient's chest is on the clinician's left, and vice versa). The left side of the patient's chest is easily identified by looking at the cardiac shadow, which is most often prominent on the left side of the chest. Also, the letters *L* and *R* identifying the patient's left and right sides may be visible to assist in identifying the correct placement. Once the film is on the view box, the nameplate should be inspected to make sure that the name on the film matches the name of the patient being evaluated.

The first step in evaluating the chest film is to determine the technical quality of the film. The adequacy of exposure can be judged by looking at the vertebral bodies. The clinician should just be able to visualize the vertebral bodies through the cardiac shadow. If the vertebral bodies are easily seen, the film

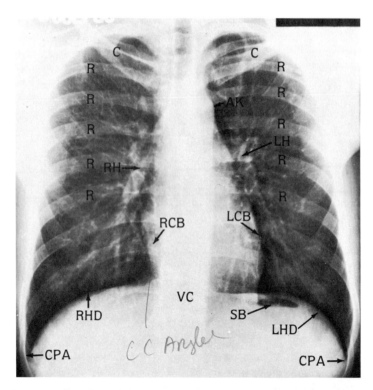

Fig. 8-9 *Posteroanterior chest x-ray film. Some important structures: right hemidiaphragm (RHD), left hemidiaphragm (LHD), costophrenic angles (CPA), right cardiac border (RCB), left cardiac border (LCB), vertebral column (VC), aortic knob (AK), stomach bubble (SB), right hilum (RH), left hilum (LH), rib (R), and clavicle (C).*

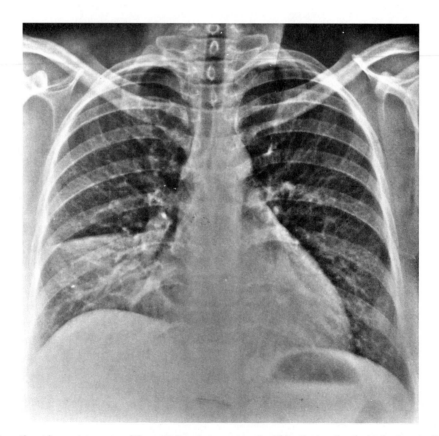

Fig. 8-10 *Note how the spinous processes of the vertebrae are centered within the tracheal air shadow indicating that the patient was not rotated when the chest film was obtained. Also note the consolidation in the patient's right lung. The infiltrate must be in the right middle lobe because the right heart border is blurred (see description of silhouette sign in text).*

is probably overexposed and the lungs will appear black. Underexposure makes identification of the vertebral bodies more difficult, and the lung fields appear whiter than on a properly exposed film. The pulmonary vascularity and some pulmonary abnormalities may be misinterpreted with overexposure or underexposure.

The film should be evaluated to make sure that the patient was not rotated when the chest film was obtained. If the patient has been rotated, uniform exposure of both lungs will not be obtained, and one side of the film will be darker than the other. Patient rotation is assessed by identifying the relationship of the spinous processes of the vertebral column to the medial ends of the clavicles or to the tracheal air shadow (Fig. 8–10). The spinous processes should be centered between the ends of the clavicles and directly behind the tracheal air shadow. If the medial end of one clavicle appears closer to the spine or if the spinous processes are to the side of the tracheal air shadow, the patient was probably rotated.

Finally, the degree of the patient's inspiratory effort is evaluated by counting the posterior ribs visible above the diaphragm. On a PA film, ten ribs indicate a good inspiratory effort. A poor inspiratory effort may cause the heart to appear abnormally enlarged and increase the density of the lung fields so that they appear too white to allow detection of certain lung abnormalities.

Interpretation

Interpretation of the chest film requires a complete understanding of the x-ray principles introduced at the beginning of this chapter. The clinician must remember that x-ray penetration of structures is inversely proportional to the density of the structure. The greater the density, the less the penetration. X-rays that do not penetrate fully are absorbed, resulting in less exposure of the film and the casting of a white shadow on the film.

Normal lung tissue has a low density (air density), and normal lung fields appear as dark shadows on the chest film. If an area of the lung consolidates (increases in density) because of pneumonia, tumor, or collapse, that area will absorb more x-rays and appear as a white patch on the film. Abnormalities that decrease lung tissue density, such as cavities and blebs, absorb fewer x-rays and result in darker areas on the film.

The heart, diaphragm, and major blood vessels are considered to have the density of water. Since water is more dense than air, water densities result in less exposure and therefore whitish-gray shadows on the film. The heart, diaphragm, and major blood vessels rarely alter in density, but may change in size, shape, and position. Evaluation of the shadows produced on the chest film by these structures allows a clear view of any deviation from normal in position or size.

The structures in the chest with the greatest density are the bones, including the ribs, clavicles, scapulae, and vertebrae. They are seen on the film as white shadows. Fractures and changes in position and density of bones may be evaluated with the chest film. A chest film should be obtained to evaluate the bony structures of the chest whenever the patient's history or physical examination suggests chest trauma. A recent history of an automobile accident or blunt chest injury from any sudden impact indicates that a chest film is needed to assess the patient.

Identification of the abnormalities visible on the chest film requires a systematic review of all the structures shown on the film. The sequence in which the structures are evaluated is not important as long as all are included. Many experts encourage beginners to develop a habit of evaluating the bony structures and peripheral areas of the chest film first. This helps prevent overlooking subtle but important abnormalities in the less conspicuous areas of the film. Once the peripheral soft tissues and bony structures have been viewed, the lung, mediastinum, heart, and diaphragms are carefully inspected. A system using the alphabet, A to Z, to remind the examiner which parts of the chest film to study has been recommended. This system, starting with *A* for *a*irway, and *B* for *b*ones, *C* for *c*ardiac shadow, and so forth, may prove useful in organizing the approach to reading the chest radiograph.

The ability to localize (identify the position of) abnormalities within the thorax is aided by special radiographic signs. Two of the most important and reliable methods are the silhouette sign and the air bronchogram.

SILHOUETTE SIGN. The silhouette sign is primarily useful in determining if a pulmonary infiltrate is in anatomic contact with a heart border. Normally, the significant difference in density between the heart and lung tissue results in sharply delineated heart borders. If the lung tissue in contact with either heart border becomes consolidated, the contrast in densities is lost and the corresponding heart border will be blurred (Figs. 8–10 and 8–11).

Since the heart is located in the anterior thorax, any infiltrate that obliterates the heart border must also be located in the anterior segments of the lungs. Infiltrates that appear to overlap the heart border on the film but do not affect its sharpness are located in posterior segments and are not in anatomic contact with the heart.

AIR BRONCHOGRAM. The air bronchogram is useful in determining if an abnormality seen on the radiograph is located within the lung. Normally the intrapulmonary bronchi are not visible on the chest film, since they contain air and are surrounded by air-filled alveoli. If the bronchi are surrounded by consolidated alveoli, they will be visible because the air

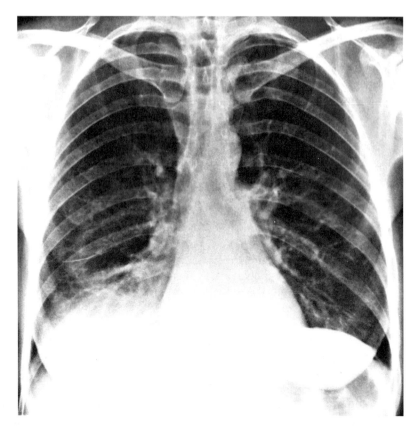

Fig. 8–11 *Right lower lobe pneumonia. Note how the right heart border is clearly seen indicating that the infiltrate must be in the lower lobe, which is posterior to the heart. Also note that the right hemidiaphragm is obscured. This provides further evidence that the consolidation is in the right lower lobe.*

within their lumina will stand out in contrast to the surrounding consolidation. In this situation the bronchi are seen as linear branching air shadows, signifying that the lesion is within the lungs and not located in the pleural space.

The air bronchogram is often seen in pneumonia and pulmonary edema. However, if the lesion fills the bronchi as well as the alveoli, air bronchograms will not be seen, since no contrast is present. Therefore the absence of the air bronchogram is of little significance.

Limitations of the Chest Radiograph

Though the chest radiograph provides important information regarding the pathologic changes within the thorax, it does have certain limitations. Small lesions and those located in "blind" areas may not be seen. Additionally, the chest film is often normal in patients experiencing significant respiratory symptoms. A typical example is the patient with asthma experiencing acute bronchospasm. Even though the patient may be experiencing cough and shortness of breath, the chest radiograph often appears normal.

Clinical and Radiographic Findings In Lung Diseases

This section reviews the radiographic findings typical of the more common respiratory disorders. Familiarity with this information is very helpful in the interpretation of chest films. In addition, this section presents the clinical findings typically associated with the different pathologic abnormalities described. In most cases the most efficient and accurate assessment is achieved when clinical and radiographic findings are used together. The following categories of chest diseases are presented:

1. Atelectasis
2. Hyperinflation
3. Interstitial lung disease
4. Congestive heart failure
5. Pleural effusion
6. Consolidation

Atelectasis

Loss of air in a portion of lung tissue results in a condition called atelectasis (Fig. 8–12). *Atelectasis* is formed from the Greek *ateles* (incomplete) and *ektasis* (extension). Atelectasis may occur as a result of changes in the transpulmonary distending pressure and in such cases is called *compressive atelectasis*. It may also be caused by obstruction of one or more airways, which allows distal gas to be absorbed (Fig. 8–12). The latter type of atelectasis may be referred to as *obstructive* or *absorption atelectasis*.

COMPRESSIVE ATELECTASIS. Compressive atelectasis is seen in patients with pleural effusion, pneumothorax, hemothorax, and any space-occupying lesion. The degree of pulmonary compromise with compressive atelectasis is dependent on the size of the lesion. Small lesions may not disrupt pulmonary function significantly; however, larger lesions may compromise cardiac function as well as lung function if the mediastinum is shifted.

OBSTRUCTIVE ATELECTASIS. Obstructive atelectasis emphasizes the blockage of an airway(s) so that ventilation of the affected region is absent. Many clinical situations can obstruct an airway leading to collapse (atelectasis). When this happens, usually entire lobes or segments are involved rather than subsegments or smaller units (microatelectasis). Tumor, aspirated foreign substances, fibrosis, mucus plugging, mechanical obstruction, and scarring are some of the more common causes of obstructive atelectasis (See Fig. 8–12).

As long as the airway obstruction remains incomplete, the distal lung will remain inflated. In fact partial obstruction of a bronchus can lead to hyperinflation of the lung if the obstruction causes a one-way valve effect, allowing air to enter the lung but not escape. Complete obstruction of a larger airway usually leads to atelectasis of the distal lung; however, collateral ventilation may occur through alveoli ventilated by unobstructed airways and thus maintain partial alveolar patency.

A related form of atelectasis occurs in patients following surgery. It is not uncommon for atelectasis to develop in the postoperative period, especially if the patient has had upper abdominal or thoracic surgery or if the patient is obese or has a history of chronic lung disease. After surgery lung secretions have a tendency to be retained in the lung because of mucociliary stasis and suppression of coughing and deep breathing. Retained secretions can obstruct multiple distal airways leading to underventilation and atelectasis of the affected region.

The physical examination findings of atelectasis vary with the amount of lung involved. With significant loss of lung volume, as occurs with lobar collapse, the findings are striking and usually include the following:

1. Rapid shallow breathing
2. Decreased to absent breath sounds
3. Decreased to absent vocal fremitus

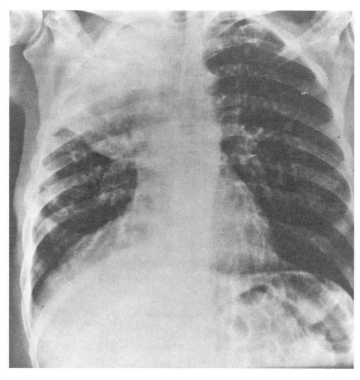

Fig. 8–12 *This patient's right upper lobe has become consolidated because of a tumor obstructing the right upper lobe bronchus. As a result, pneumonia has developed behind the obstruction. Note the well-outlined horizontal fissure, slightly rotated up and delineating the inferior boundary of the right upper lobe.*

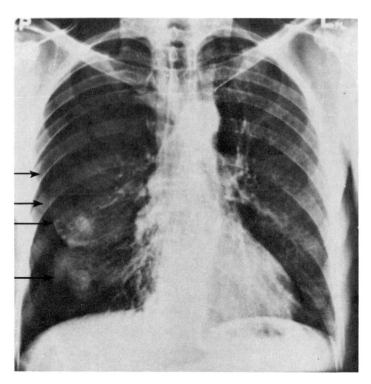

Fig. 8–13 *Good example of pneumothorax involving the right lung. Note the line along the right lateral chest wall where the lung has pulled away from the chest wall as it collapsed toward the hilum.*

4. Dullness to percussion
5. Cyanosis
6. Shift of the mediastinum toward the affected side

The chest radiograph in most cases will readily demonstrate the loss of lung volume caused by the atelectasis. With collapse of entire segments or lobes, characteristic densities will be seen. Shift of the trachea, heart, and major thoracic vessels toward the affected side is often seen. The radiographic findings seen with postoperative atelectasis are often more subtle.

Abnormalities may not be detected during physical examination of the patient with atelectasis. If an entire lobe is collapsed (atelectatic), the surrounding healthy lung tissue may expand into the space previously occupied by the atelectatic region. Thus no abnormalities may be detected over the affected region. Careful examination of the chest film and other clinical findings are needed to detect this condition. The chest radiograph may not readily demonstrate the atelectasis when the degree of atelectasis is small. In these cases more subtle signs of collapse must be looked for on the film. These signs include:

1. Shift of the fissure lines toward the collapsed area (See Fig. 8–12)
2. Movement of the hilar structures toward the area of collapse
3. Overall loss of volume in one lung
4. Hemidiaphragm elevation

Pneumothorax

Pneumothorax is an extreme form of atelectasis (Fig. 8–13). Pneumothorax is a condition in which air enters the pleural space either externally from a hole in the chest wall or internally from a hole in the lung. This leads to loss of the negative pressure normally found in the pleural space. As a result, the lung's normal elasticity, which causes it to contract, is unopposed, and the lung "collapses."

This is serious enough, but the lung can develop a potentially more serious problem called a *tension pneumothorax*. With a tension pneumothorax the hole formed has a flap on it which acts as a valve as the person breathes. The effect is to pump air into the pleural space, which now has positive pressure in it. This pressure eventually shifts the heart away from the involved lung and puts pressure on the good lung, altering blood and lymph flow. The good lung's ability to oxygenate is severely compromised, and the heart may not pump blood effectively. Not all pneumothoraces develop "tension." Clinical situations predisposing a person to pneumothorax are the following:

1. Trauma, such as an automobile accident, or stab wounds to the chest
2. Fractured ribs poking through the pleural space
3. Hospital procedures such as chest surgery thoracentesis, or placement of a CVP line, hyperalimentation line, or pulmonary artery catheters

4. Elevated mean airway pressures, as occur during positive pressure ventilation with stiff lungs
5. Spontaneous rupture of blebs along the lung margins
6. Improper placement of an oral or nasal tracheal tube, resulting in the tip of the tube coming to rest in either the right or left mainstem bronchi.

Physical findings associated with pneumothorax without tension reveal the following:

1. Chest wall—reduction in movement in the chest wall on the side where the pneumothorax has occurred
2. Auscultation of the lung—loss of breath sounds or at least distant breath sounds on the affected side
3. Percussion—increased resonance to percussion on the affected side
4. Heart—usually a rapid heart rate (tachycardia) and tachypnea
5. Other—cyanosis, an external wound, or bruising with a "sucking" noise on the involved side, usually seen when a tension pneumothorax is present
6. Absent whispered voice sounds and tactile fremitus

With a tension pneumothorax, shift of the mediastinal structures—the trachea, heart, and lung—away from the involved side results in deviation of the trachea from the affected side. In Fig. 8–13 the chest film shows a pleural line that comes down the right side of the chest wall and even shows the invagination caused by the horizontal fissure. With the lung pulled away from the chest wall it is easy to see why there is a decrease in breath sounds and increased resonance with percussion during physical examination.

Hyperinflation

The most common cause of hyperinflation is obstructive lung disease. The diagnosis of chronic obstructive pulmonary disease (COPD) does not depend solely on radiographic changes. The history, physical examination, and pulmonary function data are crucial. The chest film reveals dependable, consistent changes that help support the diagnosis of asthma, chronic bronchitis, and emphysema—the three diseases that constitute COPD. In some cases of COPD the chest film may be read as normal, especially when the disease process is mild.

The functional residual capacity (FRC), residual volume (RV), and total lung capacity (TLC) increase and are seen as hyperinflation on the chest radiograph with COPD. The specific findings of hyperinflation seen on the chest film (Figs. 8–14, *A* and *B*) are as follows:

1. Large lung volumes
2. Increased anterior airspace as seen on the lateral film (See Fig. 8–14, *B*),

3. Depressed diaphragms
4. Small narrow heart, especially with emphysema
5. Enlarged intercostal spaces

The physical examination findings that correlate with the x-ray examination include the following:

1. Large barrel chest with increased AP dimension of the chest wall
2. Increased resonance to percussion
3. Decreased breath sounds
4. Limited motion of low-set diaphragms
5. Wheezing (may not be present with fatigue)
6. Prolonged expiratory phase
7. Rapid respiratory rate
8. Use of accessory muscles to breathe

Interstitial Lung Disease

Many diseases can cause a pattern on the chest film referred to as *interstitial lung disease* (Figs. 8–15, 8–16, and 8–17). Fortunately, it occurs in a relatively small number of patients. A listing of the diseases causing this type of infiltrate is included to acquaint the reader with the terms (see accompanying box).

The basic pathologic process associated with pulmonary fibrosis is shown in Fig. 8–15. Some substance (etiologic agent) insults the lung's immune system causing the lung to scar or become fibrotic. The fibrotic process is usually progressive leading to more and more scarring of the lung with each passing year. The end result for the majority of these patients is combined cardiac and respiratory failure after many years of a slow, progressively debilitating disease. In a few instances the disease is self-limiting, and spontaneous cures have been seen.

Initially, the patient afflicted with interstitial lung diseases may notice a dry, nonproductive cough and dyspnea on exertion (DOE). This usually brings the patient in for medical care. The history is probably the most important element in helping to decide what has incited the immune response, causing the lung damage. A history of industrial exposure to silica or asbestos is crucial. A history of systemic symptoms such as swallowing disorders or joint or muscle pain may suggest a collagen-vascular disease causing the fibrosis.

The pattern seen on the chest film may give a clue to etiology (see Fig. 8–16). Upper lobe fibrosis is unusual. Most of the time the fibrotic infiltrates occur in the lower lobes; however, ankylosing spondylitis, tuberculosis, and silicosis all have a predilection for the upper lobes. If the pattern of fibrosis present is favoring the upper lung fields, the disorders just mentioned are suggested.

The term *alveolar pattern* is favored by some and disliked by others when referring to interstitial lung disease. The term has some usefulness in helping to identify the disease by looking at the pattern of the

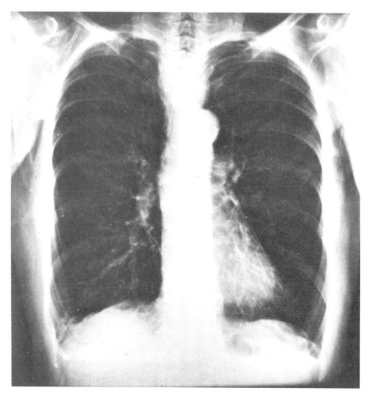

Fig. 8–14 A *Posteroanterior chest film. Marked hyperinflation with large lung volumes, low-set diaphragm, small narrow heart, and enlarged intercostal spaces.*

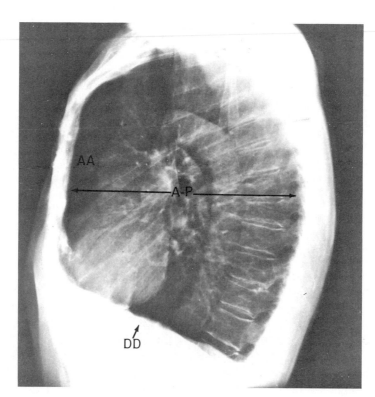

Fig. 8–14 B *Lateral view. Hyperinflation is manifested by increased anterior airspace, depressed diaphragm, and increased anteroposterior chest dimensions (barrel chest). Anterior airspace (AA), depressed diaphragm (DD), and anteroposterior dimension (A-P).*

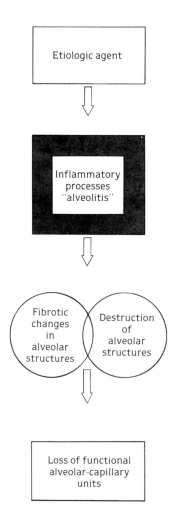

Fig. 8-15 *Theoretic explanation for development of pulmonary fibrosis. Patients who develop interstitial fibrosis are prone to develop other complications such as pneumothorax, cancer, and pneumonia. (Adapted from Simmons DH:* Current pulmonology, *New York, 1981, John Wiley & Sons.)*

INTERSTITIAL LUNG DISEASES*

Infections

Viruses: measles, chickenpox, influenza

Rickettsiae: Q fever, Rocky Mountain spotted fever

Bacteria: tuberculosis; mycoplasm, staphylococcal, and streptococcal infection; *Klebsiella*; salmonellosis; others

Fungi: histoplasmosis, coccidioidomycosis, others

Parasites

Occupational causes

Mineral dusts: asbestosis, silicosis, berylliosis, others

Chemical fumes: nitrogen dioxide, ammonia, chlorine, acetylene, many others

Neoplastic causes

Bronchioalveolar carcinoma, hematogenous metastases, lymphangitis, leukemia, lymphoma

Congenital or familial causes

Cystic fibrosis, Niemann-Pick disease, Gaucher's disease, tuberous sclerosis, familial dysautonomia (Riley-Day syndrome), pulmonary alveolar microlithiasis, familial idiopathic pulmonary fibrosis

Metabolic causes

Uremic pneumonitis

Physical agents

Postirradiation fibrosis, thermal injury, oxygen toxicity, blast injury

Circulatory causes

Thromboembolism

Hemodynamic, congestive heart failure

Immunologic causes

Hypersensitivity pneumonia: inhaled antigens, drug reactions

Collagen diseases: scleroderma, rheumatoid arthritis, lupus erythematosus, Wegener's granulomatosis, dermatomyositis, Goodpasture's syndrome

Unknown

Sarcoidosis, histiocytosis X, idiopathic hemosiderosis, pulmonary alveolar proteinosis, desquamative interstitial pneumonia, idiopathic fibrosis

*Adapted from Braunwald E and others, editors: *Harrison's principles of internal medicine,* ed 11, New York, 1987, McGraw Hill.

---

infiltrate. The alveolar pattern results when the alveoli begin to fill up with water, blood, pus, protein, or cells (see Fig. 8-17). If the patient is coughing up any of these materials or has been known to have inhaled some of these substances (e.g., near-drowning victims), the pattern on the x-ray film is better understood (see accompanying box).

The alveolar pattern of pulmonary fibrosis may lead to visualization of air bronchograms. This occurs as a result of the alveolar spaces becoming infiltrated and more dense. The air-filled airway is seen as clear and as a dark straight shadow with several attached branchings. Around the area is a whitened ground-glass–appearing area, representing affected alveolar spaces.

Physical examination of the patient with interstitial lung disease typically identifies a rapid and shallow

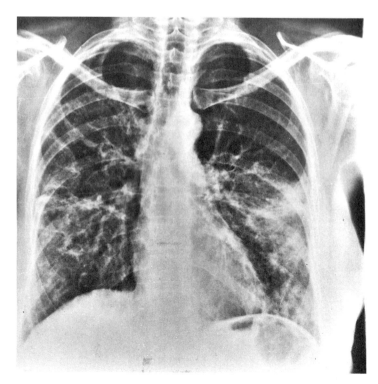

Fig. 8–16 *Severe interstitial fibrosis in the chest. Note patch of pneumonia in left lower lung field of this patient's chest.*

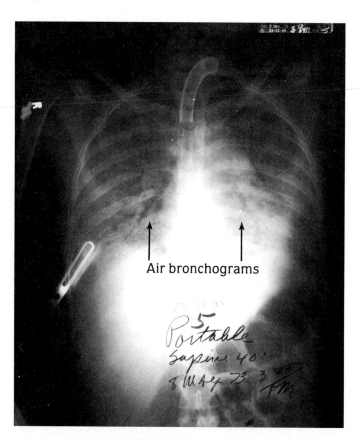

Fig. 8–17 *Typical alveolar filling pattern.*

breathing with a smaller tidal volume. As the tidal breathing pattern. The interstitial fibrosis causes a decrease in lung compliance that results in the patient volume decreases, the respiratory rate must increase to maintain adequate ventilation. Auscultation usually identifies fine inspiratory crackles that do not clear with deep breaths or changes in position. The crackles are often more noticeable over the lower lobes. If the interstitial lung disease is severe, significant hypoxemia and cyanosis may be present.

The final diagnosis of interstitial lung disease usually requires the physician to obtain a piece of lung either by open lung biopsy or transbronchial biopsy using a flexible bronchoscope. Even after a lung biopsy, the final diagnosis and determination of the cause with this group of diseases are often difficult.

Congestive Heart Failure

Pulmonary edema can be diagnosed by many different routes, but perhaps the earliest indication is obtained with the chest film. Early hidden congestive heart failure (CHF) causes definite changes in the chest film (Fig. 8–18). These changes include the following:

1. *Redistribution of pulmonary vasculature to the upper lobes. Usually the normal chest film shows the pulmonary blood vessels prominent in the lower lobes. With CHF, fluid collects in the dependent portions of the lung. The ability to exchange oxygen in these lower lung fields is impeded. To compensate for this altered physiology, the blood flow is redirected to the upper lung fields where the lung tissue is still free of edema fluid. With CHF, the chest film shows enlarged prominent blood vessels in the upper lobes where they should be small and barely noticeable.*
2. *Increase in the ratio of the width of the heart at its greatest span to the width of the thorax—the cardiothoracic (C/T) ratio. Normally, this ratio should not exceed 0.5. In CHF the heart enlarges and its width exceeds one half of the width of the thoracic cage. This enlargement (an excessive increase in the C/T ratio) is abnormal and consistent with CHF (see Fig. 8–18).*
3. *Development of of Kerley's B lines. These lines, usually seen in the right base, are 1 mm thick and approximately 1 to 2 cm in length. They are horizontal and start at the periphery, extending into the lung approximately 1 to 2 cm. They are pleural lymphatic vessels filled with fluid (see Fig. 8–18).*
4. *Miscellaneous signs.*
   a. Increased interstitial markings.
   b. Pleural effusion in the right hemithorax only.
   c. Enlarged pulmonary artery segments.

ALVEOLAR SPACE PATHOLOGY

Alveolar space fills with	Possible causes
Water	Congestive heart failure
	Drowning or near drowning
Blood	Goodpasture's syndrome
	Idiopathic pulmonary hemosiderosis
Purulent exudate (pus)	Pneumonia
Protein	Pulmonary alveolar proteinosis
Cells	Desquamative interstitial pneumonitis
	Bronchioalveolar (alveolar cell) carcinoma

The alveolar pattern exists when the following is noted on the chest x-ray film in contrast to the interstitial pattern:

Interstitial pattern	Alveolar pattern
Peripheral distribution (especially in lower lobes)	Perihilar in distribution
Small volume with contracted lungs	Minimal volume loss
Linear stranding	Early in the process small mulberry-like infiltrates are seen; later, nodules are seen that coalesce into a ground-glass appearance
No air bronchogram	Air bronchogram is seen

CHF in patients with severe hyperinflation (especially emphysema) may not result in some of the signs just mentioned. The development of an enlarged heart may be delayed in patients with emphysema because of the pathologic changes already present in the thoracic

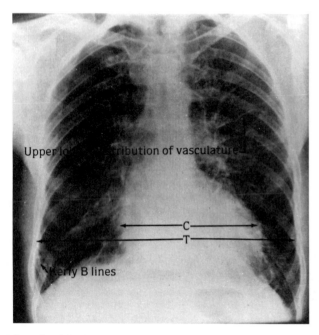

Fig. 8–18 *Congestive heart failure with upper lobe redistribution of vasculature markings, especially on the right, increased cardiothoracic (C/T) ratio, Kerley's B lines, and increased interstitial markings. Cardiac shadow should not be over half of the entire width of the thoracic cage. Here it is well over half.*

cage. With tissue destruction, common in emphysema, redistribution to the upper lobes may already have occurred before CHF develops. Also, redistribution in such cases may not occur when the vascular bed has been altered by bullae.

The physical examination findings that correlate with the x-ray findings center around crackles (rales) at the bases. The crackles may be heard in the apices in more severe cases. The patient has a rapid respiratory rate and is anxious, usually sitting upright to breathe and resisting lying down because of the dyspnea associated with reclining (orthopnea). Other important findings that relate to CHF are associated with cardiac abnormalities. The patient's neck veins are distended, and on auscultation of the heart, the following are noted:

1. Rapid heart rate, either regular or irregular in rhythm. (The rhythm regularity is vital and must be noted.)
2. Third heart sound (S_3), a consistent finding in CHF.
3. Murmurs, usually not present if CHF is the only cardiac abnormality.
4. Increased closure sound of the pulmonary component of the second heart sound.

Other findings outside the chest but related to CHF include the following:

1. Enlarged liver (hepatomegaly).
2. Pulsus alternans—on palpating the peripheral pulse, a strong pulsation alternates with a weak one. This is an indicator of severe heart failure.

3. Ankle edema (swelling) that is pronounced during the day and improves after a night of sleep. This is usually accompanied by having to get up several times each night to urinate (nocturia).

Historically, the patient complains of nocturia, orthopnea, coughing (sometimes productive of a bloody and frothy sputum), and paroxysmal nocturnal dyspnea (attacks of severe shortness of breath that awaken the patient from sleep). Fatigue and weakness are frequent complaints.

Pleural Effusion

Free fluid may form in the intrapleural space (Figs. 8–19 and 8–20). Usually 100 mL must be present before the fluid can be seen on the chest radiograph. The fluid can be a clear watery material, low in protein content (less than 3 g/L), called a *transudate,* or more commonly a fluid with a high protein content, (over 3 g/dL) called an *exudate.*

The causes of transudative pleural effusion are limited and include CHF and atelectasis. The possible causes of exudative pleural effusions are more numerous and include, among others, bacterial pneumonia, pulmonary embolism, malignancy, viral disease, tuberculosis, and fungal infections.

Other free fluids can collect in the pleural space. These include blood (hemothorax), a fatty fluid called chyle (chylothorax), and pus (empyema or pyothorax). The chest x-ray findings of pleural effusion depend on the volume of fluid collected in the pleural space. Small volume findings (see Fig. 8–19) are

1. Blunting of the otherwise sharp angle between the chest wall and the point at which the diaphragm touches the chest wall laterally—the costophrenic (CP) angle
2. Small meniscus sign. The meniscus sign is seen whenever fluid starts to track up the side of the chest wall, much as water slides for a short distance up the side of a glass container, thus forming a meniscus
3. Partially obscured diaphragm with elevation of the diaphragm from its normal position

Large (massive) volume findings (see Fig. 8–20) are

1. Complete "whiteout" of the involved side
2. Complete obscuring of the hemidiaphragm

If there is a question as to whether or not an effusion is present, or if the fluid is free to move about, a lateral decubitus film is obtained. This helpful study requires only that the patient lie on the side suspected of having the pleural effusion while the radiograph is taken. This is called the *lateral decubitus view* (Fig. 8–21). The special positioning of the patient allows for visualization of a fluid line on the chest film.

The physical findings with pleural effusion are related to the volume of free fluid in the chest. The patient may complain of pain on inspiration, a dull "heavy" feeling in the involved area, coughing, or shortness of breath. Small volumes of fluid are

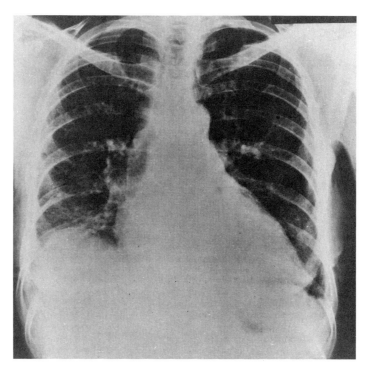

Fig. 8–19 *A small pleural effusion has developed in the right chest, resulting in a blunted right costophrenic angle and partially obscured right hemidiaphragm.*

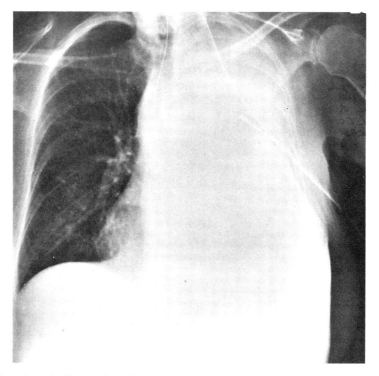

Fig. 8–20 *Large massive pleural effusion involving the left hemidiaphragm. This has caused the x-ray film to appear as a "whiteout" of the involved side, completely obscuring all structures in the left chest.*

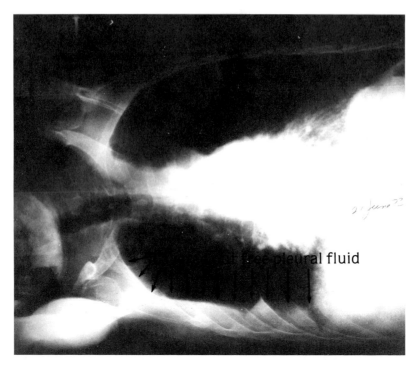

Fig. 8–21 *Patient lying on side so that pleural effusion fluid has moved by gravity to the dependent area of the chest cavity (line indicated by arrows). This is called a lateral decubitus view. Important information is available from this view: confirmation of the effusion's presence and the fact that the effusion is free and not loculated, or trapped by adhesions in one area of the chest cavity.*

symptom-free and undetectable on physical examination. However, when the size of the pleural effusion is significant, the findings may include the following:

1. Dullness to percussion in the involved area
2. Egophony just above the area of dullness
3. Decreased breath sounds on the affected side
4. Tachypnea

Consolidation

A section of lung can become airless, fill up with fluid, and not collapse. In this instance the involved lung area is said to be consolidated. The usual cause for this state is bacterial pneumonia. Many times the bacterial pneumonia is secondary to obstruction of the airways by aspirated foreign bodies (e.g., peanuts or very small toys) or tumorous growths. Figs. 8–10 and 8–11 show good examples of consolidation. The radiographic signs of consolidation include the following:

1. Minimal loss of volume
2. Usually lobar distribution
3. Homogeneous density late in the process
4. Air bronchogram if the airway leading to the consolidated area is open

The physical findings associated with a consolidated lung include the following:

1. Dullness to percussion over the involved area
2. Bronchophony and bronchial breath sounds
3. Crackles often heard over the involved area
4. Whispered voice sounds increased, and egophony present (if airway is patent)
5. Tachypnea and fever

The patient reports typical symptoms associated with pneumonia. These include a cough with sputum production, weakness, fever and chills, chest pain (pleuralin nature), and shortness of breath. If the consolidation is chronic, the patient may have mild symptoms. Surprisingly, some patients with a consolidated lung may not request medical care for some time because the symptoms are minimal.

REVIEW QUESTIONS

1. T F X-rays are produced by positron emission.

2. T F Increasing object density increases the amount of x-ray penetration.

3. Which of the following is not a radiographic density?
   a. water
   b. air
   c. mineral
   d. fat

4. T F An item that is white on the radiograph would be called radiopaque.

5. Which of the following is true regarding the distance between the x-ray source, film, and patient when taking a chest x-ray?

a. distance has no effect on the image on the film

b. as the distance between the source and the patient decreases magnification increases

c. as distance between the source and patient decreases the image becomes sharply focused

d. none of the above

6. Which of the following is the standard distance between the x-ray source and the film for a posteroanterior x-ray?
   a. 3 feet
   b. 4 feet
   c. 5 feet
   d. 6 feet

7. In which of the following situations would a chest x-ray not be indicated?
   a. during cardiopulmonary resuscitation
   b. after intubation to assess the position of the endotracheal tube
   c. to assess the progression of a patient's pneumonia
   d. to check the effectiveness of chest physical therapy

8. Which of the following is/are true regarding a posteroanterior chest x-ray?
   a. patient rotation is usually present and makes interpretation difficult
   b. heart size is subject to less magnification
   c. it is the standard for bedridden hospitalized patients
   d. all of the above

9. Which of the following views helps to evaluate for the presence of small amounts of free pleural fluid?
   a. apical lordotic
   b. expiratory
   c. oblique
   d. lateral decubitus

10. T F Chest x-rays are normally taken during a full inspiration.

11. Which of the following problems may be associated with a portable (anteroposterior) chest x-ray?
    a. poor radiographic exposure
    b. patient is not centered on the film
    c. artifactual shadows may be present on the film
    d. all of the above

12. Which of the following films is especially helpful in identifying a pneumothorax?
    a. lateral
    b. oblique

c. expiratory
d. lateral decubitus

13. Correct positioning of an endotracheal tube is confirmed if the tip of the tube is approximately ____ cm above the carina on the chest x-ray.
    a. 0–1
    b. 2–3
    c. 3–5
    d. 7–9

14. Which of the following cannot be assessed via the use of a chest x-ray?
    a. CVP line position
    b. chest tube position and effectiveness
    c. nasogastric tube placement
    d. cardiac pacemaker effectiveness

15. T F Tomography is especially useful in visualizing masses in the mediastinum and chest.

16. Which of the following is/are true regarding the use of MRI in lung disease?
    a. it is widely used
    b. it is a very useful diagnostic tool for detecting pulmonary problems
    c. it is better than CT in evaluating the hilar areas for lymph node and vascular enlargement
    d. all of the above

17. Which of the following is/are true regarding lung scanning?
    a. it can be used to detect abnormalities in ventilation compared to perfusion
    b. it utilizes radioactive tracers
    c. can be used to detect pulmonary thromboembolism
    d. all of the above

18. T F Pneumonia can cause a decrease in perfusion and ventilation on a lung scan.

19. Which of the following is the best method to evaluate for the presence of the thromboembolism?
    a. lung scan
    b. angiography
    c. CT
    d. MRI

20. T F An x-ray is considered well exposed if the thoracic vertebrae are easily visible through the heart shadow on an AP or PA film.

21. The depth of inspiration on an x-ray is adequate if 10 posterior ribs are visible above the diaphragm on a PA or AP film.

a. 5
b. 7
c. 8
d. 10

22. T F *Interpretation of the chest x-ray primarily involves identification of abnormal findings.*

23. *What is the significance of the silhouette sign?*
    a. *it allows differentiation between alveolar and interstitial infiltrates*
    b. *it can aid in detecting pleural effusion*
    c. *it helps determine the anterior or posterior position of an infiltrate based on the appearance of the heart shadow*
    d. *all of the above*

24. T F *A chest x-ray can be normal in the presence of significant pulmonary disease.*

25. *Which of the following clinical or chest x-ray findings are consistent with a tension pneumothorax?*
    a. *increased radiolucency on the affected side*
    b. *mediastinal shift toward the pneumothorax*
    c. *dullness to percussion on the affected side*
    d. *bronchial breath sounds on the affected side*

26. *Which of the following are radiographic signs of atelectasis?*
    a. *increased radiopacity*
    b. *hemidiaphragm elevation*
    c. *hilar shift toward atelectasis*
    d. *all of the above*

27. *Which of the following could be seen on a chest x-ray of a patient with congestive heart failure?*
    a. *low and flat diaphragms*
    b. *increased cardiothoracic ratio*
    c. *tracheal deviation*
    d. *increased retrosternal airspace on a lateral film*

28. *Which of the following clinical or chest x-ray findings might be found in a patient with consolidation due to pneumonia?*
    a. *lobar radiopaque pattern of the infiltrate*
    b. *increased resonance to percussion over the affected area*
    c. *stridorous breath sounds upon auscultation of the affected area*
    d. *all of the above*

29. *Which of the following chest x-ray findings is (are) consistent with hyperinflation?*
    a. *large lung volumes*
    b. *widened intercostal spaces bilaterally*

c. *small and narrow heart*
d. *all of the above*

30. *Which of the following chest x-ray findings is* not *consistent with a small pleural effusion?*
    a. *air bronchograms on the affected side*
    b. *blunted costophrenic angle*
    c. *"meniscus" sign*
    d. *partially obscured and elevated hemidiaphragm*

REFERENCES

1. Gardner D and others: CT-guided transthoracic needle biopsy, *Cardiovasc Int Radiol* 14:17–23, 1991.23.
2. Hansell DM: Computed tomographic diagnosis of diffuse lung disease, *Curr Opin Radiol* 69–78, 1992.
3. Naidich DP and McGuinness G: Pulmonary manifestations of AIDS: CT and radiographic correlations, *Radiol Clin North Am* 29:999–1017, 1991.
4. Aberle DR and Balmes JR: Computed tomography of asbestos related pulmonary parenchymal and pleural diseases, *Clin Chest Med* 12:115–131, 1991.
5. Hommeyer SH, Godwin JD, and Takasugi JE: Computed tomography of air-space disease, *Radiol Clin North Am* 29:1065–1084, 1991.
6. Westcott JL: Bronchiectasis, *Radiol Clin North Am* 29:1031–1042, 1991.
7. Sanders C: The radiographic diagnosis of emphysema, *Radiol Clin North Am* 29:1019–1030, 1991.
8. Gualdi GF, Volpe A, Polettini E, and Jula GF: Computed tomography and magnetic resonance in the TNM staging of pulmonary carcinoma [in Italian], *Clin Ter* 141:493–498, 1992.
9. Weinreb JC: Thoracic magnetic resonance imaging, *Clin Chest Med* 12:33–54, 1991.
10. *Medical knowledge self-assessment program IX, pulmonary medicine and critical care, 1992,* part C, book 3, p. 884.

BIBLIOGRAPHY

Felson B: *Chest roentgenology,* Philadelphia, 1973, WB Saunders.
Fraser R and Pare J: *Diagnosis of diseases of the chest,* vols 2 and 3, ed 3, Philadelphia, 1989, WB Saunders.
Lillington GA: Roentgenographic diagnosis of pulmonary disease. In Burton GG, Hodgkin JE, and Ward JJ, editors: *Respiratory care: a guide to clinical practice,* ed 3, Philadelphia 1991, JB Lippincott.
Murray JF and Nadel JA: *Textbook of respiratory medicine,* Philadelphia, 1988, WB Saunders.
Rau JL and Pearce DJ: *Understanding chest radiographs,* Denver, 1984, Multi-Media.
Sheldon RL and Dunbar RD: Systematic analysis of the chest radiograph. In Scanlon CL, Sheldon RL, and Spearman CB, editors: *Egan's fundamentals of respiratory therapy,* ed 5, St Louis, 1990, Mosby–Year Book.
Smith JP and Pierson DJ: Diagnostic imaging. In Pierson DJ and Kacmared RM, editors: *Foundations of respiratory care,* New York, 1992, Churchill Livingstone.

Chapter 9

Bedside Interpretation of Electrocardiogram Tracings

Robert L. Wilkins

LEARNING OBJECTIVES

Upon completion of this chapter, the reader should be able to accomplish the following:

1. *List or identify the clinical value of the electrocardiogram (ECG).*

2. *Identify the clinical findings that indicate the need for an ECG recording.*

3. *Identify the key components of the electrical conduction system of the heart and the role of each component.*

4. *Recognize a definition of depolarization and repolarization.*

5. *Identify the specific electrical activity of the heart associated with each wave and interval of the normal ECG.*

6. *Identify normal values for the P-R interval and the QRS complex.*

7. *Given a 12-lead ECG recording, identify the ventricular rate and position of the mean QRS vector.*

8. *List the steps for ECG interpretation.*

9. *Identify the criteria for each of the following abnormalities:*
   a. *sinus bradycardia*
   b. *sinus tachycardia*
   c. *sinus dysrhythmia*
   d. *premature atrial contraction*
   e. *atrial flutter*
   f. *atrial fibrillation*
   g. *premature ventricular contractions*
   h. *ventricular tachycardia*
   i. *ventricular fibrillation*
   j. *asystole*
   k. *first, second, and third degree A-V block*

10. *Identify the ECG abnormalities associated with chronic obstructive lung disease.*

Chapter Overview

This chapter describes the electrophysiology of normal and abnormal electrocardiogram (ECG) tracings. Ultimately, it is intended to teach you how to recognize basic and life-threatening ECG patterns that may occur during care of patients with cardiopulmonary disease. After a review of cardiac physiology related to the production of electrical activity within the heart, numerous abnormal rhythms (dysrhythmias) are described. Criteria for recognition and possible causes are reviewed for each abnormality presented.

What Is an ECG?

An ECG (also referred to as EKG) is a recording of the electrical currents in the heart. This recording is obtained by placing electrodes on the surface of the patient's body. The traditional ECG is made by attaching electrodes (also called leads) to each limb and to numerous locations on the chest wall to create a 12-lead ECG. The purpose of using 12 leads is to obtain 12 different views of the electrical activity in the heart and therefore a more complete picture.

In the intensive care unit, 2 leads are usually attached to the patient's chest to monitor the heart continuously. Although monitoring the heart with 2 chest leads is not an ECG by definition, in clinical practice it is referred to as *ECG monitoring.* Continuous ECG monitoring allows clinicians to identify gross changes in heart rate and rhythm rapidly; however, a 12-lead view is needed when more details are required to assess the heart. For the remainder of this chapter, *ECG* refers to the 12-lead ECG unless otherwise stated.

What Is the Value of an ECG?

The ECG can be very helpful in identifying the primary cause of the patient's symptoms or in detecting the impact disease in other body systems, such as the lungs, has had on the heart. The ECG can also indicate the severity of the problem (e.g., myocardial infarction) and, in many cases, the response to treatment. Therefore, several ECGs may be needed over the course of treatment.

It is important to note that the ECG tracing does not measure the pumping ability of the heart. It is not unusual for a patient with a low cardiac output to have a normal ECG tracing. This is because the ECG does not directly depict abnormalities in cardiac structure such as defects in the heart valves or interventricular septum. Another limitation worth noting is that the probability of any patient having an acute problem such as myocardial infarction cannot be predicted from a resting ECG tracing.

When Should an ECG Be Obtained?

Since an ECG is noninvasive and does not represent a significant risk to the patient, it is reasonable to obtain an ECG whenever the patient has signs and symptoms suggestive of an acute cardiac disorder such as myocardial infarction. The patient with a cardiac problem may have chest pain, orthopnea, paroxysmal nocturnal dyspnea, night sweats, syncope, palpitations, pedal edema, hypotension, or diaphoresis. Of course the process of obtaining the ECG should never delay the initiation of critically needed care such as oxygen therapy, airway placement, or cardiopulmonary resuscitation (CPR).

An ECG can also be used as a screening tool to determine the patient's health status prior to major surgery. An ECG is especially helpful in this situation if the patient is older or has a past history of heart disease. If an abnormality is identified, it may need to be treated before the operation is performed.

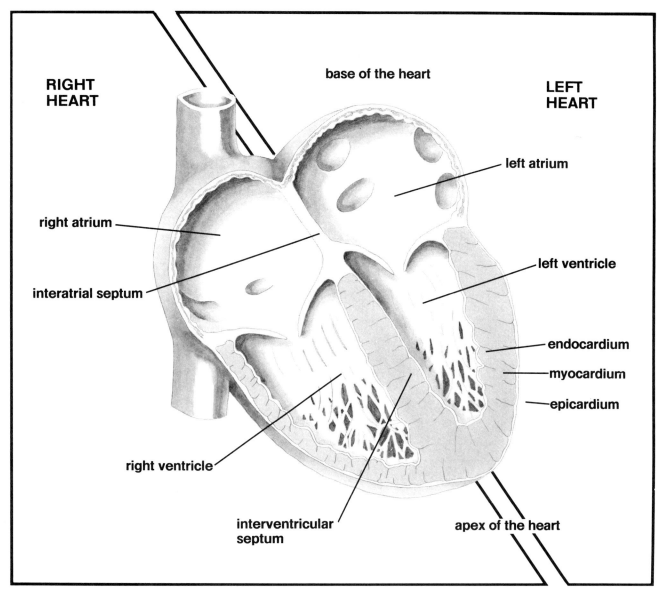

RIGHT
HEART

base of the heart

LEFT
HEART

left atrium

right atrium

interatrial septum

left ventricle

endocardium

myocardium

epicardium

right ventricle

interventricular
septum

apex of the heart

Fig. 9-1 *Anatomy of the heart. (From Huszar RH:* Basic dysrhythmias: interpretation and management, *St Louis, 1988, Mosby–Year Book.)*

Cardiac Anatomy and Physiology

A review of cardiac anatomy and the physiology related to electrical activity within the heart is helpful before discussing the interpretation of ECGs. The heart is made up of four chambers: two upper chambers called *atria* and two lower chambers called *ventricles* (Fig. 9-1). The heart is typically described as having two sides, the right side and the left side. The right side is made up of the right atrium and right ventricle. The right atrium receives deoxygenated blood from the venae cavae and directs the blood into the right ventricle. The right ventricle is responsible for pumping the blood into the pulmonary system for oxygenation. The oxygenated blood returns to the left side of the heart where the left ventricle is responsible for pumping it into the systemic circulatory system. Since the left side of the heart has to pump blood throughout the entire body it normally has a larger muscle mass than the right side.

Cardiac muscle has the ability to pump blood because it can contract in response to electrical stimulation. In order for the heart to move blood effectively, stimulation of the heart muscle must be coordinated. Initiating and coordinating the electrical stimulation of the heart muscle is the responsibility of the electrical conduction system, which is made up of special pacemaker and conducting cells (Table 9-1).

Normally the electrical activity of the heart starts in the sinus or sinoatrial (SA) node, which is located in the right atrium (Fig. 9-2). The SA node is a collection

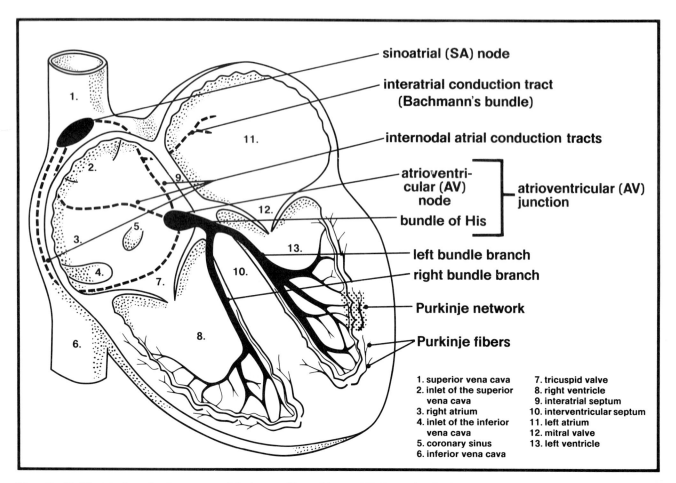

Fig. 9-2 *Electrical conduction system of the heart. (From Huszar RH:* Basic dysrhythmias: interpretation and management, *St Louis, 1988, Mosby–Year Book.)*

1. superior vena cava
2. inlet of the superior vena cava
3. right atrium
4. inlet of the inferior vena cava
5. coronary sinus
6. inferior vena cava
7. tricuspid valve
8. right ventricle
9. interatrial septum
10. interventricular septum
11. left atrium
12. mitral valve
13. left ventricle

Table 9-1	Types of Heart Cells
Pacemaker cells	Specialized cells that have a high degree of automaticity and provide the electrical power source for the heart
Conducting cells	Cells that conduct the electrical impulse throughout the heart
Myocardial cells	Cells that contract in response to electrical stimuli and pump the blood

of specialized cells capable of generating electrical signals. Cells that have the ability to generate electrical activity spontaneously are said to have *automaticity*. Because the SA node normally has the greatest degree of automaticity of all the cardiac cells, it usually controls the rate at which the heart beats. In this way, the SA node serves as the pacemaker of the heart.

The SA node is strongly influenced by the autonomic nervous system. For this reason the rate at which the SA node fires can vary significantly. Increased activity of the sympathetic system increases the heart rate, whereas vagal stimulation slows the heart rate. Stimulation of the sympathetic system and an increase in heart rate occurs with stress, anxiety, exercise, and with the administration of certain drugs.

Once the SA node initiates the electrical signal, the impulse spreads across the atria in a wavelike fashion. The electrical impulse travels through the atria by way of the internodal pathways, causing depolarization and then contraction. Contraction of the atria is helpful in filling the ventricles with blood just prior to ventricular contraction (systole).

After the electrical impulse passes through the atria it reaches the atrioventricular (AV) junction. This junction acts as an electrical "bridge" between the atria and the ventricles. The AV junction contains within it the AV node and the bundle of His (Fig. 9-2). Once the electrical impulse reaches the AV node it is delayed for approximately 0.1 second before passing on into the bundle of His. The delay is believed to serve the purpose of allowing more complete filling of the ventricles prior to ventricular contraction. In addition, the AV node can serve to protect the ventricles from excessively rapid atrial rates that the ventricles could not tolerate.

The AV node normally only guides the electrical impulse from the atria into the ventricles. Under certain circumstances, however, it can serve also as the backup pacemaker. This is because the AV node has automaticity qualities similar to those of the SA node. If the SA

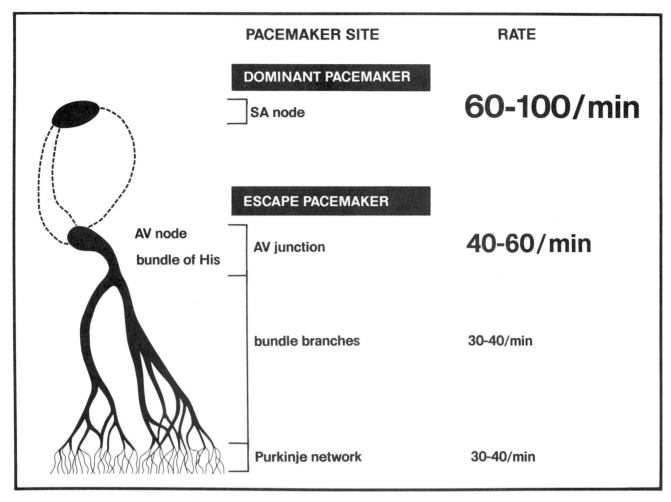

PACEMAKER SITE	RATE
DOMINANT PACEMAKER	
SA node	**60-100/min**
ESCAPE PACEMAKER	
AV junction	**40-60/min**
bundle branches	30-40/min
Purkinje network	30-40/min

AV node
bundle of His

Fig. 9-3 *Dominant and escape pacemakers. (From Huszar RH:* Basic dysrhythmias: interpretation and management, *St Louis, 1988, Mosby–Year Book.)*

node fails to function properly and does not pace the heart, the AV node can serve as the pacemaker for the ventricles. When this occurs, the ventricular rate is usually between 40 and 60 beats per minute and the ECG reveals a distinct pattern, described later in this chapter (Fig. 9–3).

After the electrical impulse leaves the AV node, it travels rapidly through the bundle of His and then into the left and right bundle branches (see Fig. 9–2). The stimulus travels simultaneously through the bundle branches into the ventricular muscle (myocardium). At the end of the bundle branches are countless fingerlike projections called *Purkinje fibers.* The Purkinje fibers pass the electrical impulse rapidly throughout the myocardium to create a coordinated contraction of the left and right ventricles.

Since most of the cardiac cells have automaticity characteristics, the heartbeat may be paced by heart tissue other than the SA node. When this occurs it often indicates that the SA node is not functioning normally or that myocardial tissue is irritated. Any impulse that originates outside the SA node is referred to as an *ectopic impulse,* and the site from which the ectopic

impulse originates is called the *focus.* Ectopic impulses can originate from foci in either the atria or the ventricles. When the ectopic impulse results from depression of the normal impulse origin, it is called an *escape beat.*

The heart muscle must receive a constant supply of oxygen and nutrients to pump blood effectively. Oxygen and nutrients are supplied to the myocardium via the left and right coronary arteries and their branches. The main coronary arteries arise from the ascending aorta, and direct arterial blood into branches which feed various regions of the heart. Blockage of one or more of the coronary vessels leads to regionalized ischemia and tissue death (infarction). The size and location of the region affected by the coronary vessel blockage determines the resulting physiologic and clinical impact. Infarction of a major portion of the left ventricle is likely to cause significant arterial hypotension, abnormal sensorium, and a backup of blood into the pulmonary circulation. Infarction of the tissues associated with pacing the heart (e.g., the SA or AV node) can lead to significant dysrhythmias and diminished blood flow to all regions of the body.

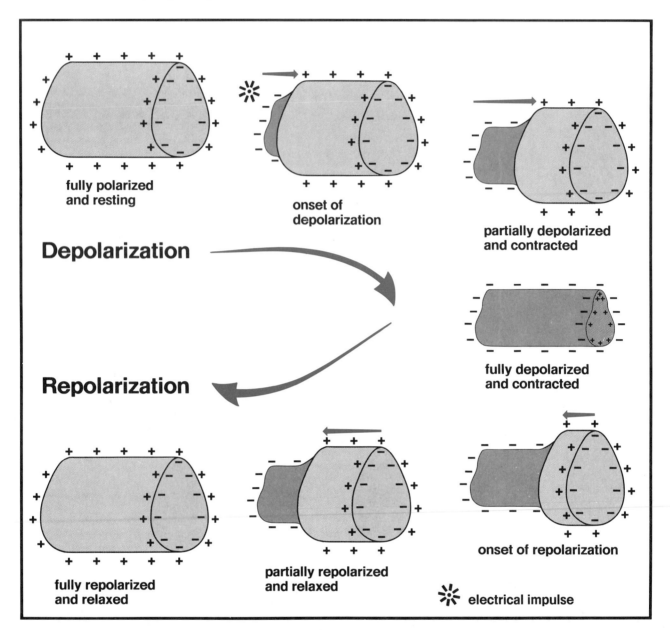

fully polarized
and resting

onset of
depolarization

partially depolarized
and contracted

Depolarization

fully depolarized
and contracted

Repolarization

onset of repolarization

fully repolarized
and relaxed

partially repolarized
and relaxed

❋ electrical impulse

Fig. 9-4 *Depolarization and repolarization of a cardiac cell. (From Huszar RH:* Basic dysrhythmias: interpretation and management, *St Louis, 1988, Mosby–Year Book.)*

Basic ECG Waves

The spread of electrical stimuli throughout the heart causes depolarization of the myocardial cells. Depolarization occurs when a polarized cell is stimulated. Polarized cells carry an electrical charge on their surface, the inside of the cell being more negatively charged than the outside of the cell. The sudden loss of the negative charge within the cell is termed *depolarization;* the return of the electrical charge (negative charge within the cell) is termed *repolarization* (Fig. 9–4). The waves of electrical activity traveling back and forth across the heart, created by the process of depolarization and repolarization, are detected by the ECG electrodes.

Depolarization of the atria creates the initial wave of electrical activity detected on the ECG tracing, known as the *P wave* (Fig. 9–5). Since the atria are usually small, the P wave is typically also small. The normal P wave is less than 2.5 mm in height and not more than 3 mm in length. Repolarization of the atria is not seen on the ECG, because it is usually obscured by the simultaneous depolarization of the ventricles.

Depolarization of the ventricles is represented by the *QRS complex.* Since the ventricular muscle mass is larger than the atria, the QRS complex is taller than the

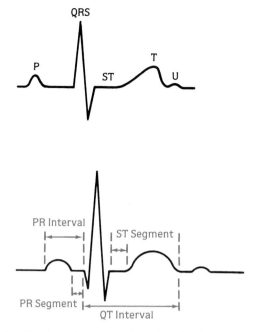

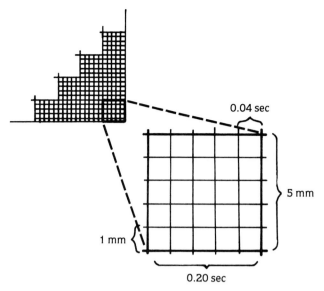

Fig. 9-7 *Gridlike boxes of ECG paper illustrating the 1-mm and 5-mm boxes.*

Fig. 9-5 *Normal configuration of the ECG waves, segments, and intervals.*

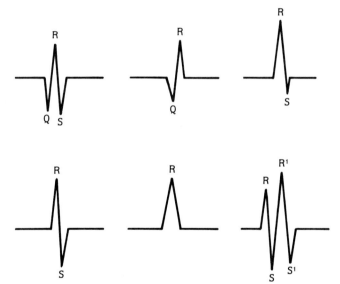

Fig. 9-6 *QRS nomenclature. See text.*

P wave in most cases (see Fig. 9-5). Ventricular repolarization is seen as the *T wave*. The T wave is normally upright and slightly rounded.

Just after the T wave and before the next P wave, a small deflection known as the *U wave* is sometimes seen. The U wave is thought to represent the final phase of ventricular repolarization. In most cases the U wave is not seen. The clinical significance of its presence or absence is not known.

QRS complexes usually consist of several distinct waves, each of which has a letter assigned to it as a label. This labeling system is needed because the

precise configuration of the QRS complex can vary from one lead to the next and from one patient to the next. To establish a standardized labeling system several guidelines have been developed. If the first deflection of the QRS complex is downward (negative) it is labeled a *Q wave*. The initial upward (positive) deflection is called an *R wave*. The first negative deflection following an R wave is called an *S wave* (Fig. 9-6). If the QRS complex has a second positive deflection it is labeled *R′* (R prime), and if a second S wave is also present it is called *S′* (S prime). A negative deflection can only be termed a *Q wave* if it is the first wave of the complex. In clinical practice, each ventricular depolarization complex is referred to as a *QRS complex* whether it has all three waves or not.

ECG Paper and Measurements

The electrical activity of the heart is recorded on special paper that has gridlike boxes with light and dark lines running horizontally and vertically (Fig. 9-7). The light lines circumscribe small boxes (1 mm × 1 mm) and the dark lines circumscribe larger boxes (5 mm × 5 mm).

Time is measured on the horizontal axis of the ECG paper. The ECG paper moves through the electrocardiograph at a speed of 25 mm/sec. Therefore each small square (1 mm) represents 0.04 second and each larger square (5 mm) represents 0.2 second. Five large boxes represent 1.0 second.

On the vertical axis, voltage, or amplitude of the ECG waves, is measured. The exact voltage of any ECG wave can be measured, because the electrocardiograph is standardized so that 1 mV produces a deflection 10 mm in amplitude. Therefore the standard for most ECG recordings is 1 mV = 10 mm.

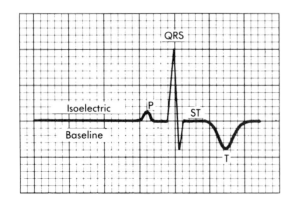

Fig. 9–8 *Isoelectric baseline used for measuring voltage of ECG waves.* (From Goldberger AL and Goldberger E: Clinical electrocardiography, *ed 3, St Louis, 1986, Mosby–Year Book.*)

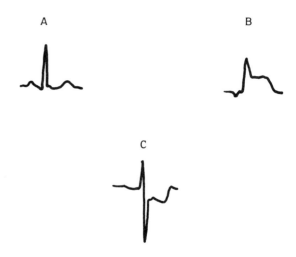

Fig. 9–9 *ST segments.* **A,** *Normal.* **B,** *Abnormal elevation.* **C,** *Abnormal depression.*

In order to measure the amplitude of a specific wave, the isoelectric baseline must be identified. This is the flat line seen just before the P wave or right after the T or U wave (Fig. 9–8). Any movement of the ECG stylus above this line is considered positive; any downward movement is considered negative. To measure the degree of positive or negative amplitude of a specific wave, the isoelectric line is used as a reference point marking zero voltage.

R waves are measured from the isoelectric line to the top of the R wave. Q and S waves are measured from the isoelectric line to the bottom of the wave (see Fig. 9–6). P waves can be either positive or negative and are also measured from the isoelectric line to the top (if positive) or bottom (if negative) of the wave.

In addition to the amplitude of any wave, the duration of waves, intervals, and segments can be measured. A *segment* is a straight line between two waves. An *interval* encompasses at least one wave plus the connecting straight line.

A common interval that is important to measure is the *P-R interval.* This interval is measured from the beginning of the P wave, where the P wave lifts off the isoelectric line, to the beginning of the QRS complex (see Fig. 9–5). The P-R interval represents the time it takes for the electrical stimulus to spread through the atria and to pass through the AV junction. The normal P-R interval is between 0.12 and 0.2 second (three to five small boxes). If conduction of the impulse through the AV junction is abnormally delayed, the P-R interval will exceed 0.2 second. A prolonged P-R interval is referred to as *first degree block* and is discussed later in this chapter.

The duration of ventricular depolarization is determined by measuring the *QRS interval.* This interval is measured from the first wave of the QRS complex to the end of the last wave of the QRS complex. Normally the QRS interval does not exceed 0.12 second (three small boxes).

A very important segment to evaluate is the *ST segment.* This segment is the portion of the ECG cycle from the end of the QRS complex (even if no S wave is present) to the beginning of the T wave (see Fig. 9–5). It measures the time from the end of ventricular depolarization to the start of ventricular repolarization. The normal ST segment is isoelectric (no positive or negative voltage) or at least does not move more than 1 mm above or below baseline. Certain pathologic abnormalities such as myocardial infarction will cause the ST segment to be elevated or depressed (Fig. 9–9). The duration of the ST segment is not as important as its configuration.

The *R-R interval* is useful in identifying the rate and regularity of ventricular contraction. The distance in millimeters is determined from one R wave to the next in successive QRS complexes. This is done for several different R-R intervals. ECG calipers can be helpful in making this measurement. The average of the measurements is determined and converted to time. Remember that each large box is equal to 0.2 second and five large boxes equal 1.0 second. If the R-R interval is 1.5 seconds, the heart rate is 40 beats per minute. If the R-R interval is 1.0 second, the heart rate is 60/min. If the R-R interval is 0.5 second, the heart rate is 120/min. This method for determining the heart rate is easy to apply if the R-R interval falls conveniently on one of the numbers just described. Unfortunately, this is not usually the case. Other methods for calculating the heart rate are described below. Marked variation in the R-R interval from one interval to the next indicates that the heartbeat is irregular and may be a sign of sinus arrhythmia, which is described in more detail later in this chapter.

The *Q-T interval* is measured from the beginning of the QRS complex to the end of the T wave (see Fig. 9–5). This interval represents the time from the beginning of ventricular depolarization to the end of ventricular repolarization. The normal values for the Q-T interval depend on the heart rate. As the heart rate increases, the Q-T interval normally shortens; as the heart rate decreases, the Q-T interval increases. As a general rule, the Q-T interval that exceeds one half of the R-R interval is prolonged provided the heart rate is 80/min or less. Common causes of an abnormally prolonged Q-T interval include hypokalemia (low potassium), hypocalcemia (low calcium), and the side effects of certain medications such as quinidine.

EVALUATING HEART RATE. If the heart rate is regular, one of the easiest ways of determining the heart rate is to count the number of large (0.2 second) boxes between two successive QRS complexes and divide this number into 300. For example, if there is one large box between successive R waves, then each R wave is separated by 0.2 second. Over the course of 1.0 second there will be 5 QRS complexes and 300 QRS complexes in 60 seconds. Therefore the heart rate is 300/min. Following this logic:

2 large boxes = rate of 150/min (300/2 = 150)
3 large boxes = rate of 100/min (300/3 = 100)
4 large boxes = rate of 75/min (300/4 = 75)
5 large boxes = rate of 60/min (300/5 = 60)
6 large boxes = rate of 50/min (300/6 = 50)

If the heart rate is irregular, this method will not be accurate, since the spacing between QRS complexes will vary from beat to beat. In such cases the average rate can be determined by counting the number of QRS complexes in a 6-second interval and multiplying the number by 10. Since the top of the ECG paper is marked with small vertical dashes every 3 seconds, 6-second intervals are easy to identify.

An increase or decrease in heart rate by more than 20% of the baseline value is a significant change and should be evaluated further. An abnormally slow heart rate may reduce cardiac performance to the point where perfusion is compromised. An abnormally rapid heart rate will increase myocardial oxygen demand, possibly to the point of inducing ischemia. An increase in heart rate above 130/min may compromise cardiac performance. Significant tachycardia reduces the ventricular filling time, and as a result cardiac output will diminish. As diastolic period shortens, coronary perfusion may diminish, since the majority of the coronary perfusion normally occurs during diastole.

ECG Leads

Since the heart is a three-dimensional organ, a more complete picture of the electrical activity in the heart will be obtained if it is viewed from several different angles. The standard ECG uses 12 different leads to provide 12 different views from different angles of the heart. Interpretation of the 12 leads is a little more difficult, but the information obtained is more complete and abnormalities are not likely to be missed.

The 12 leads can be subdivided into two groups: 6 extremity (limb) leads and 6 chest leads. To obtain the 6 limb leads, 2 electrodes are placed on the patient's wrists and 2 on the patient's ankles. The ECG machine can vary the orientation of these 4 electrodes to one another to create the 6 limb leads. The chest leads are created by attaching 6 electrodes across the patient's chest. The chest leads will be discussed after reviewing the limb leads.

Limb Leads

The 6 limb leads are called leads I, II, III, aV_R, aV_L, and aV_F. Leads I, II, and III are bipolar: each is created by comparing the difference in electrical voltage between two electrodes. For lead I the ECG machine temporarily designates the electrode on the left arm as a positive lead and the electrode on the right arm as negative. The measured difference in voltage between these two leads results in lead I. For lead II the right arm electrode remains negative and the left leg electrode is positive. Lead III is created by making the left arm negative and the left leg positive.

The other three limb leads (aV_R, aV_L, and aV_F) are called augmented leads because the ECG machine must amplify the tracings to get an adequate recording. This is because the augmented leads are created by measuring the electrical voltage at one limb lead with all other limb leads made negative. For the augmented leads the ECG machine must augment the recorded voltages by about 50% to get an adequate recording. Lead aV_R is created by making the right arm positive and all the others negative. Lead aV_L calls for the left arm to be positive and lead aV_F is created by making the left leg positive.

The 6 limb leads view the heart in a vertical plane called a *frontal plane*. Any electrical activity that is directed up or down or left or right will be recorded by the limb leads (Fig. 9–10). The frontal plane can be envisioned as a giant circle that surrounds the patient and lies in the same plane as the patient. This circle can be marked off in 360 degrees as shown in Fig. 9–10.

The angle of orientation for each of the bipolar limb leads can be determined by drawing a line from the designated negative lead to the designated positive lead. For lead I, the angle of orientation is 0 degrees; for lead II, 60 degrees; and for lead III, 120 degrees. For the augmented leads the angle of orientation can be determined by drawing a line from the average of the other three leads to the one that is designated as the positive lead. The angle of orientation is –150 degrees for lead aV_R, –30 degrees for lead aV_L, and +90 degrees for lead aV_F.

In review, the limb leads consist of 3 bipolar leads and 3 unipolar leads. The 3 bipolar leads are called leads I, II, and III. The 3 unipolar leads are called aV_R, aV_L, and aV_F. The abbreviation *a* refers to augmented; *V* to voltage; and *R, L,* and *F* to right arm, left arm, and left foot respectively. The limb leads measure the electrical activity in the heart that occurs in the frontal

FRONTAL PLANE LEADS

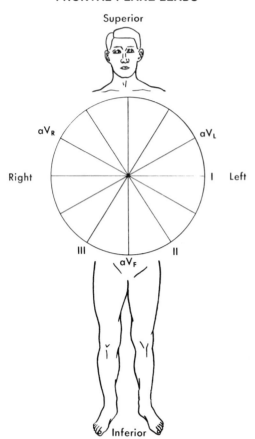

Fig. 9-10 *Frontal plane illustrated showing spatial relationships of 6 extremity leads. (From Goldberger AL and Goldberger E:* Clinical electrocardiography, *ed 3, St Louis, 1986, Mosby–Year Book.)*

CHEST LEAD PLACEMENT

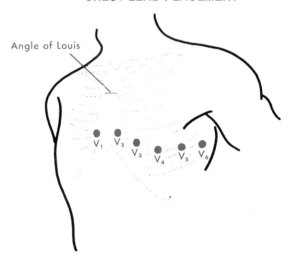

Fig. 9-11 *Position of the 6 chest leads. V_1 is located in the fourth intercostal space left of the sternum. V_2 is located in the fourth intercostal space right of the sternum. V_3 is placed between V_2 and V_4. V_4 is placed in the fifth intercostal space in the midclavicular line. V_5 is placed between V_4 and V_6. V_6 is placed in the fifth intercostal space in the midaxillary line. (From Goldberger AL and Goldberger E:* Clinical electrocardiography, *ed 3, St Louis, 1986, Mosby–Year Book.)*

plane, and each lead has its own specific view or angle of orientation to the heart.

Chest Leads

The 6 chest leads, or precordial leads, are referred to as leads V_1, V_2, V_3, V_4, V_5, and V_6. The chest leads are unipolar leads that are placed across the chest in a horizontal plane (Fig. 9-11). The chest leads define a horizontal or transverse plane and view electrical voltages that move anteriorly and posteriorly. Like the limb leads, each chest lead has its own view or angle of orientation. Under normal conditions leads V_1 and V_2 lie directly over the right ventricle; V_3 and V_4 lie over the interventricular septum; and V_5 and V_6 lie over the left ventricle. In addition, leads V_1 through V_4 are often referred to as the anterior leads since they view the anterior portion of the heart. Leads V_5 and V_6 view the left lateral portion of the heart and are therefore called the left lateral leads.

Evaluating the Mean QRS Axis

The QRS axis represents the general direction of current flow during ventricular depolarization. Even

though the depolarization stimulus spreads through the ventricles in different directions from instant to instant, an average or mean direction can be determined. Normally the mean QRS axis (vector) points leftward (patient's left) and downward, somewhere between 0 and +90 degrees in the frontal plane previously described (Fig. 9-12).

The ECG will record a positive (upward) QRS complex whenever the mean QRS axis is moving toward a positive electrode. When the mean QRS axis is moving toward a negative lead, the QRS complex is negative (downward). Since each of the 6 limb leads has its own angle of orientation as defined in the hexaxial reference system, a review of the recorded limb leads should identify the mean QRS axis in the frontal plane.

To identify the mean QRS axis, begin by sketching the hexaxial reference system, including labels for the points where the limb leads are located on the circle. Next, identify which limb lead has the QRS complex with the most voltage (positive or negative). This is accomplished by identifying the QRS complex with the largest deflection from baseline. If the most voltage is positive (R wave), the mean QRS axis points at that lead with the tallest QRS. If the most voltage is negative (Q or S wave), the mean axis points away from that lead. For example, if the most voltage is found to be in lead II and it is positive, then the mean QRS axis must be about +60 degrees, since this is where lead II is located on the hexaxial reference system (Fig. 9-12). This would be considered a normal axis since it falls between 0 and +90 degrees. If the most voltage is found

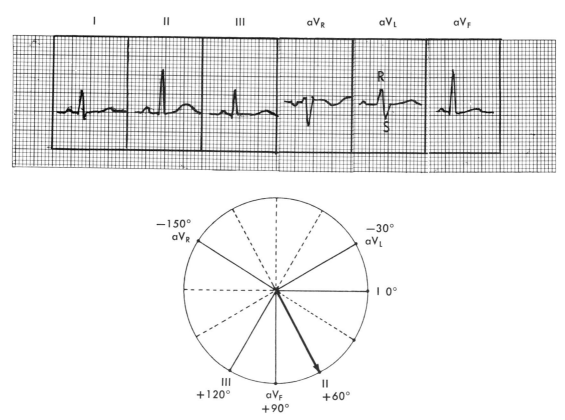

Fig. 9-12 *Normal mean QRS axis of +60 degrees. (From Goldberger AL and Goldberger E:* Clinical electrocardiography, *ed 3, St Louis, 1986, Mosby–Year Book.)*

RIGHT AXIS DEVIATION

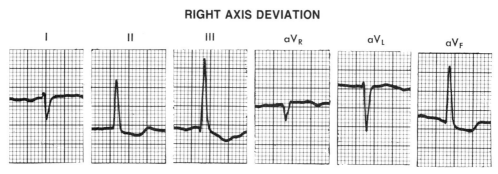

Fig. 9-13 *Sample ECG showing right axis deviation. Note the positive QRS complex (R wave) in leads II and III and the negative QRS complex (S wave) in lead I. (From Goldberger AL and Goldberger E:* Clinical electrocardiography, *ed 3, St Louis, 1986, Mosby–Year Book.)*

in lead I and is negative, then the QRS axis is approximately 180 degrees, since lead I is located at 0 degrees.

In some situations the most voltage may be equally present in two leads. If two leads exhibit equal positive voltage, then the mean axis must fall midway between the two leads. If the most voltage is equally negative in two leads, then the mean axis is opposite the midpoint between the two leads.

As mentioned, a normal QRS axis is approximately 0 to +90 degrees. If the axis is found to be between +90 and 180 degrees, right axis deviation is present. Right axis deviation is common in patients with cor pulmonale (right ventricular enlargement due to chronic lung disease). In such cases the QRS complex

will be negative in lead I but positive in lead aV$_F$. Leads II and III are both positive in most cases of right axis deviation; however, lead III will be taller than lead II (Fig. 9–13).

Left axis deviation is present when the mean axis is found to be between 0 and –90 degrees. Left axis deviation can occur in several different conditions, including left ventricular hypertrophy and blocks of the left bundle branch. In such cases the QRS complex is positive in lead I and negative in lead aV$_F$. In addition, the QRS complex in lead III will demonstrate negative voltage with left axis deviation.

If the mean QRS axis is found to be between –90 and 180 degrees, extreme left or right axis deviation is present. This condition is not common. When the ECG recording indicates that it may be present, the extremity leads should be checked to make sure they are properly attached.

The same principles of axis evaluation can be applied to the P wave as to the QRS complex. When normal sinus rhythm is present and the atria are normal in size, the P wave is positive in lead II and negative in lead aV_R. Therefore the normal P wave is directed toward lead II and away from lead aV_R, making the normal mean P wave axis about +60 degrees. In cor pulmonale, right atrial enlargement is common. The ECG will show tall, narrow P waves in leads II, III, and aV_F in such cases.

ECG Interpretation

Interpretation of the ECG recording is typically left to the cardiologist. There are certain circumstances, however, that may call for the respiratory care practitioner or nurse to identify the patient's ECG pattern. For example, in the intensive care unit where a physician is not always present, the patient's clinical condition may suddenly change and the ECG monitor may provide important data regarding the cause of the problem. The ability to review the ECG strip rapidly to identify any significant abnormalities can be essential to the patient's health. In many hospitals, recording all ECGs is the responsibility of the respiratory care personnel. They must be able to recognize the life-threatening dysrhythmias in order to know when to call for emergency measures.

Interpretation of ECGs is not difficult; however, there are numerous items to check on each recording. To make sure that a review of the ECG tracing is thorough, a systematic method is recommended. The steps outlined below provide such a method:

1. *Identify the atrial and ventricular rates. Divide the number of large boxes between two successive QRS complexes (two successive P waves for the atrial rate) into 300 if the rhythm is regular. If irregular, then count the number of QRS complexes in a 6-second interval and multiply by 10. If the rate is found to be over 100/min, tachycardia is present. Bradycardia is present if the heart rate is less than 60/min (Table 9–2).*
2. *Evaluate the rhythm. Note whether the spacing between the QRS complexes is equal by using calipers. Small variations are normal with breathing. Also decide if a sinus rhythm is present. If a sinus rhythm is occurring, each QRS complex is preceded by a P wave. If no P wave can be seen and the QRS complex is 40 to 60/min, a nodal rhythm is probably occurring.*
3. *Measure the P-R interval. The normal P-R interval is 0.12 to 0.20 second. A consistently prolonged P-R interval is first degree block.*

Table 9–2 Summary of Normal Values for the ECG Interpretation

Variable	Normal Range	Interpretation
Rate	60–100/min	Rates > 100 = tachycardia Rates < 60 = bradycardia
P-R interval	0.12–0.20/sec	>0.20 = heart block
QRS interval	<0.12/sec	>0.12 = ectopic foci
ST segment	Isoelectric	Elevated or depressed = myocardial ischemia
T wave	Upright and round	Inverted with ischemia, tall and peaked with electrolyte imbalances

4. *Identify the width of the QRS complex. The normal QRS complex is less than 0.12 second (three small boxes). Wide QRS complexes can occur with bundle-branch blocks, electrolyte imbalances, and when beats originate in the ventricles (as in premature ventricular contractions [PVCs]).*
5. *Review the P wave size. The normal P wave is less than 2.5 mm in height and less than 3 mm wide. Tall peaked P waves in leads II, III, and aV_F are typical of right atrial enlargement. Abnormally wide P waves are seen with left atrial enlargement.*
6. *Inspect the ST segments in all leads. ST segment elevation or depression indicates myocardial ischemia. The portion of the heart that is ischemic can be determined by identifying the leads in which the ST segment abnormality is present. For example, ischemia in the inferior portion of the heart will best be seen in leads II, III, and aV_F.*
7. *Inspect the T wave. Normally the T wave is positive in leads with a positive QRS complex. T wave inversions are common in the evolving phase of a myocardial infarction. Abnormally tall or depressed T waves are common with electrolyte imbalances.*
8. *Identify the mean QRS axis. To determine the QRS axis the 6 limb leads and the hexaxial reference system are helpful. With a normal axis the QRS will be positive in leads I, II, III, and aV_F since the normal axis is 0 to +90 degrees. Right axis deviation is present if the QRS complex in lead I is negative and upright in leads II and III. Also, the height of the R wave in lead III will exceed that of the R wave in lead II. Left axis deviation is present when lead I shows a tall R wave and lead III has a negative QRS complex (S wave). Lead II is often biphasic when left axis deviation is present.*
9. *All dysrhythmias should be interpreted and evaluated in light of the patient's clinical findings and medical history. Certain dysrhythmias may be tolerated well by one patient yet prove catastrophic to another. One of the questions*

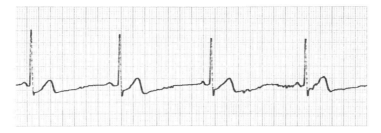

Fig. 9-14 *ECG tracing of sinus bradycardia.*

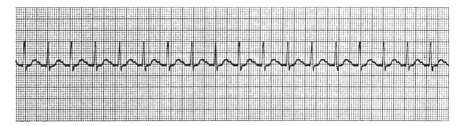

Fig. 9-15 *ECG tracing of sinus tachycardia.*

that should be asked when any dysrhythmia occurs is, How is this affecting the patient? A significant decrease in the patient's blood pressure and sensorium indicates that the dysrhythmia is a serious problem needing immediate treatment.

Identification of Common Dysrhythmias

This section discusses how to identify selected dysrhythmias that may be recognized initially on the oscilloscope during ECG monitoring in the intensive care unit. When an abnormality is seen on the oscilloscope, a paper tracing is used to study and confirm the specific dysrhythmia.

Sinus Bradycardia

Sinus bradycardia meets all the criteria for a normal sinus rhythm except for the heart rate, which is below 60/min. This dysrhythmia may be tolerated by the patient, or it may compromise cardiac performance; only close observation of the response of the patient to the dysrhythmia will determine if it is detrimental. Marked sinus bradycardia may result in hypotension, syncope, diminished cardiac output, congestive heart failure, and shock. This may predispose the patient to more serious dysrhythmias. If the bradycardia causes the patient's blood pressure to drop significantly, the bradycardia must be treated. Direct carotid massage, manipulation of tracheostomy ties or tube, the Valsalva maneuver, and tracheal suctioning can increase vagus nerve tone and may cause a transient bradycardia.

Damage to the SA node, as may occur with a myocardial infarction, can cause a long-term bradycardia.

MEASUREMENT: The ECG tracing meets the normal criteria except that the heart rate is less than 60/min. With rates less than 50/min, the heartbeat may become slightly irregular (Fig. 9-14).

Sinus Tachycardia

Sinus tachycardia is present when the heart rate is over 100/min, the SA node is the pacemaker, and all the normal conduction pathways in the heart are followed. Sinus tachycardia may be well tolerated by the patient; however, it increases myocardial oxygen demand and decreases the diastolic period, both of which can lead to myocardial ischemia. Sinus tachycardia results from sympathetic nervous system stimulation and almost always indicates a significant physiologic problem. Fever, pain, hypoxemia, hypovolemia, hypotension, sepsis, and heart failure are causes of sinus tachycardia. Tracheal suctioning, especially if it is performed without adequate oxygenation before, during, and after each catheter insertion, can cause sinus tachycardia. In addition, xanthine and the β-agonist bronchodilators often increase heart rate.

MEASUREMENT: The ECG tracing meets the normal criteria except that the heart rate is greater than 100/min (Fig. 9-15). It may be difficult to differentiate between sinus tachycardia and paroxysmal atrial tachycardia (PAT) described later, especially if the beginning of the arrhythmia was not observed. Rates over 150/min favor identification as PAT. A change in the shape of the P wave or change in the P-R interval is strongly suggestive of PAT. If possible, capturing a paper tracing of the onset or termination of the dysrhythmia can be helpful; if it is abrupt, it is PAT.

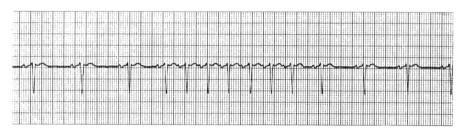

Fig. 9–16 *Short run of paroxysmal atrial tachycardia.*

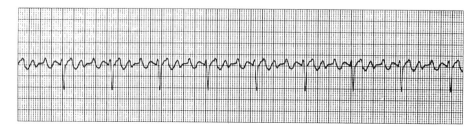

Fig. 9–17 *ECG tracing of artial flutter.*

Sinus Dysrhythmia

This is a benign dysrhythmia that meets all the criteria for normal sinus rhythm except that the rhythm is irregular. It usually does not produce symptoms in the patient and requires no treatment. In most cases of sinus dysrhythmia, no abnormality of the heart is present.

MEASUREMENT. P waves, QRS complexes, and T waves are normal in appearance and rate, but the rhythmicity is not regular. Often the irregularities are related to the respiratory pattern, suggesting that changes in intrathoracic pressure are causing changes in the tone of the vagus nerve, which may produce the irregularity.

Paroxysmal Atrial Tachycardia

PAT occurs when an ectopic focus in the atrium usurps the pacemaking function of the SA node and paces the heart, usually at an abnormally rapid rate of 180 to 280/min. It appears on the monitor as a series of normal-looking QRS complexes, each associated with a P wave. Because of the rapid rate, the P wave may be obscured by the preceding T wave.

Onset of this dysrhythmia is sudden and spontaneous; termination is similarly abrupt. PAT is seen in patients with normal hearts and in those with organic heart disease. The hazard of PAT is that it increases myocardial oxygen demand while at the same time decreasing pump effectiveness. PAT may precipitate hypotension, congestive heart failure, or an ischemic episode. PAT is especially dangerous for patients with compromised cardiovascular function, myocardial ischemia, preexisting heart failure, and recent myocardial infarction. Patients with PAT often complain of lightheadedness or palpitation. Occasionally PAT will cause the patient to faint.

MEASUREMENT: PAT is identified when the onset and termination of the tachycardia is sudden, without preceding acceleration or deceleration. The heart rate is very rapid, above 150/min, and the QRS complexes appear normal (Fig. 9–16). The P wave may be obscured by the preceding T wave, but if observable, it has a one-to-one relationship to the QRS complex. The shape of the P wave and of the P-R interval are usually somewhat different than in the preceding normal rhythm.

Atrial Flutter

Atrial flutter is a dysrhythmia that produces a very distinctive ECG pattern—a characteristic sawtooth pattern between normal-appearing QRS complexes. The sawtooth pattern of flutter waves represents the flutter of the atria and indicates that atrial assistance in filling the ventricles is minimal or absent. A secondary problem with atrial flutter is that the pattern of blood flow in the atria causes areas of diminished blood movement near the atrial walls, which promotes the formation of mural thrombi. The patient is then at risk for embolization secondary to the migration of a mural thrombus. Atrial flutter is usually a short-lived dysrhythmia; it usually deteriorates to atrial fibrillation or returns spontaneously to the patient's previous rhythm. Atrial flutter is commonly associated with pulmonary disease.

MEASUREMENT: The ECG tracing shows atrial complexes (flutter waves) with a uniform appearance, classically a sawtooth form (Fig. 9–17). The atrial complexes are rapid, around 180 to 300/min, and are regular in rhythm. The QRS complexes appear normal. The relationship between the flutter waves and the QRS complexes may be regular (e.g., four flutter waves to each QRS complex) or variable.

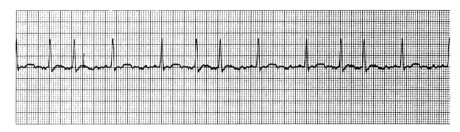

Fig. 9–18 *ECG tracing of atrial fibrillation.*

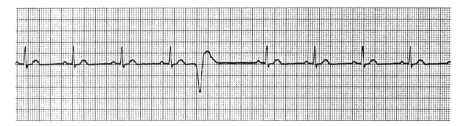

Fig. 9–19 *ECG tracing of a single premature ventricular contraction (PVC).*

Atrial Fibrillation

In atrial fibrillation, the electrical activity of the atria is completely chaotic, without coordination. This results in a quivering of the atrial myocardium and complete loss of atrial pumping ability. Since the atria provide useful assistance in filling the ventricles (sometimes called *atrial kick*), there is a decrease in ventricular filling during atrial fibrillation. In most cases, the reduction in cardiac output is not serious enough to produce symptoms, although it reduces cardiac reserve and may limit the normal activities of daily living. Atrial fibrillation carries an even higher risk of mural thrombi formation and embolization than atrial flutter.

MEASUREMENT: The ECG tracing will show a chaotic baseline between QRS complexes, with no regular pattern or organization. This irregular baseline is composed of what are termed *fibrillatory* waves. The QRS complexes have a normal appearance but occur with no regularity (Fig. 9–18).

Premature Ventricular Contractions

PVCs represent ectopic beats originating in one of the ventricles. They may occur both in persons with normal hearts and in those with serious organic heart disease. Healthy persons may have PVCs with anxiety or excessive use of caffeine. Certain medications such as isoproterenol, epinephrine, and aminophylline may also provoke PVCs in patients with normal hearts. Myocardial ischemia is a common cause of PVCs in patients with heart disease. PVCs can be recognized by five classic signs:

1. The QRS complexes are premature; i.e., they occur earlier than expected in the cardiac cycle.
2. The QRS complexes are wide (greater than 0.12 second) and bizarre in appearance.

3. There is no P wave associated with the QRS complex.
4. The T wave following the PVC is deflected in a direction opposite to that of the QRS complex.
5. There is a full compensatory pause following the PVC.

A single PVC poses no threat to the patient (Fig. 9–19), but certain configurations of PVCs may signal a serious cardiac problem that may need immediate treatment. Although the idea that PVCs are "warning" dysrhythmias has not been proved by clinical research, the following conditions warrant further investigation and indicate the need for close monitoring of the patient:

Increased frequency	More than six PVCs in 1 minute (see Fig. 9–20).
Multifocal PVCs	The QRS complexes of the PVCs have more than one configuration (Fig. 9–21); this indicates that more than one area of the ventricles is irritated and multifocal PVCs are occurring.
Couplets	Two PVCs occur in a row.
Salvos	Three or more PVCs occur in a row (sometimes called a short run of ventricular tachycardia).
R-on-T phenomenon	The PVC occurs during the T wave of the preceding beat; this poses a real danger, because it can precipitate ventricular tachycardia (Fig. 9–22).

Many coronary care units have standing orders for initiation of antiarrhythmic therapy (lidocaine) anytime one of the above conditions exists.

MEASUREMENT: PVCs are easily distinguished by the wide and bizarre shape of the QRS complex, the lack of an associated P wave, the presence of T-wave deflection opposite to that of the QRS complex, and a compensatory pause. The compensatory pause can be

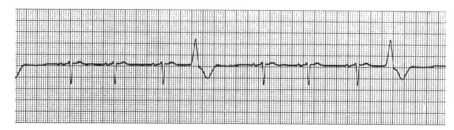

Fig. 9-20 *ECG tracing of frequent PVCs.*

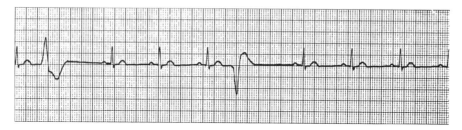

Fig. 9-21 *ECG tracing of multifocal PVCs.*

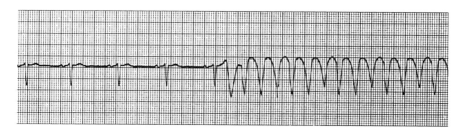

Fig. 9-22 *ECG tracing of R-on-T phenomenon.*

confirmed by measuring the interval between the normal QRS complex immediately before the PVC and the normal QRS complex immediately following the PVC; it will be double the normal R-R interval for that patient.

Ventricular Tachycardia

Ventricular tachycardia appears on the monitor as a series of broad QRS complexes, occurring at a rapid rate, without identifiable P waves. By definition, *ventricular tachycardia* is a run of three or more consecutive PVCs. It may occur as a single isolated burst or may persist for a long run. The rhythm is regular, and the rate is usually in the range of 140 to 300/min. The majority of patients deteriorate rapidly with this dysrhythmia; therefore it must be treated as an emergency. Without appropriate treatment, sustained ventricular tachycardia leads to ventricular fibrillation (described later) and ultimately to death. When ventricular tachycardia occurs, the patient may become hypotensive and be slow to respond initially. As the cardiac output deteriorates, the patient usually becomes comatose. Ventricular tachycardia is frequently caused by problems similar to those that cause PVCs. When the heart is hypoxic, as occurs with severe myocardial ischemia, ventricular tachycardia is common and is a sign that the patient is in need of immediate care.

MEASUREMENT: The ECG tracing of ventricular tachycardia shows QRS complexes that are abnormal in configuration but uniform in appearance and regular in rhythm. The QRS complex duration is greater than 0.12 second, and no P waves are associated with the QRS complexes (Fig. 9-23).

Ventricular Fibrillation

Ventricular fibrillation is the presence of chaotic, completely unorganized electrical activity in the ventricular myocardial fibers. It produces a characteristic wavy, irregular pattern on the ECG monitor. Depending on the amplitude of the electrical impulses, it can be mistaken for asystole or ventricular tachycardia. Because the heart cannot pump blood when fibrillation is occurring, the cardiac output drops to zero and the patient becomes unconscious immediately. This dysrhythmia is life-threatening and must be treated immediately (defibrillation with DC shock). Ventricular fibrillation is often caused by the same factors that precipitate ventricular tachycardia.

MEASUREMENT: No waves appear with any regularity. There may be occasional low-amplitude waves, which appear somewhat like ventricular-origin complexes, but they are sporadic in occurrence and totally irregular (Fig. 9-24).

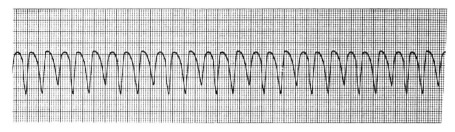

Fig. 9–23 *ECG tracing of ventricular tachycardia.*

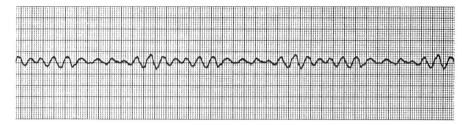

Fig. 9–24 *ECG tracing of ventricular fibrillation.*

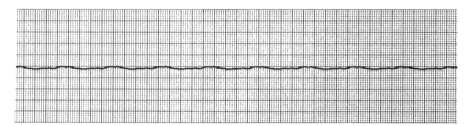

Fig. 9–25 *ECG tracing of asystole.*

Asystole

Asystole is cardiac standstill and is invariably fatal unless an acceptable rhythm is restored; in fact asystole is one of the criteria used for the determination of clinical death. Asystole is recognizable on the ECG monitor as a straight or almost straight line. The bedside clinician must take care to assess the patient with what appears to be asystole before initiating therapy, because a simple disconnection of the ECG leads can resemble asystole. Clinically, asystole is characterized by immediate pulselessness with loss of blood pressure and loss of consciousness.

MEASUREMENT: The ECG tracing shows a line that is flat or almost flat, without discernible electrical activity (Fig. 9–25).

Electromechanical Dissociation

Electromechanical dissociation (EMD) is not a discrete dysrhythmia but rather an electromechanical condition that can be diagnosed clinically. As the name implies, there is a dissociation of the electrical and the mechanical activity of the heart. In other words, the pattern that appears on the ECG monitor does not reflect the usual physical or mechanical activity associated with the heart. Fortunately, EMD is rare and does not occur without a precipitating event. Tension pneumothorax, cardiac trauma, and severe electrolyte or acid-base disturbances are among the most common causes of EMD. EMD is sometimes seen as a terminal event in an unsuccessful cardiac resuscitation effort.

MEASUREMENT: There is no relationship between the electrical pattern appearing on the oscilloscope or paper tracing and the mechanical activity of the heart. If pulses are palpable, they do not relate to any of the QRS complexes.

AV Heart Block

AV heart block is a general term that refers to a disturbance in the conduction of impulses from the atrium to the ventricles. The mildest form of heart block is first degree block, which is present when the P-R interval is prolonged more than 0.2 second. In first degree block, all the atrial impulses pass through to the ventricles but are delayed at the AV junction. The most extreme form of heart block is third degree block. This is present when there is no conduction of stimuli from the atrium to the ventricles. In this situation the ventricles and atrium beat independently of one another.

Second degree block is an intermediate form of heart block that may have two different appearances. In one type of second degree block the P-R interval becomes progressively longer until a point is reached where the stimulus from the atria is blocked completely for a single cycle. After the blocked beat, relative

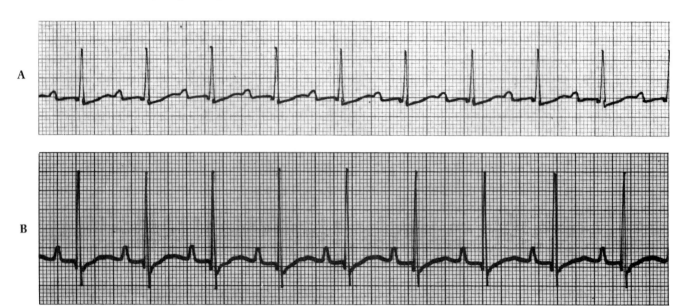

Fig. 9–26 *First degree AV block.* **A,** *P-R interval=0.30 second.* **B,** *P-R interval=0.24 second. (From Conover MB:* Understanding electrocardiography, *ed 4 St. Louis, 1984, Mosby–Year Book.)*

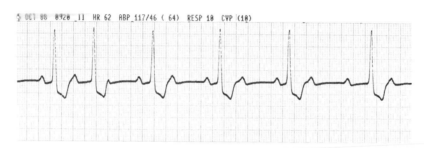

Fig. 9–27 *ECG tracing of second degree block, nonspecific.*

recovery of the AV junction occurs, and the progressive increasing of the P-R interval starts all over again. This is referred to as Mobitz type I heart block. Mobitz type II is rarer but is also classified as a second degree block. This dysrhythmia is characterized by a series of nonconducted P waves followed by a P wave that is conducted to the ventricles. Sometimes the ratio of nonconducted to conducted P waves is fixed at 3:1 or 4:1, for example.

Disturbances in AV conduction can occur as a side effect of medications such as digitalis, or when damage to the conduction system occurs with myocardial infarction. In some cases of complete heart block, the patient may develop symptoms associated with hypotension (fainting and weakness) if the ventricles are beating too slowly. In milder forms of heart block the patient is often asymptomatic.

MEASUREMENT: First degree block is recognized by identifying a P-R interval greater than 0.2 second and noting that there is a one-to-one relationship between the P waves and the QRS complexes (Fig. 9–26). Second degree block is present when the P-R interval becomes progressively longer until one P wave is not conducted

or when a series of nonconducted P waves is followed by a P wave that is conducted through to the ventricles (Fig. 9–27). Third degree block is present when there is no relationship between the P waves and the QRS complexes. Usually the P-P intervals and the R-R intervals are very regular with third degree block, and the atrial rate is greater than the ventricular rate (Fig. 9–28).

Idioventricular Rhythm

Idioventricular rhythm occurs when the normal pacemaker does not set the pace for the ventricles. This is commonly seen in third degree heart block. In this case, an ectopic focus in one of the ventricles becomes the pacemaker for the ventricles. The intrinsic rate of the ventricular tissue is usually less than 40 beats per minute, so the ventricular rate is very slow (Fig. 9–29). In idioventricular rhythm, the ECG pattern appears as a slow series of wide and bizarre QRS complexes. If P waves are present, there is no relationship between the P waves and the QRS complexes (AV dissociation). The slower ventricular rate and the loss of assistance in ventricular filling provided by the atria decrease cardiac

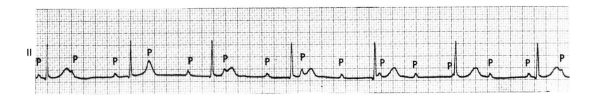

Fig. 9-28 *Third-degree heart block characterized by independent atrial (P wave) and ventricular activity. The atrial rate is always faster than the ventricular rate. (From Goldberger AL and Goldberger E:* Clinical electrocardiography: a simplified approach, *ed 3, St Louis, 1986, Mosby–Year Book.)*

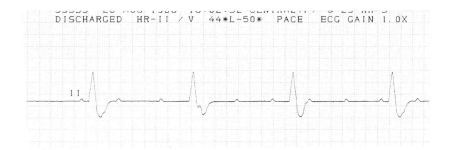

Fig. 9-29 *ECG tracing of idioventricular rhythm.*

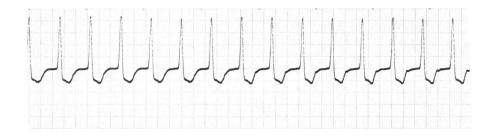

Fig. 9-30 *ECG tracing showing junctional tachycardia.*

output significantly and can lead rapidly to heart failure and more severe dysrhythmias.

There is a variation of idioventricular rhythm called *accelerated idioventricular rhythm.* In accelerated idioventricular rhythm the rate is in the normal range.

Junctional Tachycardia

In junctional tachycardia, an area in the AV junction usurps the pacemaking role and sends impulses down the normal conduction pathways in the ventricles at an abnormally rapid rate. Because the normal conduction pathways in the ventricles are being used, the QRS complexes appear normal. The P wave may be present or absent. If present, it may appear immediately after the QRS, plainly demonstrating retrograde conduction. In this case, the P wave is almost invariably inverted, indicating that depolarization of the atria followed a retrograde path. The P wave may appear before the QRS, but when it does, the P-R interval is of less than normal duration (0.12 second). This indicates that there

was not sufficient time for the P wave to be responsible for initiating the associated QRS complex (Fig. 9-30).

ST Segment Elevation or Depression

Normally the ST segment is isoelectric, meaning that it is in the same horizontal position as the baseline. Whenever the ST segment moves more than 1 to 2 mm from the isoelectric line, it may indicate myocardial ischemia. During an ischemic event such as acute myocardial infarction, the ST segment can be used as an indicator of the effectiveness of therapy in reversing ischemia. Any acute change should be reported and evaluated immediately. When ST segment elevation or depression occurs, the patient may simultaneously complain of chest pain and be diaphoretic.

MEASUREMENT: It can be helpful to identify ST segment abnormalities by drawing a straight line over the imaginary isoelectric line. This will help show whether ST segment elevation or depression is present and to what degree. If the deviation from the isoelectric line is

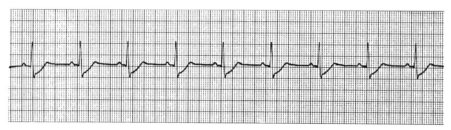

Fig. 9–31 *ECG tracing showing ST segment depression.*

greater than 1 to 2 mm, significant changes have occurred and further investigation is appropriate. The patient should be closely monitored when this abnormality is identified (Fig. 9–31).

ECG Patterns with Chronic Lung Disease

The majority of patients with chronic obstructive pulmonary disease (COPD) have ECG abnormalities caused by their lung disease. Hyperinflation of the lungs and flattening of the diaphragm are associated with a more vertical position of the heart. This causes a clockwise rotation of the QRS axis and contributes to the right axis deviation associated with COPD. In addition, chronic pulmonary hypertension is often seen in COPD patients and causes an enlargement of the right side of the heart. Enlargement of the right atrium causes rightward deviation of the P wave axis, enlarged positive P waves greater than 2.5 mm in leads II, III, and aV_F, and a prominent negative P wave in lead I. This pattern of abnormalities in the P wave associated with COPD is referred to as *P pulmonale*. Right ventricular enlargement leads to right axis deviation of the QRS axis and increased R-wave voltage in the right precordial leads (V_1, V_2, and V_3).

Reduced voltage in the limb leads is seen when severe pulmonary hyperinflation (emphysema) is present. This is seen as QRS complexes less than 5 mm in leads I, II, and III. Reduced voltage in the precordial leads V_5 and V_6 may also be present. The reduced measured voltage appears to be caused by two factors. Firstly, the lung hyperinflation associated with emphysema reduces the electrical conductivity of the lung. The electrical impulses travel poorly through the chest to the limb leads in such cases. Secondly, the mean QRS axis may be directed posteriorly and perpendicular to the frontal plane of the limb leads. As a result, decreased voltage is measured in the limb leads.

Dysrhythmias are often seen in patients with COPD and acute lung disease. Tachycardia, multifocal atrial tachycardia, and ventricular ectopic beats represent some of the more common ECG abnormalities seen in COPD. Such dysrhythmias occur as the result of hypoxemia from the lung disease and from side effects of the medications (bronchodilators) used to treat the obstructed airways. Hypoxemia often worsens during sleep in patients with COPD and increases the prevalence of nighttime dysrhythmias such as ventricular ectopic beats.

REVIEW QUESTIONS

1. ECGs are not *useful* to evaluate the:
   a. *impact of lung disease on the heart*
   b. *pumping ability of the heart*
   c. *severity of the myocardial infarction*
   d. *heart rhythm*

2. *What clinical findings are suggestive of the need for an ECG?*
   a. *headache and nausea*
   b. *orthopnea and syncope*
   c. *fever and cough*
   d. *joint pain and swelling*

3. *What is the normal pacemaker for the heart?*
   a. *SA node*
   b. *AV node*
   c. *bundle of HIS*
   d. *purkinje fibers*

4. *What is the normal back-up pacemaker for the heart?*
   a. *SA node*
   b. *AV node*
   c. *bundle of HIS*
   d. *Purkinje fibers*

5. T   F   *The sudden loss of positive charge within the cardiac cell is termed depolarization.*

6. *What does the P wave on the ECG recording represent?*
   a. *atrial depolarization*
   b. *atrial repolarization*
   c. *ventricular depolarization*
   d. *ventricular repolarization*

7. *What does the QRS wave on the ECG recording represent?*
   a. *atrial depolarization*
   b. *atrial repolarization*
   c. *ventricular depolarization*
   d. *ventricular repolarization*

8. What does the T wave on the ECG recording represent?
    a. atrial depolarization
    b. atrial repolarization
    c. ventricular depolarization
    d. ventricular repolarization

9. What is the normal P-R interval?
    a. < 0.10 sec
    b. < 0.20 sec
    c. < 0.30 sec
    d. < 0.40 sec

10. What is the length of the normal QRS complex?
    a. < 0.04 sec
    b. < 0.08 sec
    c. < 0.12 sec
    d. < 0.16 sec

11. The QRS complexes are equally spaced with three large boxes between each complex. What is the heart rate?
    a. 150/min
    b. 100/min
    c. 75/min
    d. 60/min

12. A prolonged P-R interval is indicative of:
    a. tachycardia
    b. bradycardia
    c. sinus dysrhythmia
    d. heart block

13. An early, widened QRS complex with an inverted T wave and no associated P wave is consistent with:
    a. PVC
    b. ventricular tachycardia
    c. ventricular fibrillation
    d. ventricular asystole

14. What ECG finding is suggestive of an acute myocardial infarction?
    a. prolonged P-R intervals
    b. elevated S-T segments
    c. tall, peaked T waves
    d. narrow QRS complexes

15. What ECG finding is suggestive of cor pulmonale?
    a. inverted T waves
    b. elevated S-T segments
    c. right axis deviation
    d. small QRS complexes

BIBLIOGRAPHY

Brown KR, and Jacobson S: *Mastering dysrhythmias: a problem solving guide,* Philadelphia, 1988, FA Davis.

Cherniack NS: *Chronic obstructive pulmonary disease,* Philadelphia, 1991, WB Saunders.

Conover MB: *Exercises in diagnosing ECG tracings,* ed 3, St Louis, 1984, Mosby.

Davis D: *How to quickly and accurately master ECG interpretation,* Philadelphia, 1985, JB Lippincott.

Goldberger AL, and Goldberger E: *Clinical electrocardiography,* ed 3, St Louis, 1986, Mosby.

Huszar RH: *Basic dysrhythmias: interpretation and management,* St Louis, 1988, Mosby.

Thaler MS: *The only ECG book you'll ever need,* Philadelphia, 1988, JB Lippincott.

Chapter 10

Respiratory Assessment of Neonatal and Pediatric Patients

Douglas D. Deming

LEARNING OBJECTIVES

Upon completion of this chapter, the reader should be able to accomplish the following:

1. *Identify the type of information found in the pregnancy history, labor history, and delivery history and the clinical significance of common findings.*

2. *Identify the value of the Apgar scoring system and the five physical criteria used in this scoring system.*

3. *Identify the Apgar scores that indicate normal status, moderate depression, and severe depression of the newborn.*

4. *Identify normal values for the vital signs in newborns and the clinical implications of abnormalities.*

5. *Identify the clinical implications of retractions, nasal flaring, and grunting.*

6. *Identify the normal time for capillary refill and the clinical significance of poor capillary refill in the infant.*

7. *Identify the clinical significance of abdominal distention in the infant.*

8. *Recognize true statements regarding the technique for auscultation of the infant.*

9. *Identify the clinical implications of abnormal breath sounds in the infant.*

10. *Identify potential causes of murmurs heard during auscultation of the infant precordium.*

11. *Identify normal values for the white and red blood cell count and partial differential for the infant at birth, 7 days of age, and 14 days of age.*

12. *Identify the possible causes of abnormalities in the white blood cell and red blood cell counts in the infant.*

13. *Identify the clinical implications for abnormalities in blood glucose, total protein and albumin, serum enzymes, and electrolytes.*

14. *Identify normal values for arterial pH, PO2, PCO2, HCO3, and base excess at birth, 24 hours after birth, and one month to two years after birth.*

Chapter Overview

The bases for assessing the newborn and pediatric patient are a good history, thorough physical examination, and careful attention to selected laboratory and radiographic information. Although the basic principles that apply to adult patients also apply here, certain characteristics make assessment of the newborn and pediatric patient unique. These characteristics include lack of verbal communication skills, the tendency to be afraid of strangers (particularly people in white coats), and inability or reluctance to follow directions. This chapter reviews the assessment of the newborn and pediatric patient with respiratory disease.

For the purposes of this chapter, a *young infant* is less than 3 months old, an *older infant* is between 3 and 12 months old, and a *child* is between 12 months old and adolescence. A young infant's age can be defined as either chronologic or gestational age. *Chronologic age* is the age of the infant computed from the date of birth. *Gestational age* is the age of the infant computed from the date of conception. Gestational age is usually assigned on the basis of the history and physical examination. *Term infants* are born between 38 and 42 weeks of gestational age; *preterm infants* are born at 37 weeks or less of gestational age; and *postterm infants* at 43 or more weeks of gestational age.

Assessment of the Newborn

History

The newborn's history is obtained from several sources and covers more than just the medical history of the infant. Sources include both parents, the mother's labor and delivery chart, and the infant's own chart.

MATERNAL HISTORY. The newborn's history begins with the mother's history. Was the mother healthy before she was pregnant? Does she have any chronic diseases? Is she taking any medications or illicit drugs? For example, infants born to mothers with diabetes mellitus are often maturationally delayed and may be susceptible to diseases of prematurity such as respiratory distress syndrome (RDS). Conversely, infants born to mothers who have chronic hypertension may be maturationally advanced for their gestational age.

The mother's previous pregnancy history can give the historian valuable information. Obstetricians will note this information in the mother's medical record using the terms *gravida, para,* and *abortion.* *Gravida* is a pregnant woman, *para* is a woman who delivers a live infant, and *abortion* is the delivering of a dead infant. These terms will most likely be abbreviated and followed by numbers, e.g., G2, P1, Ab0, meaning this woman is in her second pregnancy, has delivered a living infant, and has not had any abortions. Abortions can be further subdivided into therapeutic and spontaneous. These are abbreviated as TAb and SAb. If the mother has had multiple pregnancies that have ended with spontaneous abortions rather than living infants, there is the possibility of chromosomal or metabolic disease that can have serious consequences for the current pregnancy, or the mother may have an incompetent cervix that is associated with chronic preterm deliveries. If the mother has had multiple pregnancies that have ended with therapeutic abortions, the historian should think about the possibility of maternal drug abuse. Finally, for a mother that has had multiple pregnancies that have ended with the delivery of living children, the historian should inquire about the perinatal health of those previous children, because severity of diseases tends to be similar in families.

FAMILY HISTORY. It is important to inquire about family history as well as maternal history. Is there a history of prematurity? Have there been other

Table 10-1	Apgar Scores		
Sign	Score 0	Score 1	Score 2
Heart rate	Absent	< 100/min	> 100/min
Respiratory effort	Absent	Gasping, irregular	Good
Muscle tone	Limp	Some flexion	Active motion
Reflex irritability	No response	Grimace	Cry
Color	Body pale or blue, extremities blue	Body pink, extremities blue	Completely pink

infants with respiratory problems? The incidence and severity of diseases like RDS are similar among siblings. There may also be an increased tendency for the recurrence of pneumonias caused by group B β-hemolytic streptococcus in siblings.

PREGNANCY HISTORY. In evaluating the infant with respiratory disease, valuable information can be found in the pregnancy, labor, and delivery histories. In the pregnancy history the interviewer records information about the mother and the fetus. Did the mother have any illnesses during her gestation? Congenital viral infections that profoundly affect the infant may have produced only mild or even no symptoms in the mother. Did the mother have any vaginal bleeding? The mother is usually the source of vaginal bleeding, but occasionally the baby is bleeding, and these infants need to be evaluated for hypovolemia (low blood volume). Did the mother note any evidence of amniotic infection or urinary tract infection? An infant delivered in the presence of infection has an increased risk of infection-caused respiratory difficulty. Did the mother have traumatic injury? A traumatic injury may compromise the uteroplacental interface and thus decrease transfer of oxygen and other nutrients to the baby. Did the mother's uterus grow appropriately during pregnancy? If not, the infant may not have grown and could have pulmonary hypoplasia, severe malformations, or congenital infection. Any of these diseases may cause significant respiratory distress in the newborn.

Because the incidence of respiratory disease varies with different gestational ages, it is important to determine when the infant was actually due. The interviewer should attempt to identify the date of the mother's *last menstrual period (LMP)*, her estimated date of delivery (this appears as the *estimated date of confinement [EDC]* on the mother's chart), her obstetric record of uterine growth, and any reports from ultrasound examinations that she may have had.

Infants born in early gestation are more susceptible to RDS, pulmonary interstitial emphysema, intracranial hemorrhage, and bronchopulmonary dysplasia. Infants born in late gestation are more susceptible to severe perinatal asphyxia, meconium aspiration, and the development of persistent pulmonary hypertension.

LABOR HISTORY. The labor history is obtained to evaluate the well-being of the infant during the transition from intrauterine to extrauterine life. The infant must successfully deal with cyclical decreases in uterine blood flow as well as compression of his or her body. The interviewer should evaluate the available obstetric information. This might include fetal heart rate tracings, fetal activity, biophysical profile, and fetal ultrasound. Information that suggests perinatal asphyxia might include variable or late heart rate decelerations, low biophysical profile, decrease in fetal movement, presence of meconium (first feces of an infant) in the amniotic fluid, long labor, and abnormal vaginal bleeding. The interviewer should also look for information that might suggest an infection in the infant. This might include maternal fever, high maternal white blood cell count, tender uterus, rupture of the amniotic membranes for more than 24 hours, foul-smelling amniotic fluid, and fetal tachycardia.

DELIVERY HISTORY. The delivery history should include the method of delivery for the infant: vaginal or cesarean section, spontaneous or forceps or vacuum extraction, low forceps or middle or high forceps. Infants who are successfully dealing with the labor process are born by spontaneous or low forceps vaginal deliveries and are usually normal. Infants who are in trouble during the delivery process are more likely to be delivered by vacuum extraction, middle or high forceps, or cesarean delivery. (Some cesarean deliveries are done because the infant is positioned in such a manner as to be at high risk for vaginal delivery, not because the infant is in trouble.) These infants are at greater risk for respiratory disease. It is also helpful to know what type of anesthetic the mother had for delivery (e.g., narcotics, local, epidural, spinal, or general). Narcotics and general anesthetics may enter the infant's bloodstream and produce respiratory depression in the infant. Spinal anesthetics may lower the mother's blood pressure, thus compromising the oxygen supply to the infant.

At the time of delivery there is usually a great deal of excitement and tension that may hinder critical powers of observation important in determining the well-being of the newborn. The most standard objective measurement of the newborn's well-being is the *Apgar score*. This is a simple, quick, and reliable means of assessment. It assigns the infant points for the presence of five specific physical criteria (Table 10–1). Most infants are evaluated and assigned Apgar scores at 1 and 5 minutes. However, if the infant is having difficulty during the transition to extrauterine life, Apgar scores can be assigned more often and over a longer time span. For instance, a sick infant may have 1-, 2-, 5-, 10-, 15-, and 20-minute Apgar scores. Of course the process of assigning an Apgar score must not delay the initiation of resuscitative measures. If an infant is becoming asphyxiated, the signs measured by the Apgar score generally decline in a particular order (color, reflex irritability, muscle tone, respiratory effort, and heart rate). Conversely, the signs improve in a similar order (heart rate, respiratory effort, reflex irritability, color, and muscle tone) when the infant is recovering.

The Apgar score is useful in identifying infants who need resuscitation. Infants who are adjusting well to extrauterine life usually have 1-minute scores of 7 to 10. They may show acrocyanosis, irregular respirations, or *hypotonia* (lack of muscle tone). They usually require only routine newborn care such as drying, temperature maintenance, and clearing of the airway. They may occasionally require supplemental oxygen for a brief period. Moderately depressed infants have 1-minute scores of 4 to 6. They need more than routine care and frequently need an increased F_{IO_2} (fraction of inspired oxygen) with bag and mask ventilation. Most infants respond well to this therapy and improve in a few minutes. Infants who have 1-minute scores of 0 to 3 are severely depressed and need extensive medical care such as intubation and mechanical ventilation.

While the 1-minute Apgar score is a useful tool in identifying infants who might require resuscitation, the 5-minute Apgar score is a better predictor of the infant's neurologic outcome. Infants who have 5-minute Apgar scores of less than 5 have a greater risk of neurologic impairment at 1 year of age.

POSTNATAL HISTORY. After the delivery, the historian should document the magnitude of the infant's resuscitation, present diseases, treatment of the diseases, length of the hospital stay, condition at discharge, and problems that have developed since the infant was last seen. For the majority of infants, all of this information is normal, and the postnatal history is brief. All infants require some form of resuscitation. The simplest resuscitation required is clearing the airway and drying the skin. It is important to document whether the infant required only this simple intervention; a more significant intervention with oxygen, manual ventilation with bag and mask, or intubation; or chemical resuscitation with the administration of drugs to support cardiac output. How did the infant respond to resuscitation? Was the response immediate or slow?

If the infant is still hospitalized, the only further information needed for an adequate assessment is what diseases the infant has, what treatment has been initiated, and what the response to treatment has been. If the infant has been discharged and is now being readmitted, seen again in a practice office, or seen at home, the historian needs to inquire about the infant's condition since discharge. Was the infant still sick at the time of discharge? Did the infant require continuing treatment at home? How is the infant doing with the current treatment? What kind of problem does the infant have now?

Table 10–2 Ratio of Surface Area to Mass

	Surface area (m²)	Mass (kg)	Surface area/mass (m²/kg)
Adult male	1.7	80	0.02
Term infant	0.25	3.5	0.07
28-week-old infant	0.15	1.0	0.15

Physical Examination

The skills for physical examination of a newborn are not difficult to learn. As previously emphasized (Chapter 4), abnormalities can be detected only by examiners who recognize normal respiratory function. Beginning examiners should develop the techniques of physical examination on well babies to understand the complex subtleties of abnormalities in sick infants.

Examination of a newborn is based on the four classic principles of physical examination: inspection, palpation, auscultation, and percussion. Percussion is rarely used in examining newborns because of small cavity and organ sizes. Therefore, percussion is not described in this text. Transillumination, however, is a useful tool in the assessment of newborns and is discussed later in this chapter.

Careful inspection reveals clues about the type and severity of respiratory disease. It is important to inspect the overall appearance of the infant carefully because respiratory diseases in the newborn are frequently manifested by a large number of extrapulmonary signs. Palpation is useful in determining the cause of respiratory distress and the severity of side effects from the lung disease and its treatment. As in the adult, auscultation is used to define characteristics of the disease process occurring in the lung. However, statements about the internal location of the pathologic process must be made with greater caution in newborns because localization by auscultation is difficult in the small chest cavity.

VITAL SIGNS.

Body Temperature. The newborn does not differ from the adult in the range of normal body temperature. Humans maintain body temperature by balancing heat production with heat loss. The newborn loses much more heat to the environment than the older child or adult, largely because heat loss is determined by the ratio of the surface area of the body to the total body mass (Table 10–2). The average adult male has a surface area of 1.7 m² and a body mass of 80 kg. This results in a surface area-to-mass ratio of 0.02 m²/kg. The average term infant has a body surface area of 0.25 m² and a body mass of 3.5 kg, which results in a surface area-to-mass ratio of 0.07 m²/kg. This is more than three times the surface area-to-mass ratio of an adult male. For infants younger in gestational age, the problem becomes even more significant. A 28-week-

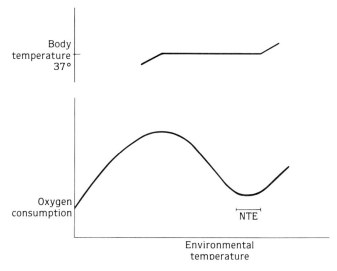

Fig. 10-1 *Effect of environmental temperature on oxygen consumption and body temperature. Neutral thermal environment (NTE).*

gestational-age infant has a body surface area of approximately 0.15 m² and a body mass of 1 kg. This results in a surface area-to-mass ratio of 0.15 m²/kg, more than six times greater than that of an adult male. Because of this, newborn term and preterm infants lose heat easily and are extremely dependent on the environment to help them maintain body temperature. Infants, like all physical objects, lose heat to the environment by one of four mechanisms: conduction (touching a cold or wet object), convection (cool gas blowing over the skin surface), evaporation (liquid evaporating from the skin surface), and radiation (attempting to warm a cold surface not in contact with the skin). All of these mechanisms must be considered when helping infants deal with their environment.

Hyperthermia is a core body temperature of more than 37.5° C. Hyperthermia in the newborn is usually caused by environmental factors. The infant may be wrapped in too many clothes, placed close to a heater, or placed in too warm an isolette or radiant warmer. It is uncommon, although not rare, for an infant with hyperthermia to have an infection. *Hypothermia* is a core body temperature of less than 36° C. Hypothermia is a more frequent sign of infection in the newborn than in the older child or adult. Hypothermia probably occurs because the infant is unable to maintain normal heat production during an acute infection. The infant, in contrast to the adult, does not shiver when hypothermic.

MEASUREMENT OF BODY TEMPERATURE. There are several methods used to obtain body temperature in infants. The most common of these are axillary and rectal temperatures. Axillary temperature is approximately 0.5° C lower than oral temperature, and rectal temperature (closest approximation of core body temperature) is approximately 0.5° C higher. Other methods of measuring skin temperature are becoming more widely available, including infrared reflectance and liquid crystal thermography. Infrared reflectance is used to measure tympanic membrane temperature, which may be an indicator of core temperature. Liquid crystal thermography measures skin heat and is useful for screening but not particularly accurate.

In addition to body temperature, the examiner should note the temperature of the infant's environment. Most sick infants are placed in a *neutral thermal environment (NTE),* or the environmental temperature at which the infant's metabolic demand and therefore oxygen consumption is the least (Fig. 10-1). If the environmental temperature leaves the neutral thermal range, the infant can usually maintain a stable body temperature but at the cost of a significant increase in oxygen consumption. Neutral thermal environments are defined for an infant based on weight and gestational and chronologic age.[1]

Pulse. The normal pulse rate for infants is between 100 and 160 beats per minute and is a function of the developmental age of the infant. The normal resting heart rate is higher in young-gestational-age infants. The resting heart rate also decreases with increasing chronologic age. Infants cannot significantly change their cardiac output by increasing stroke volume (volume of blood ejected from the heart with ventricular contraction) because their stroke volume at rest is normally more than 90% of maximal stroke volume. Infants increase their cardiac output by increasing their heart rate.

Tachycardia in the newborn is a heart rate greater than 160 beats/min, and *bradycardia* is a heart rate of less than 100 beats/min. Tachycardias in the newborn can be caused by crying, pain, decrease in the circulating blood volume, drugs, hyperthermia, and heart disease. Bradycardias can be caused by hypoxia, Valsalva maneuver (occurs frequently during crying), heart disease, hypothermia, vagal stimulation (e.g.,

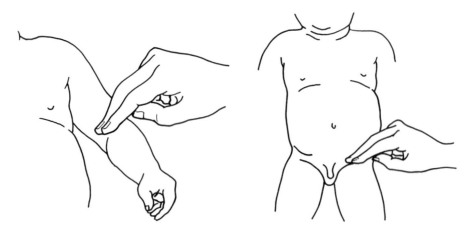

Fig. 10–2 *Position of brachial and femoral pulses in the newborn.*

passing a nasogastric tube), and certain drugs. Also, there are a few infants with *sinus bradycardia* (a normal variant) who have resting heart rates of 70 to 100 beats/min.

ASSESSMENT OF PULSE RATE. Because of the small size of the radial arteries, the pulse is usually evaluated at the brachial or femoral artery. The examiner's index finger pad is used to assess either of these pulses.

To evaluate the brachial pulse, place your index finger pad over the brachial artery on the medial superior surface of the arm just proximal to the medial epicondyle of the elbow with the baby in a supine position. The femoral artery pulse can be assessed at the groin, about halfway across the thigh, just below the inguinal ligament (Fig. 10–2).

Respiratory Rate. The normal respiratory rate for infants is between 30 and 60 breaths per minute and is a function of the developmental age of the infant. The normal respiratory rate decreases as gestational age increases. Infants' respiratory rates are higher than those of older children and adults because of mechanical properties of their chest walls and airways. *Functional residual capacity (FRC)* is maintained by the opposition of two forces: outward spring of the chest wall and recoil of the alveoli. Infants maintain a lower FRC than older children or adults because their chest walls are more compliant. This in turn places their *closing volume* (the lung volume after airway collapse) within their tidal volume. Should the infant attempt to inhale a large tidal volume with collapsed airways, the chest wall would collapse inward (retract). Conversely, a forced exhalation against collapsed airways would trap gas in the lung. Infants breathe rapidly and shallowly to avoid chest wall collapse and gas trapping in the lung. *Tachypnea* is a respiratory rate of greater than 60/min, and *bradypnea* is a respiratory rate of less than 30/min.

In newborns tachypnea can be caused by hypoxemia, metabolic and respiratory acidosis, congenital heart disease, anxiety, pain, hyperthermia, and crying. Bradypnea is not a normal physiologic response in newborns. It can be caused by certain medications

(e.g., narcotics), hypothermia, and central nervous system diseases, and it may be an important clinical sign of the imminent decompensation of the newborn with lung disease. Nonintubated infants with lung disease are usually tachypneic. As the disease progresses and the infant tires from the increasing work of breathing, bradypnea occurs just before total respiratory collapse.

Another common respiratory pattern of infants is *apnea,* or the cessation of respiratory effort. The cessation of breathing for more than 15 to 20 seconds is *long apnea;* for 6 to 14 seconds is *short apnea;* and for less than 6 seconds is a *respiratory pause.* There also exists in newborns a phenomenon known as *periodic breathing.* During periodic breathing the infant has multiple episodes of respiratory pauses or short apnea interspersed with normal-appearing ventilation. This pattern of breathing may continue for several minutes to several hours. Long apnea is always a pathologic state. Small numbers of short apnea and respiratory pauses and short spells of periodic breathing (Fig. 10–3) are normal in preterm and term infants up to 3 months of age.

ASSESSMENT OF RESPIRATORY RATE. The respiratory rate can be obtained by either visually observing chest motion or counting respiration while listening with a stethoscope. Visual observation provides a respiratory rate closer to the infant's resting rate. However, because the normal infant breathes rapidly with a small tidal volume, it may be difficult to see all of the true breaths by the visual method alone. If the examiner thinks this is a possibility, the respiratory rate should be assessed by listening with a stethoscope. The examiner must recognize that the infant is likely to respond to the touch of the stethoscope with a temporary increase in respiratory rate.

The infant's respirations are assessed not only for rate but for regularity and depth. Many immature infants have normal rates but very irregular breathing patterns, which may consist of periodic respiration or even apnea interspersed with periods of normal respiration. Also, infants with significant lung disease may

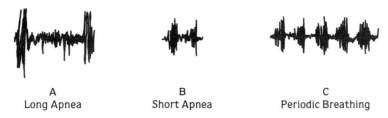

A	B	C
Long Apnea	Short Apnea	Periodic Breathing

Fig. 10–3 *Respiratory patterns showing chest wall motion during* **A,** *long apnea;* **B,** *short apnea; and* **C,** *periodic breathing.*

Table 10-3	Normal Newborn Blood Pressures*†		
Birth Weight (g)	Mean (mm Hg)	Systolic (mm Hg)	Diastolic (mm Hg)
1001–2000	38	50	30
2001–3000	42	59	35
>3000	50	66	41

*Adapted from Kitterman JA, Phibbs RH, and Tooley WH: *Pediatrics* 44:959, 1969.
†Average blood pressures at 12 hours of life.

have normal respiratory rates but tidal volumes so small that they have minimal effective ventilation.

Blood Pressure. The normal values for blood pressure depend on the size of the infant, with pressures decreasing with lower weights (Table 10–3). Usually a term infant's systolic blood pressure should be no higher than 70 mm Hg, with diastolic pressure no higher than 50 mm Hg. Normal pulse pressure (the difference between systolic and diastolic blood pressure) in a term infant is between 15 and 25 mm Hg.

MEASUREMENT OF BLOOD PRESSURE. There are two common methods of determining blood pressure in newborns: blood pressure cuff (sphygmomanometer) and direct arterial pressure. The more common method is to use a blood pressure cuff. Four techniques can be used for determining blood pressure with a cuff. The auscultatory methods used in adults are technically difficult to do in newborns and are rarely used. Two other methods that give a reflection of systolic pressure are the flush technique and the palpation technique. In the flush technique the examiner compresses the extremity beyond the blood pressure cuff, inflates the cuff to above the expected systolic pressure, and deflates the cuff, watching for the return of normal skin color to the blanched extremity. In the palpation technique the examiner palpates an artery distal to the blood pressure cuff, inflates the cuff to above the expected systolic pressure, and allows the cuff to deflate, noting when pulsations return. The fourth method, using an oscillometric noninvasive blood pressure monitoring machine, provides the most reliable blood pressure information of the four techniques mentioned.

The other common method for obtaining blood pressure in newborns is direct measurement of pressure through an arterial cannula. This is discussed in greater depth later in this chapter.

MORPHOMETRIC MEASUREMENTS. In newborns there are three important measurements that are usually not thought of in the physical examination of adults: weight, length, and head circumference. There are standard tables of normal growth for all gestational and developmental ages for these measurements.[2,3] These measurements provide important clues to assessing the infant's past nutritional environment and current state and predicting the infant's long-term growth.

LUNG TOPOGRAPHY. The infant's lungs are situated in the chest much as in the adult, but the infant's chest has a greater anteroposterior (AP) diameter than the adult's. The AP diameter of the infant's chest decreases proportionally and becomes more like the adult configuration with growth (Fig. 10–4.) The imaginary lines and thoracic cage landmarks are the same in infants as in adults (see Chapter 4).

Techniques of Examination

INSPECTION. Inspection is probably the most important and is frequently the most neglected portion of the physical examination of a newborn. The infant should be nude and in a supine position initially. The examiner should look first at the infant's overall appearance to identify level of illness, presence of malformations, and whether the infant's body position is appropriate for the gestational age (Fig. 10–5). The term infant at rest flexes arms and legs into a fetal position. Infants at earlier gestational ages have less muscle tone, and their extremities are less flexed while resting.

The examiner should look at the infant's skin to see if the infant is cyanotic. Some caution must be used in interpreting these findings. Infants with hypothermia or infants with *polycythemia* (hematocrit levels greater than 65%) may have bluish extremities (*acrocyanosis*), yet they are not really hypoxemic. Infants who are preterm and immature with thin skin can look quite pink when they are really hypoxemic. The careful examiner looks at the color of the mucous membranes in the mouth and tongue and of the nail beds in the extremities. These locations give a more reliable indication of the infant's true level of oxygenation.

The examiner must note the effort involved in breathing and the breathing pattern, noting especially

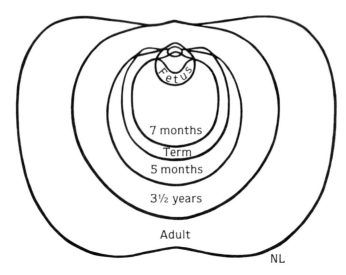

Fig. 10-4 *Changes in anterposterior (AP) chest configuration with age.*

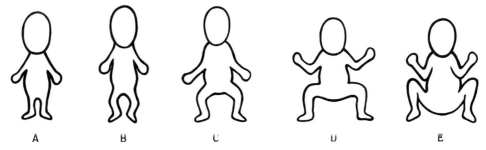

Fig. 10-5 *Progression in body position with gestational age.* **A,** *26-week infant.* **B,** *28-week infant.* **C,** *32-week infant.* **D,** *36-week infant.* **E,** *40-week term infant.*

the regularity of respirations. An infant with respiratory distress characteristically exhibits tachypnea (discussed earlier), retractions, nasal flaring, and sometimes grunting.

Retractions. *Retractions* occur when the lung's compliance is less than the compliance of the chest wall or when there is a significant airway obstruction. Thus, retractions are a sign of an increase in the work of breathing. During inspiration the diaphragm contracts, increasing the negative pressure in the intrapleural space. In the normal respiratory system the lung is the most compliant structure and will inflate to relieve this negative pressure. However, in a healthy infant the chest wall is only slightly less compliant than the lung. Any lung disease that causes a decrease in compliance can cause the lung to become less compliant than the chest wall. The chest wall then represents the most compliant structure in the respiratory system and collapses inward in response to the increasing negative intrathoracic pressure generated by diaphragmatic contraction.

Three common points of collapse are the *intercostal* area (between the ribs), the *subcostal* area (below the lower rib margin), and the *substernal* area (below the bottom of the sternum) (Fig. 10-6). A fourth point of collapse is the *supraclavicular* area (above the clavicles).

Retractions tend to be in different locations depending on the cause of the respiratory distress. Infants with lung disease tend to have retractions toward the center of the body (substernal and subcostal). Infants with heart disease tend to have intercostal retractions on the sides of their bodies, because their large hearts prevent backward motion of the sternum. Finally, infants with obstructed airways tend to have large suprasternal retractions with accessory respiratory muscle contractions.

Nasal Flaring. *Nasal flaring* is the dilation of the alae nasi during inspiration. Nasal flaring is an attempt by the infant to achieve airway dilation to decrease airway resistance, increase gas flow, and achieve a larger tidal volume. Infants are obligate nose breathers, and the minute ventilation they require must be achieved through their noses.

Grunting. *Grunting* is a sound heard at the end of expiration just before rapid inspiration. Grunting is the infant's attempt to increase the gas volume in the lung. It is typically but not exclusively heard in infants with diseases that decrease lung volume (e.g., RDS). Adults and older children with normal FRC typically increase their lung volume from their resting FRC with inspiration. However, infants who have a disease that decreases FRC attempt to increase their lung volume

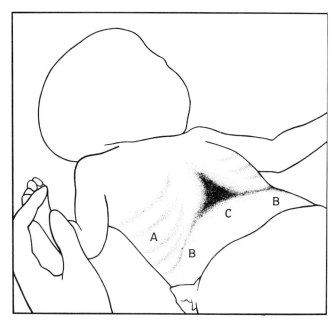

Fig. 10-6 *Retractions commonly occur in these areas.* **A,** *Intercostal.* **B,** *Subcostal.* **C,** *Substernal.*

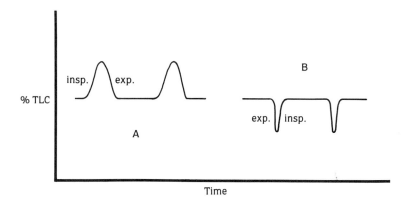

Fig. 10-7 *Comparison of lung volumes during tidal breathing.* **A,** *Adult.* **B,** *Grunting infant.*

by holding their tidal volume at end-inspiration. The infant accomplishes this by occluding the airway with glottic closure and actively exhaling against the closed glottis after the end of inspiration. The grunting sound is produced when the infant suddenly opens the glottis and quickly exhales, inhales, and again closes the glottis (Fig. 10-7).

Precordium. While observing the respiratory pattern and effort, the examiner should look at the *precordium* (area over the heart) for any increase in motion. Increased motion is present if the examiner can see the chest wall lifting or moving as the heart contracts. This increase in motion, or *hyperdynamic precordium,* is an indication of increased volume load on the heart, usually secondary to a left-to-right shunt of blood through the ductus arteriosus. When an infant has a *patent ductus arteriosus (PDA),* the anatomic connection between the aorta and pulmonary artery remains open and blood from the aorta flows into the pulmonary artery, which can cause congestive heart

failure and pulmonary edema. The presence of a hyperdynamic precordium is a clue that the infant's respiratory distress may not be completely pulmonary in origin and requires further evaluation.

PALPATION. In infants, palpation is an important tool for physical assessment. However, the use of palpation in the physical examination of infants is directed less at the lungs than at other organ systems that may influence pulmonary function.

The easiest organ to palpate is the skin. Palpation of the skin can give the examiner valuable information about the infant's cardiac output and fluid volume status, both of which are clinically important in the evaluation of the infant's pulmonary status.

The three aspects of the skin that are useful in evaluating cardiac output are the skin perfusion, the skin temperature, and the peripheral pulses. To check the skin perfusion, or capillary refill, the examiner should blanch the infant's skin with a finger and note how long it takes for the blanched skin to recover its color. Capillary refill should be checked on the trunk and extremities of the infant. Capillary refill will be longer than 3 seconds if the infant has a low cardiac output. The examiner should keep in mind that there are other pathologic states, such as acidosis, hypoxemia, hypoglycemia, and hypothermia, that can decrease blood flow to the skin and prolong capillary refill.

An approximation of the infant's skin temperature can be determined by feeling the skin. The dorsum, or backside, of the hand and fingers is more sensitive to temperature than the front side or palmar surface. Infants with low cardiac output or any abnormality that decreases skin blood flow have skin that feels cool.

Checking and comparing the central and peripheral arterial pulses gives the examiner valuable clues about the infant's cardiac output. A careful examiner should be able to palpate the pulses of the radial, brachial, posterior tibial, and dorsalis pedis arteries. The infant should be examined closely for a decrease in cardiac output if these pulses are not easily palpable or if there is a big discrepancy between them and the central arterial pulses of the femoral or axillary arteries. The examiner should also look for any discrepancies between the pulses in the upper and lower extremities. If pulses in the lower extremity are weaker than in the upper, the infant may have an aortic obstruction such as *coarctation of the aorta* or *interrupted aortic arch syndrome.*

Finally, the examiner can achieve a rough idea about the fluid volume of the infant by feeling the turgor or fullness of the infant's skin. Infants with low fluid volumes have a loss of skin turgor. This is manifest by "tenting" or gathering of the skin when it is lightly pinched together.

Palpation of the abdomen may be of help in assessing an infant's pulmonary status. An infant's abdomen and abdominal organs move significantly with respiration because the diaphragm is the major source of power for respiration and the abdominal wall musculature is relatively weak. Anything that impedes the motion of the abdomen or its organs hinders the infant's respiration. Liver or spleen enlargement (*hepatomegaly* or *splenomegaly*); enlargement of other organs such as kidneys, bladder, or bowel; or intraabdominal tumors can impede abdominal motion. Distention of the abdomen by fluid (*ascites*) or air (*pneumoperitoneum*) also impedes abdominal motion.

Gentleness is important when palpating an infant's abdomen. Many examiners fail to feel enlarged organs or masses because their vigor pushes the organ or mass away from their fingers. Examiners should gently place their second and third fingers on the skin of the lower abdomen perpendicular to the spine, then slowly slide their fingers up toward the costal margin. The liver should be soft and mobile, palpable on the right side of the abdomen parallel to and 1 to 2 cm below the costal margin. The spleen may be palpable as a soft tip below the left costal margin at the anterior axillary line. The kidney may be palpated in the immediate newborn period by compressing it between one hand placed under the posterior flank and the other hand firmly pressing in from the anterior abdominal wall.

Major central nervous system diseases, such as *intraventricular hemorrhage (IVH)* and *hydrocephalus,* are causes of respiratory problems in preterm infants. The examiner should evaluate the tautness of the *anterior fontanel,* the soft spot on top of the infant's head. Infants who have had a major IVH or hydrocephalus may have a full, tense fontanel. Also, the *cranial sutures* (junctions between two skull bones) may be widely separated in these conditions.

AUSCULTATION. The last of the classic techniques routinely used in infant examination is auscultation. Auscultation is the least definitive of the three examination techniques discussed, but this does not mean it is unimportant. Auscultation yields the best information if the infant is quiet. Because of this, auscultation is the first thing done after inspection. Auscultation should be done with a warm chest piece that has a small (1.0- to 1.5-cm diameter) diaphragm and bell. This allows for maximal localization of the findings. For auscultatory examination of the lungs the infant is ideally in the prone position. However, because most infants are in a supine position or on their side, the examiner should try to complete the majority of the examination before moving the infant. If the infant's position does not allow for an adequate examination, the examiner should gently move the infant to a more desirable position. Normal infant breath sounds are bronchovesicular in character and harsher than in the adult. The techniques for use of the stethoscope and the types of adventitious lung sounds heard are the same as in the adult (see Chapter 4).

The clinical significance of breath sounds in the infant is similar to that in the adult. Because the infant's thoracic cage is small and sound is easily transmitted, breath sounds are usually not entirely absent. A decrease in breath sounds implies a decrease in gas flow through the airways, as in RDS, atelectasis, pneumothorax, or pleural effusion. Wheezing implies gas flow through constricted airways; infants with bronchopulmonary dysplasia (BPD) may have wheezing. Crackles usually imply excess fluid or secretions in the lung (pulmonary edema) or the presence of a pneumonia. A loud ripping sound like the separation of Velcro is frequently associated with the presence of pulmonary interstitial emphysema.

In addition to the breath sounds, the examiner should listen for the presence of cardiac murmurs. The presence of a murmur does not mean that the infant has heart disease, but it may mean that the infant requires further diagnostic evaluation. Almost all infants have physiologic murmurs such as physiologic pulmonary stenosis or venous hum. The pathologic

Table 10-4 WBC Count and Partial Differential Count During the First 2 Weeks of Life*

Age	Leukocytes (mm³)	Neutrophils (mm³)			Lymphocytes (mm³)
		Total	Segmented	Band	
Birth					
Mean	18,100	11,000	9400	1600	5500
Range	9000–30,000	6000–26,000	—	—	2000–11,000
Mean %	—	61	52	9	31
7 days					
Mean	12,200	5500	4700	830	5000
Range	5000–21,000	1500–10,000	—	—	2000–17,000
Mean %	—	45	39	6	41
14 days					
Mean	11,400	4500	3900	630	5500
Range	5000–20,000	1000–9500	—	—	2000–17,000
Mean %	—	40	34	5.5	48

*Adapted from Fanaroff AA and Martin RJ, editors: *Behrman's neonatal-perinatal medicine: diseases of the fetus and infant,* ed 3, St Louis, 1982, Mosby.

murmurs that are characteristic of the newborn period are caused by PDA, ventricular septal defect, tricuspid insufficiency, and major congenital heart disease.

The abdomen is another area of the body where auscultation may help in pulmonary assessment. The abdomen should always be auscultated when there is a question about whether an infant is properly intubated. Loud sounds of air movement will be heard over the stomach during inspiration if the endotracheal tube is in the esophagus. The presence of a bruit (a murmur-like sound) in the liver should raise the question of whether the infant has an arteriovenous malformation in the liver. This type of malformation can cause respiratory distress because of high-output heart failure.

TRANSILLUMINATION. Transillumination is a technique frequently used in examining infants but not older patients. It can be used in infants because their chest wall is thin enough to shine a light through. Usually the source is a bright fiberoptic light, which is placed against the chest wall in a dark room. Normally this produces a lighted "halo" around the point of contact with the skin. In the presence of a pneumothorax or pneumomediastinum, the entire hemithorax lights up. This technique is rapid and allows for quick treatment of a serious condition. The procedure should be done by an examiner familiar with the technique because some fiberoptic lights can cause cutaneous burns and it is possible to be misled by the area of transilluminence.

Clinical Laboratory Data

Two crucial issues face anyone who wishes to use the clinical laboratory in pulmonary assessment of newborns. The first and most obvious issue is that the normal values for clinical laboratory tests may be different between newborns and adults. The magnitude of these differences depends on the laboratory test in question. However, to complicate this issue further, the normal values may be dependent on the gestational or

chronologic age of the newborn. The second, less obvious issue is the relationship between the test sample volume and the infant's blood volume.

An infant's blood volume is approximately 80 to 100 mL/kg of body weight, with young-gestational-age infants tending to have higher volume per weight. Depending on the severity of the illness, most infants can tolerate an acute blood loss of no more than 10% of their blood volume. This means that for a 1-kg infant, all of the laboratory tests should require no more than 10 mL of blood. The infant will need replacement volume should the laboratory tests require more than this amount.

A corollary of this issue is that even if the infant can tolerate the volume loss, it may not be practical or technically feasible to withdraw the sample volume. Infants have small vessels that tend to be fragile, and it is often not possible to draw large volumes by venipuncture or arterial puncture.

HEMATOLOGY. The white blood cell (WBC) count in infants tends to be higher than in older patients. Normal values vary with the chronologic age of the infant (Table 10–4). As a general rule, infants closer to delivery have higher WBC counts. Total WBCs tend to fall over the first week of life to a plateau that is just slightly higher than the normal values for adults.

Leukocytosis, or WBCs over 15,000/mm³, is usually a reflection of the infant's environment rather than of infection as in the older patient. When evaluating an infant with a high WBC count, infection should be considered, but also crying, hyperthermia from excess wrapping or high environmental temperature, and other environmental stresses. *Leukopenia,* particularly *neutropenia* (an absolute neutrophil count of less than 2000 neutrophils/mm³) is a more ominous sign. Usually neutropenia indicates an infection and implies that the infant is being overwhelmed. The neutropenia from infection can be caused by one of two mechanisms: peripheral consumption of neutrophils or failure to produce and release neutrophils from the bone marrow.

Table 10-5	Hematologic Values During Gestation*					
Age (wk)	Hemoglobin (g/dL)	Hematocrit (%)	Mean Corpuscular Volume	Mean Corpuscular Hemoglobin	Mean Corpuscular Hemoglobin Concentration	Reticulocytes (%)
24	14.0	40	123	38	31	5–10
28	14.5	45	120	40	31	5–10
34	15.0	47	118	38	32	3–10

*From Oski FA and Naiman JL: *Hematologic problems in the newborn,* ed 2, Philadelphia, 1972, WB Saunders.

There is still a great deal of debate about whether the newborn's leukocytes function as well as those of an older person. It is fair to say that even a term newborn's response to infection is not optimal, but why this is and what cellular or immunologic functions are involved are still being investigated.

The normal values for the red blood cell (RBC) count, hematocrit, and hemoglobin are dependent on chronologic age. In utero the fetus is stimulated to produce a large number of red cells by the relatively low partial pressure of arterial oxygen (Pao_2). This stimulus is withdrawn at the time of birth. The normal newborn severely limits or ceases the production of RBCs until a new stimulus is received. Anemia is the normal physiologic stimulus for this. In healthy term infants this "physiologic anemia" occurs at about 6 weeks of age. In preterm infants it usually occurs between 8 and 12 weeks of age. Infants who have received transfusions have a 4- to 6-week delay in the onset of RBC production. After an infant begins RBC production, hematocrit and hemoglobin levels rise to slightly above the level of an adult and remain there throughout childhood (Tables 10–5 and 10–6).

Platelet counts are often obtained in newborns and infants when they are being evaluated for thrombocytopenia, disseminated intravascular coagulation, or other bleeding disorders (see Table 10–6). Normal values are between 100,000 and 350,000/mm³; however, most clinicians will not transfuse infants with platelets unless the count is less than 25,000/mm³ and the infant is bleeding. *Thrombocytopenia* (platelet count less than 100,000/mm³) may be a sign of disseminated intravascular coagulation from severe infection or one of many other causes. *Thrombocytosis* (platelet count over 350,000/mm³) is usually not a clinical problem in the newborn. Thrombocytosis can be seen in infants with iron deficiency anemia, hemolytic anemia, recovery from thrombocytopenia, and in infants whose mothers have inflammatory collagen-vascular disease. A high normal value in infants is not well established, but clinical symptomatology is not seen until the platelet count exceeds 1 million.

The values for partial thromboplastin time, prothrombin time, fibrinogen, mean corpuscular volume, mean corpuscular hemoglobin, mean corpuscular hemoglobin concentration, and reticulocyte count are

Table 10-6	Hematologic Values for Low-Birth-Weight and Term Infants*		
Weight	Hemoglobin	Reticulocytes	Platelets
< 1200 g			
1–3 days	15.6	8.4	148,000
4–7 days	16.4	3.9	163,000
14 days	15.5	1.9	162,000
28 days	11.3	4.1	158,000
6 wk	8.5	5.4	210,000
8 wk	7.8	6.1	212,000
1201–1500 g			
1–3 days	20.2	2.7	151,000
4–7 days	18.0	1.2	134,000
14 days	17.1	0.9	153,000
28 days	12.0	1.0	189,000
6 wk	9.1	2.2	212,000
8 wk	9.3	2.7	244,000
2500–4000 g			
1–3 days	18.2	3–7	200,000
7 days	17.0	0–1	248,000
14 days	16.8	0–1	252,000

*Adapted from Fanaroff AA, and Martin RJ, editors: *Behrman's neonatal-perinatal medicine: diseases of the fetus and infant,* ed 3, St Louis, 1982, Mosby.

shown in Tables 10–5 and 10–7. Most of these values are close to the normal values for adults. Mean corpuscular volume and reticulocyte counts are higher in the immediate newborn period but decrease over the first few months of life to normal adult levels.

BLOOD CHEMISTRY. Blood glucose is probably the most frequent blood chemistry determination made in newborns. This relatively simple test is of tremendous importance because *hypoglycemia,* or low serum glucose, is as detrimental to the developing newborn's brain as hypoxia is. Because the exact levels and length of time necessary to cause damage to the central nervous system have not been determined, most physicians will treat an infant with a glucose level of less than 40 mg/dL. There are easy methods for approximating serum glucose at the bedside. These methods are used as screening tests, and any abnormalities found are confirmed with serum glucose levels obtained in the clinical laboratory. The normal values for glucose in the newborn period are shown in Table 10–8.

Table 10-7 Normal Coagulation Test Values*

Category	Fibrinogen (mg/dL)	Partial Thromboplastin Time (sec)	Prothrombin Time (sec)
Preterm infant (1500–2500 g)	233	90	17 (12–21)
Term infant, cord blood	216	71	16 (13–20)
Term infant, 48 hr	210	65	17.5 (12–21)
Normal child	190–420	37–50	12–14

*Adapted from Fanaroff AA and Martin RJ, editors: *Behrman's neonatal-perinatal medicine: diseases of the fetus and infant,* ed 3, St Louis, 1982, Mosby.

Table 10-8 Normal Values for Blood Chemistries*

Determination	Value
Total protein (g/dL)	4.8–8.5
Albumin (g/dL)	2.9–5.5
Random blood sugar (mg/dL)	
Preterm	21–65
Term	30–110
Child	60–105
Bilirubin (mg/dL)	
24 hr	1.0–6.0
48 hr	6.0–8.0
3–5 days	4.0–15.0

*Adapted from Fanaroff AA and Martin RJ, editors: *Behrman's neonatal-perinatal medicine: diseases of the fetus and infant,* ed 5, St Louis, 1982, Mosby; and Meites S, editor: *Pediatric clinical chemistry: a survey of normals and instrumentation,* with commentary, Washington, DC, 1992, American Association for Clinical Chemistry.

Hypoglycemia can be caused by a variety of metabolic disturbances including infection, hyperinsulinism secondary to maternal diabetes mellitus, inadequate glycogen stores secondary to being small for gestational age, and others. Although most of the time only symptomatic treatment is needed, often an extensive evaluation of the infant's glucose control mechanisms is necessary. *Hyperglycemia,* or blood glucose greater than 160 mg/dL, is most often iatrogenic. However, hyperglycemia is also one of the early signs of septicemia in infants. The problems with hyperglycemia from diabetes mellitus are very rare in this age group.

Total protein and albumin are useful tools in evaluating the nutritional status of the ill newborn. They may also give helpful clues for evaluating the cause of pulmonary edema (Table 10–8). Colloid osmotic pressure is usually not measured in infants because the sample volume required is relatively large.

The serum enzymes that are so useful in adults are much less useful in newborns and the pediatric age group. For many of the enzymes normal values have not yet been established, and the clinical significance of abnormal values is frequently unknown. *Lactate dehydrogenase (LDH), aspartate transaminase (AST,* formerly SGOT), and *alanine transaminase (ALT,* formerly SGPT) are used when evaluating liver function. *Creatinine phosphokinase (CPK)* and its isoenzymes have been used in a research setting, but currently they do not have widespread clinical use. *Alkaline phosphatase*

is useful in evaluating bone growth and the adequacy of an infant's nutrition.

Serum drug level determinations are becoming increasingly useful during the newborn period. Because infants are small, there is a narrow difference between therapeutic and toxic doses of most medications. The need for obtaining drug levels has always been present, but it has only been practical as improving technology has permitted smaller sample volumes. Drug levels for antibiotics, anticonvulsants, antiarrhythmics, and theophylline are frequently used. Gentamycin, vancomycin, and other aminoglycosides can now be used with greater margin of safety. Digitalis and cyclosporine levels are used less often, but will probably have increased use in the future.

Serum bilirubin determination is a test used frequently in evaluating newborns. Probably well over 50% of infants have a bilirubin determination made during the first week of life. There are a large number of causes for hyperbilirubinemia during the newborn period. Some abnormalities in bilirubin metabolism are likely to affect pulmonary function. First is hyperbilirubinemia from any cause that requires treatment by phototherapy. Phototherapy is associated with tachypnea in the newborn, although the exact mechanism of the tachypnea is not known. Second is hyperbilirubinemia treated with an exchange transfusion. An exchange transfusion is a procedure in which the infant's blood is replaced with donor blood by cyclically withdrawing the infant's blood and transfusing aliquots of donor blood. Usually exchange transfusions are used to treat hyperbilirubinemia caused by hemolytic diseases. Finally, the most severe and rarest is hyperbilirubinemia associated with severe hemolytic disease and hydrops fetalis. In this disorder the hyperbilirubinemia is not the fundamental problem. The infant has *anasarca* (massive total body edema) with pleural effusions and abdominal ascites that cause profound respiratory failure.

Electrolytes, blood urea nitrogen (BUN), and *serum creatinine* determinations are all useful laboratory tests for newborns. The normal values (Table 10–9) are dependent on the infant's chronologic age, nutritional status, and fluid status. They are generally similar to adult values, with serum potassium being slightly higher and BUN and creatinine levels lower. These values are useful in a wide variety of clinical situations, from assessing the infant's fluid status to evaluating renal function.

Table 10–9	Normal Electrolyte Values for Newborns*	
Determination		**Value (mEq/L)**
Sodium		133–149
Potassium		5.3–6.4
Chloride		87–114
Total carbon dioxide		19–22

*Adapted from Fanaroff AA and Martin RJ, editors: *Behrman's neonatal-perinatal medicine: diseases of the fetus and infant*, ed 3, St Louis, 1982, Mosby.

Calcium and *phosphorus* levels are of indirect importance in the evaluation of a newborn with chronic lung disease. Infants with bronchopulmonary dysplasia (BPD) or other chronic lung diseases have increased work of breathing and increased metabolic and nutritional needs. The metabolism of calcium and phosphorus is a valuable clue to the nutritional status of the chronically ill infant. A chronically ill infant with poor nutrition has low levels of calcium and phosphorus and an increased risk of developing rickets. Rickets may worsen the infant's pulmonary status by increasing the chest wall compliance secondary to a decrease in the mineralization of the ribs and decreasing the infant's depth of respiration secondary to pain from rib fractures.

MICROBIOLOGY. The sputum analysis that is useful in adults is not possible in newborns. Until a child is about 6 years old, sputum is swallowed and not expectorated. However, if the infant is intubated, samples can be obtained with sterile suction catheters through the endotracheal tube. In an older infant or young child, samples may be obtained from the stomach via nasogastric tubes. Samples obtained from the stomach should be interpreted with caution. Even samples obtained through the endotracheal tube may reflect bacterial colonization rather than infection. In addition to the gram stain, culture, and sensitivity, a polymorphonuclear neutrophil (PMN) count is useful. High PMN counts in the tracheal or stomach samples are strongly suggestive of infection rather than colonization.

NEWBORN BLOOD GASES. Monitoring the blood gas status of newborns is done either by analysis of the gas in a blood sample or by transcutaneous monitoring. Analysis of blood samples is done on blood obtained from arterial, capillary, or venous sources. Transcutaneous measurements can be made of oxygen (Po_2) and carbon dioxide (Pco_2) tension, oxygen saturation (So_2), or near-infrared niroscopy.

ARTERIAL BLOOD GASES. Arterial blood samples are the most reliable source for blood gas analysis in newborns. Normal values in newborns depend on the age of the infant when the blood is drawn (Table 10–10). Once infants are beyond the transitional period after delivery (usually 4–12 hours), their arterial oxygen (Pao_2), carbon dioxide ($Paco_2$), and pH values should be similar to those of the older child or adult. During the transitional period, Pao_2 is lower, $Paco_2$ is higher, and pH is lower as compared to later. Sick infants who require supplemental oxygenation or mechanical ventilation often have values for Pao_2, $Paco_2$, and pH that are not quite normal for this age but are accepted because of the complications that result from such treatment.

The fact that an arterial blood sample provides the most reliable source for blood gas analysis in newborns needs to be weighed against the problems associated with arterial puncture in newborns and young infants. Arterial puncture is technically possible, but it requires good technique and frequently extra assistance. Newborns and young infants have small arteries and are notoriously uncooperative, moving their extremities and making the arterial puncture difficult. This also increases the risk of arterial damage. Additionally, arterial blood does not always reflect the resting state for the newborn or young infant, since the discomfort associated with the puncture usually causes the baby to cry. Infants who are crying change their ventilation in one of two patterns: they either hyperventilate or hold their breath and stop ventilating. Either of these changes in ventilation rapidly alters the value for oxygen, carbon dioxide, and pH in the blood.

CAPILLARY BLOOD GASES. Because of the risk and the technical expertise involved, many nurseries and pediatric wards obtain their blood gas samples by capillary puncture. Although the results require special consideration, less technical expertise and fewer people are required to do a capillary puncture than an arterial puncture. Capillary samples are generally obtained by puncturing the skin of the infant's warmed heel. Fingers and earlobes are less commonly used sites for obtaining capillary samples.

When the values of capillary carbon dioxide tension (Pc_{co_2}) and pH are compared with those obtained by arterial sample, carbon dioxide is 2 to 5 mm Hg higher, and pH is 0.01 to 0.03 unit lower. These small differences are inconsequential in most clinical situations. However, when the values of the capillary oxygen tension (Pc_{o_2}) are compared with those obtained by arterial samples, the difference is not so slight. Unfortunately, there is not a fixed ratio for Pao_2 to Pc_{o_2}. An infant with a Pc_{o_2} of 50 mm Hg may have a Pao_2 of anywhere from 50 to 90 mm Hg or higher. The only statement that can be made about Pao_2 by knowing only Pc_{o_2} is that Pao_2 is no lower than Pc_{o_2}.

When capillary blood gas sampling is appropriate, the person drawing the sample and the person evaluating the results need to remember the underlying problems that must be overcome in obtaining the sample. A capillary sample that closely reflects arterial blood must be obtained from a warmed extremity (skin temperature should be approximately 103° F). Caution must be used in warming the extremity so that the

Table 10–10	Normal Values for Arterial Blood Gases in Infants*				
Age	pH	Pao$_2$	Paco$_2$	HCO$_3^-$	Base Excess
Newborn	7.25–7.35	50–70	26–40	17–23	(−10 – −2)
24 hr	7.30–7.40	60–80	26–40	18–25	(−4 – +2)
2 days–1 mo	7.32–7.43	85–95	30–40	16–25	(−6 – +1)
1 mo–2 yr	7.34–7.46	85–105	30–45	20–28	(−4 – +2)

*Unpublished data from author's laboratory; and data from Meites S, editor: *Pediatric clinical chemistry: a survey of normals, methods and instrumentation, with commentary,* Washington, DC, 1982, American Association for Clinical Chemistry.

infant is not burned and the warming device does not cool and secondarily cool the extremity. If the extremity is edematous, acrocyanotic, or not warmed or if the infant has poor peripheral circulation, all of the values will be unreliable. Also, since this procedure is painful, like arterial puncture, it reflects the infant's condition during crying, which may be vastly different from rest. Finally, if there is difficulty obtaining the sample, the results may reflect air or tissue contamination rather than the infant's true status.

VENOUS BLOOD GASES. Venous blood samples can also be obtained for gas analysis. These are useful in computing the oxygen extraction or carbon dioxide production of tissues (see Chapter 12).

NONINVASIVE MONITORS. One of the most significant recent advances in monitoring sick patients has been the development of transcutaneous oxygen and carbon dioxide monitors. These monitors give staff members up-to-date information that they otherwise would not have. In newborn intensive care units, these devices are being used around the clock to monitor sick infants.

Transcutaneous Oxygen Monitors. Transcutaneous oxygen pressure (tcPo$_2$) monitors measure electrical current that is directly proportional to the number of oxygen molecules present in the electrode. The tcPo$_2$ electrode measures oxygen present in the capillaries and tissue of the skin and not Pao$_2$, but tcPo$_2$ usually approximates Pao$_2$, with tcPo$_2$ slightly lower than Pao$_2$. Any condition that decreases blood flow under the electrode, such as acidosis, shock, hypovolemia, or hypoglycemia, can cause a tcPo$_2$ that is falsely lower than Pao$_2$.

The tcPo$_2$ monitor is a good method of evaluating the physiologic changes that occur with blood gas sampling. The pain of blood gas sampling can cause changes in the infant's resting condition. The infant can produce an increase in Paco$_2$ and a decrease in Pao$_2$ by becoming apneic. If the infant cries and hyperventilates, the Paco$_2$ might decrease and the Pao$_2$ might increase. The person obtaining the sample should note the tcPo$_2$ value three times: before disturbing the infant, at the beginning of blood flow, and 40 to 60 seconds after completion of sampling. These three values can then be used to assess the infant's resting condition, the physiologic changes the procedure caused, and the correlation between Pao$_2$ and tcPo$_2$.

TRANSCUTANEOUS CARBON DIOXIDE MONITORS. Transcutaneous carbon dioxide pressure (tcPco$_2$) electrodes are beginning to be widely used clinically. Like the tcPo$_2$ electrodes, they measure the gas present in the skin and not that in the blood. The tcPco$_2$ electrode has merit as a trend monitor for carbon dioxide, but its limitations are not yet known.

There are still problems with both tcPo$_2$ and tcPco$_2$. Both techniques use heated electrodes, which must be repositioned every 2 to 4 hours. The heater in the electrode can cause burns. The tape used to secure the electrode may tear the fragile skin of a preterm infant during repositioning. The monitors have slow response times and are subject to multiple skin perfusion artifacts.

Pulse Oximeters. Pulse oximetry has become a useful monitoring tool in the past few years. Pulse oximeters measure the changing transmission of red and infrared light through a pulsating capillary bed to identify the saturation of hemoglobin with oxygen. They overcome many of the problems of the transcutaneous monitors. The oximeter is not heated and so does not require repositioning, and does not cause burns. It has a much faster response time, and it does not require tight taping to the skin. It has its own problems, however. The early models were very sensitive to motion disruption. They are also very sensitive to background illumination. Many of these problems are being dealt with by the equipment manufacturers. (See Chapter 12 for a further discussion of pulse oximeters.)

Niroscopy. Near-infrared *niroscopy* is a monitoring technique that is being evaluated and may become important. This technique measures the oxidation-reduction state of cytochrome aa$_3$, which is thought to be a marker of tissue oxygenation status.

Pulmonary Function Testing in Newborns

VOLUMES. Pulmonary function can be tested in newborns. In the past few years, standard computerized equipment for neonatal and young infant pulmonary function testing has become available. This has taken pulmonary function testing in this age group out of the realm of the research laboratory and made it available to the clinician. While nurseries that measure pulmonary function are usually still found in major teaching and research institutions, now small institutions without major research support can be involved in pulmonary function testing. A variety of different technologies exist that compute pulmonary functions. These devices are capable of traditional lung mechanics, active and passive exhalation mechanics, and FRC measurements using either helium dilution or nitrogen washout techniques.

The fundamental difference between newborn and adult pulmonary function testing is the patient's ability to cooperate. The pulmonary function tests for adults and older children are dependent on the patient's ability to follow simple commands. The tests done on infants must be reproducible without patient cooperation.

Three volumes can be measured relatively easily in newborns independent of their cooperation: (1) FRC, (2) thoracic gas volume (TGV), and (3) crying vital capacity (CVC). A certain degree of caution must be exercised when interpreting the results of these tests, however. The range of normal values is great, and all three tests are subject to error. To compare the results of these tests for two babies or even for the same baby at different times, the results must be described against a standard unit. Usually, this is done with the body weight in kilograms (e.g., cubic centimeters of gas per kilogram) or body length in centimeters (e.g., cubic centimeters of gas per centimeter).

FRC is measured by two methods: (1) closed system helium dilution and (2) open system nitrogen washout. Both methods are becoming available with the computerized pulmonary function machines. TGV (method of DuBois[4,5]) requires the use of a plethysmograph and measures all of the gas in the thoracic cavity whether or not it is communicating with the airway. By comparing the TGV with the FRC the clinician can determine the presence of trapped gas in the thorax.

CVC is the measurement of tidal volume while the infant is crying. It is useful in following infants who have lung diseases that cause changes in FRC (e.g., RDS), in whom it is difficult to measure FRC. CVC does require that the infant be able to cry vigorously, which may be difficult for sick infants.

A method of measuring distribution of ventilation is available using a nitrogen washout curve. The pulmonary clearance delay (PCD)[6,7] divides the lung into fast, intermediate, and slow ventilating areas based on calculations from expired nitrogen concentrations obtained during a nitrogen washout. The PCD can be used to evaluate what percentage of the lung is ventilating effectively.

MECHANICS.

Compliance. *Compliance* is a measure of the distensibility of the lung. It is calculated by dividing change in volume by change in pressure and requires measurement of tidal volume and transpulmonary pressure. Tidal volume can be measured in newborns by either pneumotachography or plethysmography. Plethysmographs are tricky to use with infants because making an airtight seal around the face is difficult. Also,

plethysmographs for infants are all custom-made. Therefore, most nurseries measure tidal volume by pneumotachography. Transpulmonary pressure is the difference between airway pressure and pleural pressure. It is approximated by measuring airway and esophageal pressure in intubated infants and esophageal pressure in nonintubated infants. Either an air-filled balloon or saline-filled catheter in midesophagus can be used. Tidal volume is integrated from the pneumotachometer signal, a pressure-volume loop is constructed, and the compliance of the lung is calculated. The compliance of the chest wall can also be measured by changing the two pressure sources from airway minus esophageal to esophageal minus atmospheric pressure.

Resistance. Resistance is a measure of the inhibition of gas flow through airways. It is calculated by dividing change in transpulmonary pressure by change in flow. These measurements are obtained with the same equipment used for compliance.

Work of Breathing. The work of breathing is the cumulative product of the pressure generated and the volume at each instant of the respiratory cycle. It is usually calculated by planimetry of the pressure-volume curve or by electrically integrating the pressure and volume signals.

CHEMORECEPTOR RESPONSE. Sudden infant death syndrome has stimulated a tremendous amount of research into the way infants control respiration. Some investigators have shown that newborns have a blunted response to hypercapnia and a severely diminished or paradoxical response to hypoxia. Many nurseries have the capability of looking at carbon dioxide and oxygen responses. These studies are usually done by measuring tidal volume, minute ventilation, end-tidal oxygen and carbon dioxide, and transcutaneous oxygen. The infant's minute ventilation is then plotted against Pa_{CO_2} or F_{IO_2}.

Radiographs

Radiographic views and the methodology for obtaining radiographs are significantly different between infants and older patients. In the older patient the x-ray beam passes from the back of the patient to the front (posteroanterior [PA]). This minimizes distortion from the divergence of the x-ray beam as it passes through the body. Also, the preferred position for taking x-ray films in adults is having the patient upright. Infants cannot easily be placed upright, and they dislike being forced to lie on their stomachs; thus, most x-ray films are taken with the infant in the supine position, lying on the x-ray film. The x-ray beam passes from the front of the infant to the back (AP view).

The typical views used to evaluate an infant's lung are AP and lateral chest films. As in the older patient, these two views allow the examiner to see all areas of the lung in a standard presentation. It is important that the viewer approach the reading of these films systematically. The viewer should evaluate the airways—including the larynx, trachea, and major bronchi—for deviation from external masses or pressure, for filling defects from internal masses or hypoplasia, and for normal location in the chest.

Occasionally decubitus films of the chest and abdomen are helpful in evaluating the status of the newborn or young infant. They can be useful in detecting the presence of fluid or air in the pleural space and in evaluating the presence of fluid from a foreign body. In older patients this is done with a combination of inspiration and expiration chest films. Because newborns cannot cooperate for these views, right and left lateral decubitus views show an obstruction by not collapsing. For example, if the infant has a mechanical obstruction in the right mainstem bronchus, the left lung will collapse if the infant is lying left side down, but the right lung will not collapse when the infant is lying right side down. Decubitus films are also useful in showing the presence of pleural fluid collections.

Infants who have unexplained tachypnea, cyanosis, abnormal breath sounds, malformations of the chest or airway, or a sick appearance should have a chest x-ray examination.

Assessing Critically Ill Infants

AIRWAY. The importance of maintaining a patent airway has been emphasized. The evaluation of airway patency in newborns is not as easy as it is in adults and older children. Infants with obstructed airways still have chest wall motion, and with chest auscultation they may even have noises that could be misinterpreted as breath sounds. The examiner needs a thorough knowledge of normal newborn breath sounds and chest wall motion to be able to evaluate airway patency in infants.

Even experienced examiners can be deceived about the adequacy of the airway in intubated infants because the signs usually used in the older patient may not be reliable in the newborn. For example, an infant whose right mainstem bronchus is intubated may still have breath sounds in the left hemithorax, and left chest wall motion. This can occur because of the short tracheal lengths (less than 10 cm) and the increased compliance of the chest wall. The examiner must be careful when auscultating to compare all of the lung fields. A misplaced endotracheal tube creates a subtle difference in breath sounds, particularly in the apices, which can be picked up by the careful examiner.

The synchrony of spontaneous ventilation rate compared with a mechanical ventilation rate is more important than its frequency in the newborn. An infant who exhales during the inspiratory cycle of the ventilator can generate tremendous intrathoracic pressures,

potentially damaging the lung. Asynchronous breathing between the infant and the ventilator is usually seen during the hours and days immediately following intubation and the start of mechanical ventilation. The examiner must watch the infant's chest wall motion while listening to the ventilator cycle to document this asynchronous breathing. An inward motion of the chest or absence of an outward motion of the chest wall during mechanical inspiration may indicate that the infant is breathing asynchronously with the ventilator.

The airway pressures monitored in infants are the peak airway pressure, mean airway pressure, positive end-expiratory pressure, and occasionally esophageal pressure. These pressures are interpreted like their counterparts in the adult intensive care unit (see Chapter 12).

Static airway pressure, intrapleural pressure, lung volume, and expired gas analysis are not generally used in the clinical management of newborns. Airway resistance and lung compliance are being used clinically more frequently with the advent of reproducible, easy-to-use neonatal pulmonary function equipment. F_{IO_2} is the single gas analysis that is used in managing newborns. In a closed system, such as an intubated patient receiving mechanical ventilation, F_{IO_2} should be measured on the inspiratory side of the ventilator circuit. For an infant breathing spontaneously, F_{IO_2} should be measured close to the infant's nose. Equipment to utilize measurement of expired esophageal carbon dioxide and nitrogen pressures is being developed for use in newborns and should start making a clinical impact soon.

HEMODYNAMIC ASSESSMENTS. Hemodynamic monitoring in the critically ill infant is in some ways easier and in other ways more difficult than in the adult. The presence of patent umbilical vessels makes cannulation of the aorta and inferior vena cava quite simple. However, cannulation of the pulmonary artery is quite difficult and usually must be done in a cardiac catheterization laboratory. Also, the newborn may have varying degrees of right-to-left shunt, depending on the pulmonary vascular resistance, with the presence of a PDA and a patent foramen ovale. This makes calculation of a cardiac output difficult if not impossible.

Cannulation of the umbilical artery and vein is routine practice in almost every nursery in the country. The technique for such a cannulation is easy, and although there are risks to indwelling central catheters, they can be minimized by using a good technique and appropriate indications. Additionally, many nurseries are now utilizing percutaneous puncture to cannulate radial arteries and subclavian veins. The indications for umbilical artery catheterization include (1) a source for frequent arterial blood gas sampling, (2) continuous blood pressure monitoring, and (3) large-scale blood replacement (e.g., exchange transfusion). The indications for umbilical venous catheterization include (1) central venous pressure monitoring and (2) large-scale

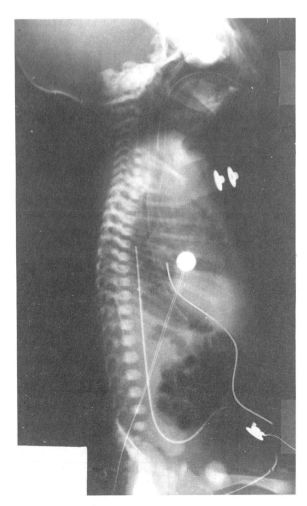
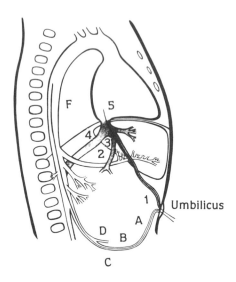

Fig. 10-8 *Lateral radiograph and diagram of the course of umbilical venous and arterial catheters. Umbilical venous catheter enters through umbilicus, passes through* **1,** *umbilical vein,* **2,** *portal vein,* **3,** *ductus venosus, and* **4,** *inferior vena cava and stops in* **5,** *right atrium. Umbilical arterial catheter enters through umbilicus, passes through* **A,** *umbilical artery,* **B,** *hypogastric artery,* **C,** *internal iliac artery,* **D,** *common iliac artery, and* **E,** *abdominal aorta and stops in* **F,** *thoracic aorta.*

blood replacement. The course of the umbilical artery and vein is shown in Fig. 10-8.

These two methods of hemodynamic monitoring are susceptible to many of the same problems that exist in adults and older children. Signal damping is a major concern for several reasons: (1) the small internal lumina of the catheters involved; (2) softer materials used in catheter production; and (3) development of fibrin sleeves. Infections, thrombus formation, embolization, and arteriospasm are also major concerns when using these monitoring methods.

Assessment of the Older Infant and Child

History

The history of the older infant and the child combines that of the newborn and the adult. The parents remain the major source of information about the infant or child until adolescence. Until the age of 2 years, it is important to include the birth history as part of the evaluation of these patients. The historian assessing the patient must begin to include a review of systems in the historical assessment at 3 months of age. The review of systems is not of great benefit before this.

It is important to differentiate acute from chronic problems. When did the symptoms begin? How rapidly have the symptoms progressed? Is the child truly sick or just not feeling well?

The historian inquiring about the pulmonary symptoms in an older infant or child is limited to those signs that are visible or audible to the parent. Historical information about coughing, wheezing, cyanosis, purulent nasal discharge, frequent colds or infections, and change in behavior is easy to obtain. Dyspnea, chest pain, night sweats, and other symptoms that are not observable by the parent may be impossible to document. It should be remembered that hemoptysis and sputum expectoration do not occur in children. Most children swallow any mucus, blood, or purulent material that might be generated by the upper or lower airway.

In addition to the usual respiratory symptoms, the older infant and child frequently have extrapulmonary symptoms caused by pulmonary disease. The careful historian queries parents for these. The most obvious of these signs is general activity. Infants and children who are sick act differently from well babies and children. The parents or guardians are the best judges of an infant's or child's normal behavior. The clinician must be alert to a parent's statement that the child is acting differently. Similarly, infants and children who are sick do not eat well. The interviewer should inquire about the infant's feeding habits if the parents do not bring this up.

Gastrointestinal upset is a frequent complaint with the infant and child. Vomiting and diarrhea are major causes for hospitalization in this age group. Many people who take care of infants and children forget that vomiting and diarrhea may be manifestations of pneumonia or other pulmonary diseases. Also, diseases such as cystic fibrosis and gastroesophageal reflux may have gastrointestinal and pulmonary symptoms.

Finally, an infant or child who does not maintain growth appropriate for developmental age (failure to thrive) should be investigated for an underlying chronic pulmonary disease. In this age group such diseases would be asthma, cystic fibrosis, gastroesophageal reflux, foreign body aspiration, chronic infection (e.g., sinusitis, cytomegalovirus, tuberculosis, sarcoidosis, histoplasmosis, coccidioidomycosis, bronchiectasis, lung abscess, and empyema), nonasthmatic allergic pulmonary diseases, neuromuscular disease affecting the chest wall, immotile cilia syndrome, and others.

Physical Examination

The components of the physical examination discussed in Chapter 4 are the basis for the physical examination of an older infant or child. Observation, palpation, percussion, and auscultation should be used to localize the disease process within the patient's body. The uniqueness of the physical examination in the older infant or child is in the order of the examination. It is most important to gain the infant or child's trust and cooperation. The examiner should first examine the parts that upset or frighten the infant or child the least, saving for last those parts of the examination that are upsetting or frightening. If possible, the clinician should make a game out of the examination.

Clinical Laboratory

Older infants, children, and adolescents tend to have a narrower range of normal values on both clinical laboratory and blood gas laboratory tests. Their normal values tend to reflect the normal values seen in adults.

Although some laboratory tests show a wide divergence from adult values (e.g., growth hormone and others), in most clinical situations the normal values for adults can also be used for the pediatric population.

Other special tests are occasionally used in this age group for the diagnosis of diseases that have a major pulmonary component. Sweat chloride is the most prominent of these. This test is used to make the diagnosis of cystic fibrosis. It is relatively simple to do, but laboratories frequently obtain erroneous results because of poor methodology or technique.

Blood Gases

The older infant and child present a unique problem in obtaining and interpreting blood gases. Their arteries are still small and arterial puncture is not easy. Most of these patients vigorously object to having an arterial puncture done even if they are relatively sick. Because of this, more than one person is usually required to obtain the sample. Like the newborn, the older infant and child can quickly change arterial blood gas (ABG) values by crying and hyperventilating. The clinician interpreting the ABG sample should be aware not only of the patient's disease but of what conditions existed when the sample was obtained.

Pulse oximetry is more reliable in this age group than transcutaneous monitoring. Because of the increased thickness of the skin and subcutaneous tissue, there is a greater difference between arterial and transcutaneous gas values. However, transcutaneous monitoring is still useful as a trending device, to identify changes in the patient's status. It is also useful in estimating the true arterial gas value, since the value may have changed during the sampling process. The greatest problem with pulse oximeters in this age group is motion artifact. Manufacturers are currently working on solutions to this problem.

Pulmonary Function Testing

Beyond the newborn and young infant stage, standard pulmonary function testing is not possible until the child is between 5 and 6 years of age. There are two important points to remember when doing pulmonary function tests on a child. First, the validity of the results is directly related to the child's cooperativeness. Children in the 5- to 8-year range can have remarkably short attention spans and be frustratingly uncooperative. Second, the lungs of the child are still growing, and the results of pulmonary function tests must be adjusted to body size. Some exciting new techniques are being tested in research centers that will allow pulmonary function testing in older infants and younger children to be done. Although these techniques are not yet commercially available, they do provide hope for the future care of these patients.

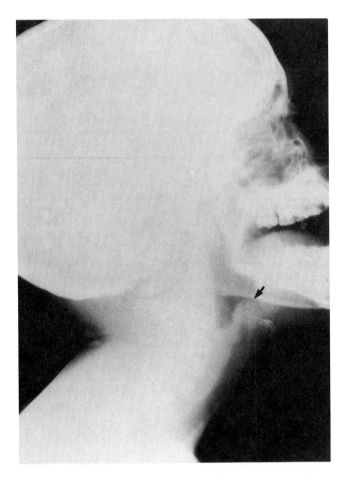

Fig. 10-9 *Lateral neck radiograph demonstrating an enlarged epiglottis (arrow). (Courtesy of Lionel Young, MD, Loma Linda University Medical Center, Loma Linda, Calif.; reproduced with permission from Wilkins RL and Dexter JR: Respiratory disease: principles of patient care, Philadelphia, 1993, FA Davis.)*

Radiographs

As the infant becomes older and progresses through childhood, radiographs become easier to obtain and interpret. After the child can sit erectly, it becomes possible to take a PA chest film. One of the major problems in the young ambulating child is foreign body aspiration. When a child can follow simple instructions, after the age of 2 to 3 years, inspiratory-expiratory films can be taken to evaluate this problem. Before the age of 2 to 3 years, right and left lateral decubitus films can be obtained that yield essentially the same information as inspiratory-expiratory films.

Two other major respiratory but nonpulmonary diseases that are common to young children are croup and epiglottitis. It is important to distinguish croup or laryngotracheobronchitis from epiglottitis because the treatment and clinical course are significantly different. Both of these diseases have a prominent inspiratory stridor. The radiographic view that helps distinguish between these two diseases is a lateral view of the neck. Subglottic narrowing is present in laryngotracheobronchitis, and supraglottic narrowing with a large

thumb-shaped epiglottis is present with epiglottitis (Fig. 10-9).

REVIEW QUESTIONS

1. *Infants born in late gestation are more susceptible to*
   a. *respiratory distress syndrome*
   b. *pulmonary interstitial emphysema*
   c. *intracranial hemorrhage*
   d. *meconium aspiration*

2. *What Apgar parameter usually deteriorates first in the hypoxic infant?*
   a. *respiratory effort*
   b. *heart rate*
   c. *muscle tone*
   d. *skin color*

3. *Infants needing extensive medical resuscitation at birth will have Apgar scores in the range of*
   a. *7-10*
   b. *4-6*
   c. *0-3*
   d. *none of the above*

4. T F *Hypothermia is a frequent sign of infection in the newborn.*

5. T F *Hyperthermia in a newborn is usually caused by environmental factors.*

6. *What is the upper limit of normal range for heart rate in the newborn?*
   a. *120 beats/min*
   b. *140 beats/min*
   c. *160 beats/min*
   d. *180 beats/min*

7. *Which of the following is* not *a typical cause of tachypnea in the newborn?*
   a. *hypothermia*
   b. *hypoxemia*
   c. *respiratory acidosis*
   d. *pain*

8. *What is the upper limit for normal systolic blood pressure in the term newborn?*
   a. *60 mmHg*
   b. *70 mmHg*
   c. *80 mmHg*
   d. *90 mmHg*

9. *What is indicated by the presence of retractions in the newborn?*
   a. *a stiff chest wall*
   b. *stiff lungs*
   c. *reduced airways resistance*
   d. *heart failure*

10. What is indicated by a capillary refill greater than 3 seconds in the infant?
    a. normal cardiopulmonary function
    b. respiratory failure
    c. circulatory failure
    d. renal failure

11. What effect does abdominal distention have on respiration?
    a. impedes diaphragm movement
    b. increases the chance of ventilatory failure
    c. may cause respiratory failure
    d. all the above

12. What abnormal finding during chest auscultation is associated with bronchopulmonary dysplasia in the infant?
    a. bronchial breath sounds
    b. inspiratory fine crackles
    c. wheezing
    d. stridor

13. What is the normal leukocyte count for newborns?
    a. 5,000 to 10,000
    b. 9,000 to 30,000
    c. 15,000 to 40,000
    d. 21,000 to 35,000

14. What is indicated by leukopenia in the infant?
    a. overwhelming infection
    b. chronic infection
    c. acute infection
    d. local infection

15. What clinical problem is associated with low serum levels of calcium and phosphorus?
    a. acute hypoxia
    b. liver failure
    c. poor nutrition
    d. renal failure

16. What is the normal range for PaO_2 at birth?
    a. 40 to 60 mmHg
    b. 50 to 70 mmHg
    c. 60 to 80 mmHg
    d. 70 to 90 mmHg

17. What parameter(s) demonstrate(s) the largest difference when comparing capillary blood to arterial blood?
    a. PO_2
    b. PCO_2
    c. pH
    d. none of the above

18. Which of the following conditions is least likely to cause a falsely low tcPO2 reading?
    a. acidosis
    b. shock

    c. hypovolemia
    d. hyperthermia

19. What lung volume is not easily measured in the newborn?
    a. thoracic gas volume
    b. residual volume
    c. functional residual capacity
    d. crying vital capacity

20. Which of the following clinical findings suggest the need for a chest radiograph in the infant?
    a. cyanosis
    b. unexplained tachypnea
    c. abnormal breath sounds
    d. all the above

REFERENCES

1. Klaus MH and Fanaroff AA, editors: *Care of the high-risk neonate,* ed 4, Philadelphia, 1993, WB Saunders.
2. Smith DW: *Growth and its disorders,* Philadelphia, 1977, WB Saunders.
3. Fanaroff AA and Martin RJ, editors: *Behrman's neonatal-perinatal medicine: diseases of the fetus and infant,* ed 5, St Louis, 1992, Mosby.
4. DuBois AB, Botelho SY, and Comroe JH: A rapid plethysmographic method for measuring thoracic gas volume: a comparison with a nitrogen washout method for measuring functional residual capacity in normal subjects, *J Clin Invest* 35:322, 1956.
5. Klaus MH and others: Lung volume in the newborn infant, *Pediatrics* 30:111, 1962.
6. Strang LB and McGrath MW: Alveolar ventilation in normal newborn infants studied by air wash-in after oxygen breathing, *Clin Sci* 23:129, 1962.
7. Fowler WS, Cornish ER, Jr, and Kety SS: Lung ventilation studies VIII: analysis of alveolar ventilation by pulmonary N_2 clearance curves, *J Clin Invest* 31:40, 1952.

BIBLIOGRAPHY

Burgess WR and Chernick V: *Respiratory therapy in newborn infants and children,* New York, 1982, Thieme-Stratton.
Fanaroff AA and Martin RJ, editors: *Neonatal-perinatal medicine: disease of the fetus and infant,* ed 5, St Louis, 1992, Mosby.
Forester RE and others: *The lung,* ed 3, St Louis, 1986, Mosby.
Kendig EL and Chernick V, editors: *Disorders of the respiratory tract in children,* ed 5, Philadelphia, 1990, WB Saunders.
Kitterman JA, Phibbs RH, and Tooley WH: Aortic blood pressure in normal newborn infants during the first 12 hours of life, *Pediatrics* 44:959, 1969.
Meites S, editor: *Pediatric clinical chemistry: a survey of normals, methods and instrumentation, with commentary,* Washington, DC, 1982, American Association for Clinical Chemistry.
Nathan DG and Oski FA: *Hematology of infancy and childhood,* ed 3, Philadelphia, 1987, WB Saunders.
Streeter NS, editor: *High-risk neonatal care,* Aspen, Colo, 1986, Aspen Publications.
Thibeault DW and Gregory GA: *Neonatal pulmonary care,* ed 2, Menlo Park, Calif, 1986, Addison-Wesley.
Wilkins RL, Hodgkin JE, and Lopez B: *Lung sounds: a practitioner's guide,* St Louis, 1988, Mosby. (This book includes an audiocassette with normal and abnormal lung sounds in infants.)

Section Two

Advanced Assessment Techniques

Identification of the Critically Ill Patient

A critically ill patient is one who has developed, or is at high risk for developing, failure of one or more organs. Because of the presence of these real or potential life-threatening problems, the patient requires continuous observation and intervention to prevent complications and restore health.

Critically ill patients are usually cared for in critical care units, also called *intensive care units (ICUs)*. ICUs vary greatly in size, degree of specialization, level of patients' conditions, and sophistication of monitoring. They have in common an immediate availability of emergency life-support equipment, supplies, ancillary services, and a patient care team trained for continuous patient assessment and rapid intervention.

Critical Care Assessment

Critical care assessment is a continuous process: gathering data, analyzing relationships, looking for trends, making educated guesses about cause-and-effect relationships, obtaining results from tests or interventions, making predictions, and reevaluating.

Baseline assessment in critical care refers both to the initial collection and analysis of history, physical examination, and laboratory data on admission, and to the periodic reassessment of the patient's condition and all available data. Baseline assessments are usually performed at the beginning of each shift and after a major procedure or a change in the patient's condition.

Trends are comparisons of what is happening now to what happened 10 minutes ago, 1 hour ago, yesterday, 2 days ago, etc. For most physiologic measurements—in fact for most of the evaluations made in the ICU—the *trends are far more important than any single measurement.* Past history plus physiologic trends plus current clinical status suggests the physiologic cause and treatment of the current problem and predicts potential problems.

A *high index of suspicion* means that certain problems may be expected because of the patient's previous or current condition or because of the therapeutic modalities being used. For the critically ill patient, *prediction, prevention,* and *early recognition of potential problems* are as important to survival as the correct treatment of the current condition. Problems that place a patient at risk for developing acute respiratory failure are listed in the table below.

Acute Respiratory Failure: Who Is at Risk?*[†]

Patients With	Associated Diseases or Disorders
Pulmonary disorders	COPD, restrictive airway diseases, pulmonary embolism, high-altitude pulmonary edema
Impaired airway function	Acute airway obstruction: epiglottitis, croup, bronchiolitis, aspiration of foreign body, laryngeal edema or masses, vocal cord paralysis, excessive mucus production
Airway irritation: asthma, inhaled irritants
Infection: bronchitis, bronchiectasis, pneumonias
Retained secretions, atelectasis	Inadequate pulmonary toilet especially due to immobility, weakness, debilitation, chest pain, abdominal distention/pain, restrictive binders, and chest dressings
Increased pulmonary capillary wedge pressures	Fluid overload, pulmonary venous disease
Cardiogenic pulmonary edema: LV failure, mitral valve stenosis
Increased capillary permeability, ARDS	Transfusion reaction, drug overdose (especially opiates like heroin), fat emboli, DIC, chemical or smoke inhalation, infection, septic shock, tuberculosis, pneumonias
Humoral substances (histamine, endotoxin, kinins, prostaglandins, myocardial depressant factor) released with: anaphylaxis, sepsis, shock, pancreatitis
Chest surgery/trauma	Fractured ribs, flail chest, lung or cardiac contusion, hemothorax, pneumothorax, cardiopulmonary bypass
Extrathoracic surgery/trauma	Especially head, spine, abdomen
Impaired central nervous system	Sedatives, narcotics, tranquilizers, anesthetic drugs, sleep disorders (sleep apnea syndrome), cerebral vascular accident, tumors, increased ICP, neurogenic pulmonary edema
Impaired neuromuscular transmission or muscle function	Neuromuscular disease: poliomyelitis, tetanus, Guillain-Barré syndrome, muscular dystrophies, myasthenia gravis, multiple sclerosis, amyotrophic lateral sclerosis, botulism
Spinal cord injury, curarelike drugs, hypokalemia, organic phosphate poisoning
Hypophosphatemia resulting from: inadequate nutrition, alcoholism, combined use of hyperalimentation and antacids, hemodialysis, diabetic ketoacidosis
Chronic conditions	Smoking, severe obesity, pickwickian syndrome, old age

* Data from references 1–4.
† COPD = chronic obstructive pulmonary disease; LV = left ventricular; ARDS = adult respiratory distress syndrome; DIC = disseminated intravascular coagulation; ICP = intracranial pressure.

Respiratory Assessment of the Critically Ill Patient

Respiratory assessment of the critically ill patient is a continuous comparative analysis of data obtained by history and physical examination, clinical tests, mechanical and invasive physiologic monitoring, and calculated indices to evaluate the following:

1. Ability of the airway-lung-thorax to move air into and out of the lung (ventilation)
2. Ability of oxygen and carbon dioxide to diffuse across the alveolar-capillary membrane (pulmonary gas exchange)
3. Ability of the blood to carry the gases from the lungs to the body tissues and back to the pulmonary circulation (oxygen transport)
4. Ability of the heart and vascular system to move blood between the heart and lungs and body tissues (hemodynamics)
5. Ability of the transport system to adjust to the changing demands of the body tissues
6. Ability of the tissues to receive and use nutrients and oxygen (oxygen uptake)

In keeping with this definition, the following chapters discuss assessment of cardiopulmonary function and measures used to evaluate ventilation, hemodynamics, oxygen transport and tissue oxygenation, and nutrition. Patient interviewing and physical examination, chest films, electrocardiography, arterial blood gases and other laboratory measurements, also mainstays of respiratory assessment in the ICU, have been discussed in previous chapters.

REFERENCES

1. George RB: Pathophysiology of acute respiratory failure. In Bone RC, George RB, Hudson LD: *Acute respiratory failure,* New York, 1987, Churchill Livingstone.
2. Adler SN, Lam M, Connors AF, Jr: *A pocket manual of differential diagnosis,* Boston, 1982, Little, Brown.
3. Morris AH: Acute respiratory failure: therapeutic strategies. In Parrello JE: *Current therapy in critical care medicine,* Philadelphia, 1987, BC Decker.
4. Johanson WG and Peters JI: Respiratory failure. In Murray JF and Nadel JA: *Textbook of respiratory medicine,* Philadelphia, 1988, WB Saunders.

Chapter 11

Physical Assessment of the Critically Ill Patient

Susan Jones Krider

LEARNING OBJECTIVES

Upon completion of this chapter, the reader should be able to accomplish the following:

1. *Identify the importance of the physical assessment in the critically ill patient.*

2. *Recognize the factors that can cause airway occlusion.*

3. *Recognize the conditions that can predispose patients to aspiration.*

4. *Identify the signs of partial and complete airway obstruction.*

5. *Identify factors which may cause airway obstruction of an artificial airway.*

6. *Recognize the significance of evaluating the following items in regards to artificial airways:*
   a. *position and depth*
   b. *security of tube in the airway and equipment connections*
   c. *health of tissue around site of insertion*
   d. *cuff pressure*
   e. *ventilator alarms*
   f. *signs of problems associated with long term intubation*
   g. *relationship between size of airway and work of breathing*

7. *Identify the indications and hazards of extubation.*

8. *Recognize the significance and factors that affect respiratory rate, rhythm, and lung sounds in a critically ill patient.*

9. *Recognize the significance of asymmetrical and paradoxical chest wall movement and paradoxical abdominal movement.*

10. *Recognize a definition, cause(s), physical assessment findings, and significance of the following problems:*
    a. *pleural effusion*
    b. *pneumothorax*
    c. *tension pneumothorax*
    d. *subcutaneous emphysema*
    e. *pneumomediastinum*
    f. *reexpansion pulmonary edema*

11. *Identify the methods used to drain the pleural space and complications associated with those methods.*

12. *Identify the purpose and correct function of one-, two-, or three-bottle closed chest drainage systems.*

13. *Identify the normal findings/values, and the significance of the following parameters as they relate to the assessment of circulation:*
    a. *peripheral skin temperature*
    b. *capillary refill time*
    c. *cyanosis*
    d. *urine output*
    e. *level of consciousness*
    f. *heart rate and rhythm*
    g. *arterial pressure*
    h. *jugular venous pressure, hepatomegaly, and peripheral edema*

Chapter Outline

Airway
Aspiration
Airway Obstruction
Artificial Airways
Extubation

Breathing
Respiratory Rate and Rhythm
Lung Sounds
Changes in Chest Wall Movement
Barotrauma and Pleural Fluid Collection
Chest Drainage

Circulation
Peripheral Skin Temperature
Capillary Refill Time
Cyanosis
Urine Output
Level of Consciousness
Heart Rate and Rhythm
Palpitations
Pulses
Cardiac Tamponade and Pericardial Effusion
Arterial Pressure
Jugular Venous Pressure
Hepatomegaly and Peripheral Edema

Chapter Overview

The purpose of the intensive care unit (ICU) is to provide an environment where potential problems can be prevented and emergent problems immediately recognized and managed. It must be remembered that the *ICU patient is at risk for failure of one or more organ systems and requires continuous observation.* Assessment of the patient for distress that requires immediate therapeutic intervention should become second nature to every member of the ICU team and should be a part of every interaction with the patient.

Most new critical care staff members become so concerned with equipment, numbers, procedures, and what to do if something happens that they forget to look at the most important thing, the patient. Placing information on physical examination first in this book makes a statement about priorities. *The patient is most important, not the machinery.* Computers and machines are tools; humans are the assessors and decision makers.

Machines are only capable of providing reliable information if they are constantly maintained and used with the utmost attention to proper technique. In fact one study showed that 37% of all adverse events in an intensive care setting were related to equipment malfunction.[1] Therefore the reliability of numbers must be questioned in light of the patient's condition. When the patient is sitting up in bed and talking with a heart rate of 70 beats per minute, a respiratory rate of 12 breaths per minute, a urine output of 50 mL/hr, and warm and pink feet, and the monitor displays an arterial pressure of 60/30 mm Hg, the monitor is wrong! (The bed may have been put down to low position without moving the transducer.) When the patient is "straight-lining" on the electrocardiographic (ECG) monitor while rearranging bedcovers and asking for a pillow, look for a detached lead. Reattaching the lead does more for the patient's well-being than a precordial thump. Anyone who has worked in an ICU for even a short time can relate many stories of minor to major catastrophies occurring because someone looked at the monitors first and the patient second.

There are other reasons for emphasizing physical assessment. Even in the most mechanized and computerized ICUs, there are times when the patient is not connected to the monitors: admission, equipment change in preparation for transport (ideally not *during* transport), equipment failures, and the last few hours before discharge from the ICU. The patient's survival at such times is dependent on the staff's ability to recognize subtle changes.

Humans, unlike machines, have the capacity to gather information from multiple sources simulta-

Table 11–1 Conditions Predisposing the Patient to Aspiration Syndromes*

Condition	Possible Cause of Condition†
Altered level of consciousness	Cardiac arrest, stroke, seizure, coma, CNS trauma General anesthesia, especially emergency or close to eating Sedatives, narcotics
Pharyngeal or laryngeal dysfunction	Laryngospasm Neuromuscular disorders, stroke Inflammation/edema secondary to extubation procedure, trauma Vocal cord paralysis from recurrent laryngeal nerve damage, compression, or intubation
Presence of an artificial airway	Endotracheal tube, tracheostomy
Improper placement of an artificial airway	Intubation of the trachea with an esophageal obturator airway Intubation of the esophagus with an endotracheal tube or nasopharyngeal airway that is too long
Esophageal dysfunction and procedures	Surgery, dilation, prosthesis, stent Reflux, varices, bleeding
Gastrointestinal disorders	Hiatus hernia, nasogastric tube placement, reflux Ileus secondary to bowel obstruction or decreased bowel perfusion Abdominal compression (e.g., inflation of "MAST suit") Insufflation of the stomach (e.g., CPR, misplaced airway)
Vagal nerve stimulation	Suctioning, choking, gagging, vomiting Cholinergic stimulants (e.g., ipecac)
Resumption of oral or nasogastric feeding following anesthesia, trauma, or prolonged period without feeding	

* Data from references 4, 5.
† CNS = central nervous system; MAST = military antishock trousers; CPR = cardiopulmonary resuscitation.

neously, check it for accuracy, evaluate its significance to the patient, and take action. Humans can perceive the unspoken or unmeasured: when it's time for the kids to visit (even if they are only 4 and 5 years old), when undisturbed rest will be the best healer, when "the patient just doesn't look right" or has "lost the will to live." Although some patients live when the numbers say they should die, others "crash" when the numbers say they should be fine. It is human perception that provides the first clue that all is not well and that immediate intervention is necessary. These "gut feelings," as they are called in the ICU, come from a complex interaction of observation, experience, and caring. No machine or computer can ever replace caring, observant, persistent people who can see when something is going wrong and get help before it is too late.

Physical assessment usually provides the first clue. The ABCs of cardiopulmonary resuscitation—*ai*rway, *b*reathing, and *c*irculation—can provide a framework for learning as well as performing physical assessment in the ICU. This chapter describes the signs and symptoms used to assess the adequacy of these three elements.

Airway

Maintenance of an open airway has the highest priority.[2] The airway may be occluded by any of the following[3]:
- Aspiration of food or vomitus
- Foreign objects (including dentures)
- Loss of tonicity of the submandibular muscles, which support the tongue

- Excessive production of secretions
- Constriction of the airway smooth muscles (as in asthma)
- Bilateral vocal cord paralysis
- Spasms of the larynx or bronchi
- Swelling of the larynx or internal neck tissues (as may occur with a submucosal and retropharyngeal hemorrhage, epiglottitis, allergic reactions, head and neck trauma, subcutaneous emphysema in infants, or following extubation)

Aspiration

The presence of a nasogastric (NG) tube does not negate the possibility of vomiting with aspiration, especially during tube placement or while the tube is connected to gravity drainage rather than suction. The risk of vomiting with aspiration is very high during emergency anesthesia and catastrophic events such as trauma, myocardial infarction, or cardiac arrest. Additionally, patients experiencing altered states of consciousness, vagal nerve stimulation, or dysfunction of the pharynx, larynx, or esophagus are at increased risk for aspiration. Table 11–1 lists situations and disease processes that should alert the clinician to watch carefully for signs of aspiration.

Airway Obstruction

The airway may be partially or totally occluded. *Partial airway obstruction* produces noisy airflow, which may be accompanied by an increased effort to breathe; suprasternal and intercostal muscle retraction; nasal flaring; tachypnea; and tachycardia. *Stridor* or *crowing* suggests laryngospasm, *wheezing* indicates bronchial narrowing, *gurgling* points to the presence of excessive secretions or foreign matter in the airway, and *snoring* suggests partial occlusion of the pharynx.

When the *airway is totally occluded,* no sound is heard; obstruction is recognized by the patient's extreme efforts to move air with deep sternal and intercostal retractions, nasal flaring, diaphoresis, cyanosis, anxiety progressing to panic, and respiratory arrest.

Artificial Airways

The presence of an artificial airway does not negate the possibility of airway obstruction. All artificial airways must be monitored continually for patency. Airways containing valves (e.g., Kirschner valves or speaking tracheostomy tubes) may become occluded when the excess moisture or secretions cause the valves to stick or otherwise work improperly. In general the smaller the tube, the higher the risk of obstruction. Kinking mucus plugs, rapid mobilization of secretions from the lung, tracheal tissue protruding through the hole of a fenestrated tracheostomy tube, or obstruction of the tip of the tube by the tracheal wall, carina, or a piece of dislodged cuff can obstruct ventilation through an ET or tracheostomy tube. When a patient with atelectasis or large amounts of retained secretions is placed on a Roto-Rest (kinetic therapy) bed or begins intensive chest physiotherapy, secretions may be mobilized so rapidly that suctioning is required every 10 minutes (or more often) to keep the airway patent. In such a situation, even a patient on continuous ventilation may show signs of hypoxia if the artificial airway is not modified to permit continuation of mechanical ventilation during suctioning.

The following example points out the importance of checking for airway obstruction in the patient with an artificial airway.

Following a routine tracheostomy cleaning procedure, the patient became increasingly restless and began showing signs of tachypnea and tachycardia, using accessory muscles for breathing and "fighting the ventilator." Suctioning was performed without obtaining secretions, and breath sounds were clear with auscultation. The intercannula of the tracheostomy tube was again removed for cleaning, and no foreign material was found; however, the patient immediately relaxed. When the intercannula was reinserted, the patient panicked, threw a liter bottle of saline solution (the closest thing he could reach) through a nearby window, and pulled out his tracheostomy tube. Another tracheostomy tube was inserted, the patient was reconnected to a ventilator, and he relaxed and went to sleep. On examination of the first tube, silastic-like mucus was found surrounding the inside of the tube. When the inner cannula was inserted, the mucus plug was pushed down and occluded the end of the tube. Because of the consistency of the mucus, a suction catheter would pass through the plug but could not aspirate it from the tube.

In addition to airway patency, the following should be checked and documented on each shift:

1. *Position and depth of an artificial airway.* The angle and movement of the tube, the ease of suctioning, the ease of replacing the inner cannula of a tracheostomy tube, and centimeter or other markings on the tube can be used as reference points. The actual position is verified by the chest film.
2. *Security of both the tube in the airway and the connections.* Accidental or self-extubation may have disastrous consequences.
3. *Health of the tissue around the tube insertion site.* Tissue breakdown (necrosis) from the constant pressure of the tube occurs most commonly in the nose and at the corners of the mouth. Necrosis is best prevented by careful hygiene and slight variations in the tube position.
4. *Pressure of the cuff on the tracheal wall.* Ensuring that there is air movement around the cuff with each breath and using a high-volume, low-pressure cuff decrease the risk of tracheal necrosis. A *minimal leak* is verified by placing a stethoscope over the trachea and hearing air movement around the cuff during the last third of a positive pressure inspiration. Two alternative methods may be used to control the amount of pressure in the cuff. When *minimal occlusive volume (MOV)* is used, a minimal leak is verified, then just enough air is put back into the cuff to eliminate the sound of the leak, thus providing a seal in the airway. Alternatively, the pressure in the cuff can be monitored with a manometer and maintained at or below a pressure of 20 mmHg so that the intracuff pressures do not exceed mucosal perfusion pressure. An *increasing cuff pressure* while the cuff volume remains constant is indicative of tissue swelling around the cuff. Conversely, *increasing cuff volumes* required to reach MOV may indicate tracheal dilation and tracheolmalacia.
5. *Ventilator disconnect and apnea alarms.* These should be set as appropriate for continuous mechanical ventilation.
6. *Signs of problems associated with long-term tracheal intubation.* These signs include infection, vocal cord paralysis, tracheoesophageal fistula, tracheal stenosis, and tracheal errosion. Sudden hemoptysis or a pulsating tracheostomy tube suggest that the tube is eroding through the anterior wall of the trachea and into a major vessel, usually the innominate or subclavian artery or the aortic arch. Erosion of a tube through the trachea into either a vessel or the esophagus is a life-threatening complication.
7. *Relationship of the size of the tube to the work of breathing.* Normally the largest tube that

fits into the airway without causing excessive pressure on the vocal cords or tissues is selected to reduce airway resistance and the work of breathing. Although the ventilator can deliver adequate gas volumes and pressures to offset the use of an airway that is too small, the patient may not be able to perform the same task without becoming exhausted during the weaning process. On the other hand, using a fenestrated tube that is too large in the patient being weaned from an artificial airway can result in partial obstruction of the airway and increased work of breathing when the tube is occluded. The signs of partial airway obstruction were discussed earlier.

Extubation

In general, the patient is ready for extubation when:

1. The original reason for intubation has been resolved.
2. The effects of anesthesia and other respiratory depressant medications no longer exist.
3. The patient is able to mobilize and cough up secretions without repeated suctioning.
4. Ventilator weaning criteria have been met.
5. A trial of spontaneous continuous positive airway pressure (CPAP) or T-tube breathing has been successfully completed.

There are no specific measurements to predict a patient's readiness for extubation beyond those used to assess readiness for ventilator weaning (see Chapter 12.) However, the longer the patient has been intubated, the more carefully the appropriate time for extubation must be selected. Ideally, it will be during the day at a time when the patient is most rested. Adequate personnel and equipment must be readily available for reintubation.

The patient should not be left unattended until it is clinically evident that reintubation will not be necessary. Mild apprehension and discomfort during the extubation as well as hoarseness and some dysphagia (difficulty swallowing) immediately following extubation are expected. However, following extubation, patients may also experience laryngospasm, laryngeal edema, glottic injury, vomiting, or aspiration. Bleeding, tracheal stenosis, dysrhythmias, or even cardiac arrest can accompany or follow the traumatic removal of any artificial airway and are reasons for emergent intervention.

Breathing

Spontaneous breathing depends on the following factors:

1. Patent airway
2. Intact and mobile thoracic cage
3. Maintenance of pleural contact and normally negative intrapleural pressure
4. Normally functioning respiratory muscles
5. Intact and normally functioning nervous system control of ventilation
6. Adequate amount of functioning lung tissue
7. Reasonable elasticity (compliance) of the lung
8. Will to breathe and live

When any of these factors are disrupted, breathing can become inadequate or cease entirely. The physical examination techniques used to evaluate a patient's breathing in the ICU are the same as those used in chest physical diagnosis: measurement of respiratory rate, rhythm, and pattern; auscultation of lung sounds; and inspection and palpation of the chest (see Chapter 4). A high index of suspicion (an expectation that secondary problems will occur because of the patient's history and current therapies) helps immensely in early recognition of emerging respiratory complications.

Respiratory Rate and Rhythm

The rate, depth, and rhythm of breathing are controlled by the respiratory centers in the pons and medulla of the brainstem. Increases in carbon dioxide production and the metabolic rate, hypoxemia, and acidosis stimulate both the rate and depth of breathing. An increased metabolic rate occurs with exercise, anxiety, stress, infection, fever, heart failure, pulmonary edema, hepatic coma, and early hypoglycemia. *Kussmaul's breathing,* characterized by rapid deep respirations that resemble sighs, is seen with metabolic acidosis, particularly diabetic ketoacidosis.

Rapid shallow breathing is usually associated with restrictive lung disorders and is also seen when the diaphragm is elevated, as may occur with abdominal distention or phrenic nerve damage. Patients that cannot be successfully weaned from mechanical ventilation tend to adopt a pattern of rapid shallow breathing immediately on discontinuation of mechanical ventilation.[6,7] Despite initial evidence of increased drive and maintenance of minute ventilation, this pattern of breathing leads to inefficient gas exchange, hypoxemia, and hypercapnia.[8] (See the discussion in Chapter 12.)

Injury to the CNS and lesions that result in increased intracranial pressure also alter the rate and pattern of respiration. Altered respiratory patterns resulting from increased intracranial pressure include yawns, sighs, apnea, Biot's (atactic) breathing, sustained hyperventilation (central neurogenic hyperventilation or hyperpnea [CNH]), and Cheyne-Stokes respiration.[9] (Cheyne-Stokes respiration also occurs with heart failure, uremia, drug-induced respiratory depression, sleeping at a high altitude,[10] and in sleeping children.)

Depression of the respiratory centers results in *slowing of the respiratory rate* and occurs in the following situations:

1. Arterial pH above 7.45 (alkalosis)
2. Severe hypoxemia and hypercapnia

Table 11-2   Conditions Associated with Altered Chest Wall Movement

Condition	Possible Causes of Condition*
Abdominal paradox, sometimes with respiratory alternans	Splinting after abdominal surgery COPD, diaphragmatic paralysis Respiratory muscle fatigue with impending respiratory failure
Accentuated abdominal breathing	Restrictive disease Low cervical spinal cord lesions
Inward motion of thorax during inspiration	Lower cervical cord transection
Paradoxical chest wall movement	Flail chest
Accessory muscles augmenting inspiration and sometimes expiration	Obstruction, COPD
Unilateral decrease in chest expansion	Tension pneumothorax, pleural effusion, pulmonary resection Ball-valve obstruction of major bronchus, parenchymal infiltrate Atelectasis, consolidation, splinting secondary to pain Intubation of right mainstem bronchus

*COPD: chronic obstructive pulmonary disease

3. Hypothermia
4. Severe hypoglycemia and diabetic coma
5. Drug overdose
6. Administration of narcotic, sedative, or anesthetic agents

The respiratory depression effect of narcotics is not a problem with the patient on continuous mechanical ventilation. Even use of thoracic nerve block or continuous intravenous (IV) infusion of morphine following chest injury does not present a problem with respiratory depression in the patient receiving mechanical ventilation. However, the patient not receiving mechanical ventilation who is given adequate pain relief to permit sleep requires close observation for bradypnea resulting from respiratory depression. Intravenous injection of pain medication is preferred following thoracic trauma and surgery because the medication is immediately and completely available for pain relief and any potential respiratory depression can be readily assessed. When the intramuscular route is used in patients with decreased tissue perfusion, the medication may be only partially absorbed, giving incomplete pain relief. Later, when tissue perfusion is increased, the retained narcotic may be absorbed, resulting in respiratory depression.

Lung Sounds

In the ICU, listening to lung sounds over all areas of the patient's chest may be difficult, but in many cases the extra effort to do so is beneficial. Lung sounds are most thoroughly assessed by rolling the patient onto one side or, if possible, having the patient sit up. This allows auscultation of the posterior lung fields where the initial abnormalities often appear first in the recumbent patient. Careful attention to the patient's artificial airway (if present) and its connection to a ventilator, chest tubes, catheters, and IV lines is essential when moving the patient to assess the posterior chest.

Lung sounds may be different in patients receiving mechanical ventilation than in spontaneously breathing patients. It is commonly accepted that the breath sounds heard during a positive pressure breath are as useful as those heard with spontaneous breathing in determining the quality of gas movement into the underlying lung. The greatest variation in breath sounds occurs in patients on intermittent mandatory ventilation (IMV) when the patient is breathing spontaneously as well as receiving mechanical breaths. Patients on jet ventilation have decreased lung sounds over all areas of the chest.

In the ICU, *decreased breath sounds and late inspiratory crackles* in the dependent regions of the lungs occur most often because of atelectasis. The abnormal lung sounds are sometimes accompanied by fevers when atelectasis is present. The combination of fever and diminished breath sounds over the bases or late inspiratory crackles suggest that the patient could benefit from lung expansion therapies.

Unilateral decreased or absent breath sounds occur when one of the following exists:

- Accidental movement of an ET tube into a mainstem bronchus
- Unilateral airway obstruction
- Air (pneumothorax), blood (hemothorax), or other fluids (pleural effusion or hydrothorax) collecting in the pleural space (Fig. 11–1).

The appearance of any of these problems may be delayed following blunt trauma to the chest or abdomen.

Diminishing or absent breath sounds in conjunction with chest pain, subcutaneous emphysema, and a mediastinal shift away from the affected side suggest tension pneumothorax. Precipitating factors include mechanical ventilation, especially with high inspiratory pressures and positive end-expiratory pressure (PEEP), chest trauma, and improperly functioning chest tubes.[11]

Changes in Chest Wall Movement

Visual inspection and physical examination of the patient's thorax and abdomen offer valuable information to the critical care clinician. Each hemithorax should be

Table 11–3 Clinical Conditions Associated with Tracheal Deviation

Trachea Deviates Toward Affected Side	Trachea Deviates Away From Affected Side
Atelectasis	Pleural effusion
Pneumonectomy	Tension pneumothorax
	Unilateral hyperinflation secondary to ball-valve obstruction of main bronchus

compared with the other to assess whether movements are symmetric. Abnormalities of chest wall and abdominal movement should be appreciated. Changes in chest wall movement associated with airway obstruction have been discussed. Table 11–2 lists conditions associated with altered chest wall movement.

ASYMMETRIC MOVEMENT OF THE HEMITHORACES. *Asymmetric movement of the hemithoraces* is seen with unilateral disease processes. Decreased expansion of one lung can occur because of consolidation, atelectasis, intubation of a main bronchus, air or fluid in the pleural space, or collapse or removal of a lung. This assessment is especially important in the critically ill patient who has central venous catheters placed and is intubated, mechanically ventilated, and at risk for barotrauma. In addition to unilateral chest wall movement, patients who develop tension pneumothorax develop tracheal deviation. Tension pneumothorax pushes the mediastinum and therefore the trachea away from the affected side. Table 11–3 lists the clinical conditions associated with tracheal deviation.

Pain causes the patient to splint or guard (bend toward or hold) the tender section, resulting in a decrease of both pain and chest wall movement on the affected side. If the pain involves the entire chest, the patient will splint by taking shallow breaths at a faster rate. Atelectasis develops if pain relief is not adequate to stop splinting and permit mobility, deep breathing, and coughing. *A patient who is splinting his or her chest and refusing to breathe deeply, cough, or turn is not receiving adequate pain relief.* An important point to remember is that the patient receiving paralyzing agents (such as pancuronium bromide or succinylcholine) has total awareness of pain even though muscle paralysis prevents observable signs of chest pain.

PARADOXICAL (FLAIL) CHEST WALL MOVEMENT. *Paradoxical (flail) chest wall movement* most often occurs after three or more adjoining ribs are fractured in two or more places (see Fig. 11–1). Negative intrathoracic pressure during each inspiratory effort pulls the fractured segment inward. On expiration the broken chest wall segment moves outward. This to-and-fro motion of paradoxical respiration was thought by some to cause air to move uselessly between the right and left bronchi; the German word

pendelluft (pendulum air) is also used to describe paradoxical chest movement.

Paradoxical chest wall movement and lung contusion, like other problems secondary to blunt chest trauma, are not always apparent when the patient is admitted. Later, when the patient becomes tired from the increased effort required to keep the chest moving as a unit, the paradoxical motion appears. Except in young, previously healthy persons with a relatively small area of chest wall damage, flail chest is treated with volume ventilation. It is not uncommon for paradoxical chest wall movement to reappear several hours following initial attempts to wean a patient from mechanical ventilation. The reappearance of paradoxical chest wall movement in conjunction with increased respiratory rate and use of accessory muscles for breathing indicates that the patient is not ready to be weaned from the ventilator.

Blunt trauma (collision of the patient with another object such as the ground or a steering wheel) commonly causes simultaneous injury to the chest, head, spinal cord, and abdomen, but symptoms may not be apparent on admission. Intubation of a patient with a fracture of the cervical spine can result in spinal cord damage. The respiratory complications of spinal cord injury depend on the initial level of cord involvement, the completeness of the lesion, and the degree of recovery over time. Cord damage at C2-3 results in respiratory paralysis. Damage at C3-5 involves the phrenic nerve and results in partial or complete paralysis of the hemidiaphragm in addition to loss of intercostal and abdominal muscle function; patients inspire only with their accessory muscles. Damage at or below C6 does not impair diaphragmatic innervation. Pneumothorax, hemothorax, and cardiac tamponade are other potentially delayed sequelae of blunt trauma (see Fig. 11–1).

PARADOXICAL ABDOMINAL MOVEMENT. *Paradoxical abdominal movement* occurs with dyspnea and paralysis of the hemidiaphragm, suggesting respiratory muscle fatigue. With normal breathing, the diaphragm, as the primary muscle for inspiration, contracts downward, increasing abdominal pressure and pushing the abdomen outward while the chest wall expands. On expiration, the diaphragm relaxes and the abdomen and chest wall recoil inward. When the diaphragm is fatigued or paralyzed, intercostal and accessory muscles take over the task of inspiration. As the rib cage expands and moves outward, negative intrathoracic pressure pulls the relaxed diaphragm upward into the rib cage, resulting in an inward movement of the abdomen. This *asynchronous movement of the thorax and abdomen* during spontaneous breathing is frequently seen in patients following upper abdominal surgery; however, when seen in other contexts, it is a *good indicator of inspiratory muscle fatigue.*[6,8]

Hypoxemia, anemia, poor nutrition, and reduced cardiac output can result in inefficient respiratory

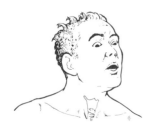

Upper airway (laryngeal) obstruction

Marked restlessness
Anxious facies
Ashen-gray color or cyanosis
Stridor (crowing respiration)
Indrawing at suprasternal notch, around
    clavicles, in intercostal spaces,
    and at epigastrium

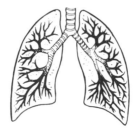

Secretional obstruction of lower
airways (signs of laryngeal
obstruction absent)

Cyanosis
Marked dyspnea
Frequent, ineffective cough
Audible wheezes and rhonchi
Signs of atelectasis may be present

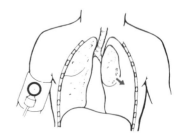

Tension pneumothorax

Progressive cyanosis
Respiratory embarrassment
Tracheal displacement away from affected side
Hyperresonant percussion note
Distant or absent breath sounds
Shock

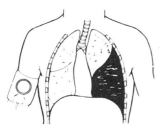

Massive hemothorax

Cyanosis
Respiratory embarrassment
Severe chest wall pain
Paradoxical motion of chest wall
Bony crepitation at sites of fracture
Shock

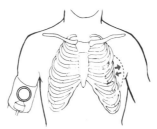

Flail (stove-in) chest

Cyanosis
Respiratory embarrassment
Dullness of percussion
Absent or distant breath sounds
Unrelenting shock if hemothorax increases

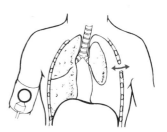

Open pneumothorax

Cyanosis
Respiratory embarrassment
Sucking wound of chest
Shock

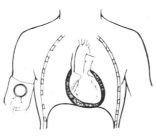

Cardiac tamponade

Neck veins distended
Falling or absent blood pressure
Patient in variable degrees of shock
Venous pressure elevated (pathognomonic)
Muffled or distant heart tones
Paradoxical pulse

Fig. 11-1 *Pertinent clinical findings. A brief survey in each case usually suggests the presence and nature of life-endangering abnormalities. (From Naclerio RA:* Chest injuries: physiologic principles and emergency management, *New York, 1971, Grune & Stratton.)*

Table 11-4 Disorders Associated with Pleural Effusions*

Type of Pleural Effusion	Associated Disorders
Transudative	
Increased pressure or low serum protein causing low protein fluid to leak out of the capillaries into the pleural space	Congestive heart failure, pericardial disease Pulmonary embolism Cirrhosis, hypoalbuminemia Nephrotic syndrome, hydronephrosis, acute glomerulonephritis, peritoneal dialysis
Exudative	
High protein fluid actively secreted into the pleural space	Pneumonia, tuberculosis, other pulmonary infections Malignancy; primary lung cancer (adenocarcinoma), metastatic (breast, lung, lymphoma), mesothelioma Pulmonary embolism with infarction Gastrointestinal: esophageal rupture/perforation, pancreatitis, subphrenic abscess, postabdominal surgery Collagen-vascular disease: lupus, rheumatoid, etc. Trauma, iatrogenic disorder, radiation therapy, uremia Drug-induced: nitrofurantoin, dantrolene, methysergide, bromocriptine, procarbazine

muscle function. Contractility of the diaphragm is also reduced by hypercapnea, hypophosphatemia, and shortening of the respiratory muscle fibers, which occurs with hyperinflation secondary to obstructive lung disease. When respiratory muscle fatigue supervenes in the course of acute or chronic lung dysfunction, it may identify impending respiratory failure.[12-14]

Barotrauma and Pleural Fluid Collection

Critically ill patients receiving positive pressure ventilation are at high risk for development of barotrauma. Additionally, the disease process that brought them to the ICU or to therapeutic procedures (such as central line placement) can put them at high risk for developing pleural effusion, pneumothorax, tension pneumothorax, subcutaneous emphysema, pneumomediastinum, or reexpansion pulmonary edema.[15-17] Assessment of breathing should include the ruling out of these disorders.

PLEURAL EFFUSION. Normally fluid does not accumulate in the pleural space, because it is removed by the lymphatics. Excess fluid in the pleural space is called a *pleural effusion*. Multiple disorders associated with pleural effusions are listed in Table 11-4. The most common causes of pleural effusion experienced by critically ill patients are congestive heart failure, pulmonary embolism, cirrhosis, pneumonia, malignant disease, and gastrointestinal disease.[18-20]

Symptoms of pleural effusion are related to the following conditions:

1. Inflammation of the pleura
2. Compromise of the pulmonary mechanics
3. Interference with gas exchange
4. The underlying process and coexisting disease

The most common symptoms are dyspnea, pleuritic or dull chest pain, and occasionally a dry, nonproductive cough. Dyspnea becomes more pronounced as the size of the effusion increases. Diminished tactile fremitus, dullness to percussion, and fullness or even bulging of the affected hemithorax may be noted. Lung sounds are usually decreased; however, because the fluid usually moves freely in the pleural space, these signs may change when the patient changes position. If the fluid is trapped (fixed) in one location by adhesions it is said to be *loculated*. Some patients experience no effusion-related signs or symptoms when effusions are loculated or small (less than 500 mL). On the other hand, in patients with coexisting pulmonary disorders or with effusions that are large or accumulating rapidly, symptoms and respiratory failure may occur rapidly.

Confirmation of pleural effusion is made by chest film. Sampling the fluid for study and evacuating the effusion to decompress the lung are accomplished by either *thoracentesis* (needle aspiration) or placement of chest tubes (discussed later in this chapter). Once the type of fluid causing the effusion has been identified, more specific descriptions may be used: *hydrothorax* (serous fluid), *hemothorax* (blood), *pyothorax* or *empyema* (pus), or *chylothorax* (chyle).

PNEUMOTHORAX. When a communication develops between the pleural space and the atmosphere or between the pleural space and an alveolus, air flows into the pleural space until the pressure is equal or the opening is closed. This equalization of intrapleural pressure coupled with disruption of the cohesion between the two pleural membranes allows the lung to recoil inward. The lung's collapse may be partial or complete.

This violation of the pleural space can be caused by a surgical opening or wound in the chest wall, by spontaneous rupture of a bleb in the lung (*spontaneous pneumothorax*), or by puncture of the lung or chest wall secondary to medical procedures such as needle aspiration of the pleural space or an open chest catheter (*iatrogenic pneumothorax*). If there is an opening in the chest wall (*open pneumothorax*) that is larger in diameter than the trachea, airflow into the thorax may take the path of least resistance and move back and forth through the wound rather than through the trachea (see Fig. 11–1). To sustain ventilation and life, the wound must be occluded or at least be made smaller than the diameter of the trachea.

The main physiologic consequences of pneumothorax are decreased vital capacity and arterial oxygen pressure (Pa_{O_2}). If the pneumothorax is small (less than 50% decrease in lung size), these changes may be well tolerated in the otherwise healthy patient. However, if lung function was compromised before the pneumothorax, even a small pneumothorax may result in a decrease in vital capacity significant enough to result in respiratory insufficiency with alveolar hypoventilation and respiratory acidosis. Therefore, pneumothorax or pleural effusion of any size must be monitored very closely and must usually be treated in patients with coexisting pulmonary disorders.

Dyspnea and chest pain on the side of the pneumothorax are the two primary symptoms. The physical examination reveals tachycardia with a hyperresonant percussion note and an enlarged hemithorax on the affected side while breath sounds and tactile fremitus are decreased or absent.

TENSION PNEUMOTHORAX. Tension pneumothorax is said to be present, when the intrapleural pressure exceeds the atmospheric pressure throughout expiration. This can only occur when air enters the pleural space from the lung or atmosphere with each inspiration and cannot escape; therefore pressure builds up, resulting in positive pressure (tension) in the pleural space.

As pressure increases, it pushes the contents of the mediastinum against the contralateral lung, causing the trachea to deviate *away* from the affected side (*mediastinal shift*) (see Fig. 11–1). As a consequence, the opposite lung may also be compressed and the venae cavae distorted enough to partially obstruct systemic venous return and decrease cardiac output. The patient exhibits distress, labored respirations, cyanosis, marked tachycardia and profuse diaphoresis. Additionally, the high pressures may force air into the tissues, resulting in subcutaneous and mediastinal emphysema (discussed below).

Precipitating factors include chest trauma, CPR, invasive chest procedures, insertion of lines in the central veins, improperly functioning chest tubes, and mechanical ventilation with high pressures, especially in patients with emphysematous blebs. *Tension pneumothorax should be suspected in patients who are difficult to ventilate during CPR or who deteriorate clinically while being ventilated,* especially when high peak pressures and PEEP are being used. *Treatment of a tension pneumothorax should be on an emergency basis.*

SUBCUTANEOUS EMPHYSEMA. The presence of air in the subcutaneous tissues is referred to as *subcutaneous emphysema.* When the tissue is palpated, the movement of air within the tissue sounds like the rattle of cellophane; therefore subcutaneous emphy-

sema is occasionally referred to as *crepitus.* The most common origin for this type of emphysema is air escaping from a hole or laceration in the lung or chest wall secondary to trauma or surgery. It is a common finding with tension pneumothorax. In patients with preexisting inflammatory pleural disease, the lung remains adherent to the chest wall; therefore air leaking from the lung escapes into the surrounding tissues rather than producing a massive pneumothorax. Mechanical ventilation of a patient with a fresh tracheostomy commonly results in collections of subcutaneous emphysema around the face, neck, and shoulders.

Subcutaneous emphysema looks and feels abnormal to the patient but rarely causes serious problems in adults. In male patients, rapidly progressing subcutaneous emphysema can result in severe scrotal enlargement. Severe subcutaneous emphysema in the neck of a child can cause tracheal compression, necessitating intubation or tracheostomy.

PNEUMOMEDIASTINUM. Air in the mediastinum is also known as *mediastinal emphysema* or *pneumomediastinum.* It most commonly results from alveolar rupture but can also result from injury to the upper respiratory tract, intrathoracic airways, or gastrointestinal tract and is occasionally seen following violent coughing or straining. Air can also be introduced into the mediastinum by trauma, surgery, chest tube insertion, or infections caused by gas-producing organisms.

Substernal pain resulting from stretching of the mediastinal tissue is the most common symptom. Other symptoms may include dyspnea, dysphagia, dysphonia (change in voice), cyanosis, and neck vein distention. Crackling sensations are usually only felt with palpation of the supraclavicular area. Confirmation is made by chest film. *When pneumomediastinum occurs in a patient receiving positive pressure ventilation, the patient should be watched closely for rapid progression to tension pneumothorax.*

REEXPANSION PULMONARY EDEMA. Pulmonary edema may occur when the lung is rapidly reinflated following pneumothorax or pleural effusion. Patients may exhibit varying degrees of coughing, chest tightness, hypoxia, hypotension, and on occasion bilateral pulmonary edema. On rare occasions, the syndrome results in cardiac arrest and can be fatal. The vast majority of these events occur when negative pressure is used to evacuate the pleural space.[21]

Chest Drainage

The presence of even a small amount of air or fluid in the pleural space can seriously compromise the oxygenating capacity of the lungs when the patient has limited pulmonary reserve (e.g., COPD), low oxygen availability (e.g., high altitude), ventilation-perfusion ($\dot{V}/\dot{Q}$) mismatch (e.g., atelectasis), or stiff lungs (e.g., adult respiratory distress syndrome, or ARDS). When patients become symptomatic (dyspnea, chest pain, arterial hypoxemia), it is necessary to drain the pleural space and reexpand the lung.

THORACENTESIS. Thoracentesis is removal of fluid or air from the thoracic cavity by a needle or catheter placed through the chest wall. Evacuation of the pleural space relieves symptoms, allows a collection of specimens for laboratory analysis, and may prevent the need for a chest tube and continuous drainage.

Following thoracentesis, the patient must be observed closely for signs of reoccurring pneumothorax or pleural effusion or iatrogenic injury. If there is concern that the source of the fluid or air may still be active, serial chest films (usually every 4–6 hours) are also performed to monitor the state of the pleural space.

Iatrogenic pneumothorax may be caused by puncture of the lung with the aspirating needle, especially if a metal needle rather than an IV catheter is used for the procedure. Additionally, if a low posterior tap (eighth intercostal space or below) is performed with the patient sitting and leaning forward, it is possible to puncture the diaphragm, liver, spleen, colon, or stomach, resulting in hemorrhage or infection, or both. A chest film must be obtained following the procedure to rule out these complications.

THORACIC CATHETERS. When the source of air or fluid in the pleural space is still active or the volume large, continuous thoracic drainage is preferred to thoracentesis. The location, size, and number of the catheters used depends on what is to be drained. The anterior chest (second interspace in the midclavicular line) is used for draining a pneumothorax; the axillary area (fourth, fifth, or sixth costal interspace in the midaxillary line) is used for fluid drainage. It is common for a patient to have more than one catheter in the same pleural space: one for air, another for fluid, or two or more for drainage of an active bleed. Mediastinal chest tubes may be placed instead of or in addition to pleural tubes following chest trauma, cardiac surgery, and other mediastinal events.

Chest tubes vary in size and style. Large IV catheters, NG tubes, urinary catheters, or suction catheters may be used for air and serous drainage, but they must be watched carefully so they do not kink or become occluded by the drainage.[22,23] More commonly, clear, flexible vinyl *trocar catheters* are used for closed chest *thoracostomy* (placing a tube through the closed chest). The pointed metal rod (trocar) inside facilitates insertion, but it can also puncture the lung or surrounding organs.[24] When large thoracic catheters with multiple holes are placed through the closed chest, the last one or two holes can end up in the tissue instead of the pleural space, causing fluid to seep out and air to be aspirated into the chest around the tube. Laceration of the intercostal artery or vein during insertion is also possible. A chest film is always obtained to verify tube placement and drainage of the pleural space and to rule out complications.

CLOSED CHEST DRAINAGE. The purpose of a closed chest drainage system is to remove air or fluid while keeping the pleural cavity closed to the atmosphere.[24–33] Ideally the system should be able to remove air and fluid rapidly enough to reestablish and maintain normal pleural pressures and lung expansion. Once a chest tube has been put in place and attached to a chest drainage system, the system becomes an extension of the patient's chest. Its function must also be regularly assessed.

Closed chest drainage can be accomplished in an emergency by attaching a finger cot or balloon to the catheter, then cutting a slit in the end. Air under pressure could escape through the slit; however, the soft rubber would collapse and occlude the catheter, preventing air from entering the pleural space during inspiration (negative intrapleural pressure). Fig. 11–2 illustrates the *Heimlich valve*,[22,23] a commercially available device that functions in the same manner. It is frequently used on chest tubes during transport and is often found with trocar catheters on "crash carts," since pneumothorax can be either a cause of cardiac arrest or the result of CPR.

Water Seal. The water seal is the most common method used to allow positive pressure to be expelled while preventing air from reentering the pleural space. It is used with one-, two-, three-, or four-bottle glass chest drainage systems or with commercially available systems of molded plastic. The patient's chest tube is connected by tubing to another tube that extends approximately 2 cm under water (Fig. 11–3). The water acts as a one-way valve, allowing air to exit by bubbling through the water. When negative pressure is created by inspiration, water is pulled up into the tube, thus preventing air from entering the pleural space.

Normally the water level in the water seal tube fluctuates 5 to 10 cm with respiration, rising with the negative pressure of inspiration and falling with expiration. This fluctuation, termed *tidaling,* is more dramatic during forced respiration or mechanical ventilation. With forced inspiration, water is drawn up the tube to a height equal to the negative intrapleural pressure, which rarely exceeds –20 cm H_2O but may approximate –60 cm H_2O with upper airway obstruction.

If air is present in either the pleural space or the system, the water will be pushed out of the water seal tube and bubbles will appear in the bottle or in the water seal chamber of a plastic system (*air leak*). When the system seal is set up, bubbling will appear in the water seal chamber until all the air has been removed from the system. *Continuous bubbling* thereafter is an indication that air is being continuously supplied to the system. The source of the air could be either a large active pneumothorax such as a bronchopleural fistula or a leak in the system. *Intermittent bubbling* with expiration, coughing, or bearing down is seen until the patient's pneumothorax is resolved and the lung is reexpanded.

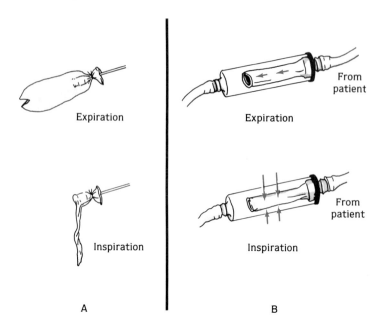

Expiration

Inspiration

A

From patient

Expiration

From patient

Inspiration

B

Fig. 11-2 *Emergency chest drainage systems.* **A,** *Finger cot with a slit attached to a needle.* **B,** *Heimlich valve connected to a chest tube, which can be used to allow positive pressure and fluid to escape from the pleural space. During inspiration, the negative intrapleural pressure collapses the flexible rubber, preventing outside air from entering the pleural space (see text).*

An air leak is described as inspiratory, expiratory, intermittent, or continuous. The volume of the leak is assessed by the speed of the bubbling as large, medium, or small. Some commercially made systems include a flowmeter, so the exact volume of the air leak can be measured. With a properly calibrated ventilator, the difference between the delivered and exhaled gas volumes may also be used to quantify the air leak.

No air leak indicates that the lung is totally reexpanded. However, when there is inadequate water in the water seal to cover the end of the tube, no bubbles will appear and air can be sucked through the tube and into the pleural space during inspiration. Bubbles will not be seen or will be intermittent when knots, kinks, clots, clamps, or fluid trapped in the tubes obstructs the system. When pressure cannot escape, tension pneumothorax can develop even though chest tubes are in place; therefore, *the chest tubes of patients with active pneumothorax should not be clamped.*

For patients with pneumothorax, the activity in the water seal determines when the chest tubes can be discontinued. Usually tubes are left in place until there is no air leak with cough for 48 hours.

When a one-bottle water seal system is used for drainage of fluids, the fluid level in the bottle continues to rise. As the tube extends deeper into the fluid, the resistance to drainage for both fluid and air increases with the distance of the tube under the water. Thus when the tube is 25 cm below the surface of the water, 25 cm H_2O of positive pressure is required to empty air or fluid from the pleural space. This problem can be overcome by frequent checking and withdrawal of the water seal tube so that the tip is never more than 2 cm

below the surface of the water, or by adding a collection bottle (chamber).

Collection Chamber. When a two- or three-bottle system is used, the patient's tubing is connected to the collection chamber and the collection chamber is connected to the underwater seal (Fig. 11-4). A two-bottle system consists of a collection chamber and an underwater seal. Fluids fall into the collection bottle where they can be accurately measured. Air rises and exists from the top of the container via the connection to the underwater seal. Air can escape by bubbling through the water seal, but the water seal still prevents air from flowing backward into the system. Commercially available molded plastic chest drainage systems are two-bottle drainage systems when they are not connected to suction. The short tube that connects the system to suction functions as the vent to atmosphere when suction is not used; therefore, it should never be clamped.

Ideally the collection chamber should be marked in small increments: 5 mL or less for adults, 1 mL for infants and children. Initially, following trauma or surgery, the volume of drainage should be checked at least every 15 minutes. Large volumes (500-1000 mL/hr) of free-flowing, bright-red, warm blood with few clots is evidence of active bleeding and should be reported immediately. Surgical intervention to stop the bleeding may be required in addition to administration of extra IV volume or blood, or both.

Sudden cessation of active bleeding is *not* a sign that bleeding has decreased. Rather, it is suggestive that kinks or clots are obstructing the tubing. To prevent clotting, the tubes should be milked by squeezing or

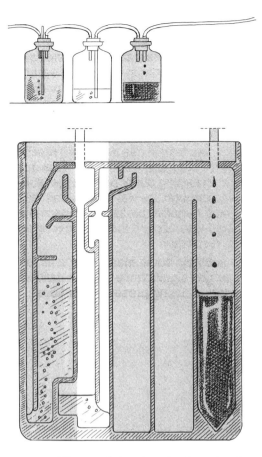

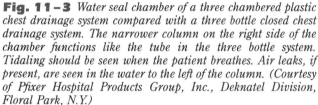

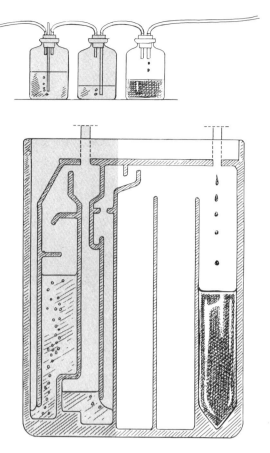

Fig. 11-3 *Water seal chamber of a three chambered plastic chest drainage system compared with a three bottle closed chest drainage system. The narrower column on the right side of the chamber functions like the tube in the three bottle system. Tidaling should be seen when the patient breathes. Air leaks, if present, are seen in the water to the left of the column. (Courtesy of Pfixer Hospital Products Group, Inc., Deknatel Division, Floral Park, N.Y.)*

Fig. 11-4 *Collection chamber of a three chambered plastic chest drainage system compared with a standard three bottle system. The V at the bottom of the chamber makes it possible to measure in small increments. Fluids spill over and fill the two other channels so that increments of measurement remain small (Courtesy of Pfixer Hospital Products Group, Inc., Deknatel Division, Floral Park, N.Y.)*

twisting and drained each time the volume of drainage is checked. When anticoagulants are given to stop active bleeding, it may be necessary to milk tubes continuously to prevent clotting in the tubes. Stripping chest tubes, a technique in which the rubber tubing is held tightly pressed between the thumb and forefinger of one hand while the other hand stretches the tubing flat before letting go, can create negative pressures to −400 cm H_2O and can dislodge tissue or vasculature and result in hemorrhage. Therefore, chest tubes should not be stripped except possibly as a last-ditch effort to keep a patient from returning to surgery because of clotted tubes, and then only under the direction of a physician.[34-38]

Within 24 hours following surgery or trauma, chest drainage should be serosanguineous if bleeding is controlled. A sudden surge of dark-red blood with clots that does not persist is frequently associated with changes in the patient's position and drainage of previously dependent areas. It may also occur with sudden increases in pleural pressure, as with cough or the

Valsalva maneuver. Chest tubes left in place for drainage of blood or fluids can usually be removed when drainage is serous and less than 25 mL per shift, provided no air leak is present and there is no sign of pleural infection.

Suction Control Chamber. One- and two-bottle drainage systems, like Heimlich valves, permit positive pressure and fluid to exit from the pleural space, thus preventing tension pneumothorax. However, when a large amount of air is entering the pleural space from the patient's lung, the amount of air removed is not sufficient to reestablish negative pleural pressure and reexpand the lung. Suction hastens expansion of the lung and expedites the evacuation of blood and other fluids.

The suction control bottle (chamber) is a sealed container connected between the water seal and a vacuum source. An open tube has one end submerged in water within the chamber while the other end extends out of the chamber and is open to the atmosphere (atmospheric vent) (Fig. 11-5). As the vacuum is increased, air is sucked into the tube and the water in

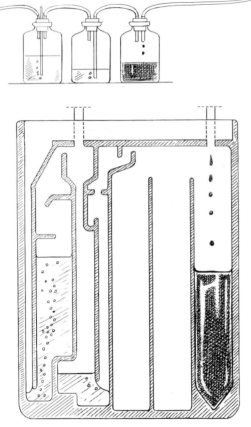

Fig. 11-5 *Suction control chamber of a three-chambered plastic chest drainage system compared with a standard three-bottle system. The weight of water in the column to the left determines the amount of suction exerted on the pleural space when the system is connected to a suction source. (Courtesy of Pfixer Hospital Products Group, Inc., Deknetel Division, Floral Park, N.Y.)*

the tube is pulled downward. Suction in the chamber increases until all the water is displaced and air is pulled through the tube, creating bubbles in the suction control chamber. Once air enters the system, suction cannot be increased; therefore the amount of suction in the system is determined by how far the vent tube is in the water. Normally the suction control chamber is filled to approximately 20 cm H_2O. Once bubbling occurs in the chamber, 20 cm of suction is present in the system. Increasing the amount of vacuum only increases the speed of bubbling and the water loss by evaporation; it does not change the amount of suction. If additional suction is required, more fluid must be placed in the suction control chamber. The water level must be routinely checked to ensure that the prescribed suction is maintained.

A chest drainage system is an extension of the patient's pleural space. An improperly functioning system can prevent removal of fluid or air from the pleural space, or worse, add air or fluid to it.[39] Assessment of the chest drainage system must therefore be a part of routine patient assessment.

Circulation

In general the flow of blood through the body per minute (cardiac output) is regulated by the tissues' need for oxygen. Blood flow in the skin is also largely governed by body temperature and the body's need to conserve or release heat. When body temperature increases or when the tissues' need for oxygen increases, the vessels dilate. Vasodilation decreases the resistance to blood flow; if pressure remains adequate, blood flow to the area increases. Maintenance of blood pressure is crucial for maximal augmentation of blood flow in any organ system or the body as a whole. Therefore, the body regulates flow by vasodilation in tissues where maximal flow is needed, while vasoconstriction in other organs controls blood pressure.[40]

If the heart or vascular tree is damaged or when there is an inadequate amount of blood (hypovolemia), the heart is not able to pump enough blood to meet the increased tissue demand. In essence, vasodilation causes the size of the container to increase while the volume stays the same, resulting in a fall in arterial pressure. When arterial pressure falls, the body immediately sets up a series of compensatory responses to maintain arterial pressure and the supply of blood to the vital organs: the brain, heart, and lungs. Peripheral vasoconstriction shunts blood to the vital organs. Closure of precapillary sphincters (on the arteriolar side of the capillary) causes fluid to be absorbed from the interstitial space. Retention of sodium and water also conserves blood volume. Sympathomimetic stimulation causes the rate and strength of the heartbeat to increase. This series of events results in the following predictable changes, which can be recognized on physical examination and used to assess circulation: increased heart rate, cold extremities, decreased urine output, and changes in pulses, pressure, cardiac rhythm, and level of consciousness. Two crucial concepts for noninvasive monitoring of the circulation must be remembered[41]:

- Hemodynamic processes change to maintain a normotensive state.
- "Normal" blood pressure does not guarantee adequate perfusion.

Peripheral Skin Temperature

Cold feet indicate hypoperfusion. Common sense must be used in considering the effects of body core temperature and environmental temperature as well as the possibility of decreased perfusion to a single extremity. However, differences between the toe and ambient (room) temperature have been shown to be not only good estimators of peripheral perfusion but also good prognostic indicators.[42,43] Normally, toe temperature should be at least 2° C warmer than ambient temperature. Less than 2° C difference indicates hypoperfu-

CLINICAL SIGNS OF DECREASING CARDIAC OUTPUT

Altered level of consciousness
Decreased mentation, mood changes
Dizziness, syncope with position change
Color may be pale and dusky
Skin and extremities become cool
Diaphoresis
Cold, clammy skin suggests impending shock
Heart rate increases
Respiratory rate increases
Urine output decreases *(< 0.5 mL/Kg/hr)*
Intestinal peristalsis slows
Nausea, vomiting as fluids back up into
    stomach
Abdominal pain due to visceral fluid
    engorgement
Blood glucose increases due to stress
    response
Carbon dioxide tension (Pco_2) decreases as
    result of tachypnea
Decreasing peripheral perfusion results in:
- ↓ Po_2
- ↓ pH, acidosis
- ↑ C(a–v) o_2 (unless septic or ↓$\dot{V}o_2$)
- ↑ Blood lactate

sion; less than 0.5° C difference indicates a life-threatening situation resulting from reduced perfusion. These temperature changes have been shown to be better indicators of survival than either cardiac output or blood pressure during shock.[44,45]

In the absence of a toe–ambient temperature gradient monitor, changes in temperature can be assessed using touch. Although touch does not provide an exact measurement of the temperature gradient, it may provide a better indicator of the effect of therapy on cardiac output and peripheral perfusion than the measurement of temperature in a single peripheral location. When perfusion to the extremities is decreased, a point of temperature change can be identified by moving your hand slowly up the leg from the foot. The point of temperature change (often more easily felt using the backs of the fingers rather than the palmar aspect of the hand) can be marked on the skin. If therapy is successful in improving peripheral blood flow, the line of temperature change moves down the leg toward the foot; if perfusion is not increased, the line stays in the same place or advances up the leg and thigh as vasoconstriction increases; therefore, it is easily assessed regardless of skin color. Remember, *cold and clammy skin* occurs as a result of sympathetic

stimulation, a compensatory mechanism for cardiac output decline, and *may indicate impending shock.*

Capillary Refill Time

As mentioned in Chapter 4, following a 5-second compression of the nail beds, the pink color should return to the blanched area within 3 seconds. When the peripheral circulation is too vasoconstricted to shunt blood to the vital organs, capillary refill time is increased: longer than 3 seconds is considered sluggish; longer than 5 seconds is clearly abnormal. Like all other physical examination measurements of peripheral perfusion, capillary refill time must be assessed in light of both the body's core temperature (rectal, blood, esophageal, or urinary bladder temperature) and environmental temperature, since cold also causes vasoconstriction. Assessments of peripheral perfusion must also include comparison of the two extremities, since decreased blood flow to an extremity may result from a clot or vascular spasm occluding blood flow to the area.

Capillary refill time has been evaluated as a technique for assessment of hypovolemia; however, loss of a unit of blood does not significantly alter capillary refill time. Therefore, capillary refill time does not appear to be a useful test for detecting mild-to-moderate hypovolemia.[46]

Cyanosis

Dyspnea, tachycardia, and cyanosis constitute the classic triad of signs indicating hypoxia of either cardiac (low perfusion) or pulmonary (poor oxygenation) origin. However, cyanosis can occur without hypoxia (as in hypothermia), and hypoxia can occur without cyanosis (as in patients with anemia). Additionally, detection of cyanosis is subjective and often it is not recognized visually until the arterial oxygen saturation is lowered to about 80% in previously healthy adults.

Assessment of cyanosis is made more difficult by lighting conditions, the patient's preexisting skin color, and the possibility of pseudocyanosis. Interestingly, fluorescent lighting aids in the detection of cyanosis, whereas the broad spectrum of sunlight may make the identification of cyanosis more difficult.[47] Variations in skin thickness and color occurring as a result of age and race leave only the *tongue* as a reliable location for observing cyanosis.[48]

Pseudocyanosis (false cyanosis), a permanent discoloration of the skin caused by some drugs and metals, must be ruled out. Characteristics of pseudocyanosis which differentiate it from true cyanosis include
- Normal pink coloration of the tongue
- Absence of blanching of the skin with pressure
- Absence of respiratory and cardiac signs and symptoms of hypoxia.

True cyanosis may be central, peripheral, or both. *Peripheral cyanosis* occurs in the extremities when regional blood flow is decreased resulting in increased extraction of oxygen from the blood. If hemoglobin is within normal limits, peripheral cyanosis represents at least 5 g/L of reduced (unoxygenated) hemoglobin in the *capillary* blood. This may occur as a result of vasoconstriction or vascular obstruction. However, unless central cyanosis is also present, peripheral cyanosis does not indicate hypoxemia.

Central cyanosis, identified by bluish discoloration of the tongue and sublingual area, almost always indicates hypoxic crisis and should be treated as a medical emergency. Like peripheral cyanosis, central cyanosis becomes visible when there is more than 5 g/L of reduced (unoxygenated) hemoglobin in the *capillary* blood. Apparently, when the amount of reduced hemoglobin in *arterial* blood reaches somewhere between 2.6 g/dL and 3.4 g/dL, medical personnel are able to see that central cyanosis is present.[46,49] Patients with anemia may not be cyanotic even when hypoxemia is severe.

Urine Output

Urine output is one of the best indicators of the adequacy of both cardiac output and arterial pressure. When arterial pressure falls to 60 mm Hg, urine output falls to near zero.[50] Decreased glomerular filtration rate as well as the effects of aldosterone and ADH (antidiuretic hormone, vasopressin) reduce renal output of water and salt. Retention of water increases blood volume and helps return cardiac output and arterial pressure to normal. Conversely, elevation in arterial pressure increases the kidney's excretion of water and salt, thereby moving blood volume, cardiac output, and arterial pressure back toward normal.

In the ICU setting, a urine output greater than 30 mL/hr or 0.5 to 1.0 mL/Kg/hr is considered adequate.[51] In children, 1 mL/Kg/hr is considered normal.[52] A decreasing urine output indicates inadequate perfusion of the kidney, low blood volume, or onset of acute renal failure.[53] On the other hand, over an extended period of time, output must equal intake. Therefore urine outputs greater than 50 mL/hr, in patients who have not received diuretics or who are not in the diuretic phase of recovery from shock or renal failure, suggest overhydration (fluid intake that is higher than necessary).[54]

Level of Consciousness

A change in the patient's level of consciousness may be one of the first clues to a perfusion problem. Level of consciousness (sensorium, mentation) describes where the patient is on the continuum from awake and alert to nonresponsive. When the patient becomes hypoxic or the flow of blood to the brain is decreased, either from an acute event (like cerebral vascular occlusion [stroke]) or because the heart can no longer pump an adequate blood supply, the brain cells do not receive an adequate supply of oxygen. The result is decreasing awareness and ability to respond appropriately. As an adequate supply of oxygen is supplied to the brain, the patient becomes more alert and oriented to time, place, and person. If delivery of oxygen to the brain does not improve, the patient's sensorium will continue to deteriorate to the point of coma and eventually death.

RESPONSIVENESS. Since a sleeping patient and a comatose patient look the same, the first step in assessing level of consciousness is to rouse the patient. Calling them by name rouses most patients. If it does not, a touch or gentle shake should be tried. Shaking a patient awake without speaking first has an irritating effect on the patient. Speaking to the patient should always come first.

If the patient cannot be roused by speech or touch, a progression of stimuli from light to deep pain (noxious stimuli) is used. The noxious stimuli usually used include squeezing the trapezius muscle (top of the shoulder), placing pressure on the supraorbital ridge (bone just above the eye), or putting pressure at the base of the fingernail. Other methods such as rubbing the sternum with the knuckles or pinching or sticking the patient are often suggested but should be avoided because of bruising or danger to the patient.

When assessing the patient's responsiveness, it is important to be aware of medications the patient is receiving. If the patient is not yet awake from anesthesia or is receiving a paralyzing drug, a response will be impossible even though the patient can hear and is fully aware of any pain.

ORIENTATION. The second part of assessing level of consciousness is checking for orientation and ability to follow commands. If patients do not have an artificial airway, orientation can be assessed by asking them their name (person), where they are (place), what happened to them, and the date (time). (If the patient has not had access to a calendar or been able to see when it is day or night, even an alert patient will not be able to give the date.)

When assessing cerebral perfusion, the patient should be asked to perform a task that is objective, specific, and takes his or her physical limitations into account. Commands such as "Squeeze my hand" or "Wiggle your toes" can elicit a reflex or accidental response. Asking the patient to do something that requires conscious effort such as "Raise your left hand" will provide a much better indicator of cerebral perfusion. Of course, a patient who has no function of the left hand because of stroke or paralysis could not raise the

Table 11–5 Glasgow Coma Scale	
Eye opening	
Spontaneous	4
To speech	3
To pain	2
None	1
Best verbal response	
Oriented	5
Confused conversation	4
Inappropriate words	3
Incomprehensible sounds	2
None	1
Best motor response	
Obeys commands	6
Localizes*	5
Withdraws	4
Abnormal flexion	3
Extends	2
None	1

*Localizing to pain requires the patient to move a limb in an appropriate attempt to remove the painful stimulus.

hand. Be sure that the patient is capable of doing what you request.

There are reasons other than decreased perfusion for lack of orientation and changes in sensorium in the patient in an ICU. Inadequate sleep, constant noise, lack of privacy, and the effects of anxiety and pain medications produce responses varying from inability to concentrate to paranoia, nightmares, and frank hallucinations. This so-called *ICU psychosis* is seen most often in patients who are extremely fearful but deny their fear before surgery.[55,56] Patients who have heart surgery (postcardiotomy psychosis) and prolonged ICU stays also show this form of psychosis.[57,58] Ideally, all caregivers should be able to assess and interpret a patient's level of consciousness in the same way. The Glasgow coma scale (see Chapter 4) is a quantitative assessment tool that can be used by all ICU team members to describe the patient's level of alertness (Table 11–5).

The current Glasgow coma scale is not a prognostic scale. As health care shifts its attention to predicting outcomes, more precise prognostic scales and outcome indicators are being developed. The Glasgow coma scale is now one of the scored items used with other prognostic scoring systems such as the trauma scoring system[59] which includes four other categories: respiratory rate, respiratory effort, systolic blood pressure, and capillary refill. A new coma–near-coma scale which uses eight patient responses (auditory, olfactory, tactile, pain, vocalization, threat, visual, and command) has been proposed for use in predicting the potential for rehabilitation in patients that have been categorized as near-vegetative.[60] Variations of the Glasgow coma scale and other prognostic indicator tools are expected to be introduced in the next few years.

Heart Rate and Rhythm

Hypoxemia or decreased blood flow results in stimulation of the sympathetic nervous system causing a reflex increase in heart rate. *Sinus tachycardia* is the most common dysrhythmia seen in patients with pulmonary disease. Pain, anxiety, fever, dehydration, congestive heart failure, acute myocardial infarction, and various drugs also cause sinus tachycardia.

Bradycardia may be seen in patients with hypothermia, profound hypoxemia, and anesthetic toxicity following surgery and following vagal nerve stimulation. Vagal nerve stimulation may occur from pressure on the carotid sinus in the neck, stimulation of internal organs (during surgery), nausea and vomiting, eyeball pressure (occulocardiac reflex), and stimulation of the nerves in the upper airways by intubation or suctioning. Bradycardia, tachycardia, and arrhythmias (especially atrial fibrillation) may decrease cardiac output.

Irregular heart rates suggest cardiac dysrhythmia, respiratory alteration in cardiac function, or heart failure. Auscultation (see Chapter 4) or palpation of an irregular heart rate requires documentation of the rhythm by ECG, rhythm strip, or continuous cardiac monitoring. The most common dysrhythmias seen in patients with pulmonary disease include sinus tachycardia, atrial arrhythmias, and premature ventricular contractions (PVCs). These are also the most common dysrhythmias occurring after cardiac surgery. The risk of dysrhythmia is increased with advancing age, extensive intrathoracic surgery, preexisting heart or lung disease, and the degree of hypoxemia.[61] Dysrhythmias were described in Chapter 9.

Palpitations

Palpitations is the term used to describe the patient's unpleasant awareness of his or her heartbeat. Patients describe the feeling with words like "throbbing," "pounding," "skipping," "fluttering," and "flopping." Perception of heartbeat is normal during strenuous exercise and aroused emotional states when the heart rate and strength of cardiac contraction are increased, but most resting patients are unaware of their heartbeat. Development of palpitations suggests that the heart may be in a hyperkinetic state, as occurs with fever, anemia, hypoglycemia, hypervolemia with elevated blood pressure, high anxiety states, thyrotoxicosis, administration of cardiopulmonary stimulant medications, or ingestion of caffeine or other stimulant drugs.

Sudden onset of palpitations can be related to the initiation of compensatory mechanisms to protect the patient from low-volume states associated with hemorrhage, hypovolemia, or postural hypotension. Irregularity of cardiac rhythm as a consequence of dysrhythmia must also be suspected and verified by ECG or cardiac monitoring. Palpitations are most frequently associated with extrasystoles, ectopic beats, paroxysmal atrial tachycardia (PAT), and premature atrial or ventricular contractions and mitral valve prolapse (see Chapter 9).

Pulses

Pulses are checked to assure that there is adequate blood flow to a specific body part and to assess the function of the heart. Examination of the pulse was described in Chapter 3.

The presence of any catheter in a vein or artery creates the possibility of obstruction to blood flow by the catheter, dressing, blood clot, or vascular spasm. Additionally, removal of a catheter, especially arterial, places the patient at risk for vascular obstruction by clot or dressing, bleeding, or even hemorrhage. Bilateral comparison of pulses clarifies whether decreased pulses are due to alternation of flow to the specific body part (usually an extremity) or as a result of more generalized peripheral hypoperfusion.

What is felt as the arterial pulse is not the blood pulsing through the arteries (as commonly thought) but rather a shock wave that travels along the walls of the arteries as the heart contracts. The shock wave is generated by the pounding of the blood as it is ejected from the heart under pressure; therefore, the arterial pulse gives an indication about the strength of the cardiac contraction and the stroke volume (amount of blood ejected with each heartbeat). Irregular pulse patterns suggest dysrhythmia or heart failure.

PULSE DEFICIT. A *pulse deficit* is present when there is a significant difference between the auscultated heart rate and palpated pulse rate counted over the same minute (yes, it takes two people to detect it: one to count the pulse and one to auscultate the heart rate). A pulse deficit is an indication of left-sided heart failure. Tachycardia and a gallop rhythm in which all four of the heart sounds are heard on auscultation (lubb-dupp-dupp-dupp) also suggests serious cardiac decompensation.

PULSUS ALTERNANS. Pulsus alternans refers to a regular, alternating pattern of weak and strong pulses. It usually indicates that the volume of blood ejected by the ventricle is alternately larger on one beat and smaller the next. This pattern commonly occurs in patients with severe left ventricular failure. It may also indicate a bigeminal cardiac dysrhythmia such as PVCs.

PARADOXICAL PULSE. *Pulsus paradoxus,* a pulse that is felt to be weaker on inspiration and stronger on expiration, is clinically measurable when it is accompanied by a fall in systolic pressure at inspiration that exceeds 10 mmHg. A slight reduction in blood flow during inspiration followed by an increase in flow during expiration is normal and occurs because of the alterations in intrathoracic pressure that accompany spontaneous respiration. This pattern is exaggerated when compression of the heart by pericardial or mediastinal contents or when extremes in intrathoracic pressure alter cardiac filling and ejection. Paradoxical pulse is seen in patients with *pericardial effusion* (fluid, blood, or air between the pericardium and the heart) and in approximately 50% of patients with *pericarditis* (inflammation of the pericardium). It is not uncommon in patients with congestive heart failure, or severe obstructive pulmonary disease and may also occur in patients with acute pulmonary embolism, hypovolemia, or shock. There is a close correlation between the degree of pulsus paradoxus and the degree of airway obstruction in asthma.[62,63]

The development of paradoxical pulse in a patient following trauma or cardiothoracic surgery, especially in connection with increasing venous pressure and heart rate, suggests *cardiac tamponade.* When fluid or blood collects between the heart and the nonelastic pericardium, the heart is compressed and its ability to pump is severely compromised; immediate intervention is necessary. Cardiac tamponade, pericardial effusion, and methods of pericardial and mediastinal drainage are discussed below.

REVERSED PULSUS PARADOXUS. *Reversed pulsus paradoxus*[64] looks the same as paradoxical pulse on the monitor and may feel the same on palpation. However, on close observation the pressure is noted to *increase* during inspiration (just the opposite of paradoxical pulse). The phenomenon is seen most commonly in patients receiving mechanical ventilation with PEEP following cardiac surgery. It is thought to indicate hypovolemia and usually disappears when appropriate volume therapy is instituted. This pattern is also seen in patients receiving IMV in the presence of left ventricular failure. The presence of reversed pulsus paradoxus may also mask the inspiratory fall in pressure expected secondary to cardiac tamponade.

Cardiac Tamponade and Pericardial Effusion

Signs and symptoms of cardiac tamponade and pericardial effusion are determined by two factors: speed of fluid accumulation and competence of the myocardium. To compress the heart significantly, the pericardial or mediastinal contents must increase at a rate exceeding the rate of stretch to the pericardium or rate of mediastinal drainage (in the post–cardiac surgery patient). A rapid accumulation of a large amount of fluid produces serious and emergent circulatory embarrassment. Conversely, a slow accumulation of a large amount of fluid (1–2 L) may be well tolerated if the myocardium is intact. However, even a slow accumulation of a relatively small amount of fluid may result in serious circulatory failure if the extent of myocardial damage is significant.

Cardiac tamponade is said to exist when the cardiac compression caused by the accumulating fluid or air becomes hemodynamically significant and exceeds compensatory mechanisms. Signs of cardiac tamponade include venous distention, tachycardia, pulsus paradoxus, quiet or distant heart sounds, dyspnea, dizziness, and even syncope (signs of reduced cardiac output). Hypotension with peripheral vasoconstriction does not usually occur until the body's compensatory mechanisms have been defeated, and then blood pressure falls.

PERICARDIAL DRAINAGE. Decompression of the heart must be accomplished immediately once tamponade develops. This may be done surgically by creating a *pericardial window* (a hole in the pericardium created through a subxiphoid incision) or by *pericardiocentesis* (needle or catheter drainage of the pericardium). Until pericardial drainage can be accomplished, the patient needs to receive large amounts of IV fluid in an attempt to keep the cardiac filling pressures greater than the pericardial pressure and thus maintain cardiac output.

Emergency pericardiocentesis may be done "blindly" using a long metal cardiac needle connected to an ECG lead by metal alligator clips. An ECG signal will be seen as soon as the needle is in contact with the heart.[65] Needless to say, this procedure is not without risk of myocardial puncture but it can be accomplished immediately at the bedside and relatively safely when there is a large amount of fluid between the pericardium and the heart. When time allows, an IV catheter or percutaneous balloon pericardial catheter[66,67] can be placed under echocardiographic or radiographic guidance.[68] Whether the catheter will be left in place or removed is dependent on the type of fluid (or air) and the probability of a significant effusion recurring. Complications of pericardial drainage include perforation of the ventricle, leakage into the pleural space, pleural pain, cardiac arrhythmias, arterial bleeding, pneumothorax, infection, and vasovagal reaction.

PERICARDIAL CATHETERS. Pericardial catheters, unlike chest tubes, are small and periodically aspirated rather than being left to continuous drainage. They have been used successfully in both adults and children[69] and left in for weeks. Rarely, the catheter may be used for instillation of antibiotics, cytotoxic substances, or steroids. Potential risks associated with indwelling pericardial catheters include occlusion, infection at the catheter site, and pericardial infection. Continued patency via a semiclosed system can be safely maintained using a continuous flush device (Intraflo, Sorenson Research)[70] like those used for invasive monitoring. These systems deliver 3 mL/hr (72 mL/day) and permit intrapericardial pressure monitoring. Removing or disabling the fast-flush mechanism prevents accidental administration of flush solution, which could result in tamponade. Addition of a stop-cock to the system allows administration of medication and periodic aspiration of pericardial fluid. Pericardial catheters are usually removed when less than 100 mL of true pericardial fluid (total fluid minus flush fluid) is obtained in 24 hours.

MEDIASTINAL DRAINAGE TUBES. Mediastinal drainage tubes were discussed with chest tubes previously in this chapter. When a pericardial window and mediastinal drainage tubes are used, as is frequently done with cardiac surgery, the mediastinum, tubes, and drainage system become, in effect, an extension of the pericardium. Obstruction of the tubes by clot, kink, or improper drainage can cause the patient to develop cardiac tamponade secondary to drainage fluid collection in the mediastinum. Massive bleeding or bleeding that clots and obstructs the tube will necessitate a return to the operating room.

Arterial Pressure

Arterial pressure is the most frequently measured hemodynamic parameter. It must be remembered, however, that a *falling arterial pressure is a late sign of decreased cardiac output*. Since arterial pressure is dependent on the multiple factors controlling both cardiac output and peripheral vascular resistance (Fig. 11–6), a compensatory increase in any or all of these factors maintains or increases arterial pressures even when the amount of blood or effectiveness of the pump is decreased. Unless an acute catastrophic event such as hemorrhage or massive pulmonary embolism has occurred, if a patient's arterial pressure is falling, earlier clues to decreasing cardiac output have been missed.

Arterial pressure in the patient in an ICU may be assessed indirectly—using a sphygmomanometer (as outlined in Chapter 3), an ultrasonic device, or an oscillometric detection device[71]—or directly—using an invasive technique. Since peripheral vasoconstriction can cause variations of as much as 30 to 40 mm Hg between the pressure in the aorta and cuff pressures measured at the peripheral arteries, invasive pressure monitoring is used for most patients with cardiopulmonary problems in the ICU.

CUFF PRESSURE MEASUREMENTS. Whenever a blood pressure cuff is used to obtain an arterial pressure reading in a critically ill patient, erroneous pressure readings may be obtained for any of the reasons listed in Table 11–6. Attention to the following details will result in more accurate and reliable assessment[72] and therefore less error in blood pressure–based therapy:

1. Select the proper cuff size. Cuff and bladder width must[73,74] cover two-thirds the distance from the elbow to the shoulder *or* be 20% wider than the diameter of the arm *or* encircle 40% of the circumference of the arm.[75]

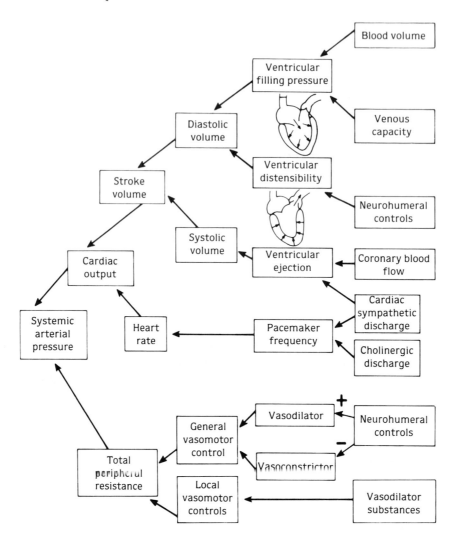

Fig. 11–6 *Factors determining systemic arterial pressure. (From Rushmer RF:* Cardiovascular dynamics, *ed 3, Philadelphia, 1970, WB Saunders.)*

Table 11–6	Errors in Indirect Blood Pressure Measured by Cuff
False high reading	Cuff too narrow Patient's arm below heart level Patient's arm not supported during measurement Talking during pressure measurement Physical activity within 5 minutes of measurement Pain, anxiety, discomfort
False low reading	Cuff too large Arm above heart level
Diminished or altered sound transmission	Stethoscope: excessive pressure during reading; using diaphragm rather than a shallow bell Cuff applied too tightly Peripheral edema or vascular disease, obesity
Misreading	Mercury manometer: meniscus not at eye level; clogged air vent at top of chamber Aneroid manometer: needle not zeroed Applying cuff too tightly

2. Apply the cuff properly; deflate at 2 to 3 mm Hg per heartbeat.
3. Use a shallow, large-diameter bell on the stethoscope[76] and light pressure.
4. Support the patient's arm at heart level.
5. Keep the top of the meniscus of the mercury column at eye level.
6. Deflate the cuff at a rate of 2 to 3 mmHg per heartbeat.
7. Use the *same cuff* on the *same arm* with the patient in the *same position*.

COMPARING CUFF AND INTRAARTERIAL BLOOD PRESSURE MEASUREMENTS. Discrepancy between cuff and intraarterial measurement is expected and in the presence of vasoconstriction often exceeds 30 mmHg. When a comparison of cuff and intraarterial pressure measurements is wanted, the cuff pressure must be taken on the extremity with the arterial catheter (arterial pressure is normally different in the two arms). Variations of up to 20 mmHg are considered within the normal range as long as the intraarterial pressure exceeds the cuff pressure. Pressure variations of more than 20 mmHg and an intraarterial pressure less than the cuff pressure indicate the need for reevaluating pressure measurement technique and rebalancing and recalibrating the transducer-monitor system (see the section on technical considerations for invasive hemodynamic monitoring in Chapter 14).

PALPATED ARTERIAL PRESSURE. When a cuff pressure cannot be auscultated and an arterial catheter has not yet been placed, arterial pressure may be measured using a blood pressure cuff and palpation, a pulse oximeter pulse signal, a Doppler flow probe, or flush pressure.

Palpated arterial pressure is obtained by pumping the cuff 20 to 30 mmHg above the expected systolic pressure and then deflating the cuff approximately 2 mmHg per heartbeat while palpating the radial pulse. The pressure at which the radial pulse is first palpated represents systolic arterial pressure. When the pressure is difficult to palpate, a Doppler flow probe or the pulse signal from a pulse oximeter can be used to obtain systolic pressure. With the probe positioned over the radial artery, the cuff is inflated, obstructing the blood flow and stopping the pulse sound. The pulse is heard again when the cuff is deflated to systolic pressure. *Flush pressure,* most frequently used with infants, was discussed in Chapter 10.

AUTOMATIC INDIRECT BLOOD PRESSURE. *Automatic indirect blood pressure* can now be measured as often as every minute using automatic oscillometry. However, because this technique uses a double bladder cuff, it too is subject to errors resulting from cuff size and fit. The proximal bladder is automatically inflated, then the distal bladder senses oscillations in the arterial wall as the proximal bladder deflates in a stepwise fashion. A microprocessor is used to analyze the oscillations and determine heart rate and systolic, diastolic, and mean arterial pressures.

The device's algorithms are based on Korotkoff or oscillometric vibrations and require two oscillations of the same size before a step deflation. If similar oscillations are not sensed within a prescribed period of time, the device will abort, vent the cuff to prevent injury to the patient, and produce an error message. Dysrhythmias that are associated with a variable pulse waveform may cause variation in the size of oscillations. Therefore, *an automatic noninvasive blood pressure monitor may not be able to compute a pressure reading in a patient with dysrhythmia.* The intermittent drop in blood pressure associated with an arrhythmia such as ventricular trigeminy may be interpreted by the device as an air leak rather than alerting the operator to its inability to obtain a pressure.[77]

There is no significant difference between mean arterial pressure obtained by automatic noninvasive blood pressure monitors and directly measured arterial pressure. However, systolic pressure is slightly underestimated and diastolic pressure slightly overestimated by this technique.[78,79] Nevertheless, this is a noninvasive technique that can be used for nearly continuous blood pressure measurement in critically ill patients who are not receiving titrated cardiopulmonary drugs, are not experiencing a dysrhythmia associated with intermittent drops in blood pressure, and who do not have a high systemic vascular resistance (see Chapter 13).

NONINVASIVE FINGER ARTERIAL PRESSURE. The Finapress device uses a finger cuff to provide continuous blood pressure and arterial waveform display. A rapidly responding servomechanism controls the circumferential pressure applied by the cuff so that the pressure in the cuff is maintained at zero transmural pressure. The computer then uses the stored cuff pressures to calculate heart rate and mean, systolic, and diastolic pressures.[80] Although accurate readings are obtained most of the time, some evaluations of the device have found it to be inconsistent at times without apparent clinical cause.[81] Few comparison studies have been done to find out if the accuracy of the device is affected by low cardiac output, hypothermia, low blood pressure, vasospasm, and vasoconstrictor drugs. The ability of the device to measure an arterial waveform has prompted increased interest in improving the Finapress and using it to obtain continuous noninvasive cardiac output measurements using the pulse contour curve.[82]

HEMODYNAMIC ASSUMPTIONS MADE FROM BLOOD PRESSURE MEASUREMENTS. *Rate-pressure product,* a simplified approach to evaluating cardiac work, is obtained by multiplying heart rate and systolic blood pressure. Values greater than 12,000 are thought to indicate increased myocardial work and increased myocardial oxygen demand.

Pulse pressure, the difference between the systolic and diastolic blood pressure, can be used as a rough estimate of the heart's pumping ability. *Stroke volume,* the amount of blood ejected by the heart with each beat, is the major determinant of pulse pressure. As stroke volume increases, pulse pressure increases. Cardiac output is the product of stroke volume and heart rate.

Jugular Venous Pressure

Failure of the right ventricle to adequately move blood through the lungs results in a backup of blood in the systematic venous system. This venous congestion causes the jugular venous pressure (JVP) to rise and increases the hydrostatic pressure in the systemic capillary bed, resulting in both liver congestion and peripheral edema. Damage to the right ventricle (e.g., myocardial infarction), stenosis of the heart valves, compression or occlusion of the major vessels by clot or other mass, or failure of the left ventricle will cause these symptoms to appear progressively over time. When pulmonary hypertension results in right ventricular failure, it is called *cor pulmonale.*

Severe right ventricular failure, constrictive pericarditis, and cardiac tamponade can be associated with JVPs above 30 cm H_2O and marked neck vein distention to the ear or temporal region while the patient is sitting. Increasing JVP with paradoxical pulse, tachycardia, and distant heart sounds, especially in a trauma or cardiac surgery patient, should alert the examiner to the probability of cardiac tamponade and the need for emergency intervention.

In the absence of cardiopulmonary disease, JVP provides information about the volume status of the patient. However, an increasing JVP over time suggests increasing vascular volume, and a downward trend suggests volume loss, even when cardiac or pulmonary disease is present. When no jugular distention is observed, horizontal compression of the base of the internal jugular vein at the level of the clavicle will occlude venous drainage and cause the veins to distend. If the jugular veins collapse when pressure is released, the pressure is low. The head of the bed can then be lowered until venous pulsations are seen. An estimate of central venous pressure can be obtained by measuring the vertical distance in centimeters between the right atrial level and the pulsations in the internal jugular vein.

Hepatomegaly and Peripheral Edema

Although peripheral edema and hepatomegaly are frequently associated with neck vein distention and increased JVP, the ICU patient may be edematous and gaining weight but have a very low venous pressure. In fact, the patient could be severely hypovolemic. This occurs when the Starling forces at the capillary level are disrupted. Normally the forces moving fluid into and out of the capillary are approximately equal (Fig. 11–7). When more fluid leaves the capillary than is pulled back in, the fluid is retained (sequestered) in the interstitial space. Edema occurs when capillary dynamics are disrupted by one or more of the following:

1. *Hydrostatic pressure is increased, usually because of venous obstruction or heart failure. More fluid moves out of the capillary and cannot return against the increased pressure in the venule.*
2. *Serum proteins and other colloids are decreased, so serum oncotic pressure is decreased; less fluid is pulled back into the capillary.*
3. *Capillary permeability is altered (as occurs in sepsis, shock, trauma, etc.), allowing excess fluid and protein to leak out of the capillary.*
4. *Obstruction of the lymphatics prevents removal of excess fluids from the tissues.*

This "third spacing" of fluid may be extremely pronounced in septic shock, low protein states, trauma, and following abdominal surgery. The patient's weight rises because total body water increases, and edema may become clinically visible. However, because much of the fluid is not pulled back into the venule end of the capillary, the patient's circulating blood volume decreases. Fluids must be administered, sometimes in huge amounts, to maintain ventricular filling pressure and prevent hypoperfusion and hypovolemic shock. JVP, as it reflects central venous pressure, can be used to monitor these fluid challenges as outlined in Chapter 14 and Tables 14–10 and 14–11.

Summary

The purpose of the ICU is to provide an environment where potential problems can be prevented and emergent problems immediately recognized and managed. Because the ICU patient is at risk for failure of one or more organ systems, assessing the patient for distress and the need for immediate therapeutic intervention must become second nature. A high index of suspicion (the expectation that secondary problems will occur because of the patient's history and current therapies) helps immensely in early recognition of problems.

Skill in assessment, or sorting the normal from the abnormal and grading its significance, is the hallmark that sets the health professional apart from the nonprofessional. Physical assessment usually provides the first clue that something is wrong. The ABCs of cardiopulmonary resuscitation—*a*irway, *b*reathing, and *c*irculation—provide a framework for learning as well as performing physical assessment in the ICU. A patent airway is the highest priority. Respiratory rate and rhythm, chest wall movement, and lung sounds are used to evaluate ventilation (breathing). The adequacy of per-

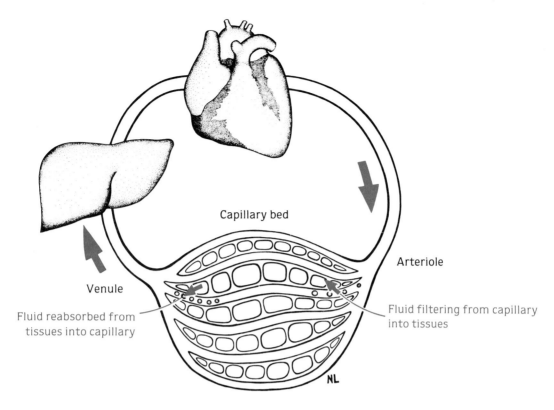

Venule mm Hg	Force tending to move fluid out of the capillary:	Arteriole mm Hg
10.0	Capillary hydrostatic (blood) pressure	28.0
6.3	Negative interstitial (tissue) fluid pressure	6.3
5.0	Interstitial (tissue) colloid osmotic pressure	5.0
21.3	TOTAL OUTWARD FORCES	36.3

Force tending to move fluid into the capillary:

Venule		Arteriole
28.0	Plasma colloid oncotic pressure	28.0
28.0	TOTAL INWARD FORCE	28.0
6.7 Inward	NET FORCES	8.3 Outward

Fig 11–7. *Schematic of fluid exchange through a systemic capillary bed. Differences in pressure forces cause fluid to filter out of the capillary at the arteriolar end, flow through tissues, and be reabsorbed into the venous system at the venule end of the capillary. Normally the small amount of fluid remaining in the tissue is removed by the lymphatic system. Abnormal collection of fluid in soft tissue is known as edema. (Pressure values from Guyton AC:* Textbook of medical physiology, *ed 7, Philadelphia, 1988, WB Saunders)*

fusion (circulation) can be evaluated by the temperature, color, and capillary refill time of the extremities; the level of consciousness; and the urine output. Heart rate and rhythm, JVP, and arterial pressure provide additional information about cardiac function.

The presence of an artificial airway does not negate the possibility of aspiration or airway obstruction, nor does the presence of a chest tube negate the possibility of pneumothorax or tamponade. Once tubes, ventilators, and other mechanical devices are connected to the patient, they must be considered as extensions of the patient. Assessment must include validation of their proper functioning and monitoring for problems they may create.

REVIEW QUESTIONS

1. T F   *The most accurate critical care assessment uses sophisticated, technical evaluation tools and equipment to monitor patient's status.*

2. *Which of the following can cause airway occlusion?*
    a. laryngospasm
    b. foreign body aspiration
    c. dried secretions
    d. all of the above

3. Which of the following would predispose a patient to aspiration?
   a. decreased level of consciousness
   b. vagal nerve block
   c. administration of beta adrenergic drugs
   d. increased pressure in the cuff of a patient's artificial airway

4. Which of the following is a sign of complete upper airway obstruction?
   a. "noisy" respiratory efforts
   b. deep intercostal retractions
   c. wheezing
   d. stridor

5. T F   Obstruction is more likely with larger diameter artificial airways.

6. Which of the following could help verify endotracheal tube position and depth?
   a. auscultation
   b. centimeter markings on tube
   c. chest x-ray
   d. all of the above

7. Which of the following methods of cuff management would insure minimal cuff pressure?
   a. using 15 mL of air to fill the cuff
   b. using minimal leak technique
   c. keeping cuff pressure at 35 mmHg
   d. all of the above

8. T F   Large artificial airways reduce work of breathing compared to smaller airways.

9. Which of the following is (are) hazards of extubation?
   a. dysphagia
   b. vomiting
   c. aspiration
   d. all of the above

10. Which of the following would cause respiratory center depression?
    a. diabetic ketoacidosis
    b. fear and anxiety
    c. alkalosis
    d. hyperglycemia

11. T F   Position-dependent late inspiratory crackles suggest atelectasis.

12. Which of the following could cause asymmetrical chest wall movement?
    a. emphysema
    b. tension pneumothorax
    c. asthma
    d. congestive heart failure

13. Which of the following is (are) true regarding paradoxical chest wall movement?
    a. it is also called flail chest
    b. it results in inward chest wall movement during expiration and outward movement during inspiration
    c. it can occur with one fractured rib
    d. none of the above

14. T F   Paradoxical abdominal movement may signify inspiratory muscle fatigue.

15. Which of the following are characteristic findings or symptoms of pleural effusion?
    a. increased resonance to percussion
    b. dyspnea
    c. bronchial breath sounds
    d. increased tactile fremitus

16. Which of the following is (are) true regarding pneumothorax?
    a. it will decrease vital capacity
    b. it results in an increased resonance to percussion
    c. common symptoms include dyspnea and chest pain
    d. all of the above

17. T F   Subcutaneous emphysema is commonly a result of airway or lung laceration from trauma or surgery.

18. The use of a needle to drain the chest cavity is a description of which of the following?
    a. thoracotomy
    b. pericardiocentesis
    c. thoracentesis
    d. none of the above

19. Which of the following is (are) true regarding a one-bottle chest drainage system?
    a. air escape during exhalation signifies a resolved pneumothorax
    b. the bottle can function as a one-way valve to prevent air entry into the chest
    c. the bottle can act as a collection chamber for pleural fluid drainage
    d. b and c

20. T F   A three-bottle chest drainage system incorporates the use of negative pressure (vacuum) to aid in reexpansion of the lung.

21. Which of the following indicates adequate tissue perfusion?
    a. warm temperature of the extremities
    b. reduced urinary output

c. *capillary refill time of 7 seconds*
d. *mental confusion*

22. *What is the minimum urinary output in the ICU setting that is considered adequate?*
    a. *10 mL/hr*
    b. *20 mL/hr*
    c. *30 mL/hr*
    d. *40 mL/hr*

23. *Which of the following are findings associated with right ventricular failure?*
    a. *hepatomegaly*
    b. *increased jugular venous pressure*
    c. *peripheral edema*
    d. *all of the above*

REFERENCES

1. Abramson NS and others: Adverse occurrences in intensive care units, *JAMA* 244:1582, 1980.
2. Adjuncts for airway control, ventilation, and supplemental oxygen. In *Textbook of advanced cardiac life support,* ed 2, Dallas, 1987, American Heart Association.
3. Pierson DJ: Upper airway obstruction. In Luce JM and Pierson DJ: *Critical care medicine,* Philadelphia, 1988, WB Saunders.
4. Zimmerman GA: Syndromes caused by the aspiration of gastric contents. In Parrillo JE, *Current therapy in critical care medicine,* Philadelphia, 1987, BC Decker.
5. Pierson DJ: Aspiration. In Luce JM and Pierson DJ: *Critical care medicine,* Philadelphia, 1988, WB Saunders.
6. Tobin MJ and others: The pattern of breathing during successful and unsuccessful trials of weaning from mechanical ventilation, *Am Rev Respir Dis* 143:1111, 1986.
7. Pardee NE, Winterbauer RH, Allen JD: Bedside evaluation of respiratory distress, *Chest* 85:203, 1984.
8. Cohen CA and others: Clinical manifestations of inspiratory muscle fatigue, *Am J Med* 73:308, 1982.
9. Drislane FW and Samuels MA: Update on CNS-induced cardiorespiratory problems, part 2: neurogenic pulmonary edema and respiratory rhythm abnormalities, *J Res Pir Dis* 9:33, 1988.
10. Strahl KP: Periodic breathing and sleep hypoxemia. In Sutton JR, Jones JL, Houston CS: *Hypoxia: man at high altitude,* New York, 1981, Thieme-Stratton.
11. Fishman NH: *Thoracic drainage: a manual of procedures,* St Louis, 1983, Mosby.
12. Collett PW, Roussos C, Macklem PT: Respiratory mechanics. In Murray JF and Nadel JA: *Textbook of respiratory medicine,* Philadelphia, 1988, WB Saunders.
13. Johanson WG and Peters JI: Critical care. In Murray JF and Nadel JA: *Textbook of respiratory medicine,* Philadelphia, 1988, WB Saunders.
14. Leasa DJ and Sibbald WJ: Respiratory monitoring in a critical care unit. In Simmons DH, editor: *Current pulmonology,* vol 9, St Louis, 1988, Mosby.
15. Strieter RM and Lynch JP III: Complications in the ventilated patient, *Clin Chest Med* 9:127, 1988.
16. Fleming WH and Bowen JC: Early complications of long-term respiratory support, *J Thorac Cardiovasc Surg* 64:729, 1972.
17. Mathru M, Tao TL, Venus B: Ventilator-induced barotrauma in controlled mechanical ventilation versus intermittent mandatory ventilation, *Crit Care Med* 11:359, 1983.
18. Light RW: *Pleural disease,* Philadelphia, 1982, Lea & Febiger.

19. Broaddus C and Stab NC: Pleural liquid and protein turnover in health and disease, *Semin Respir Med* 9:7, 1987.
20. Light RW: Disorders of the pleura: general principles and diagnostic approach. In Murray JF and Nadel JA: *Textbook of respiratory medicine,* Philadelphia, 1988, WB Saunders.
21. Light RW: Pneumothorax. In Murray JF and Nadel JA: *Textbook of respiratory medicine,* Philadelphia, 1988, WB Saunders.
22. Guyton SW, Paull DL, Anderson RP: Introducer insertion of minithoracostomy tubes, *Am J Surg* 155:693, 1988.
23. Conces DJ and others: Treatment of pneumothoraces utilizing small caliber chest tubes, *Chest* 94:55, 1988.
24. Fraser RS: Lung perforation complicating tube thoracostomy: pathologic description of three cases, *Hum Pathol* 19:518, 1988.
25. Farley J: Myths and facts about chest tubes, *Nursing* 18:16, 1988.
26. Cohen S and Stack M: How to work with chest tubes, *Am J Nurs* 80:685, 1980.
27. Erickson R: Chest tubes: they're really not that complicated, *Nursing* 11:34, 1981.
28. Fishman N: *Thoracic drainage: a manual of procedures,* St Louis, 1983, Mosby.
29. Fuchs C: The ins and outs of chest drainage systems, *Nursing* 16:26, 1986.
30. Kersten L: Chest-tube drainage system—indications and principles of operation, *Heart Lung* 3:97, 1974.
31. Miller K and Sahn S: Chest tubes—indications, technique, management and complications, *Chest* 9:258, 1987.
32. von Hippel A: *Chest tubes and chest bottles.* Springfield, Ill, 1970, Charles C Thomas.
33. Kersten LD: Chest tube drainage systems and post-thoracotomy care. In Kersten LD: *Comprehensive respiratory nursing,* Philadelphia, 1989, WB Saunders.
34. Duncan C, Erickson R, Weigel R: Effect of chest tube management on drainage after cardiac surgery, *Heart Lung* 16:1, 1987.
35. Isaacson J, George L, Brewer M: The effect of chest tube manipulation on mediastinal drainage, *Heart Lung* 15:601, 1986.
36. Knauss P: Chest tube stripping: is it necessary? *Focus Crit Care* 12:41, 1985.
37. Lim-Levy F and others: Is milking and stripping chest tubes really necessary? *Ann Thorac Surg* 42:77, 1986.
38. Duncan C and Erickson R: Pressures associated with chest tube stripping, *Heart Lung* 11:166, 1982.
39. Erickson R: Solving chest tube problems, *Nursing* 11:62, 1981.
40. Clemmer TP, Orme JF, Thomas FO: Physiology and management of failure of oxygen transport and utilization. In Fallat FJ, and Luce JM, editors: *Clinics in critical care medicine: cardiopulmonary critical care management,* New York, 1988, Churchill Livingstone.
41. Murphy TG and Bennett EJ: Low-tech, high-touch perfusion assessment, *Am J Nurs* :366 1992.
42. Vincent JL, Moraine JJ, van-der-Linden P: Toe temperature versus transcutaneous oxygen tension monitoring during acute circulatory failure, *Intensive Care Med* 14:64, 1988.
43. Kholoussay A and others: Central peripheral temperature gradient: its value in the management of critically ill surgical patients, *Am J Surg* 140:609, 1980.
44. Joly HR and Weil MH: Temperature of the great toe as an indicator of the severity of shock, *Circulation* 39:131, 1969.
45. Henning RJ and others: Measurement of toe temperature for assessing the severity of acute circulatory failure, *Surg Gynecol Obstet* 149:1, 1979.
46. Schriger OL and Baraff LJ: Capillary refill—is it a useful predictor of hypovolemic states?, *Ann Emerg Med* 20:601, 1991.
47. Barnette HB and others: When does central cyanosis become detectable?, *Clin Invest Med* 5:39, 1990.
48. Carpenter KD: A comprehensive review of cyanosis, *Crit Care Nurs* 13:68, 1993.
49. Martin L and Khalil H: How much reduced hemoglobin is necessary to generate central cyanosis?, *Chest* 97:182, 1990.
50. Guyton AC: *Textbook of medical physiology,* ed 7, Philadelphia, 1986, WB Saunders.

51. Peitzman A: Principles of circulatory support and the treatment of hemorrhagic shock. In Snyder JV and Pinsky MR: *Oxygen transport in the critically ill,* St Louis, 1987, Mosby.

52. Levin DL and Perkin RM: Postoperative care of the pediatric patient with congenital heart disease. In Shoemaker WC, Thompson WL, and Holbrook PR: *Textbook of critical care,* ed 2, Philadelphia, 1989, WB Saunders.

53. Shoemaker WC: Monitoring of the critically ill patient. In Shoemaker WC, Thompson WL, Holbrook PR: *Textbook of critical care,* ed 2, Philadelphia, 1989, WB Saunders.

54. Berk JL: Multiple organ failure. In Berk JL and Sampliner JE: *Handbook of critical care,* ed 2, Boston, 1982, Little, Brown.

55. Janis IL: *Psychological stress,* New York, 1958, John Wiley & Sons.

56. Hay D and Oken D: The psychological stresses of intensive care units, *Psychosom Med* 24:109, 1972.

57. Layne OL and Yudofsky SC: Postoperative psychosis in cardiotomy patients: the role of psychiatric factors, *N Engl J Med* 284:518, 1971.

58. Lasater KL and Grisanti DJ: Postcardiotomy psychosis indications and interventions, *Heart Lung* 4:724. 1975.

59. Ducey JP and Lamiell JM: Surgical scoring system for trauma, *Probl Crit Care* 3:528, 1989.

60. Caine RL: New coma scale targets patients in low level states. *Headlines* January/February 1993, p. 22.

61. Cordell RA and Ellison RG: *Complications of intrathoracic surgery,* Boston, 1979, Little, Brown.

62. Rebuck AS and Pengelly LD: Development of pulsus paradoxus in the presence of airways obstruction, *N Engl J Med* 288:66, 1973.

63. Robtham JL: Cardiovascular disturbances in chronic respiratory insufficiency, *Am J Cardiol* 47:941, 1981.

64. Massumi RA and others: Reversed pulsus paradoxus, *N Engl J Med* 289:1272, 1973.

65. Kirland LL and Taylor RW: Pericardiocentesis, *Crit Care Clin* 8:699 1992.

66. Ziskind AA and others. Percutaneous balloon pericardiotomy for the treatment of cardiac tamponade and large pericardial effusions: description of technique and report of the first 50 cases, *J Am Coll Cardiol* 21:1, 1993.

67. Hajduczok ZD and Ferguson DW: Percutaneous balloon pericardiostomy for non-surgical management of recurrent pericardial tamponade: a case report. *Intensive Care Med* 17:299, 1991.

68. Gatenby RA, Hartz WH, Kessler HB: Percutaneous catheter drainage for malignant pericardial effusion, *J Vasc Intervent Radiol* 2:151, 1991.

69. Zahn EM and others: Percutaneous pericardial catheter drainage in childhood, *Am J Cardiol* 70:678, 1992.

70. Patel AK and others: Catheter drainage of the pericardium: practical method to maintain long-term patency, *Chest* 92:1018 1987.

71. Saidman LJ, Smith NT, Bendixen HH: *Monitoring in anesthesia,* ed 2, Boston, 1983, Butterworth.

72. Anderson FD, Cunningham SG, Maloney JP: Indirect blood pressure measurement: a need to reassess, *Am J Crit Care* 2:272 1993.

73. Burch GE and Shewey L: Sphygmomanometeric cuff size and blood pressure recordings, *JAMA* 225:1215, 1973.

74. Kirkendall WM, Burton AC, Epstein FH: *Recommendations for human blood pressure determinations by sphygmomanometers,* New York, 1951, American Heart Association.

75. Frolich ED and others: *Recommendations for human blood pressure determination by sphygmomanometers, V,* Dallas, 1987, American Heart Association, AHA publications no. 70-1005(SA):i-34.

76. Londe S and Klitzner TS: Auscultatory blood pressure measurement: effect of pressure on the head of the stethoscope, *West J Med* 141:193, 1984.

77. Weinger M, Scanlon T, Miller L: A widely unappreciated cause of failure of an automatic noninvasive blood pressure monitor, *J Clin Monit* 8:291, 1992.

78. Venus B and others: Direct versus indirect blood pressure measurements in critically ill patients, *Heart Lung* 14:228, 1985.

79. Manolio TA and others: Evaluation of the Dinamap continuous blood pressure monitor, *Am J Hypertens* 1:161S, 1988.

80. Bochmer RD: Continuous real-time, noninvasive monitoring of blood pressure: Penaz methodology applied to the finger, *J Clin Monit* 3:282 1987.

81. Gibbs NM, Larach DR, Derr JA: The accuracy of Finapress noninvasive mean arterial pressure measurements in anesthetized patients, *Anesthesiology* 74:647, 1991.

82. Grazt I and others: *J Clin Monit* 8:20 1992.

BIBLIOGRAPHY

Bone RC, George RB, Hudsom LD: *Acute respiratory failure,* New York, 1987, Churchill Livingstone.

Cain SM: Assessment of tissue oxygenation, *Crit Care Clin* 2:537, 1986.

Carroll GC: Blood pressure monitoring, *Crit Care Clin* 4:411, 1988.

Clements FM and deBruijn NP: Noninvasive cardiac monitoring, *Crit Care Clin* 4:435, 1988.

Daily EK and Schroeder JS: *Techniques in bedside hemodynamic monitoring,* ed 4, St Louis, 1989, Mosby.

Darovic GO: *Hemodynamic monitoring: invasive and noninvasive clinical application,* Philadelphia, 1987, WB Saunders.

Deknatel Pleur-evac: *Understanding chest drainage systems. Nos. 1, 2, 3, and 4.* Floral Park, NY, Deknatel Division of Pfizer Hospital Products Group.

Fishman NH: *Thoracic drainage: a manual of procedures,* St Louis 1983, Mosby.

Kersten LD: *Comprehensive respiratory nursing care,* Philadelphia, 1989, WB Saunders.

Kreit JW and Eschenbacher WL: The physiology of spontaneous and mechanical ventilation. In Morganroth ML, editor: Mechanical ventilation, *Clin Chest Med* 9(1), 1988.

Luce JM and Pierson DJ: *Critical care medicine,* Philadelphia, 1988, WB Saunders.

Morganroth ML, editor: Mechanical ventilation, *Clin Chest Med* 9: 1988.

Murray JF and Nadel JA: *Textbook of respiratory medicine,* Philadelphia, 1988, WB Saunders.

Naclerio EA: *Chest injuries: physiologic principles and emergency management,* New York, 1971, Grune & Stratton.

Shoemaker WC and others: *Textbook of critical care,* ed 2, Philadelphia, 1989, WB Saunders.

Textbook of advanced cardiac life support, ed 2, Dallas, 1987, American Heart Association.

Vender JS, editor: Intensive care monitoring, *Crit Care Clin* 4: 1988.

Chapter 12

Respiratory Monitoring in the Intensive Care Unit

Tom Malinowski

LEARNING OBJECTIVES

Upon completion of this chapter, the reader should be able to accomplish the following:

1. Identify the methods, normal values, and significance of measuring the following lung volumes and flows in the intensive care unit:
   a. tidal volume
   b. vital capacity
   c. functional residual capacity

2. Recognize the methods, normal values, and significance of measuring the following airway pressures or related indices in the intensive care unit:
   a. peak pressure
   b. static pressure
   c. compliance
   d. airway resistance
   e. mean airway pressure
   f. maximum inspiratory pressure

3. Recognize the methods and significance of measuring the F_{IO_2} and exhalted carbon dioxide in the intensive care unit.

4. Identify the components of oxygen transport and their significance.

5. Identify the components involved in the clinical evaluation of oxygenation and their significance.

6. Recognize how the following parameters can be used to evaluate tissue oxygen delivery and utilization:
   a. oxygen delivery/availability
   b. oxygen consumption
   c. mixed venous oxygen tension ($P\bar{v}O_2$)
   d. venous saturation ($S\bar{v}O_2$)
   e. arterial to mixed venous oxygen content difference
   f. oxygen extraction ratio
   g. blood lactate

7. Recognize the value of the following noninvasive methods of monitoring oxygenation and oxygen delivery:
   a. pulse oximetry
   b. transcutaneous monitoring
   c. conjunctival monitoring

Chapter Overview

Monitoring has been defined as "repeated or continuous observations or measurements of the patient, his or her physiologic function, and the function of life support equipment, for the purpose of guiding management decisions, including when to make therapeutic interventions, and assessment of those interventions..."[1]

Respiratory monitoring refers to the process of continuously evaluating the cardiopulmonary status of patients for the purpose of improving clinical management. The goals of monitoring include alerting clinicians to changes in the patient's condition and improving our understanding of pathophysiology, diagnosis, and cost-effective clinical management. This is accomplished through the use of physical examination, measurements and calculations, and alarms.

The goals of this chapter are to introduce the instruments or tools available for the most common forms of respiratory monitoring, describe the information they can provide, and say when they should and should not be used. This chapter will primarily describe *ventilatory* and *oxygenation assessment*. Some of the information that would normally be included under respiratory monitoring, such as physical assessment and blood gas interpretation, is reviewed in other chapters of this book.

Ventilatory Assessment

Arterial blood gases are traditionally[2] thought of as the standard for assessing ventilation and oxygenation (see Chapter 6). However, changes in the patient's metabolism, lung mechanics, ventilatory efficiency, and equipment function will occur before changes are seen in the blood gases. It is therefore important to monitor the ventilatory parameters in addition to the blood gases.

The ventilatory measurements that can be monitored at the bedside in the intensive care unit (ICU) routinely include the following:

- Lung volumes and flows
- Airway pressures
- Fractional gas concentrations

Lung Volumes and Flows

Ventilation is the process of moving gases between the atmosphere and the lung. These gases occupy spaces commonly referred to as *lung volumes*. Lung volumes have been described and their measurement discussed in Chapter 7, but their importance to the critical care clinician is emphasized here.

WHY MONITOR LUNG VOLUMES? There are four reasons why lung volumes are important to the clinician:

1. *Changes in lung volumes have a direct effect on gas exchange in the pulmonary-capillary bed.*
2. *Changes in lung volumes reflect the mechanical function of the patient-ventilator interface, especially when the ventilator has malfunctioned.*
3. *Changes in lung volume frequently occur when there is improvement or deterioration in the patient's pulmonary status.*
4. *Changes in lung volume can reflect the patient's response to therapy.*

WHO SHOULD BE MONITORED FOR LUNG VOLUMES? Following is a list of the most common circumstances in which patients will benefit from the monitoring of lung volumes:

A. Intubated patients.
   1. Patients being considered for mechanical ventilation.
   2. Patients receiving mechanical ventilation.
   3. Patients with an abnormal breathing pattern.

B. Nonintubated patients.
   1. Preoperative evaluation (especially upper abdominal and thoracic surgery).
   2. Adult patients with respiratory rates greater than 30 breaths per minute.
   3. Patients with neuromuscular disease.
   4. Patients with central nervous system (CNS) depression.
   5. Patients with deteriorating blood gases.

WHAT DO WE MEASURE?

Tidal Volumes. *Tidal volume* (V_T) is defined as the volume of air inspired or passively exhaled in a normal respiratory cycle. V_T for a healthy person varies with each breath, but is usually 5 to 7 mL/Kg of ideal body weight.

V_T has two components: (1) alveolar volume (V_A), or the portion of V_T that effectively exchanges with alveolar-capillary blood; and (2) dead space volume (V_D), the portion of V_T that does not exchange with capillary blood. The V_D is normally about 2 mL/Kg of ideal body weight, or about 25% to 30% of the V_T, and consists of the conductive airways and alveolar units that are ventilated but not perfused. This is the true or physiologic dead space.

In healthy, spontaneously breathing persons, the V_T occasionally increases to three or four times normal levels. These larger tidal breaths are known as *sighs* and normally occur about six to ten times each hour. In acutely ill patients there is often a loss of the sigh, and the size of the patient's V_T tends to diminish. In addition, the V_T does not vary from breath to breath.[3] If shallow breathing without occasional sighing is maintained for prolonged periods of time, atelectasis and pneumonia may result, especially in patients breathing high oxygen concentrations or in patients with a compromised mucociliary clearance mechanism.

Conditions that may cause the V_T to be reduced include pneumonia, atelectasis, the postoperative period following chest and abdominal surgery, chest trauma, acute exacerbation of chronic obstructive pulmonary disease (COPD), congestive heart failure (CHF), pulmonary edema, acute restrictive diseases such as adult respiratory distress syndrome (ARDS), neuromuscular diseases, and CNS depression (especially of the respiratory centers).

Larger-than-normal tidal volumes may be seen with metabolic acidosis or severe neurologic injury.

Critically ill patients without an artificial airway may not tolerate the measurement of V_T. To get accurate measurements, the use of a face mask or mouthpiece is required. Frequently patients change their breathing pattern when a mask or mouthpiece is applied, thereby altering their V_T.[4]

Patients receiving continuous mechanical ventilation (CMV) are routinely ventilated with tidal volumes of 10 to 15 mL/Kg, two to three times the normal spontaneous V_T (5–7 mL/Kg).[5] When normal spontaneous V_T is used during CMV without positive end-expiratory pressure (PEEP), there is a reduction in functional residual capacity (FRC), an increase in intrapulmonary shunt, and a fall in partial pressure of arterial oxygen (Pao_2). These potentially harmful conditions can be reversed in part or totally by increasing the V_T to 10 to 15 mL/Kg or by applying PEEP.[6]

Unfortunately the use of large V_T ventilation can induce complications. There is considerable experimental evidence to suggest that lung injury may occur with peak alveolar pressures of as little as 30 cm H_2O.[7–9] The use of large V_T ventilation may predispose patients to higher alveolar pressures.

The application of PEEP in combination with smaller tidal volumes maintains FRC and prevents the fall in Pao_2. This may suggest that an increase in mean lung volume is more important than larger tidal volumes.[6,10,11]

Monitoring the V_T of the mechanically ventilated patient is crucial. Discrepancies in set vs. measured V_T may be due to (1) pneumothorax, (2) leaks in the ventilator circuit, (3) a leaky endotracheal tube cuff, or (4) a poorly calibrated spirometer. A low measured V_T can also be due to "stacking," a problem seen with severe airways obstruction. If not enough time is allowed for exhalation before the next breath is initiated by the ventilator, the subsequent V_T will "stack" on top of the previous breath. Reduction of ventilator rate, increased inspiratory flows, and decreased tidal volumes will help resolve the problem, which, if not corrected, can lead to severe barotrauma.

Where V_T is monitored often plays an important role in data interpretation. Proximal volume monitoring eliminates the compressible volume factor of tubing circuits and may more accurately reflect delivered V_T than expiratory limb monitoring. This is particularly true during conditions of low V_T, low lung compliance, and high airway resistance. Proximal monitoring is not without drawbacks. Proximal sensing makes the measuring device more susceptible to condensate and secretions, potentially reducing reliability and accuracy. It may also increase circuit resistance and dead space, increasing the respiratory work for the patient to breathe.

Air trapping and dynamic hyperinflation frequently occur in mechanically ventilated patients with severe airway obstruction. One technique that can measure the degree of dynamic hyperinflation is to measure the volume of gas exhaled during a prolonged apnea (20–40 seconds) following a tidal breath from the ventilator.[12] This maneuver measures the additional trapped gas above the patient's normal FRC. Ventilatory adjustments that reduce $\dot{V}_E$ and lengthen expiratory time will reduce the degree of air trapping.

Patients receiving intermittent mandatory ventilation (IMV) and synchronized IMV (SIMV) are allowed to breathe spontaneously through the ventilator circuit between mechanical breaths. As a result, their spontaneous V_T may differ in size from the mechanical V_T being delivered by the ventilator. It is important for the clinician to distinguish between spontaneous and mechanical V_T during the weaning process so that a true assessment of the patient's ventilatory status can be made.

Before and during the process of weaning the patient from mechanical ventilation, spontaneous V_T should be monitored frequently.[13] The adult patient's spontaneous V_T should be at least 300 mL if weaning is to be successful.[14] If V_T falls more than 25% during weaning, the clinician should be alerted to the possibility of impending respiratory muscle fatigue. This finding is frequently accompanied by a concurrent rise in the respiratory rate.

The rapid shallow breathing index (RSB) incorporates this spontaneous breath rate change, and measures the ratio of respiratory frequency (f) to V_T.

$$RSB = F(breaths/min)/V_T (L)$$

RSB values greater than 100 are strong prognostic indicators of weaning failure.

Minute Ventilation. Minute ventilation ($\dot{V}_E$) is the product of V_T and respiratory rate or frequency and represents the total volume of gas inspired or exhaled by the patient in 1 minute. The average $\dot{V}_E$ for a normal healthy adult is 4 to 8 L/min. As with V_T, approximately 25% to 30% of $\dot{V}_E$ is in the form of dead space ventilation. $\dot{V}_E$ is frequently increased in the early stages of respiratory failure; it is not until later stages of failure that $\dot{V}_E$ begins to fall.

If the arterial carbon dioxide pressure ($Paco_2$) is considered an indicator of the *adequacy* of ventilation, the relationship of $\dot{V}_E$ to $Paco_2$ indicates the *efficiency* of ventilation. A $\dot{V}_E$ of 6 L/min is usually associated with a $Paco_2$ of approximately 40 mmHg in a normal healthy person with a normal metabolic rate. If a higher-than-normal $\dot{V}_E$ is associated with a normal $Paco_2$ in a patient with a normal metabolic rate, there must be an increase in wasted or dead space ventilation. This is usually associated with hypovolemia, a decrease in lung perfusion as seen with pulmonary embolism, or reduced V_T.

An increase in carbon dioxide production caused by an increased metabolism (as occurs with trauma or fever) or high carbohydrate loading accompanying glucose administration via parenteral feedings may cause an increase in $\dot{V}_E$ with a normal $Paco_2$ (see Chapter 15). The elevated production of carbon dioxide requires an increase in ventilation to maintain the $Paco_2$ in normal range. The $Paco_2$ of patients mechanically ventilated in the control mode varies with changes in metabolism. Patients with varying metabolic rates should be ventilated with modes that allow them to set their own respiratory rate and thereby increase $\dot{V}_E$ to clear higher levels of carbon dioxide produced.

When a $\dot{V}_E$ greater than 10 L/min is needed for a mechanically ventilated patient to maintain a normal $Paco_2$, weaning is not likely to be successful. The elevated $\dot{V}_E$ indicates that the patient's respiratory muscles will probably fatigue when the mechanical ventilation is discontinued.[15] In addition, a resting spontaneous $\dot{V}_E$ of 10 L/min or less during a T-piece trial is considered an acceptable weaning criterion.[16] While spontaneous $\dot{V}_E$ is frequently used as a weaning criterion, it is often unreliable.[17]

$\dot{V}_E$ may fluctuate widely both during traditional T-piece weaning and during IMV and therefore should be monitored frequently before and during the weaning procedure. A rapid rise or a sudden drop in $\dot{V}_E$ should be quickly investigated, as both may signal ventilatory failure.[13,14]

Many therapeutic activities directed toward the patient's care can alter $\dot{V}_E$. A good example is the administration of opiates postoperatively to control pain. Opiates can blunt the respiratory drive sufficiently to cause a sudden onset of hypoventilation.

Vital Capacity. *Vital capacity* (*VC*) is the maximal volume of gas that can be expired from the lungs following a maximal inspiration. Normal values for healthy persons range from 60 to 80 mL/Kg of ideal body weight. The VC maneuver is position-dependent, the largest values usually being recorded with the patient in the upright position.[18]

The VC is an excellent measurement of ventilatory reserve in the cooperative patient. It reflects the respiratory muscle strength and volume capacity of the lung while the patient is performing a sustained maximal inspiratory or expiratory maneuver. These are of paramount importance in maintaining an adequate cough to clear secretions and in guaranteeing periodic inflation of alveoli that may be prone to collapse.

VC can be measured as either a forced maneuver (forced vital capacity [FVC]) or a slow expiratory maneuver (slow vital capacity [SVC]). An FVC maneuver also provides expiratory flow values and an indication of airway resistance (Raw). The SVC maneuver may be much easier for the patient to perform, especially if the patient is lethargic, medicated, experiencing pain, or has obstructive airways disease.

The accuracy and repeatability of the values are dependent on the patient's effort and the coaching skills of the clinician. It is important that the patient understand how to perform the maneuver correctly. A tight seal around the mouthpiece or mask is crucial. The patient may perform better if able to observe the tracing generated by the effort or to receive some similar visual feedback (incentive spirometry).

During preoperative evaluation of a patient's lung function, findings of a reduction in forced expiratory volume in 1 second (FEV_1/FVC%) to less than 50% of normal, or a FVC of less than 20 mL/Kg, because of nonreversible obstructive or restrictive disease, indicate that the patient is at high risk for developing pulmonary complications in the postoperative period. Factors that influence the degree of decrease in VC during the postoperative period and the incidence of postoperative pulmonary complications include (1) the surgical site, (2) smoking history, (3) age, (4) nutritional status, (5) obesity, (6) pain, (7) type of anesthesia, and (8) type of narcotics used for pain control.

Although many factors can contribute to a reduction in VC postoperatively, one of the most important is the incision site. Thoracoabdominal incisions are associated with the highest incidence of postoperative morbidity, followed by upper abdominal incisions, then transsternal surgery. Thoracic and upper abdominal surgery produce a significant fall in VC within the first day postoperatively. This reduction may persist for up to 2 weeks.[19] Operative procedures below the umbilicus are associated with fewer pulmonary complications, even in patients with preexisting pulmonary disease.

A VC of 10 to 15 mL/Kg is usually needed for effective deep breathing and coughing. Values of less than 10 mL/Kg are usually associated with impending respiratory failure. Values greater than 10 to 15 mL/Kg usually indicate adequate ventilatory reserve and the possibility of discontinuing CMV and extubation.

VC is also measured in order to follow the responsiveness of the patient to various respiratory therapies such as incentive spirometry or intermittent positive pressure breathing (IPPB). A common goal of both these maneuvers is to promote lung expansion.

Functional Residual Capacity. FRC is the volume of gas remaining in the lungs at the end of a normal passive exhalation. The FRC is continuously in contact with pulmonary capillary blood and thereby undergoing gas exchange. It is composed of a combination of residual volume (RV) and expiratory reserve volume (ERV). Normally, FRC is about 40 mL/Kg of ideal body weight, or approximately 35% to 40% of total lung capacity (TLC).[18]

FRC can vary from breath to breath by as much as 300 mL in healthy persons.[20] Changes in body position affect FRC, with the greatest values being recorded in the upright position.[21-23] Using lung models, it has been estimated that 25% of a 500-mL V_T comes in contact and mixes with the FRC during each breath, thereby continuously supplying fresh oxygen-enriched air to the gas exchange units.[24] Prolonged changes in FRC can have a dramatic impact on gas exchange.

When alveolar volume falls, as with atelectasis, FRC is reduced and there are regional changes in alveolar pressure–volume curves. Initially, as FRC decreases, dependent alveoli collapse and require higher distending pressures to reinflate. Since the apical alveoli remain at least partially open, they are more compliant and require less pressure to reinflate. Subsequently during mechanical ventilation, the inspired volumes are preferentially distributed to the apices. Unfortunately these apical alveoli are poorly perfused with blood. This distribution of inspired volumes to nondependent, poorly perfused alveoli contributes to the abnormal gas exchange seen in patients with decreased FRC.[25] Experimental evidence now demonstrates that repeated collapse and reinflation of alveoli lead to alveolar damage, capillary rupture, and considerable lung injury. The application of PEEP prevents alveolar collapse and may reduce the extent of acute lung injury.[26-28]

Therapeutic modalities such as PEEP or continuous positive airway pressure (CPAP) increase FRC.[29,30] This is a primary benefit to patients with atelectasis and

refractory hypoxemia. The increase in FRC occurs within seconds of the application of PEEP, but the Pao_2 may take longer to increase.[31]

In healthy adults, 5 cm H_2O of PEEP results in a total increase in FRC of approximately 400 to 500 mL.[32] In patients with restrictive lung diseases (low compliance), the increase in FRC with 5 cm of PEEP is much lower. Some patients may require an FRC that exceeds the predicted normal volumes to achieve adequate oxygenation.[30]

The FRC measurement in patients with acute respiratory failure indicates the severity of alveolar collapse and identifies improvement in lung volume as a result of PEEP therapy. This can reduce the time needed to adjust PEEP to the appropriate therapeutic levels. FRC is traditionally measured in the pulmonary function laboratory by the technique of nitrogen washout, helium dilution, or body plethysmography (see Chapter 7). Techniques incorporating the traditional methods as well as sulfur hexafluoride (SF_6) have been used with mechanically ventilated patients.[33-43] However, FRC is rarely measured in the ICU because of the difficulty of applying these techniques to the critically ill.

DEVICES FOR MEASURING LUNG VOLUME. A wide variety of devices exists for measuring volumes and flows (Table 12–1). Devices that measure gas volume are known as spirometers. Spirometers vary in their operation and performance characteristics. They can be classified into smaller subgroups based on their principle of operation, such as *volume displacement, turbine-driven, flow transducers,* and *anemometers.*

Volume displacement devices are considered the gold standard and are commonly used in the pulmonary function laboratory but not as frequently in the ICU setting. Examples are the (1) water-sealed, (2) wedge, and (3) dry-rolling seal spirometers. These devices are accurate and unaffected by variations in flow rates, humidity, and gas density, but generally have the disadvantage of being too bulky for use in the ICU. Two exceptions to this are the Hudson disposable Venti-comp bag (Hudson Oxygen, Temecula, Calif.) and the Bennett Monitoring spirometer (Bennett Respira-

Table 12–1	Flow Measuring Devices for Critical Care Monitoring
Device	**Example**
Metal screen (pneumotachograph)	Flow sensors in Siemens 900B and 900C ventilators
Variable orifice (pneumotachograph)	Hamilton Veolar Flow Sensor, Bicore, Ventrak
Fixed orifice (pneumotachograph)	Monaghan RVM 761
Mass flow (anemometer)	Bear Neonatal Volume Monitor
Turbinometer	Boehringer Spirometer
Vortex spirometer	Bear LS75 and LS80

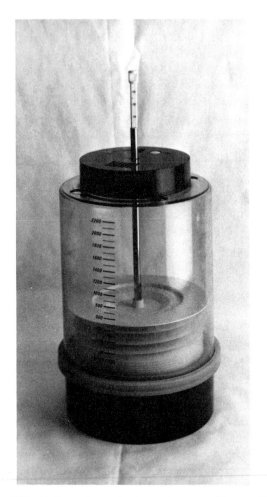

Fig. 12-1 *Bennett monitoring spirometer (Bennett Respiration Products, Inc., Santa Monica, Calif.)*

tion Products, Inc., Santa Monica, Calif.). The Venticomp bag is a 4.8-L graduated plastic bag that can be used to measure exhaled tidal volumes during assist/control ventilation and for SVC or FVC maneuvers. It is also convenient and compact enough to be carried, which makes it suitable for transport situations. The Bennett spirometer indicates each exhaled V_T by the filling of bellows within a clear, graduated plastic jar (Fig. 12-1). The Bennett spirometer is accurate only to ±100 mL. It is generally accurate when the rate of breathing is less than 30/min and when the V_T is greater than 400 to 500 mL.

Spirometers that calculate volume by dividing flow by time ($V = F/t$) are known as *flow transducers.* Some flow transducers calculate flow by measuring the pressure drop across a known resistance (Fig. 12-2). The accuracy of these devices in measuring volume is dependent on their ability to accurately measure flow.

Mass flow anemometers incorporate a single or a set of heated wires within a flow tube. As gas flows over the wires, the temperature in the wires is reduced. The greater the gas flow, the greater the temperature loss. The electric current necessary to maintain the temperature of the wires is proportional to the flow.

Vortex ultrasonic spirometers (Bear Medical Systems, Inc., Riverside, Calif.) incorporate two struts (a triangular protrusion) that extend across the inner lumen of the sensor. As flow occurs through the sensor, the struts create a *vortex* (a swirl of turbulent flow). These vortices interrupt an ultrasonic beam being pulsed through the tube from a transmitter to a receiver

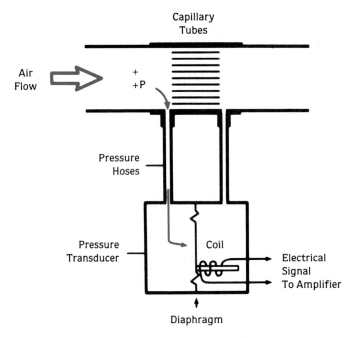

Fig. 12-2 *Fleisch pneumotachograph and differential pressure transducer. (Reprinted, with permission, from Daedalus Enterprises, Sullivan WJ, Peters GM, and Enright PL: Pneumotachographs: theory and clinical application,* Respir Care *29:736-749, 1984.)*

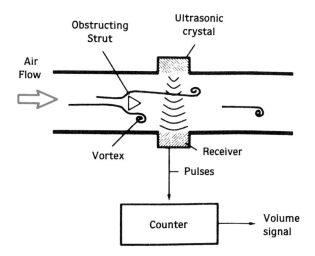

Fig. 12-3 *An ultrasonic flow sensor (Bear Medical Systems, Inc., Riverside, Calif.) incorporating the vortex principle. (Reprinted, with permission, from Daedulus Enterprises, Sullivan WJ, Peters GM, and Enright PL: Pneumotachographs: theory and clinical application,* Respir Care 29:736–749, 1984.)

(Fig. 12–3). Each vortex disturbance is associated with 1 mL of gas moving through the sensor tube. The number of vortex disturbances is counted during each period of gas flow and the total volume of gas determined. The manufacturer claims an accuracy of ± 4% over a flow range of 5 to 250 L/min (Table 12–2).

Variable orifice pneumotachographs usually consist of two chambers separated by a variable orifice flow element. The flow element is constructed from material that retains shape and returns to its original position in the orifice (memory). The flow element bends in the direction of flow and creates a small pressure difference between the two chambers. The difference in pressure is directly related to the amount of flow passing through the transducer. The element readily sheds water and mucus, and some units are suitable for continuous placement in the proximal dead space of a mechanical ventilator circuit. Variable orifice pneumotachographs have been incorporated into stand-alone monitors (Bicore, Irvine, Calif.; Ventrak, Wallingford,

Conn.) and also into ventilators (Hamilton, Reno, Nev.; Bird, Palm Springs, Calif.). These units are disposable, lightweight, easy to use, and allow for integration of multiple respiratory parameters including flow, pressure, volume, and time.

Turbine-driven spirometers such as the Wright respirometer (Ferraris Medical, Inc., Holland, N.Y.) incorporate miniature vanes or rotors that revolve when exposed to gas flow (Fig. 12–4). They may use an analog gauge or a digital display. Some turbine-driven units incorporate an infrared light-emitting diode (LED) to measure the revolutions of the vanes and thereby calculate flow and volume. These devices are not affected by gas viscosity, temperature, or water vapor, but they are affected by inertia and friction. If flow is too low (less than 3 L/min), the turbine may not spin, causing volume to be underestimated. Excessively high flow rates (over 200–300 L/min) can cause the turbine to spin after exhalation is over, resulting in overestimation of volume. These devices are small and easily used to measure V_T, $\dot{V}_E$, and nonforced or slow VC and therefore are clinically useful.

Most of the newer spirometers feature a sequential display of values that have traditionally been limited to the pulmonary function laboratory, such as FEV_1, FVC, and peak expiratory flow (PEF), in addition to V_T and $\dot{V}_E$. This has led to an increased use of these spirometers in the ICU and the emergency room as a substitute for standardized pulmonary function testing. Nevertheless, their accuracy may be questionable. Very few of the handheld spirometers meet established minimal acceptable limits for pulmonary function testing equipment in terms of instrument stability, linearity, freedom from hysteresis, and appropriate frequency response.[44] A recent report suggests that 50% of the commercially available spirometers do not meet the revised standards of the American Thoracic Society.[45] Therefore these devices should be used for screening or predicting trends rather than for obtaining absolute values.

The noninvasive *inductive plethysmograph* is gaining increased acceptance in the ICU for monitoring

Table 12-2	Types of Volume and Flow Measuring Devices and Their Range of Accuracies*	
Type	**Example**	**Accuracy†**
Volume-displacing	Wet-bell spirometer	± 3%–5%
	Dry-rolling seal	± 3%–5%
	Wedge	± 3%–5%
	Bellows	± 10%–20%
Turbine	Rotating vane	± 2%–15%
	Rotating cogs	± 2%–15%
Pneumotachometer	Pressure differential	± 2%–15%
	Fixed resistor	
	Variable resistor	
	Heated thermistor bead	± 5%–10%
	Heated wire anemometer	± 5%–10%
	Ultrasonic vortex shedder	± 2%–4%

* From Wilkins, RL, and Hicks G: Gas volume, flow, pressure, and temperature monitoring. In Hicks G, editor: *Problems in respiratory care: applied noninvasive monitoring,* vol 2, no 2, Philadelphia, 1989, JB Lippincott.
† Percent accuracy of full-scale reading

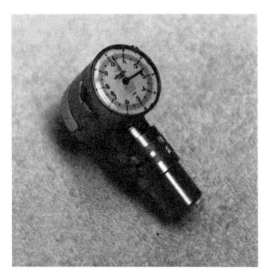

Fig 12–4 *Turbine-type Wright respirometer (Ferraris Medical, Inc., Holland, N.Y.).*

acutely ill and chronic difficult-to-wean patients. The system is composed of a transducer, oscillator, and calibrator. It uses insulated wire coils attached to a vest that fits closely over the patient's chest and upper abdomen. The coils form the inductive element of a simple transistor oscillator that measures changes in the cross-sectional volume of the rib cage and abdomen during breathing. Respiratory rate, V_T, and breathing pattern can be conveniently monitored with the unit. The system needs occasional recalibration, and proper positioning of the transducer bands is important (Fig. 12–5).

Airway Pressures

It is important to monitor airway pressures for the following reasons:

1. To help determine the need for mechanical ventilation and the patient's readiness for weaning
2. To help determine the site and thereby the cause of Raw to mechanical ventilation
3. To evaluate elastic recoil and compliance of the intact thorax
4. To help estimate the amount of positive airway pressure being transmitted to the heart and great vessels
5. To help assess the patient's respiratory muscle strength

Airway pressures should be measured as closely as possible to the endotracheal (ET) tube. This prevents resistance caused by the ventilator circuit from influencing the peak pressure measurement. On certain occasions, as when using high-frequency ventilation, the pressure should be measured at the distal tip of the ET tube.

Distal ET tip measurements may prove useful in triggering inspiratory and expiratory cycling during

---

POTENTIAL CAUSES OF INCREASED PEAK PRESSURE

Resistance factors

Patient airways	Artificial airway
Bronchospasm	Internal diameter of
Peribronchiolar	tube too small
edema	Kinking of ET tube
Retained secretions	Mucus plugging
Airway obstruction	Cuff herniation
caused by foreign	Tube impinging on
body	tracheal wall

Ventilator circuit
Water in tubing
Kinking of circuit tubing
High inspiratory flow rates (mechanical)

Elastic recoil

Thoracic cage	Lung involvement
Chest wall deformity	Acute respiratory
Obesity	failure
Abdominal distention,	Pneumonia
compression, or	Adult respiratory
herniation	distress syndrome
Diaphragmatic and	Atelectasis
intercostal muscle	Pneumothorax
discoordination	Fibrosis
Active expiration,	
restlessness, pain	
Patient placement in	
lateral or prone	
position	
Chest wraps or casts	

---

pressure support ventilation. Distal measurement will eliminate sensing problems associated with the added Raw of the ET tube.

PEAK PRESSURE. Peak pressure is the maximal pressure attained during the inspiratory phase of mechanical ventilation. It reflects the amount of force needed to overcome opposition to airflow into the lungs. Causes of this opposition to flow can be (1) resistance generated by the ventilator circuit, the artificial airway (ET tube), or the patient's airways and (2) elastic recoil of the thoracic cage and the lungs. Sudden increases in peak airway pressure should alert the clinician to the presence of a patient-ventilator interface problem. Potential causes of an increase in peak pressure appear in the accompanying box.

If the peak pressure increases while the static pressure (explained later) is unchanged, an increase in Raw is probably occurring. Common causes include bronchospasm, airway secretions, and mucus plugging.

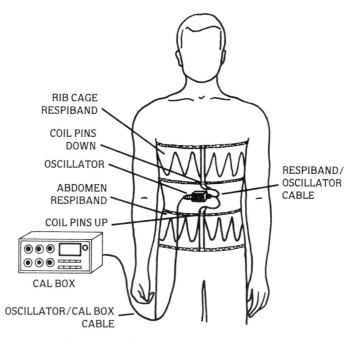

Fig. 12–5 *Inductive plethysmograph using chest and abdominal bands (Respitrace Corp.; courtesy of Ambulatory Monitoring, Ardsley, N.Y.).*

As a result of the relationship between peak pressure and Raw, monitoring the peak pressure provides valuable information about the bronchodilator-induced changes in lung function of the mechanically ventilated patient.[46] It is important to note that whenever changes in the peak pressure are used for evaluating Raw, no changes in the inspiratory flow, flow pattern, or V_T should be made.

High peak airway pressure is often considered to be the cause of barotrauma.[47] Evidence supports, however, the concept that high peak alveolar pressures leads to alveolar rupture.[48] Conditions that raise the peak airway pressure may not affect alveolar pressure owing to increased inspiratory resistance during mechanical ventilation. Static pressure more accurately reflects alveolar pressure than does peak pressure and should be used as the primary indicator for the risk of alveolar rupture.[48]

STATIC PRESSURE. One way to determine the cause of an elevated peak pressure is to separate the resistance component from the elastic recoil of the combined lung and chest wall. This can be done by measuring the *static pressure*. The static pressure is the pressure required to maintain a delivered V_T in a patient's lungs during a period of no gas flow. Static pressure is measured by occluding an exhalation valve immediately after the onset of the inspiratory breath and holding the exhalation valve closed throughout a portion of the expiratory phase until a plateau pressure is observed. In patients with airway obstruction, plateau pressure may take several seconds to be achieved.[49] Another technique incorporates a shutter valve that intermittently stops flow during the expiratory phase.[50]

During the period of no gas flow, the Raw component of ventilation is eliminated, leaving the elastic recoil component as the force required to maintain inflation. If the volume maintained inside the lungs during this plateau period is known, the effective static compliance can be determined.

Mechanically ventilated patients with status asthmaticus may have low levels of measured auto-PEEP (see discussion below) despite obvious signs of dynamic hyperinflation. Static pressure has been suggested to be superior to auto-PEEP for determining the degree of dynamic hyperinflation in these patients.[51] Consequently, patients with severe dynamic hyperinflation at risk of barotrauma who demonstrate low auto-PEEP may be better evaluated by using static pressures.

Compliance. *Compliance* is defined as volume change per unit of pressure change, or the amount of lung volume achieved per unit of pressure. Two forms of compliance are commonly reported: effective dynamic compliance and static compliance. *Dynamic compliance* represents the total impedance to gas flow into the lungs, and is determined by dividing mechanical V_T by the peak airway pressure minus PEEP:

$$\text{Dynamic compliance} = \frac{V_T - [(Ppk - PEEP) \times CV]}{Ppk - PEEP}$$

where

$$V_T = \text{tidal volume}$$
$$Ppk = \text{peak airway pressure}$$
$$PEEP = \text{set PEEP or auto-PEEP, whichever is higher}$$
$$CV = \text{tubing compliance correction factor}$$

Dynamic compliance incorporates both the flow-resistive characteristics of the airways and ventilator circuit, and the elastic components of the lung and chest wall. *Static compliance* is the measurement of the lung volume change per unit of pressure during a period of no gas flow. It is calculated clinically by dividing V_T by the plateau pressure minus PEEP:

$$\text{Static compliance} = \frac{V_T - [(Pplateau - PEEP) \times CV]}{Pplateau - PEEP}$$

where

$$
\begin{aligned}
V_T &= \text{tidal volume} \\
Pplateau &= \text{plateau pressure} \\
PEEP &= \text{set PEEP or auto-PEEP, whichever is higher} \\
CV &= \text{tubing compliance correction factor}
\end{aligned}
$$

In practice, static calculations should be based on at least three breaths. The measured values include not only the lung-thorax unit but the compliance of the ventilator circuit as well. Compliance of the adult ventilator circuit varies with the structure and diameter of the tubing but is generally 2 to 3 mL/cm H_2O/L of the circuitry volume. If the patient is being ventilated with high airway pressures, a significant portion of the V_T is "lost" to tubing expansion, and erroneous compliance measurements can be computed if this phenomenon is not considered.

The effective static compliance measurements can be valuable in monitoring patients receiving mechanical ventilation.[52,53] Lung diseases such as pulmonary edema, pneumothorax, pneumonia, and ARDS increase lung recoil and the observed static pressure. As a result, the static compliance is reduced in such situations.

The textbook normal values for thoracic compliance of 100 mL/cm H_2O are rarely seen in mechanically ventilated patients because even patients with normal lungs usually develop a decrease in lung volume and compliance after receiving positive pressure ventilation for a few hours.[49] Thus normal compliance values in patients receiving mechanical ventilation range from 60 to 80 mL/cm H_2O. Compliance values of less than 25 mL/cm H_2O are usually not associated with successful weaning attempts[2,14] or PEEP withdrawal.

Auto-Peep. Mechanically ventilated patients with higher ventilatory rates may develop a condition termed *auto-PEEP*. This can be seen if airway obstruction is present.[46,49,53,54] If there is insufficient time for exhalation, the lung is unable to return to its relaxed state prior to the next mechanical breath. Therefore exhalation of each successive V_T will be incomplete, and a positive alveolar pressure will occur. The alveolar pressure will slowly rise and result in a PEEP-like effect, thus the term *auto-PEEP*. Auto-PEEP is not detected by the ventilator pressure manometer unless the expiratory limb is occluded. When the flow is stopped at end-exhalation, pressure will equilibrate throughout the closed system and register on the ventilator manometer.

When auto-PEEP is due to dynamic airways compression the patient may be unable to trigger ventilator breaths despite spontaneous efforts. Forceful inspiratory efforts or inability to trigger the ventilator will be seen. Titrating PEEP in this case may reduce the inspiratory efforts needed to trigger inspiratory breaths. There will be negligible increases in peak inspiratory pressure during application of PEEP in such cases.

Auto-PEEP varies with the time allowed for exhalation, the elastic recoil of the lung, and the resistance to flow of the airways, ET tube, and expiratory limb (exhalation valve) of the ventilator circuit. Bronchodilator therapy, higher ventilator inspiratory flow rates, and a reduction in the mechanical rate have been shown to reduce the auto-PEEP effect.[46,53] The most effective method to reduce auto-PEEP during conventional ventilation is through the reduction of $\dot{V}_E$. Strategies which alter V_T, ventilator rate, or inspiratory time without reducing $\dot{V}_E$ do little to reduce auto-PEEP.[12]

AIRWAY RESISTANCE. Raw is the opposition to airflow by the nonelastic forces of the lung. True Raw is not measured routinely in the ICU. A reliable estimate of the flow-restrictive components of Raw can be made by subtracting the static or plateau pressure from the peak pressure. Raw can be estimated by subtracting static pressure from peak pressure and dividing by flow in liters per second. Normal values are 2 to 3 cm H_2O/L/sec.

$$\text{Raw} = \frac{\text{peak pressure} - \text{static pressure}}{\text{flow (L/sec)}}$$

Raw can be elevated by numerous factors (see above). Increased Raw can cause problems not only during positive pressure breathing but also during spontaneous breathing. A small-diameter ET tube will significantly increase the work of breathing for a spontaneously breathing patient.[55] High flow rates from a continuous flow IMV system can increase expiratory work by forcing the patient to exhale the mechanically delivered V_T against the expiratory valve of both the machine and the continuous flow of the IMV system.

MEAN AIRWAY PRESSURE. *Mean airway pressure (MAP)* is the average pressure recorded during the positive pressure and spontaneous phases of a respiratory cycle. MAP is calculated to determine the average airway pressure being applied to the lungs. Ventilator measurements affecting MAP include CPAP and PEEP levels, inspiratory time (flow rate, flow patterns), peak pressure, and rate. Increases in MAP are usually associated with an improvement in Pa_{O_2}, but can cause barotrauma and a reduction in cardiac output. Some studies indicate that PEEP and CPAP levels affect oxygenation more than variation in inspiratory flow rates and inspiratory times do, even though they both increase MAP.[56] MAP is often considered to be equivalent to mean *alveolar* pressure, but these values are not always equal. Discrepancies between the two values may be due to imbalances in inspiratory and expiratory resistance, variable flow resistance, leakage of gas volume, and measurement error.[57] Despite the absence of reported studies that show a correlation between specific levels of MAP and barotrauma, MAP levels greater than 30 cm H_2O appear to greatly enhance the risk for the development of lung injury. Currently, no studies have shown a correlation between specific levels of MAP and barotrauma in the adult population.

MAXIMUM INSPIRATORY PRESSURE. The *maximum inspiratory pressure (MIP),* sometimes called the *negative inspiratory force (NIF),* is the maximum inspiratory pressure the patient's ventilatory pump is capable of generating against a closed airway. Multiple factors influence the patient's ability to produce a normal MIP:

1. Respiratory muscle strength
2. Patient effort
3. Ventilatory drive
4. Lung volume
5. Phrenic nerve function
6. Nutritional status
7. Oxygenation status
8. Acid-base status

Since MIP is intended to be a measure of respiratory muscle strength, these variables must be considered when interpreting MIP (also called PImax).

MIP can be measured even if an artificial airway is not in place by using a mask or mouthpiece and an external pressure manometer. The alert patient should be asked to exhale to a volume between FRC and residual volume (RV) because this will improve the mechanical advantage of the inspiratory muscles. At the end of exhalation, the airway is occluded while the patient makes a maximal inspiratory effort.

Marini and associates[58] have reported a standardized approach to measuring MIP in uncooperative critically ill patients. The patient is prepared for the maneuver by careful explanation of the procedure, proper positioning, and thorough suctioning with hyperoxygenation. Next, a one-way valve is placed in the expiratory path of a rigid T-tube to allow exhalation but not inhalation. This technique reduces lung volume to a level between RV and FRC. MIPs are usually generated within 20 seconds of occlusion. Careful explanation of the procedure is important because occlusion of the airway can be frightening.

A normal MIP is approximately 80 to 110 cm H_2O. An MIP of 30 cm H_2O has been shown to be a predictor of successful weaning[2,16]; however, there is some debate as to its usefulness.[59] Although MIP is useful in measuring the patient's respiratory muscle strength, it provides little information regarding muscle endurance

or Raw. MIP should not be the sole respiratory factor used to predict the patient's ability to wean.

Fractional Gas Concentrations

The ability to monitor delivered oxygen concentrations is crucial for many respiratory procedures, and exhaled gases, sampled either intermittently or continuously, provide information about changes in equipment function, blood gases, tissue perfusion, ventilation-perfusion ($\dot{V}/\dot{Q}$) relationships, and metabolic rate. This section deals with oxygen concentration and carbon dioxide analysis and their use in the ICU.

FRACTION OF INSPIRED OXYGEN CONCENTRATION (F_{IO_2}). The measurement of F_{IO_2} is essential to the modern ICU. Various oxygen delivery devices require at least intermittent analysis of F_{IO_2} to ensure that the appropriate oxygen concentration is being delivered and to interpret blood gases. If the F_{IO_2} is inappropriately low, hypoxia may result; an inappropriate elevation of F_{IO_2} may lead to oxygen toxicity. Variations in delivered oxygen concentrations may make metabolic evaluations impossible.[60]

EXHALED CARBON DIOXIDE. Carbon dioxide is one of the by-products of tissue metabolism, and its elimination is a prime function of ventilation. Monitoring of exhaled carbon dioxide (capnometry) can detect changes in the following:

1. Metabolic rate as a result of cardiac output and body temperature changes, shivering, seizures, trauma, and high carbohydrate infusion
2. Ventilator function such as a patient disconnection or apnea
3. Efficiency of ventilation (by looking at the increase and decrease in alveolar and dead space ventilation)
4. Transport of carbon dioxide as a result of changes in perfusion

Carbon dioxide elimination is dependent on cardiac output and on the regional $\dot{V}/\dot{Q}$ ratios and the "emptying times" of different regions of the lung. Nondependent lung regions (so-called *type A* alveoli) open first and empty last and usually have high $\dot{V}/\dot{Q}$ ratios and subsequently low alveolar carbon dioxide concentrations. Dependent lung regions (so-called *type B* alveoli) have low $\dot{V}/\dot{Q}$ ratios, with alveolar carbon dioxide values approaching mixed venous values. Exhaled alveolar carbon dioxide concentrations are frequently at their highest at the end of exhalation, and therefore the term *end-tidal* P_{CO_2} (P_{ETCO_2}) may be used to indicate the highest exhaled carbon dioxide concentrations attained. In normal subjects, the P_{ETCO_2} is an accurate estimate of P_{aCO_2}, but conditions that alter $\dot{V}/\dot{Q}$ relationships, such as mechanical ventilation, pulmonary disease, and a decrease in perfusion increase the arterial-P_{ETCO_2} gradient.[61]

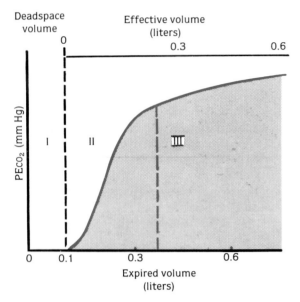

Fig. 12-6 *Single breath tracing for exhaled carbon dioxide.*

Capnometry has also been applied in the operating room,[62] emergency department, and prehospital care setting[63] for determination of ET tube placement,[64] airway disconnect, and systemic perfusion monitoring during cardiopulmonary resuscitation (CPR).[65] The last application may prove to be useful as a noninvasive prognostic indicator of CPR effectiveness.

Analysis may be done on a breath-by-breath basis or by sampling mean concentration. The systems currently used include infrared analysis, which detects absorption of a specific wavelength of infrared radiation, partial pressure analyzers, and mass spectrometry. Sampling may be done either by aspiration through a sample line or by placement of the sensor around the dead space of a ventilator circuit. Carbon dioxide tracings can be plotted against time or, by incorporating a flow transducer, volume. The latter technique allows the practitioner to measure breath-by-breath dead space.

A single breath tracing for carbon dioxide concentration vs. time is illustrated (Fig. 12-6). The tracing has three phases. Phase I contains no carbon dioxide (pure dead space). Phase II shows a rapid increase in carbon dioxide concentration. Phase III rises as a result of sequential lung emptying and the continual release of carbon dioxide into the alveoli during expiration.

Carbon Dioxide Production. Carbon dioxide production ($\dot{V}_{CO_2}$) is the carbon dioxide produced and excreted over 1 minute. The $\dot{V}_{CO_2}$ values provide information concerning changes in metabolic rate and transport of carbon dioxide. The formula for calculating $\dot{V}_{CO_2}$ is as follows:

$$\dot{V}_{CO_2} = F\bar{E}_{CO_2} \times \dot{V}_E$$

where

$F\bar{E}_{CO_2}$ = mean fraction of expired carbon dioxide
$\dot{V}_E$ = minute volume exhaled at STPD*

The formula assumes that there is no carbon dioxide in inspired air. $\dot{V}_{CO_2}$ is frequently increased in fever (10% increase per 1° C increase), trauma, peritonitis (25%–50% increase), head trauma, rewarming after hypothermia, and high carbohydrate loading with total parenteral nutrition.[66] $\dot{V}_{CO_2}$ increases with carbohydrate loading as a result of oxidation of carbohydrates and carbohydrate conversion to fats (lipogenesis). $\dot{V}_{CO_2}$ may increase by 75% because of carbohydrate "overloading" (see section on respiratory quotient in Chapter 15.)

A rapid decrease in $\dot{V}_{CO_2}$ or elimination accompanies a low cardiac output and a fall in tissue perfusion, decreased right ventricular output, decreased venous return, or pulmonary embolism.

Dead Space–Tidal Volume Ratio. V_D is that inspired volume that does not come in contact with pulmonary capillary blood. The V_D/V_T ratio expresses the relationship between V_D and total V_T, or the portion of the V_T that is "wasted." V_D has two components: anatomic dead space and alveolar dead space. *Anatomic dead space* is made up of the conducting airways and is normally about 2 mL/Kg of ideal body weight. *Alveolar dead space* is classically defined as alveoli that are ventilated but not perfused. The combination of anatomic and alveolar dead space is called *physiologic dead space.* V_D/V_T is traditionally calculated by the Englehoff modification of the Bohr equation, as follows:

$$V_D/V_T = \frac{Pa_{CO_2} - P\bar{E}_{CO_2}}{Pa_{CO_2}}$$

where

Pa_{CO_2} = arterial P_{CO_2}
$P\bar{E}_{CO_2}$ = P_{CO_2} of mixed exhaled gas

The patient is stabilized for 20 minutes, and arterial blood and exhaled gases are sampled simultaneously. The exhaled gases may be either collected in a Douglas bag or sampled at the outlet of a mixing box. Factors that may contaminate or dilute the $P\bar{E}_{CO_2}$, such as compressible gas volume from the patient ventilator circuit or gases from a continuous flow IMV system, should be eliminated by double exhalation valves.[67] A correction factor for patients on the assist/control mode of CMV can also eliminate compressible volume. The correction factor does not work during IMV because spontaneous and mechanical tidal volumes can vary in IMV modes.[67]

$$P\bar{E}_{CO_2} \text{ corrected} = \frac{V_T}{V_T - CV} \times P\bar{E}_{CO_2}$$

where

CV = compressible volume in tubing
V_T = mechanical tidal volume

*A volume of gas at standard temperature and pressure that contains no water vapor.

CAUSES OF IMPAIRED OXYGENATION IN CRITICALLY ILL PATIENTS*

Equipment-related problems, low/high flow oxygen delivery devices
Loose tubing connection, cannula
Loose humidifier, nipple connector
Inadequate flow to meet patient peak inspiratory flow, air entrainment
Blender malfunction

Ventilator-related problems
Endotracheal: tracheostomy tube malfunctions
Ventilator and circuit malfunctions
Improper settings, modes of ventilation

Progression of underlying disease process
ARDS
Cardiogenic pulmonary edema
Pneumonia
Airway obstruction, asthma/COPD

Onset of a new clinical problem
Pneumothoraces: simple, tension, loculated
Lobar atelectasis
Gastric aspiration
Artificial airway problems: stenosis, fistula, malacia
Nosocomial pneumonia
Fluid overload

Onset of a new clinical problem (cont.)
Microatelectasis
Bronchospasm
Retained secretions
Shock
Sepsis
Additional organ failure

Interventions and procedures
Endotracheal suctioning
Position changes
Chest physiotherapy
Bronchoscopy
Thoracentesis
Peritoneal dialysis
Hemodialysis
Transport
Diagnostic procedures
Line/tube placement

Medications
Bronchodilators
Vasodilators
Inotropic agents

Miscellaneous
Leukocytopenia
Intralipids

*Data from Glauser R and others: Worsening oxygenation in the mechanically ventilated patient, *Am Rev Respir Dis* 138:458, 1988.

The use of the V_D/V_T in patients on IMV may be misleading as a result of variations in PE_{CO_2} between mechanical and spontaneous breaths.

The normal V_D/V_T for healthy persons is between 25% and 35% and is position-dependent. Patients receiving positive pressure ventilation usually have a higher V_D/V_T while they are upright or in the lateral position than when they are in the supine position.[68] During anesthesia, V_D/V_T is usually increased because of an overall reduction in lung volume. In patients receiving mechanical ventilation, faster inspiratory flow rates or small tidal volumes are usually associated with an increase in V_D/V_T.[11,61,69] Variations in the inspiratory waveforms, tapered wave, sine waves, and end-inspiratory pause maneuvers may decrease V_D/V_T.[70] Changes in the pulmonary perfusion caused by emboli, hypoperfusion, and precapillary constriction may result in an increased V_D/V_T.

Evaluation of Oxygenation and Estimates of Oxygen Transport

Inadequate oxygenation is a common occurrence in patients in the ICU. The recognition and correction of this problem is crucial to the patient's well-being. Respiratory care maneuvers, pharmacologic and fluid support, and diagnostic procedures frequently affect tissue oxygenation. The bedside clinician must be able to monitor and determine the impact of these activities.

This section describes the concepts and techniques used in the assessment of oxygenation: first the components of oxygen transport and the measurements used to monitor oxygenation, then the indices of pulmonary gas exchange and indicators of systemic oxygenation and when they should be used.

The potential causes of hypoxemia and hypoxia are diverse. Hypoxic episodes can be iatrogenic in origin, as with suctioning or equipment failure. Progressive disease or a new problem can make oxygenation more difficult. Therefore the bedside clinician must be able to identify the causes of these problems, select the appropriate therapy or therapies, and monitor the outcome. Haldane, the physiologist, said it best almost a century ago: "Anoxia not only stops the machine but wrecks the machinery."

Oxygen Transport

Oxygen transport is the mechanism by which oxygen is carried from the lungs to the capillary bed for use by cellular mitrochondria, primarily for the production of adenosine triphosphate (ATP). Following are the crucial factors that determine oxygen availability to the tissues:

1. Oxygen content of the blood
2. Cardiac output
3. Distribution of the cardiac output
4. Oxyhemoglobin dissociation curve

In the clinically normal person, an increase in oxygen demand or an impairment in oxygen delivery to the tissues is compensated[71] for by an increase in one or more of four systems:

1. Circulatory (increase in cardiac output)
2. Blood (increase in hemoglobin concentration)
3. Chemical (oxyhemoglobin affinity factors)
4. Ventilatory (hyperventilation to increase alveolar oxygen tension [P_{AO_2}] and thus increase Pa_{O_2})

Patients in the ICU frequently have compromised reserve systems. Low cardiac output (shock), blood flow maldistribution, anemia, and ventilatory failure do not allow for adequate compensation to occur. As the abnormal situation persists, it becomes more difficult to correct. The longer oxygenation is compromised, the more profoundly the "machinery" is damaged.

Components of Oxygen Transport

OXYGEN CONTENT. *Oxygen content* is defined as the total amount of oxygen carried in the blood and is the sum of oxygen bound chemically to hemoglobin (Hb) plus oxygen dissolved in plasma. Under normal conditions hemoglobin is responsible for carrying 99% or more of the oxygen in blood. The remaining oxygen (less than 1%) is carried dissolved in plasma and is measured as Pa_{O_2}. Pa_{O_2} is important because it reflects the degree of saturation of hemoglobin and the driving pressure of oxygen between systemic capillary blood and the tissues:

$$O_2 \text{ content} = (Hb \times 1.34 \times \% \text{ saturation}) + (Pa_{O_2} \times 0.003)$$

CARDIAC OUTPUT. The techniques used to assess cardiac output are described in Chapter 13. Oxygen delivery is extremely dependent on cardiac output and systemic distribution of blood flow. The major determinant of cardiac output is metabolic activity, whereas peripheral distribution of blood flow is dependent on regional oxygen consumption, temperature, humoral agents, and other factors.[72] Cardiac output is not sensitive to moderate changes in oxygen tension (P_{O_2}) and usually does not increase until the Pa_{O_2} drops below 50 mmHg.[71] In the patient with shock, blood flow to the low oxygen consuming regions of the body (i.e., the skin) is reduced as a protective mechanism in response to an increase in sympathetic tone.[73,74] Clinically, the practitioner should be able to use the simple physical signs to assess perfusion as described in the previous chapter.

OXYHEMOGLOBIN DISSOCIATION CURVE. Another factor influencing oxygen delivery is the oxyhemoglobin dissociation curve (ODC). The ODC graphically depicts the relationship between Pa_{O_2} and either the oxygen content or hemoglobin saturation. The clinical significance of the curve is that large changes in Pa_{O_2} may have little effect on the oxygen content or hemoglobin saturation of arterial blood on the upper, flat portion of the curve (Pa_{O_2} greater than 70 mmHg), but dramatic changes occur in oxygen content or hemoglobin saturation at the steep portion of the curve (Pa_{O_2} = 40–70 mmHg). At this part of the curve large volumes of oxygen can be unloaded at the cellular level with small changes in Pa_{O_2}. Shifting the curve to the right or left may profoundly affect oxygen availability to the tissues.[71,73–81]

Clinically the position of the curve is measured by tonometry or calculated[79,80] at a point where the oxygen's partial pressure has saturated 50% of the hemoglobin (P-50). The normal P-50 value is approximately a P_{O_2} of 27 mmHg. Many factors can affect the position of the curve. A shift to the left will decrease the P-50. This indicates an increase in oxygen affinity or a tendency for the hemoglobin not to release oxygen to the tissues. A shift to the right (increased P-50) indicates a reduction in oxygen-hemoglobin affinity, resulting in oxygen being released more readily to the tissues.

A left-shifted ODC can be caused by massive transfusion of acid citrate dextrose (ACD)–stored blood, rapid correction of acidosis that has been present for hours or days, or severe hyperventilation resulting in respiratory alkalosis. Other less commonly seen causes of a left-shifted ODC are hypothermia and hypophosphatemia.

The normal compensatory mechanism for a left-shifted curve is an increase in the cardiac output. Patients with compromised reserve systems who are not capable of increasing cardiac output or who cannot tolerate a further reduction in tissue oxygenation are at great risk for hypoxia if they have a significantly left-shifted ODC.

To show how efficient the position of the ODC is in improving oxygen delivery, consider the following theoretical clinical situation. A patient with a normal fixed oxygen consumption of 250 mL/min, a cardiac output of 5.4 L/min, a mixed venous oxygen tension ($P\bar{v}O_2$) of 36 mmHg, and a P-50 of 27 mmHg develops a clinical condition in which the ODC shifts to the left and reduces P-50 so severely that P-50 falls to 20 mm Hg. This patient would need to increase cardiac output by 50% to deliver the equivalent volume of oxygen to the tissues. However, if P-50 were increased from 27 mmHg to 30 mmHg, the patient would require 20% less cardiac output.[24] If this theoretical patient had a damaged heart and was unable to increase cardiac output, the significant shift to the left of ODC could be very serious.

In most patients, a rightward shift of the ODC is advantageous for oxygen transport except under the most extreme hypoxemic conditions (PaO_2 = 30–35 mmHg).

Evaluation of Oxygen Transport

Traditional respiratory care has focused on the physiologic mechanisms that result in inadequate oxygenation of the pulmonary capillary blood. These mechanisms are the following:

1. $\dot{V}/\dot{Q}$ mismatch (most common cause)
2. Diffusion block (rare cause)
3. Hypoventilation
4. Shunt (an extreme case of $\dot{V}/\dot{Q}$ mismatch)

Not all tissue oxygenation problems are the result of lung problems. Changes in tissue oxygenation may also occur because of variations in oxygen consumption or cardiac output. It is critical to determine the reasons for oxygenation changes. The accompanying box lists the clinical conditions that frequently cause a worsening of oxygenation in both the pulmonary capillary blood and the tissues in critically ill patients.[82]

PARTIAL PRESSURE OF ARTERIAL OXYGEN (PaO_2).

PaO_2 is universally used in the ICU as a measure of pulmonary gas exchange, but it is not specific or sensitive enough to be used exclusively in the estimation of oxygen transport. This must be kept in mind when managing the critically ill patient who is hemodynamically unstable. When managing a pulmonary gas exchange problem, such as asthma, that is not associated with other complications, PaO_2 is an excellent value to follow to identify which therapies are effective. It should not be relied on when attempting to assess systemic oxygen transport for the following reasons. First, it is a gas tension and does not directly reflect delivered oxygen. Second, PaO_2 reflects partial pressure available at the systemic bed, not what is used. Third, factors that may actually improve oxygen transport by improving cardiac output may cause PaO_2 to fall because of an increase in intrapulmonary shunt.[83,84] It is not uncommon for multiple deficiencies to exist that adversely affect the oxygen transport system but that are not directly related to pulmonary gas exchange.

Under most clinical conditions, PaO_2 should be kept within a range of 60 to 80 mmHg. This usually ensures an arterial saturation of at least 90%. PaO_2 values greater than 80 mmHg are usually unnecessary except in situations such as carbon monoxide poisoning and during periods of severe anemia or cardiogenic shock. Hyperoxic PaO_2 does not necessarily improve oxygen transport. A PaO_2 in excess of 125 mmHg has been shown to cause a reduction of blood flow to both the kidneys and the brain, probably as a result of vasoconstriction.[81]

ALVEOLAR-ARTERIAL OXYGEN TENSION DIFFERENCE [$P(A-a)O_2$]. $P(A-a)O_2$ has commonly been used as an indication of gas exchange efficiency. Its major limitation is that it changes with adjustments in FIO_2.[85] See Chapter 6 for a description of how $P(A-a)O_2$ is calculated.

ARTERIAL-ALVEOLAR TENSION RATIO (PaO_2/PAO_2 or a/A). The PaO_2/PAO_2 ratio is a more useful index of pulmonary gas exchange than the $P(A-a)O_2$ because it remains more stable with changes in FIO_2. It is most stable when FIO_2 is greater than 0.30 and PaO_2 is less than 100 mmHg. It can also be used to predict the FIO_2 required for a desired PaO_2.[86]

PaO_2/FIO_2 RATIO. The PaO_2/FIO_2 ratio is similar to the PaO_2/PAO_2 ratio but easier to use since it does not require calculation of PAO_2. This may lead to an increase in error since it does not compensate for changes in $PaCO_2$. A PaO_2/FIO_2 ratio of 200 or greater has been identified as an indication that the patient may be ready for a reduction in the PEEP level.[87]

OXYGENATION INDEX (OI). The OI was initially developed as an index of ventilatory-oxygenation support for a human surfactant trial[88] and was more recently adapted as a prognostic index for morbidity and mortality for infants requiring extracorporeal membrane oxygenation (ECMO).[89] The OI is calculated by the following formula:

$$\frac{MAP \times FIO_2 \times 100}{PaO_2}$$

where

MAP = mean airway pressure
FIO_2 = fraction of inspired oxygen
PaO_2 = postductal PaO_2

The advantage of the OI over other indices is that it incorporates MAP, a ventilation value that is strongly related to the degree of ventilatory support (and lung injury) and oxygenation. Infant ECMO candidates with severe respiratory failure often have OI values greater than 40, indicative of a high predicted mortality (greater than 80%). OI values greater than 20 to 25 indicate a predicted mortality greater than 50%.[89]

INTRAPULMONARY SHUNT. *Intrapulmonary shunt* ($\dot{Q}S/\dot{Q}T$) is a major contributor to hypoxemia in most ICU patients. It is defined as perfusion without ventilation and theoretically should be differentiated from another cause of hypoxemia: low $\dot{V}/\dot{Q}$ ratios, or perfusion in excess of ventilation. Clinical states that frequently produce an increase in $\dot{Q}S/\dot{Q}T$ are atelectasis, pneumonia, ARDS, pulmonary edema, and, rarely, congenital heart anomalies or arteriovenous anastomosis. The $\dot{Q}S/\dot{Q}T$ and $\dot{V}/\dot{Q}$ relation may be measured by tracer gas techniques[29] or radioactive gas and microsphere techniques,[23] but the calculation most often used in the ICU is the following classic shunt equation:

$$\dot{Q}S/\dot{Q}T = \frac{C\dot{c}o_2 - Cao_2}{C\dot{c}o_2 - C\bar{v}o_2}$$

where

$C\dot{c}o_2$ = end-capillary oxygen content
Cao_2 = arterial oxygen content
$C\bar{v}o_2$ = mixed venous oxygen content

The shunt formula is a mathematical method that separates blood into two components: the component that carries oxygen and the component that does not. If no shunt existed, $C\dot{c}o_2$ would equal Cao_2. The normal anatomic shunt is 3% to 5% and is the result of bronchial and thebesian vein drainage from the pulmonary artery to the left atrium.

The value of $C\dot{c}o_2$ is derived from the assumption that somewhere in the lung end-capillary blood leaving an alveolus has a Po_2 equal to Pao_2. The theoretic end-capillary blood value is calculated from the alveolar air equation:

$$C\dot{c}o_2 = [(Hb \times 1.34)(100\% \text{ saturated} - COHb\% - MetHb\%)] + (Pao_2 \times 0.003)$$

The percentage of "total" saturation of end-capillary blood is amended to include the effects of carboxyhemoglobin (COHb) and methemoglobin (MetHb). These hemoglobins are incapable of carrying oxygen, and therefore modifications to the calculations must be made.[90] Cao_2 is calculated from the following standard formula:

$$Cao_2 = (Hb \times 1.34)(\%Sao_2) + (Pao_2 \times 0.003)$$

where

Sao_2 = arterial oxygen saturation

Cvo_2 is calculated by the following formula:

$$C\bar{v}o_2 = (Hb \times 1.34)(\%S\bar{v}o_2) + (P\bar{v}o_2 \times 0.003)$$

where

$S\bar{v}o_2$ = mixed venous oxygen saturation

Both the arterial and mixed venous samples should be directly measured with a co-oximeter and not calculated. This reduces errors in estimations resulting from calculations.

Shunt Fraction Determination With 100% Oxygen. $\dot{Q}S/\dot{Q}T$ is frequently measured while the patient is breathing 100% oxygen. However, breathing 100% oxygen for 30 minutes can lead to nitrogen washout and collapse of low $\dot{V}/\dot{Q}$ units.[91-95] This phenomenon of alveolar collapse appears to be caused by poor ventilation of low $\dot{V}/\dot{Q}$ units so that oxygen uptake by the blood exceeds oxygen delivery to the alveoli via ventilation. The resulting microatelectasis increases shunt. Regional blood flow is usually reduced to areas of the lung with low $\dot{V}/\dot{Q}$ as a protective mechanism.[94] Breathing 100% oxygen alters this natural autoregulation,[95,96] causing increased shunt.

Pulmonary vasodilation[96] and inotropic agents such as dopamine increase cardiac output but can also increase intrapulmonary shunt.[83,84,97] If oxygen transport is improved with this pharmacologic support, its use may be indicated regardless of the increased shunt.

Estimated Shunt. In patients without pulmonary artery catheters, an estimation of intrapulmonary shunt can be made by substituting the measured arteriovenous difference in the denominator with the value 3.5 vol%. This is a "typical" value in a critically ill patient with acceptable cardiac reserves.

The estimated shunt has been compared to the other oxygen tension indices described and to the gold standard, the measured shunt. The estimated shunt fraction has a stronger correlation to measured shunt than the other indices.[98]

Clinical Evaluation of Tissue Oxygen Delivery and Utilization

Oxygen Delivery/Availability

Oxygen delivery is calculated by the following equation:

$$\text{Cardiac output} \times Cao_2 \times 10^* = O_2 \text{ delivery}$$

The delivered oxygen value reflects the total amount of oxygen carried in the blood per unit of time. Normal values range from 550 to 650 mL/min/m². The delivered oxygen is frequently elevated with hyperdynamic states such as septic shock and ARDS.[99,100] Reduced values indicate low cardiac output, decreased Cao_2, or both. Increases in mean airway pressure may increase oxygen content but decrease cardiac output. Measuring oxygen delivery is one way to see if the overall effect of a specific therapy is positive or negative. It could be argued that oxygen delivery as defined above does not accurately reflect the oxygen made available to the tissues. For example, oxygen bound to hemoglobin at a partial pressure of less than 20 mmHg is typically considered to be unavailable to support aerobic metabolism.[77] This occurs because, at a Pao_2

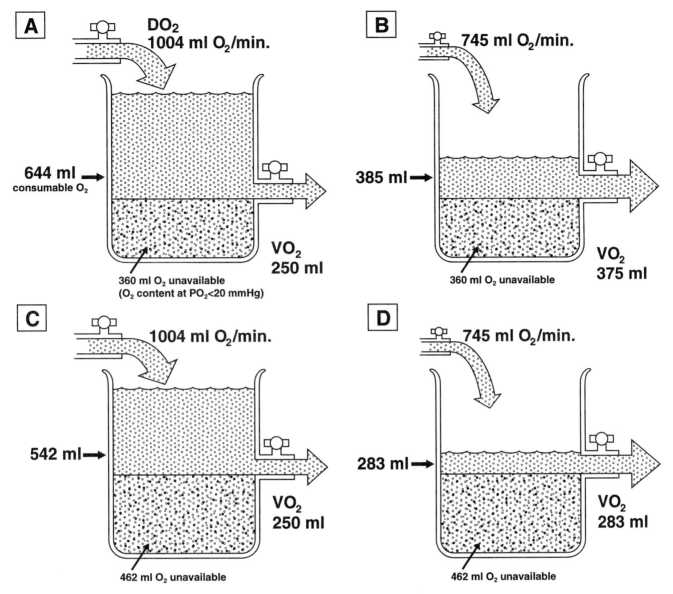

Fig. 12–7 *Interactions of oxygen delivery, oxygen consumption, and consumable oxygen. DO_2 = delivered oxygen; VO_2 = oxygen consumption; Cons O_2 = oxygen available at a PO_2 > 20 mmHg (see text). In figure A, DO_2(cardiac output × CaO_2) and VO_2 (metabolic rate) are normal. The amount of O_2 carried in blood but not available to tissues for aerobic metabolism (O_2 carried at a PO_2 <20 mmHg) is represented by the hatched area below the spigot. Consumable oxygen (DO_2- unavailable O_2) exceeds VO_2. Figure B illustrates a typical occurrence in trauma. There is a reduction in DO_2 (fall in Hb, PaO_2/SaO_2, cardiac output) and an increase in VO_2 (tissue injury, sepsis, etc.). Despite the fall in DO_2, Cons O_2 exceeds VO_2, ensuring adequate oxygen availability. Figure C illustrates an increase in oxygen unavailable for consumption (i.e., left-shift in ODC). Consequently, there is a reduction in Cons O_2, but sufficient O_2 remains available to exceed VO_2. Figure D illustrates the collapse of oxygen reserves (reduced DO_2, low Cons O_2). VO_2 is limited by Cons O_2. VO_2 may rise if Cons O_2 is increased, either by increasing DO_2 or by "right shifting" the ODC. If metabolic demands continue to exceed O_2 availability, lactic acidosis results.*

less than 20 mmHg, there is an insufficient partial pressure gradient for oxygen to diffuse to the tissues. Hence, the total amount of oxygen carried in the blood at a Po_2 of 20 mmHg is *unavailable* for tissue consumption. The amount of oxygen *available* would be the oxygen that could be extracted by the tissues. Therefore:

$$O_2 \text{ available} = CO \times (Cao_2 - C_{20}o_2)$$

where

CO = cardiac output
Cao_2 = arterial oxygen content
$C_{20}o_2$ = oxygen content at a Po_2 of 20 mmHg

The amount of $C_{20}o_2$ is significantly influenced by the position of the ODC as measured by the P-50. Left shifts in the ODC (low P-50) will result in higher levels of $C_{20}o_2$, and less oxygen available to the tissues (Fig. 12–7).

OXYGEN CONSUMPTION. *Oxygen consumption* ($\dot{V}o_2$) is defined as the oxygen consumed by the

*Change vol % to mL = L.

entire body in milliliters per minute. The normal range is 2.86 to 4.29 mL/min/Kg at STPD or 100 to 140 mL/min/m^2 of body surface area. If one thinks of oxygen delivery as *supply,* then $\dot{V}_{O_2}$ is *utilization.* Adequate supply does not always ensure proper utilization.

Many factors determine tissue $\dot{V}_{O_2}$. $\dot{V}_{O_2}$ can be limited by decreased oxygen availability[97,100–102] because of a decrease in regional perfusion or a decrease in oxygen content. Demand may exceed supply, as in a hypermetabolic state, or cellular metabolism may be impaired as in cyanide poisoning.

$\dot{V}_{O_2}$ can be measured directly, through the analysis of inspired and exhaled gas volumes and concentrations, or indirectly, by multiplying the cardiac output by the arteriovenous oxygen content difference (Fick calculation).

The formula for the calculation of $\dot{V}_{O_2}$ using the direct method is as follows:

$$\dot{V}_{O_2} = \left(\left[\left(\frac{1 - FE_{O_2} - FE_{CO_2}}{1 - F_{I_{O_2}}} \right) \times F_{I_{O_2}} \right] - FE_{O_2} \right) \times \dot{V}_E$$

All volumes are converted to STPD conditions. FE_{O_2} is measured directly. The formula assumes that nitrogen is an inert (nonreactive) gas and that no other gases are present. The presence of nitrous oxide (a gas used in surgery by anesthesiologists) may introduce a considerable error if the patient's $\dot{V}_{O_2}$ is measured immediately after anesthesia.

Another direct technique requires that the patient breathe a specific concentration of gas through a closed circuit system that incorporates a carbon dioxide absorber. $\dot{V}_{O_2}$ can be measured by the following formula:

$$\dot{V}_{O_2} = \text{change in volume at STPD} \times F_{I_{O_2}}$$

Direct $\dot{V}_{O_2}$ measurement techniques are extremely demanding. The circuit must be completely free of leaks, gas volumes, and concentrations accurately collected and measured, and $F_{I_{O_2}}$ stable with minimal fluctuation. Recent technologic advances allow $\dot{V}_{O_2}$ to be monitored continuously in critically ill patients during continuous mechanical ventilation.[103]

The indirect calculation of $\dot{V}_{O_2}$ is based on the Fick principle:

$$\dot{V}_{O_2} = \text{cardiac output} \times C(a - \bar{v})_{O_2}$$

The Fick principle is used frequently in the ICU more because of its convenience than its accuracy. Variations between Fick calculations and direct measurement of $\dot{V}_{O_2}$ may be as high as 20%, primarily because of errors in venous gas sampling and cardiac output analysis.[104] This error is greatest in patients with high cardiac output.

Interpretation of $\dot{V}_{O_2}$. When oxygen delivery is adequate, $\dot{V}_{O_2}$ is determined by the metabolic demands

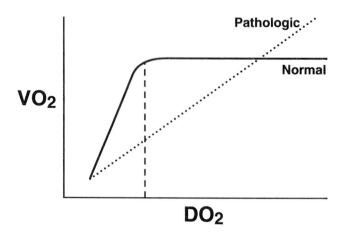

Fig. 12–8 *Supply dependence of oxygen consumption. Under normal conditions (solid line), VO$_2$ will increase until a critical threshold (dashed line) of DO$_2$ is reached. Beyond this critical threshold. VO$_2$ will remain stable, despite the increase in DO$_2$. In pathologic conditions (dotted line) such as ARDS, VO$_2$ may not plateau, but will continue to rise as DO$_2$ increases, until well past the normal critical threshold.*

of the patient. $\dot{V}_{O_2}$ will stay constant as long as the delivered oxygen is greater than a *critical threshold* of approximately 8 to 10 mL/min/Kg in anesthetized humans.[105] This critical threshold is significantly elevated in ARDS and in sepsis[106] (Fig. 12–8). In patients with ARDS, $\dot{V}_{O_2}$ is linearly related to oxygen delivery up to 21 mL/min/Kg.[107]

ICU patients frequently exhibit alterations in $\dot{V}_{O_2}$ due to trauma, sepsis, shock, changes in body temperature, anesthesia, therapeutic modalities such as chest physiotherapy, and ventilator settings. $\dot{V}_{O_2}$ has been shown to be an excellent predictor of survival in patients with trauma and shock and is helpful in determining the adequacy of resuscitation.[99,102,106] It has also been advocated as an index of the cost of breathing in terms of oxygen use and is therefore useful in predicting the patient's ability to be weaned from mechanical ventilation.[108]

$\dot{V}_{O_2}$ values of 100% to 150% of normal following trauma or shock are associated with a better prognosis and have been identified as appropriate therapeutic goals for the high-risk surgical patient.[109] Values less than 100% may be the result of decreased oxygen availability, as with low cardiac output or oxygen content, or with decreased use, as in hypothermia. In patients with severe injury, values greater than 150% may indicate a poor prognosis. If oxygen delivery is increased for any reason, increased availability may lead to increased consumption. This phenomenon has been observed in patients with ARDS, cardiogenic pulmonary edema, COPD, and pneumonia.[100,101,110]

MIXED VENOUS OXYGEN TENSION ($P\bar{v}_{O_2}$). $P\bar{v}_{O_2}$ is a measure of the partial pressure of oxygen in mixed venous blood and is an indication of oxygen usage by the entire body. Factors that influence oxygen

Table 12-3	Basal Tissue Oxygen Exchange*	
	P$\bar{\text{v}}$o$_2$ (mmHg)	Arteriovenous Oxygen Difference (vol%)‡
Heart	23	11.4 (11)
Muscle	34	8.4 (30)
Brain	33	6.3 (20)
Viscera	43	4.1 (25)
Kidney	56	1.3 (7)
Skin	60	1.0 (2)

*Modified with permission from Finch CA and Lenfant C: *N Engl J Med* 286:407, 1972.
‡The number in (parentheses) represents the percentage of total oxygen delivery.

Table 12-4	Interpretation of Venous Saturation (S$\bar{\text{v}}$o$_2$)
S$\bar{\text{v}}$o$_2$	Interpretation
68%–77%	Normal
>77%	Sepsis, left-to-right shunt, excessive cardiac output, hypothermia, cell poisoning, wedged catheter
<60%	Cardiac decompensation
<50%	Lactic acidosis
<30%	Unconsciousness
<20%	Permanent damage

transport and consumption invariably affect P$\bar{\text{v}}$o$_2$. The normal range is 38 to 42 mmHg.

Low P$\bar{\text{v}}$o$_2$ may result from the following:

1. Inadequate cardiac output
2. Anemia
3. Significant hypoxia
4. "Affinity" hypoxia (low P$\bar{\text{v}}$o$_2$ with increased S$\bar{\text{v}}$o$_2$)

A P$\bar{\text{v}}$o$_2$ of less than 27 mmHg is usually associated with lactic acidosis.

Increased P$\bar{\text{v}}$o$_2$ (greater than 45 mmHg) may result from the following:

1. Poor sampling technique
2. Left-to-right shunt
3. Septic shock
4. Increased cardiac output
5. Cyanide poisoning

Because P$\bar{\text{v}}$o$_2$ reflects the components of the supply-demand balance in perfused tissues, it is possible to have normal values of P$\bar{\text{v}}$o$_2$ and still have inadequate oxygen delivery to certain organs (e.g., kidneys). Organs with poor perfusion make a minimal contribution to venous return; therefore, P$\bar{\text{v}}$o$_2$ may remain in the normal range even though an oxygen deficit exists, as in the vasodilated, septic patient with normal cardiac output.

P$\bar{\text{v}}$o$_2$ may not reflect changes in oxygen delivery and cardiac output. Since variations in $\dot{\text{V}}$o$_2$ also affect the balance between supply and demand, elevated P$\bar{\text{v}}$o$_2$ may indicate inadequate tissue oxygen utilization and marked maldistribution in systemic blood flow. This is common in septic shock. Low P$\bar{\text{v}}$o$_2$ may be expected when the tissues are using the available oxygen effectively but the supply is inadequate.[111]

Table 12-3 shows that $\dot{\text{V}}$o$_2$ is high for the heart and the brain, and therefore the P$\bar{\text{v}}$o$_2$ of these organs is extremely critical. A fall in perfusion would require a compensatory mechanism to maintain blood flow and oxygen to these organs.

The mixed venous sample is obtained by slowly aspirating, over approximately 1 minute, 3 to 5 mL of blood from the distal port of a pulmonary artery catheter. Central venous blood samples may trend well if the catheter is properly positioned, but generally there is a difference of from 2 to 3 mmHg between the Po$_2$ of central venous and pulmonary artery samples.[112] The technique used for mixed venous gas analysis is important, since errors in sampling may result in erroneous readings. The pressure waveform should be inspected before aspirating the sample to ensure that the catheter is not wedged. Wedging may result in aspirating post-capillary blood and so produce an erroneously high measurement of P$\bar{\text{v}}$o$_2$. Air bubbles in the sample are also a possible cause of falsely elevated values.

MIXED VENOUS OXYGEN SATURATION

(S$\bar{\text{v}}$o$_2$). S$\bar{\text{v}}$o$_2$ is measured from a mixed venous blood sample. Small changes in P$\bar{\text{v}}$o$_2$ lead to large changes in S$\bar{\text{v}}$o$_2$ and therefore large changes in C$\bar{\text{v}}$o$_2$. As a result, the S$\bar{\text{v}}$o$_2$ measurement is a sensitive index of cardiac output and tissue perfusion if $\dot{\text{V}}$o$_2$ is stable[113] (Table 12-4). Like P$\bar{\text{v}}$o$_2$, S$\bar{\text{v}}$o$_2$ is a means of monitoring the general supply and demand differences in oxygen delivery, not the use of oxygen at a specific site.

S$\bar{\text{v}}$o$_2$ may be continuously monitored through a fiberoptic reflectance oximetry system incorporated in a five-lumen pulmonary artery catheter. The system incorporates the principle of reflection spectrophotometry. Traditional oximetry uses transmission spectrophotometry. An optical module transmits light through the blood via a fiberoptic monofilament. Reflected light is transmitted by a separate monofilament to a photodetector in the module. Because reduced hemoglobin and oxygenated hemoglobin absorb different wavelengths of light, a microprocessor can quantify the reflected wavelengths and calculate S$\bar{\text{v}}$o$_2$[114] (Fig. 12-9). When the catheter is properly positioned and calibrated, values correlate well with benchmark saturation measurements.[115-117] Continuous monitoring has the advantage of providing immediate feedback for purposes of evaluating therapy.

Various factors such as suctioning, shivering, pharmacologic intervention, extubation, weaning, and positive pressure therapy[114-118] can decrease the S$\bar{\text{v}}$o$_2$ measurement, signifying a deterioration in pulmonary

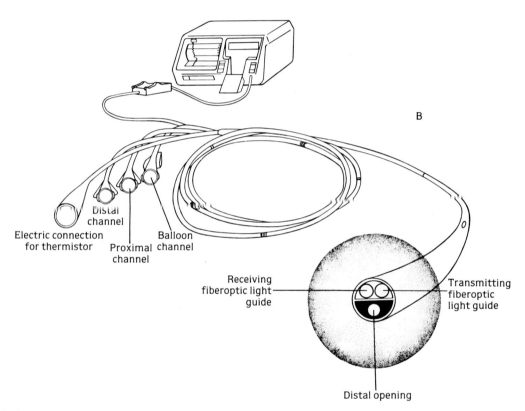

Fig. 12-9 A, *Principles of reflection spectrophotometry.* **B,** *Fiberoptic catheter system used for continuous monitoring of venous oxygen saturation. (Courtesy of Oximetric, Inc., Mountain View, Calif.)*

gas exchange, an increase in $\dot{V}O_2$, or a reduction in cardiac output.

ARTERIAL–MIXED VENOUS OXYGEN CONTENT DIFFERENCE. The arterial–mixed venous oxygen content difference, $C(a-\bar{v})O_2$, reflects the difference in oxygen content between arterial and venous blood. It is derived after simultaneous arterial and mixed venous blood gases are drawn. Normal range is 4 to 6 vol%.

Values greater than 6 vol% may be the result of the following:

1. Low cardiac output
2. Increasing $\dot{V}O_2$

Values less than 4 vol% may be the result of the following:

1. Septic shock
2. Increased cardiac output
3. Anemia
4. Increased oxygen affinity due to a left-shifted ODC

The $C(a-\bar{v})O_2$ is useful in determining the effects of mechanical ventilation and PEEP on cardiac output[119] and in evaluating the need for additional circulatory support. It has a slight advantage over the $P\bar{v}O_2$ measurement in that it reflects content differences instead of partial pressure.

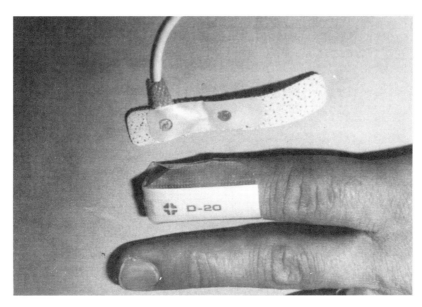

Fig. 12-10 *Pulse oximetry finger probe.*

OXYGEN-EXTRACTION RATIO. The oxygen-extraction ratio $C(a–v)_{O_2}/Ca_{O_2}$ expresses the relation between available oxygen (oxygen content of arterial blood) and oxygen extracted $[C(a–v)_{O_2}]$. The normal value is 25% to 30%. Values greater than 30% indicate one of the following:

1. Increased extraction caused by low cardiac output
2. Increased $\dot{V}_{O_2}$
3. Decreased oxygen availability caused by decreased Ca_{O_2}

Values less than 25% indicate that supply is out of proportion to demand, which may be a result of the following:

1. High cardiac output
2. Sepsis with systemic shunts

The oxygen-extraction ratio identifies the portion of the delivered oxygen actually consumed and is therefore an index of the efficiency of circulation.

BLOOD LACTATE. If oxygen transport or its use by the tissues is insufficient for metabolic demands, anaerobic metabolism occurs and lactic acid is produced. Clinically this is seen as a metabolic acidosis with an elevation in blood lactate concentrations. The degree of lactic acidosis corresponds to the severity of oxygen deficit and is therefore a good indicator of prognostic outcome in patients with shock.[120,121] Normal values for blood lactate are less than 1.7 to 2.0 mM/L. In patients with shock, lactate levels greater than 3.83 mM/L are associated with 67% mortality, and values greater than 8 mM/L are associated with greater than 90% mortality.[121,122] β-adrenergic stimulator drugs increase lactate levels because of glycolysis, and β blockers decrease blood lactate levels.[123] Patients with lactic acidosis are frequently treated with alkaline solutions such as sodium bicarbonate. This alkalinization

may increase blood lactate levels because of a redistribution of extracellular and intracellular lactate levels but does not indicate a worsening metabolic acidosis.[124]

Patients with cirrhosis have a reduced ability to clear peak lactate concentrations after periods of increased production. As a result, lactate is useful in confirming the presence of tissue hypoxia in these patients, but it is not a useful prognostic index.[125]

Noninvasive Monitoring of Oxygenation and Oxygen Delivery

PULSE OXIMETRY. Oximetry is a noninvasive technique for measuring oxygen saturation of hemoglobin in the blood. The oximeter uses the spectrophotometric principle of light absorption. Oximeters transmit two wavelengths of light—red and infrared—through arterialized capillary beds, such as the ear lobe[126] or digit[127] (Fig. 12–10). Some of the light is absorbed by skin, fat, muscle, and venous blood, which are constant sources of absorption. Some of the light is absorbed by the blood that flows through the arterioles in a pulsatile manner typical of arterial blood flow. As a result, there is a variable source of absorption. The pulse oximeter ignores the constant sources and focuses on the pulsatile absorption. The light absorption of oxygenated hemoglobin is different from that of reduced hemoglobin, and the pulse oximeter reads the differences to determine the degree of oxygen saturation. This process is very rapid and provides measurement of heart rate as well as oxygen saturation.

The co-oximeters that are commonly used in blood gas laboratories transmit four wavelengths of light and can detect the amount of methemoglobin, carboxyhemoglobin, deoxyhemoglobin, and oxyhemoglobin. Pulse oximeters and co-oximeters therefore measure saturation differently. The pulse oximeter value is called *functional saturation* because it only looks at hemoglobins capable of binding with oxygen. It compares the amount of hemoglobin that is saturated with the amount of hemoglobin that is capable of being saturated:

$$\text{Pulse oximeter saturation} = \frac{\text{Hb saturated}}{\text{Hb saturated} + \text{Hb unsaturated}}$$

The co-oximeter value is called *fractional saturation*. It compares the amount of hemoglobin that is saturated with the total amount of hemoglobin present, including those forms of hemoglobin that do not bind with oxygen, the dyshemoglobins (e.g., COHb, MetHb):

$$\frac{\text{Cooximeter}}{\text{saturation}} = \frac{\text{Hb saturated}}{\text{Hb saturated} + \text{Hb unsaturated} + \text{dyshemoglobins}}$$

As a result, in clinical conditions where dysfunctional hemoglobin levels are elevated (carbon monoxide poisoning, increased MetHb), the pulse oximeter will overestimate the true saturation.

Because pulse oximetry is quick, noninvasive, and can be used for continuous monitoring, it has become extremely popular in recent years. As many as 28 companies manufacture pulse oximeters. Many studies have been performed to compare the accuracy and responsiveness of these different oximeters to directly measure saturation.[128,129] Studies of healthy and critically ill patients with adequate cardiac outputs generally show a high degree of accuracy and correlation when compared to direct arterial saturation, as long as saturation is greater than 65%. The ability of oximeters to accurately measure severe desaturation (less than 65%) varies widely between instruments. Conditions that can cause erroneous values include abnormal perfusion levels from low cardiac output or peripheral shunting, hypothermia, elevated bilirubin concentrations (greater than 10 mg/dL), elevated COHb or MetHb levels, and indocyanine green (Cardio-Green) or methylene blue dye.

Oximetry has been shown to be helpful in multiple settings, including the operating room, emergency room, during transport, and during special procedures such as bronchoscopy, computed tomography (CT) scanning, sleep studies, exercise testing, weaning from supplemental oxygen and mechanical ventilation, and in pulmonary rehabilitation.[130,131] Oximetry can also be helpful in prescribing home oxygen therapy.

Pulse oximetry can be a useful tool in the ICU, but it is also prone to overuse and misinterpretation. Normal pulse oximetry values do not guarantee adequate oxygen delivery to the tissues. The anemic patient may be adequately saturated, but hypoxia may be present because of the low CaO_2.

TRANSCUTANEOUS MONITORING IN ADULTS. Use of a miniaturized heated Clark electrode to measure skin surface oxygen tension and transcutaneous oxygen tension ($tcPo_2$) was a major breakthrough in noninvasive respiratory monitoring techniques. The development of a pH electrode has enabled investigators to monitor transcutaneous carbon dioxide tension ($tcPco_2$) as well.

Initially, clinicians using cutaneous monitors were concerned with the correlation between arterial and cutaneous values. Investigators anticipated that $tcPo_2$ should closely follow Pao_2. This assumption is essentially true in the newborn with adequate circulatory status, but evidence shows that a variety of factors may be involved.[132] One of the more important factors is cardiac output or perfusion. Studies using a $tcPo_2$ index ($tcPo_2/Pao_2$) showed that when the cardiac index was relatively normal (greater than 2.2 L/min/m^2), the ratio was approximately 70% ± 12%, and the $tcPo_2$ values were reliable as noninvasive monitors of Pao_2.[133] In moderate and severe shock, the $tcPo_2$ index dropped to less than 50% and the correlation between Pao_2 and $tcPo_2$ was poor.

Current data indicate that $tcPo_2$ reflects oxygen availability at the sample site.[132-135] In patients with adequate cardiovascular reserves, $tcPo_2$ correlates well with Pao_2 in both hypoxic and normoxic conditions. It is not necessarily the same as Pao_2, but the ratio is consistent, and therefore Pao_2 can be adequately predicted based on the cutaneous value.[133] Transcutaneous values vary from arterial values because of rightward shifts in the ODC, resistance to oxygen permeability by the skin, increases in regional $\dot{V}o_2$ at the sensor site, and changes in blood flow at the sample site.[136]

Transcutaneous measurements are adversely affected by cutaneous vasoconstriction due to low cardiac output, vasoconstricting agents, hypothermia, and elevated cutaneous vascular resistance due to hypovolemic or cardiogenic hypotension.[136,137]

Studies seem to indicate that the general causes of hypoxia (pulmonary or cardiac) can be differentiated by the amount of power required to maintain the electrode at temperature.[132,137] Unfortunately, about 60% of the energy required to heat the electrode is lost to the environment and only about 20% is lost to blood flow, thereby limiting the sensitivity of the sensor to changes in blood flow.[137]

$tcPco_2$ measurements were first reported by Severinghaus in 1960.[138] Present techniques and equipment have updated the reliability and accuracy of some transcutaneous sensors, including both $tcPco_2$ and $tcPo_2$ capability. The $tcPco_2$ values are consistently higher than $Paco_2$ values because of a decrease in the solubility of carbon dioxide and an increase in metabolic rate. Both factors are caused by heating of the sample site. Hypoxia and acidosis may decrease the gradient between $tcPco_2$ and $Paco_2$. There is a strong correlation between $tcPco_2$ and $Paco_2$ in infants and adults, but the $tcPco_2$ response time is greatly affected by sensor temperature. $tcPco_2$ is not as sensitive to changes in hemodynamic status as $tcPo_2$ but does vary depending on sensor temperature and car-

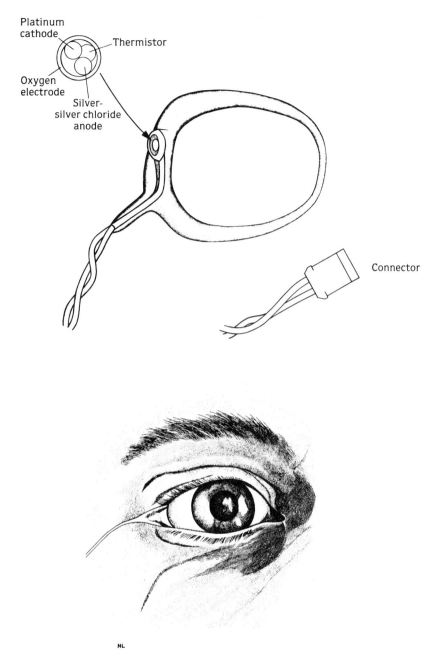

Fig. 12-11 **Top,** *Diagram of conjunctival Po_2 sensor with Clark-type electrode.* **Bottom,** *Conjunctival electrode in place. Eye is normally taped closed during surgery to maintain lubrication and prevent irritation of palpebral conjunctiva. (Courtesy of Orange Medical Instruments, Costa Mesa, Calif.)*

diac output. Higher sensor temperatures shorten the response times.[137]

Another potential application of transcutaneous monitoring is in the analysis of Pao_2 and $Paco_2$ in emergency situations. Blood samples can be directly placed on the electrodes and stabilized values obtained within 50 to 90 seconds. These values have shown excellent correlation with those obtained by blood gas analysis techniques.[139,140]

CONJUNCTIVAL MONITORING. This system uses a Clark-type electrode mounted in an ophthalmic conformer eyepiece that measures oxygen tension in the capillary bed of the palpebral conjunctiva. A thermistor in the electrode measures conjunctival temperature (Tcj). With normal perfusion, conjunctival Po_2 monitoring (cjPo_2) tracks Pao_2 during hypoxia, normoxia, and hyperoxia.[141-143] The thermistor is affected by environmental temperature, but because the electrode is not heated it may be better than the heated sensor in transcutaneous oxygen monitors for the differentiation of low cjPo_2 values associated with hypoxemia or low perfusion. The device can be left in place for as long as 3 or 4 days if the eye is properly lubricated and taped shut. The potential advantage of this device over a transcutaneous monitor is that it has no heater and therefore does not have to be moved from site to site (Fig. 12-11).

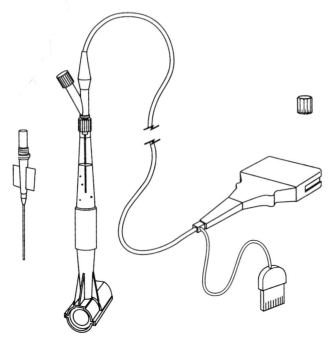

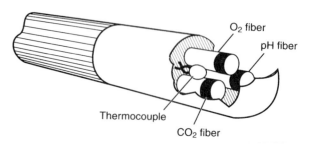

Fig. 12-13 *Fluorescent optode. An example of a fluorescence-based intra-arterial blood gas sensor. The three optical fibers, one each for pH, Pco₂, and Po₂, contain a specific fluorescent dye at the sensor tip. These dyes are activated when exposed to the appropriate analyte, and return a light signal to the monitor. (Courtesy of Puritan-Bennett Corp, Carlsbad, Calif.)*

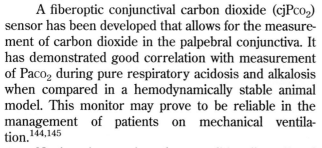

Fig. 12-12 *Continuous intraarterial blood gas sensor. A four-parameter (pH, Pco₂, Po₂, and temperature) intra-arterial blood gas catheter/sensor residing within a buffer solution cuvette. The sensor is calibrated and protected within the sterile buffer solution and then placed into an artery for continuous blood gas monitoring. (Courtesy of Puritan-Bennett Corp, Carlsbad, Calif.)*

A new technology incorporating fluorescent optodes may significantly enhance our continuous in vivo monitoring capabilities (Figs. 12–12 and 12–13). Fluorescent optodes are optical fibers with a fluorescent dye at the sensor tip. These dyes are activated when exposed to an appropriate light. The dye modifies the colors of the light and returns the light signal to the monitor. The dyes are specifically modified by oxygen, carbon dioxide, and hydrogen ions.[148]

A fiberoptic conjunctival carbon dioxide (cjPco₂) sensor has been developed that allows for the measurement of carbon dioxide in the palpebral conjunctiva. It has demonstrated good correlation with measurement of Paco₂ during pure respiratory acidosis and alkalosis when compared in a hemodynamically stable animal model. This monitor may prove to be reliable in the management of patients on mechanical ventilation.[144,145]

Noninvasive monitors have traditionally suffered from a lack of understanding and consequent misinterpretation of delivered data. Transcutaneous and conjunctival measurements are proving to be valuable in the ICU, not because they correlate with Pao₂ or Paco₂ but because they measure something more important: overall oxygen and carbon dioxide transport. Monitoring peripheral circulation may be ideal because it is the first to be shut down in the face of inadequate oxygen delivery and gives early warning before inadequate oxygen delivery to the brain and heart can occur.

Continuous Intraarterial Blood Gas Monitors

The technology of in vivo electrodes for continuous monitoring of arterial blood gases has been around since 1958.[146] Unfortunately, clinical application of the electrode systems has been limited by problems with probe size, drift, accuracy, and thrombogenicity.[147]

REVIEW QUESTIONS

1. *Which of the following is true regarding the measurement of tidal volume as a means of ventilatory assessment in the intensive care unit?*
   a. *it is normally 3-4 mL/Kg of ideal body weight*
   b. *it should be at least 450 mL prior to weaning from mechanical ventilation*
   c. *it may decrease after abdominal or thoracic surgery*
   d. *all of the above*

2. *Which of the following would minimize the chance of "stacking" of mechanical tidal volumes (air trapping) during mechanical ventilation?*
   a. *increasing inspiratory flow*
   b. *increasing mechanical respiratory rate*
   c. *increasing the set tidal volume*
   d. *none of the above*

3. *An increased $\dot{V}_E$ with a normal PaCO₂ indicates which of the following?*
   a. *shunt*
   b. *decreased metabolic rate*
   c. *increased deadspace*
   d. *atelectasis*

4. T F An increased metabolic rate results in an increased production of carbon dioxide.

5. Which of the following is (are) true regarding the measurement of vital capacity in the intensive care unit?
    a. the value obtained is dependent on patient position and effort
    b. it reflects the ventilatory reserve of the patient
    c. a value of less than 10 mL/Kg suggests pending respiratory failure
    d. all of the above

6. Which of the following modalities increases functional residual capacity?
    a. prolonging expiratory time (expiratory retard)
    b. PEEP/CPAP
    c. pressure-controlled ventilation
    d. volume-controlled ventilation

7. T F Flow transducers are the "gold standard" for measuring lung volumes.

8. Which of the following would cause peak airway pressures to increase on a mechanical ventilator?
    a. partial obstruction of an artificial airway
    b. tension pneumothorax
    c. high inspiratory flow setting
    d. all of the above

9. T F The measurement of static pressure during mechanical ventilation is a better index of the elastic recoil of the lung than peak pressure.

10. Given a peak pressure of 50 cm H_2O, a static pressure of 35 cm H_2O, a PEEP of 5 cm H_2O, and a measured tidal volume of 850 mL, what is the effective static compliance?
    a. 12 mL/cm H_2O
    b. 18 mL/cm H_2O
    c. 24 mL/cm H_2O
    d. 28 mL/cm H_2O

11. Which of the following is (are) true regarding auto-PEEP?
    a. it is normally not detected on the ventilator manometer
    b. it can be reduced by decreasing inspiratory flow
    c. bronchodilators exacerbate the condition
    d. all of the above

12. Given a peak airway pressure of 40 cm H_2O, a static pressure of 32 cm H_2O, a PEEP of 7 cm H_2O, a tidal volume of 675 mL, and an in-spiratory flow of 60 LPM, what is the airway resistance?
    a. 2 cm H_2O/L/sec
    b. 5 cm H_2O/L/sec
    c. 8 cm H_2O/L/sec
    d. 12 cm H_2O/L/sec

13. T F Increases in mean airway pressure usually cause a reduction in Pao_2.

14. Which of the following is true regarding the measurement of V_D/V_T in the intensive care unit?
    a it is calculated using the Pao_2 and $PaCo_2$
    b. it is frequently increased during mechanical ventilation
    c. it is normally 50% to 60%
    d. none of the above

15. Which of the following would cause a decrease in oxygen transport?
    a. cardiac output of 6 LPM
    b. arterial saturation of 75%
    c. hemoglobin level of 15 g/dL
    d. all of the above

16. T F A left-shifted oxyhemoglobin dissociation curve may result in a decreased oxygen delivery to the tissues.

17. Which of the following clinical indices denotes poor oxygenation?
    a. Pao_2 of 80 mmHg
    b. Pao_2/FIO_2 ratio of 400
    c. $P(A-a)Do_2$ of 95 on 21% oxygen
    d. all of the above

18. T F Oxygen consumption is an excellent predictor of survival in patients with shock and trauma.

19. Which of the following would cause a low $P\bar{v}O_2$?
    a. left to right shunt
    b. increased cardiac output
    c. lactic acidosis
    d. hypoxia

20. T F A $C(a-v)o_2$ of 8 vol% could be caused by a reduced cardiac output.

21. Which of the following is true regarding the measurement of blood lactate?
    a. it corresponds to the level of oxygen deficit
    b. it is usually a result of anaerobic metabolism
    c. it can be increased by the administration of beta adrenergic agonist drugs
    d. all of the above

22. What does pulse oximetry measure?

a. Pa_{O_2}
b. saturation
c. oxygen content
d. blood pH

23. *What parameters can be evaluated via transcutaneous monitoring?*
    a. Pa_{O_2}
    b. Pa_{CO_2}
    c. Sa_{O_2}
    d. a and b

REFERENCES

1. Hudson LD: Monitoring of critically ill patients: conference summary, *Respir Care* 30:628, 1985.
2. Tobin MJ: Respiratory monitoring in the intensive care unit, *Am Rev Respir Dis* 138:1625, 1988.
3. Askanazi J and others: Patterns of ventilation in postoperative and acutely ill patients, *Crit Care Med* 7:41, 1979.
4. Gilbert R and others: Changes in tidal volume, frequency and ventilation induced by their measurement, *J Appl Physiol* 33:252, 1972.
5. Kacmarek RM and Venegas J: Mechanical ventilatory rates and tidal volumes, *Respir Care* 32:466, 1987.
6. Hedley-Whyte J and others: The response of patients with respiratory failure and cardiopulmonary disease to different levels of constant volume ventilation, *J Clin Invest* 45:1543, 1966.
7. Carlton DP and others: Lung overexpansion increases pulmonary microvascular protein permeability in young lambs, *J Appl Physiol* 69:577, 1990.
8. Dreyfuss D and others: High inflation pressure pulmonary edema, respective effects of high airway pressure, high tidal volume, and positive end-expiratory pressure, *Am Rev Respir Dis* 137:1159, 1988.
9. Hernandez LA and others: Chest wall restriction limits high airway pressure-induced lung injury in young rabbits, *J Appl Physiol* 66:2364, 1989.
10. Sykes MK and others: Oxygenation during anaesthesia with controlled ventilation, *Br J Anaesth* 37:314, 1965.
11. Visick WC and others: The effect of tidal volume and end expiratory pressure on pulmonary gas exchange during anaesthesia, *Anesthesiology* 39:285, 1973.
12. Tuxen DV and Lane S: The effects of ventilatory pattern on hyperinflation, airway pressures, and circulation in mechanical ventilation of patients with severe airflow obstruction, *Am Rev Respir Dis* 136:872, 1987.
13. Morganroth ML and others: Criteria for weaning from prolonged mechanical ventilation, *Arch Intern Med* 144:1012, 1984.
14. DeHaven CB and others: Evaluation of two extubation criteria: attributes contributing to success, *Crit Care Med* 14:92, 1986.
15. Pierson DJ: Weaning from mechanical ventilation in acute respiratory failure: concepts, indications, and techniques, *Respir Care* 28:646, 1983.
16. Sahn SA and Lakshminarayan S: Bedside criteria for discontinuation of mechanical ventilation, *Chest* 63:1002, 1973.
17. Yang KL and Tobin MJ: A prospective study of indexes predicting the outcome of trials of weaning from mechanical ventilation, *N Engl J Med* 324:1445, 1991.
18. Comroe JH: *The lung*, ed 2, St Louis, 1962, Mosby.
19. Craig DG: Postoperative recovery of pulmonary function, anaesthesia and analgesia, *Anaesthesia* 60:46, 1981.
20. Wessell HV and others: Breath-by-breath variation of FRC: effect on V_{O_2} and V_{CO_2} measured at the mouth, *J Appl Physiol* 46:1122, 1979.
21. Kaneko JK and others: Regional distribution of ventilation and perfusion as a function of body position, *J Appl Physiol* 21:767, 1966.
22. West JB: *Regional differences in the lung*, New York, 1977, Academic Press.
23. West JB: Regional differences in the lung, *Chest* 74:426, 1978.
24. Scadding JG and Cumming G: *Scientific foundations of respiratory medicine*, Philadelphia, 1981, WB Saunders.
25. Pontoppidan H and others: Acute respiratory failure in the adult, *N Engl J Med* 287:690, 1972.
26. Webb H and Tierney D: Experimental pulmonary edema due to intermittent positive pressure ventilation with high inflation pressures: protection with PEEP, *Am Rev Respir Dis* 110:556, 1974.
27. Corbridge T and others: Adverse effects of large tidal volume, and low PEEP in canine acid aspiration, *Am Rev Respir Dis* 142:311, 1990.
28. Muscedere J and others: Tidal ventilation at low airway pressures can cause pulmonary edema (abstract), *Am Rev Respir Dis* 145:A454, 1992.
29. Dantzker DR and others: Ventilation-perfusion distributions in the adult respiratory distress syndrome, *Am Rev Respir Dis* 120:1039, 1979.
30. Shapiro BA and others: Positive end expiratory pressure therapy in adults with special reference to acute lung injury: a review of the literature to suggested clinical correlations, *Crit Care Med* 12:127, 1984.
31. Rose DM and others: Temporal responses of FRC and oxygen tension to changes in PEEP, *Crit Care Med* 9:79, 1981.
32. Gherini S and others: Mechanical work on the lungs and work of breathing with PEEP and CPAP, *Chest* 76:251, 1979.
33. Neaver LJ and others: A practical procedure for measuring FRC during mechanical ventilation with or without PEEP, *Crit Care Med* 9:873, 1981.
34. Ibanez J and others: A simple method for measuring the effect of PEEP on FRC during mechanical ventilation, *Crit Care Med* 10:332, 1982.
35. Laws AK: Effect of induction of anaesthesia and muscle paralysis on FRC of the lungs, *Can Anaesth Soc J* 15:325, 1968.
36. Suter PM and Scholbohn RM: Determination of FRC during mechanical ventilation, *Anesthesiology* 41:605, 1974.
37. Heldt GP and Peters RM: A simplified method to determine FRC during mechanical ventilation, *Chest* 74:492, 1978.
38. Hylkema BS and others: Measurement of FRC during mechanical ventilation for acute inspiratory failure: a comparison between closed and an open-circuit helium dilution technique, *Chest* 81:27, 1982.
39. Paloski WH and others: A system to measure FRC in critically ill patients, *Crit Care Med* 9:342, 1981.
40. Mitchell RR and others: Oxygen wash-in method for monitoring FRC, *Crit Care Med* 10:529, 1982.
41. Adriano KP, East TD, Pace NL: Automated measurement of FRC during PEEP by SF_6 washout (abstract), *Anesthesiology* 63:A167, 1985.
42. Jonmarker and others: Measurement of FRC by sulfur hexafluoride washout, *Anesthesiology* 63:89, 1985.
43. Hewlett AM and others: Functional residual capacity during anaesthesia: methodology, spontaneous respiration and artificial ventilation, *Br J Anaesth* 46:479, 1974.
44. American Thoracic Society: Standardization of spirometry, *Am Rev Respir Dis* 119:831, 1979.
45. Gardner RM: Pulmonary function laboratory standards, *Respir Care,* 34:651, 1989.
46. Gay PC and others: Evaluation of bronchodilator responsiveness in mechanically ventilated patients, *Am Rev Respir Dis* 138:880, 1987.

47. Haake R and others: Barotrauma: pathophysiology, risk factors, and prevention, *Chest* 91:608, 1987.

48. Pierson DJ: Alveolar rupture during mechanical ventilation: role of PEEP, peak airway pressure, and distending volume, 33:472, 1988.

49. Broseghini C and others: Respiratory mechanics during the first day of mechanical ventilation in patients with pulmonary edema and chronic airway obstruction, *Am Rev Respir Dis* 138:355, 1988.

50. Gottfried SB and others: Interrupter technique for measurement of respiratory mechanics in anaesthetized humans, *J Appl Physiol* 59:647, 1985.

51. Leatherman J and others: Does measured auto-PEEP accurately reflect the degree of dynamic hyperinflation during mechanical ventilation of status asthma? (abstract), *Am Rev Respir Dis* 147:A877, 1993.

52. Bone RC: Compliance and dynamic characteristics curves in acute respiratory failure, *Crit Care Med* 4:173, 1976.

53. Rossi A and others: Measurement of static compliance of the total respiratory system in patients with acute respiratory failure during mechanical ventilation, *Am Rev Respir Dis* 31:672, 1985.

54. Marini JJ: The role of the inspiratory circuit in the work of breathing during mechanical ventilation, *Respir Care* 32:419, 1987.

55. Nunn JF: *Applied respiratory physiology,* Boston, 1977, Butterworth.

56. Berman LS and others: Inspiration: expiration ratio: is mean airway pressure the difference?, *Crit Care Med* 9:775, 1981.

57. Marini JJ and Ravenscraft SA: Mean airway pressure: physiologic determinants and clinical importance—part 2: clinical implications, *Crit Care Med* 20:1604, 1992.

58. Marini JJ and others: Estimation of inspiratory muscle strength in mechanically ventilated patients: the measurement of maximal inspiratory pressure, *Crit Care Med* 1:32, 1986.

59. Tahvanai J and others: Extubating criteria after weaning from IMV and CPAP, *Crit Care Med* 11:702, 1983.

60. Browning JA and others: Effect of a fluctuating FIo_2 on metabolic measurement in mechanically ventilated patients, *Crit Care Med* 10:82, 1982.

61. Fletcher R: *The single breath test for carbon dioxide,* Lund, Sweden, 1980, University of Lund.

62. Eichorn JH and others: Standards for patient monitoring during anesthesia at Harvard Medical School, *JAMA* 266:1017, 1986.

63. Gerald J and others: Verification of endotracheal intubation using a disposable end-tidal Co_2 detector, *Prehosp Disaster Med* 4:74, 1989.

64. Owen RL and Cheney FW: Use of an apnea monitor to verify endotracheal intubation, *Respir Care* 30:974, 1989.

65. Gazmuri RJ and others: Arterial Pco_2 as an indicator of systemic perfusion during cardiopulmonary resuscitation, *Crit Care Med* 17:237, 1989.

66. Covelli HD: Respiratory failure precipitated by high carbohydrate loads, *Ann Intern Med* 95:579, 1981.

67. Craig K and Pierson DJ: Expired gas collections for deadspace calculations: a comparison of two methods, *Respir Care* 24:435, 1979.

68. Reidek K and others: Regional intrapulmonary gas distribution in awake and anaesthetized paralyzed man, *J Appl Physiol* 42:391, 1977.

69. Fairley HB and Blenkarm GD: Effect on pulmonary gas exchange of variations in inspiratory flow rate during IPPV, *Br J Anaesth* 38:320, 1966.

70. Dammann JF and others: Optimal flow pattern for mechanical ventilation of the lungs, *Crit Care Med* 6:293, 1978.

71. Woodson RD: Physiological significance of oxygen dissociation curve shifts, *Crit Care Med* 368, 1979.

72. Finch CA and Lenfant C: Oxygen transport in man, *N Engl J Med* 286:407, 1972.

73. Hechtman HB and others: Importance of oxygen transport in clinical medicine, *Crit Care Med* 7:419, 1979.

74. Bryant-Brown CW: Tissue blood flow and oxygen transport in critically ill patients, *Crit Care Med* 3:103, 1975.

75. McConn R: The oxyhemoglobin dissociation curve in acute disease, *Surg Clin North Am* 55:627, 1975.

76. Jalonen J: Oxygen transport in the blood, *Ann Clin Res* 33:39, 1981.

77. Bryant-Brown CW and others: Consumable oxygen: availability of oxygen in relation to oxyhemoglobin dissociation, *Crit Care Med* 1:17, 1973.

78. Valeri CR and others: Improved oxygen delivery to the myocardium during hypothermia by perfusion with 2,3-DPG enriched cells, *Ann Thorac Surg* 30:527, 1980.

79. Aberman A and others: Blood P50 calculated from a single measurement of pH, Po_2, and So_2, *J Appl Physiol* 38:171, 1975.

80. Muller-Plathe O: A nomogram for the calculation of P50 from a single equilibration, *Crit Care Med* 7:399, 1979.

81. Bryant-Brown CW: Blood flow to the organs: parameters for function and survival in critical illness, *Crit Care Med* 16:170, 1988.

82. Glauser R and others: Worsening oxygenation in the mechanically ventilated patient, *Am Rev Respir Dis* 138:458, 1988.

83. Berk JL and others: The use of dopamine to correct the reduced cardiac output resulting from positive end expiratory pressure, *Crit Care Med* 5:269, 1977.

84. Jardin F and others: Dobutamine: a hemodynamic evaluation in human septic shock, *Crit Care Med* 9:329, 1981.

85. Kanber GJ and others: The alveolar-arterial oxygen gradient in young and elderly men during air and oxygen breathing, *Am Rev Respir Dis* 97:376, 1968.

86. Maxwell C and others: Use of the arterial/alveolar oxygen tension ratio to predict the inspired oxygen concentration needed for a desired arterial oxygen tension, *Respir Care* 29:1135, 1984.

87. Luterman A and others: Withdrawal from positive end-expiratory pressure, *Surgery* 83:328, 1981.

88. Hallman M and others: Exogenous human surfactant for treatment of severe respiratory distress syndrome: A randomized prospective clinical trial, *J Pediatr* 106:963, 1985.

89. Bartlett H and others: Extracorporeal membrane oxygenation (ECMO) in neonatal respiratory failure, *Ann Surg* 204:236, 1986.

90. Cane RD: Minimizing errors in intrapulmonary shunt calculations, *Crit Care Med* 8:294, 1980.

91. West JB: Pulmonary gas exchange in the critically ill patient, *Crit Care Med* 2:171, 1974.

92. Douglas ME and others: Change in pulmonary venous admixture with varying inspired oxygen, *Anesth Analg* 55:688, 1976.

93. Reines HD and Civetta JM: The inaccuracy of using 100% oxygen to determine intrapulmonary shunt in spite of PEEP, *Crit Care Med* 7:301, 1979.

94. Suter PM and others: Shunt, lung volume and perfusion during short periods of ventilation with oxygen, *Anesthesiology* 43:617, 1975.

95. Quan SF and others: Changes in venous admixture with alterations of inspired oxygen concentration, *Anesthesiology* 52:477, 1980.

96. Domino KB and others: Influence of mixed venous oxygen tension on blood flow to atelectatic lung, *Anesthesiology* 59:428, 1983.

97. Jardin F and others: Venous admixture in human septic shock, *Circulation* 60:159, 1979.

98. Cane RD and others: Unreliability of oxygen tension-based indices in reflecting intrapulmonary shunting in critically ill patients, *Crit Care Med* 16:1243, 1988.

99. Rackow EC and others: Cellular oxygen metabolism during sepsis and shock: relationship of oxygen consumption to oxygen delivery, *JAMA* 259:1989, 1988.

100. Dorinsky PM and others: Relationships of oxygen uptake and oxygen delivery in respiratory failure not due to the adult respiratory distress syndrome, *Chest* 93:1013, 1988.

101. Mohsenifar Z and others: Dependence of oxygen consumption on oxygen delivery in patients with chronic congestive heart failure, *Chest* 92:447, 1987.

102. Shoemaker WC and others: Tissue oxygen debt as a determinant of lethal and nonlethal postoperative organ failure, *Crit Care Med* 16:1117, 1988.

103. Nelson LD and others: Clinical validation of a new metabolic monitor suitable for use in critically ill patients, *Crit Care Med* 15:951, 1987.

104. Nelson LD and others: V_{O_2} and PEEP in acute respiratory failure, *Crit Care Med* 10:857, 1982.

105. Cain SM: Peripheral oxygen uptake and delivery in health and disease, *Clin Chest Med* 4:139, 1983.

106. Astiz ME and others: Relationship of oxygen delivery and mixed venous oxygenation to lactic acidosis in patients with sepsis and acute myocardial infarction, *Crit Care Med* 16:655, 1988.

107. Moshsenifar Z and others: Relationship between O_2 delivery and O_2 consumption in ARDS, *Chest* 84:267, 1983.

108. Harpin RP and others: Correlation of the oxygen cost of breathing and length of weaning from mechanical ventilation, *Crit Care Med* 15:807, 1987.

109. Shoemaker WC and others: Prospective trial of supranormal values of survivors as therapeutic goals in high-risk surgical patients, *Chest* 94:1176, 1988.

110. Danek SJ and others: The dependence of oxygen uptake on oxygen delivery in ARDS, *Am Rev Respir Dis* 122:387, 1980.

111. Dantzker DR: Oxygen transport and utilization, *Respir Care* 33:874, 1988.

112. Tahuanainen J and others: Can central venous blood replace mixed venous blood samples?, *Crit Care Med* 10:758, 1982.

113. Jamieson WRE and others: Continuous monitoring of mixed venous oxygen saturation in cardiac surgery, *Can J Surg* 25:538, 1982.

114. Schweiss JF: *Continuous measurement of blood oxygen saturation in the high risk patient,* vol 1, San Diego, 1983, Beach International.

115. Waller JL and others: Clinical evaluation of a new fiberoptic catheter oximeter during cardiac surgery, *Anesth Analg* 61:676, 1982.

116. Divertie MB and McMichan JC: Continuous monitoring of mixed venous oxygen saturation, *Chest* 85:423, 1984.

117. Baele PL and others: Continuous monitoring of mixed venous oxygen saturation in critically ill patients, *Anesth Analg* 61:513, 1982.

118. Carroll GC: A continuous monitoring technique for management of acute pulmonary failure, *Chest* 92:467, 1987.

119. Downs JB and others: The effect of incremental PEEP on Pa_{O_2} in patients with respiratory failure, *Anesth Analg* 52:210, 1973.

120. Broder G and Weil MH: Excess lactate: an index of reversibility of shock in human patients, *Science* 143:1457, 1964.

121. Rashkin MC and others: Oxygen delivery in critically ill patients: relationship to blood lactate and survival, *Chest* 87:580, 1985.

122. Cady LD and others: Quantitation of severity of critical illness with special reference to blood lactate, *Crit Care Med* 1:75, 1973.

123. Berk J and Sampliner JE: *Handbook of critical care medicine,* ed 2, Boston, 1982, Little, Brown.

124. Pichette C and others: Elevation of the blood lactate concentration by alkali therapy without requiring additional lactic acid accumulation: theoretical considerations, *Crit Care Med* 10:323, 1982.

125. Rinke C: Controversies in lactic acidosis: implications in critically ill patients, *JAMA* 258:497, 1988.

126. Burki NK and others: Noninvasive monitoring of arterial blood gases: a report of the ACCP section on respiratory pathophysiology, *Chest* 83:666, 1983.

127. Swedlow DB and Stern S: Continuous non-invasive oxygen saturation monitoring in children with a new pulse-oximeter. Paper presented at the meeting of the Society of Critical Care Medicine, March 1983.

128. Severinghaus JW and Naifeh KH: Accuracy of response of six pulse oximeters to profound hypoxia, *Anesthesiology* 67:551, 1987.

129. Nickerson BG and others: Bias and precision of pulse oximeters and arterial oximeters, *Chest* 93:515, 1988.

130. Chapman KR and others: The accuracy and response characteristics of a simplified ear oximeter, *Chest* 83:860, 1983.

131. Scoggin C and others: Clinical evaluation of a new ear oximeter, *Heart Lung* 6:121, 1977.

132. Shoemaker WC and Vidyasagar D: Physiological and clinical significance of Pt_{CO_2} and Pt_{CCO_2} measurements, *Crit Care Med* 9:689, 1981.

133. Tremper KF and Shoemaker WC: Transcutaneous oxygen monitoring of critically ill adults with and without low flow shock, *Crit Care Med* 9:706, 1981.

134. Nolan LS and Shoemaker WC: Transcutaneous O_2 and CO_2 monitoring of high risk surgical patients during the perioperative period, *Crit Care Med* 10:762, 1982.

135. Shoemaker WC: Transcutaneous and conjunctival measurement of oxygen tension for assessment of tissue perfusion. Summary proceedings of the twenty-first annual symposium of critical care medicine, Los Angeles, March 1983.

136. Beran AV and others: Cutaneous blood flow and its relationship to transcutaneous O_2/CO_2 measurements, *Crit Care Med* 9:736, 1981.

137. Ebherard P and others: Cutaneous blood gas monitoring in the adult, *Crit Care Med* 9:702, 1981.

138. Severinghaus JW: Methods of measurements of blood and gas carbon dioxide during anaesthesia, *Anesthesiology* 21:717, 1960.

139. Shukla A and others: A bedside technique for measuring Pa_{CO_2} using a $PtcCO_2$ monitor, *Crit Care Med* 11:376, 1983.

140. Applebaum R and others: Emergency Pa_{O_2} estimates in one minute with a transcutaneous oxygen sensor, *Crit Care Med* 9:742, 1981.

141. Fink SE and others: A new device for measuring conjunctival oxygen tension and its application to hyperoxic and hypoxic states, *Crit Care Med* 11:224, 1983.

142. Kwan M and Fatt I: A noninvasive method of continuous arterial oxygen tension estimation from measured palpebral conjunctival oxygen tension, *Anesthesiology* 35:309, 1971.

143. Gottrup F and others: Continuous monitoring of tissue oxygen tension during hyperoxia and hypoxia: relation of subcutaneous, transcutaneous, and conjunctival oxygen tension to hemodynamic variables, *Crit Care Med* 16:1229, 1988.

144. Healey CJ and others: Comparison of noninvasive measurement of carbon dioxide tension during withdrawal from mechanical ventilation, *Crit Care Med* 15:764, 1987.

145. Kram HB and others: Noninvasive measurement of tissue carbon dioxide tension using a fiberoptic conjunctival sensor: effects of respiratory and metabolic alkalosis and acidosis, *Crit Care Med* 16:280, 1988.

146. Kreuzer F and Nessler CG: Method of polarographic in vivo continuous recording of blood oxygen tension, *Science* 128:1005, 1958.

147. Bratanow N and others: Continuous polarographic monitoring of intra-arterial oxygen in the perioperative period, *Crit Care Med* 13:859, 1985.

148. Shapiro B: In-vivo blood gas monitoring. *Respir Care* 37:166, 1992.

Chapter 13

Cardiac Output Assessment

Susan Jones Krider

LEARNING OBJECTIVES

Upon completion of this chapter, the reader should be able to accomplish the following:

1. *Define cardiac output and venous return.*

2. *Recognize the following regarding cardiac output:*
   a. *method of calculation*
   b. *range of normal values*
   c. *effect of sympathetic nervous stimulation*

3. *Recognize the following regarding the distribution of blood flow:*
   a. *effect of metabolism and reduced oxygen availability on the regulation of blood flow through organs*
   b. *percent of total blood volume in venous system*
   c. *effect of blood loss (hypovolemia) on circulatory function*
   d. *basal distribution of blood flow to organs vs. distribution during cardiac failure*
   e. *effect of mechanical ventilation*

4. *Identify the normal values, method of calculation, and significance of the following indicators of cardiac output:*
   a. *cardiac index*
   b. *ejection fraction*
   c. *stroke volume*
   d. *end-diastolic volume*
   e. *cardiac work*
   f. *ventricular stroke work*

5. *Recognize the following regarding preload:*
   a. *definition*
   b. *values used to measure preload of the left and right ventricles*
   c. *factors affecting*
   d. *clinical value of ventricular function curves*
   e. *effect of mechanical ventilation*

6. *Recognize the following for afterload:*
   a. *definition*
   b. *factors affecting*
   c. *how it is measured*
   d. *effect of vasodilators*
   e. *how to calculate systemic and pulmonary vascular resistance*
   f. *effect of mechanical ventilation*

Chapter Overview

The adequacy of perfusion is the most important factor in the assessment of the cardiovascular system's ability to meet the metabolic demands (need for nutrients and oxygen) of the body. The physical (noninvasive) indicators of perfusion (urine output, peripheral skin temperature, mentation, etc.) have been discussed in Chapter 11. The indicators available for direct (invasive) measurement of cardiovascular functioning include systolic, diastolic, and mean arterial and pulmonary artery pressures; cardiac filling pressures (central venous pressure and pulmonary capillary wedge or left atrial pressure); and cardiac output. Once these measurements have been obtained, calculation of cardiac index, stroke work index, pulmonary vascular resistance, and systemic vascular resistance can be made. Various diagnostic and treatment decision-making tools, such

as hemodynamic subsets, ventricular function curves, and decision-making trees, have been designed to assist the clinician in making sense of all the available information.

One cannot separate cardiac output and hemodynamics in clinical practice; they work together and control each other. However, it is easier for the student to first study the specifics of each individually and then combine the concepts. Throughout this chapter, various hemodynamic pressures and their relationship to cardiac output are discussed. The novice may need to refer to both Chapters 11 and 14 while studying this chapter.

Cardiac Output

The amount of blood pumped out of the left ventricle in a minute is known as *cardiac output*. The average cardiac output for men and women of all ages is approximately 5 L/min at rest; however, the normal cardiac output for an individual varies with age, sex (10% higher in men), body size, blood viscosity (hematocrit), and the tissue demand for oxygen.[1,2]

The normal heart, when not stimulated by the autonomic nervous system, is capable of pumping about 10 to 13 L/min, and can pump about double that amount when stimulated by the sympathetic nervous system. A well-trained athlete's heart enlarges sometimes as much as 50% and is capable of pumping up to 35 L/min.[1,2] Under normal conditions, the heart plays a passive role in cardiac output and pumps whatever amount of blood is returned to it. When the heart is diseased or damaged so that it can no longer pump the amount of blood returned to it, it is said to be *failing*.

Venous Return

The volume of blood returning to the right atrium is known as the *venous return*. Venous return is the sum of all the local blood flow through all the individual

Table 13-1 Distribution of Blood Flow*						
	Basal		**Cardiac failure**		**Exercise**	
	L/min	%	L/min	%	L/min	%
Brain	0.75	13	0.5	15	0.75	3.0
Heart	0.25	4	0.3	9	1.0	4.0
Muscle	1.2	21	1.2	35	22.0	88.0
Liver	1.4	24	0.8	24	0.3	1.2
Kidney	1.1	19	0.35	10	0.25	1.0
Skin	0.5	9	0.05	1	0.6	2.4
Other	0.6	10	0.2	6	0.1	0.4
	5.8		3.4		25.0	
O₂ uptake	240 mL/ min		300 mL/ min		2000 mL/ min	

*Adapted from Finch CA, and Lenfant C: Oxygen transport in man. *N Engl J Med* 286:407, 1972.

tissues of the body. The resting blood flow through an organ is determined by the metabolic needs of the organ. The greater the need for oxygen, the greater the blood flow through the organ. Table 13-1 shows that the muscles, liver, and kidneys receive the greatest amount of blood flow in the resting state because of their high metabolic needs. When the metabolic activity of the tissue increases (as in muscles during exercise) or when the availability of oxygen to the tissues decreases (as occurs at high altitudes or with carbon monoxide or cyanide poisoning), vasodilation allows more blood to flow to the tissues.

The muscle fibers of the precapillary sphincters and the metarterioles in the capillary beds are controlled by the concentration of oxygen, carbon dioxide, hydrogen ions, electrolytes, and other humoral substances. When oxygen is low and hydrogen ions and carbon dioxide levels are increased at the tissue level, vasodilation occurs. The greater the vasodilation, the more blood flows to the area. (Hypoxia has the opposite effect on the pulmonary vasculature, causing vasoconstriction, which shunts the greatest amount of blood flow to the oxygenated alveoli, thus maintaining the best oxygenation.)

In addition to providing tissue control of cardiac output, the venous system acts as a reservoir of blood to maintain flow to the vital organs when blood volume is lost. Approximately 64% of the total blood volume is in the venous system normally.[2] When blood volume decreases, the veins as well as the venous reservoirs (spleen, liver, abdominal veins, and even heart and lungs) constrict and redistribute volume to maintain venous return and cardiac pressures. In fact, 20% to 25% of the total blood volume can be lost without altering circulatory function and pressures.[2] When blood flow is decreased to the point that central nervous system (CNS) compensatory mechanisms come into play, sympathetic stimulation causes vasoconstriction and the blood flow to certain organs is further decreased. Table 13-1 shows that flow to the kidneys, liver, and other body areas is significantly decreased to maintain perfusion to the heart and brain with heart failure.

Measures of Cardiac Output and Pump Function

Cardiac output is the product of heart rate (HR) and *stroke volume* (SV), the volume of blood ejected by the ventricle with each beat. Normal stroke volume for adults is 60 to 130 mL/beat and is approximately the same for the right and left ventricles unless one of the ventricles is malfunctioning or there is an intracardiac shunt. Since the normal heart rate is 60 to 100 beats/min, the normal adult range for cardiac output (HR × SV) is 4 to 8 L/min.

Cardiac Index

Because cardiac output, like most other hemodynamic measurements, varies with body size, cardiac index may be used to describe flow output. *Cardiac index (CI)* is cardiac output divided by body surface area (BSA) and is reported as liters per minute per square meter (L/min/m²). A normal resting cardiac index for patients of all ages is 2.5 to 4.0 L/min/m², with the average for adults approximately 3.0 L/min/m². The cardiac index is highest at 10 years of age and decreases with age to approximately 2.4 L/min/m² at age 80 years.[2]

Body Surface Area and Indices

Body surface area (BSA) is calculated using the patient's weight and height and a nomogram (Fig. 13-1). When a straight line is drawn connecting the patient's weight and height, it intersects the center line and shows the patient's BSA in square meters. BSA can also be calculated using weight. The advantage of using an indice is that the normals are standardized and comparisons can be made between patients of different heights and weights.

Stroke volume, end-diastolic volume (EDV), ejection fraction (EF), ventricular stroke work (SW), and cardiac work (CW) are other measures of ventricular function commonly reported as indices. The normal hemodynamic values and formulas are listed in Table 13-2.

Ventricular Volumes

End-diastolic volume is the amount of blood in the ventricle at the end of filling (diastole). *End-systolic volume* is the amount of blood in the ventricle following ejection (systole).

Ejection Fraction

Ejection fraction represents the percentage of the end-diastolic volume that is ejected with each beat. A

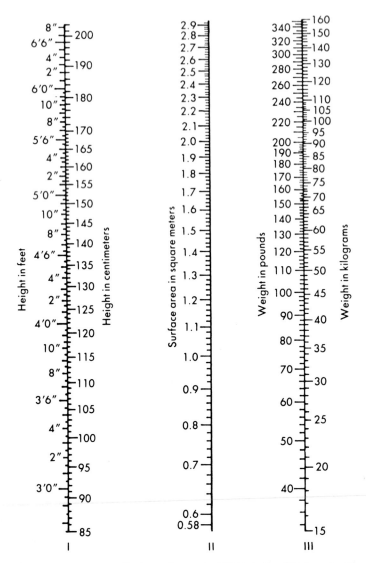

Fig. 13-1 *DuBois body surface area nomogram. Body surface area (BSA) is found by locating the patient's height on scale I and weight on scale III and placing a straightedge between the two points. The line intersects scale II at patient's BSA. (From DuBois EF: Basal metabolism in health and disease. Philadelphia, 1936, Lea & Febiger.)*

normal ejection fraction is 65% to 70%. Ejection fraction is either measured directly or calculated from the following formula:

$$EF = \frac{SV}{EDV}$$

The ejection fraction declines as cardiac function deteriorates. When the ejection fraction falls to the 30% range, a patient's exercise tolerance is severely limited because of the heart's inability to maintain adequate cardiac output.

Cardiac Work

Cardiac work is a measurement of the energy the heart uses to eject blood against the aortic or pulmonary pressures (resistance). Cardiac work correlates well with the oxygen requirements of the heart. Although the left

(LV) and right (RV) ventricles eject the same volume of blood, the LV must eject against the mean aortic pressure (MAP), which is about six times the mean pulmonary artery pressure (MPAP); therefore, the measures of cardiac work are much higher for the left ventricle. The *cardiac work index* (CWI) measures the work per minute per square meter and is calculated from the following formulas:

$$LCWI = CI \times MAP \times 0.0136 = 3.4\text{--}4.2 \; Kg/min/m^2$$
$$RCWI = CI \times MPAP \times 0.0136 = 0.4\text{--}0.66 \; Kg/min/m^2$$

where 0.0136 is a conversion factor for changing pressure to work.

Ventricular Stroke Work

Ventricular stroke work is a measure of myocardial work per contraction. It is the product of the stroke volume

Table 13-2 Hemodynamic Variables, Normal Values, and Formulas*

Variable	Normal Range†	Formula‡
Cardiac output (CO)	4–8 L/min	CO = direct measurement
Cardiac index (CI)	2.5–5.0 L/min/m²	CI = CO/BSA
Stroke volume (SV)	60–130 mL/beat	SV = CO/HR or EDV – ESV
Stroke index (SI)	30–50 mL/m²	SI = CI/HR or SV/BSA
Ejection fraction (EF)	65%–75%	EF = SV/EDV or direct measurement
End-diastolic volume (EDV)	120–180 mL/beat	EDV = direct measurement
End-systolic volume (ESV)	50–60 mL	ESV = direct measurement
Rate-pressure product (RPP)	<12,000 mmHg	RPP = systolic BP × HR
Coronary perfusion pressure (CPP)	60–80 mmHg	CPP = diastolic BP – PCWP
Left cardiac work index (LCWI)	3.4–4.2 Kg/min/m²	LCWI = CI × MAP × 0.0136§
Right cardiac work index (RCWI)	0.4–0.66 Kg/min/m²	RCWI = CI × MPAP × 0.0136§
Left ventricular stroke work index (LVSWI)	50–62 g/min/m²/beat	LVSWI = SI × MAP × 0.0136‖
Right ventricular stroke work index (RVSWI)	7.9–9.7 g/min/m²/beat	RVSWI = SI × MPAP × 0.0136‖
Pulmonary vascular resistance (PVR)	<2 units	PVR = (MPAP – PCWP)/CO
	110–250 dynes/sec/cm⁵	PVR = (MPAP – PCWP)/CO × 80¶
Pulmonary vascular resistance index (PVRI)	225–315 dynes/sec/cm⁵/m²	PVRI = (MPAP – PCWP)/CI × 80¶
Systemic vascular resistance (SVR)	15–20 units	SVR = (MAP – CVP)/CO
	900–1400 dynes/sec/cm⁵	SVR = (MAP – CVP)/CO × 80¶
Systemic vascular resistance index (SVRI)	1970–2400 dynes/sec/cm⁵/m²	SVRI = (MAP – CVP)/CI × 80¶

*Data from references 3–5. †Normal values for adults. Sources vary in normal values reported, but values are within the same general range. ‡BP=blood pressure; MAP=mean arterial pressure in mmHg; CVP=central venous pressure in mmHg; MPAP=mean pulmonary artery pressure in mmHg; PCWP=pulmonary capillary wedge pressure in mmHg. §Conversion factor to convert L/mmHg to Kg/min/m²; 0.0144 is used by some sources.[3] ‖Conversion factor to convert mL/mmHg to g/min/m²; 0.144 is used by some sources.[3] An alternative version of the formula includes subtraction of the filling pressures: LVSWI = SV × (MAP – PCWP) × 0.0136; RSWI = SV × (MPAP – CVP) × 0.0136.[2,4] ¶Conversion factors of 79.92 and 79.96 may also be used.[3,4]

times the pressure across the vascular bed. The *ventricular stroke work index* is most commonly calculated as follows:

$$LVSWI = SI \times (MAP - PCWP) \times 0.0136 = 43–61 \text{ g/min/m}^2/\text{beat}$$
$$RVSWI = SI \times (MPAP - CVP) \times 0.0136 = 7–12 \text{ g/min/m}^2/\text{beat}$$

where

PCWP = pulmonary capillary wedge pressure
CVP = central venous pressure

A simplified form of the ventricular stroke work equation is listed in Table 13–2.

Decreased stroke work values indicate decreasing ability of the heart to perform work and are usually accompanied by decreasing stroke volume and ejection fraction. Conversely, increasing stroke work indicates that the ventricle is performing better but also that it is using more oxygen. When myocardial oxygen supply is decreased, as occurs with angina, keeping cardiac work in the low normal range enhances the ratio of myocardial oxygen supply to demand.

Determinants of Pump Function

The performance ability of the heart (cardiac output) is determined by both heart rate and stroke volume. Stroke volume has been found to be determined by three factors: preload, afterload, and contractility (Fig. 13–2).

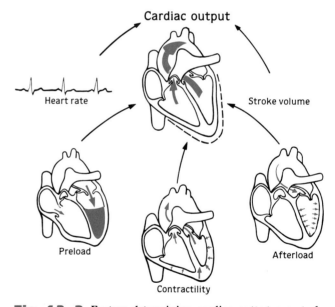

Fig. 13-2 *Factors determining cardiac output are stroke volume and heart rate. Stroke volume is determined by preload, afterload, and contractility.*

Heart Rate

Heart rate normally does not play a large role in control of cardiac output in the adult except when it is outside the normal range or when arrhythmia is present.

Bradycardia is a heart rate less than 60 beats/min in an adult. Low heart rate does not drop cardiac output if the heart can compensate with increased stroke volume; the best example is the well-trained athlete with a resting pulse rate below 50 but a normal blood pressure. However, if a patient has a damaged heart that cannot alter stroke volume to compensate for bradycardia, cardiac output will fall.

Tachycardia (adult heart rate in excess of 100 beats/min) is the body's compensation to maintain cardiac output when compensatory mechanisms to increase stroke volume are inadequate. In the resting patient, cardiac output may begin to decline at rates of 120 to 130 beats/min. Because diastole is shortened by increased rates, the time for ventricular filling is decreased with tachycardia. In addition, maintaining the higher rate requires an increased oxygen consumption that the patient with coronary artery disease may not be able to provide. With exercise and sympathoadrenal stimulation, cardiac output does not decline until approximately 180 beats/min. *Premature heart beats* (premature ventricular [PVCs] and atrial [PACs] contractions) also alter the time for ventricular filling and may decrease cardiac output.

Preload

Preload is the stretch on the ventricular muscle fibers before contraction. *Preload* is created by the *end-diastolic volume*. In 1914, Starling found that up to a critical limit, the strength of contraction of myocardial muscle fiber was directly related to the amount of stretch on the fiber before contraction. His theory has come to be known as *Starling's law* of the heart. Simply stated, the greater the stretch on the resting ventricle, the greater the strength of contraction within physiologic limits. A rubber band or a toy balloon can be used as an analogy. The tighter the rubber band is stretched, the farther it flies when it is released; or the more a balloon is inflated, the faster the flow rate when the balloon deflates.

VENTRICULAR FUNCTION CURVES. Figure 13–3 shows *ventricular function curves* (often called *Starling curves*) for both the right and left ventricles. The horizontal axis represents the volume (preload), and the vertical axis is a measure of the heart's output: cardiac output, cardiac index, stroke volume, stroke index, or ventricular stroke work index. It can be seen that increasing volume increases output. When the pump is no longer able to eject all of its blood efficiently because it is overstretched, cardiac output begins to fall.

Continuously measured end-diastolic volume is the ideal way to assess preload. However, most critical care units can only measure ventricular volumes on a periodic basis using echocardiography or radionuclide imaging. Therefore, atrial pressures, which can be measured continuously, are used to reflect end-diastolic volume. During diastole the atrioventricular valves (tricuspid and mitral) are open. If there is no narrowing or dysfunction of the valves, the pressures

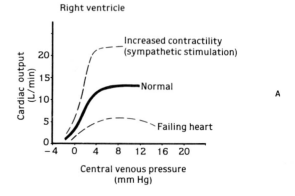

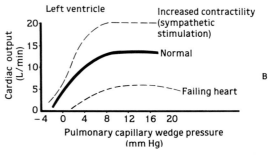

Fig. 13–3 *Ventricular function curves for right and left ventricles. Note that filling pressures are used to represent end-diastolic volume. **A,** Family of ventricular function curves for right ventricle. Upstroke of curve shows rapid change in cardiac output for small change in end-diastolic volume initially, but curve then plateaus, with little change in output for large changes in right atrial pressure. Dashed curves show change in output for given pressure occurring with altered contractility from sympathetic stimulation (as occurs with exercise or fear) and heart failure. **B,** Family of ventricular function curves for left ventricle. End-diastolic volume can be used for plotting horizontal axis. Cardiac index, stroke volume, or left ventricular stoke work index can be graphed on vertical axis rather than cardiac output. Output begins to decline after pulmonary capillary wedge pressure of 20 mmHg unless ventricular compliance is altered.*

in the atrium and ventricle should be the same at end-diastole. The filling pressure for the right heart is right atrial pressure, commonly measured as *central venous pressure (CVP)*. The filling pressure for the left heart is left atrial pressure, but it is more commonly measured as *pulmonary capillary wedge pressure (PCWP)*. How these pressures are measured and used to represent preload is discussed in Chapter 14. It must be remembered, however, that *filling pressure does not always reflect ventricular volume in the critically ill patient.*[6,7] This is especially true when ventricular compliance is altered.

VENTRICULAR COMPLIANCE. It is important to understand that pressure is the result of the volume, space, and compliance of the chamber the volume is entering. Forcing 100 mL of water into a small, rigid chamber takes more pressure than filling a

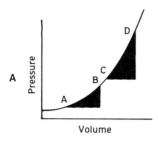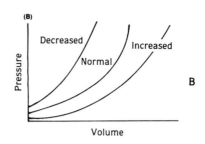

Fig. 13-4 *Compliance can be altered along a single pressure-volume relationship or by a change in the rate of rise of diastolic pressure.* **A,** *Small rise in pressure (point A to point B) for given change in end-diastolic volume is in contrast to large increase in pressure seen from point C to point D with the same (or smaller) change in end-diastolic volume. Therefore, the ventricle described by A to B is more compliant than the ventricle described by C to D.* **B,** *"Family" of ventricular compliance curves. Not only may compliance fall along the ascending curve but disease and drugs may also effect a change in the compliance curve up and to the left (reduced compliance) or down and to the right (increased compliance). (From Sibbald WJ and Driedger AA: Right and left ventricular preload and diastolic ventricular compliance: implications for therapy in critically ill patients. In Shoemaker WC and Thompson WL, editors:* Critical care state of the art, *vol 3, Fullerton, Calif, 1982, Society for Critical Care Medicine.)*

balloon with 100 mL of water. Figure 13–4 shows how ventricular pressure is affected by changes in volume and ventricular compliance (elasticity, stretchability, distensibility). When compliance is reduced, a much higher pressure is generated for a given volume. Pressure also increases more rapidly as the ventricle fills; thus, ends of the curves rise more abruptly as the ventricle becomes full and tension is developed in the ventricular walls.

Factors that *decrease ventricular compliance*[6,8] (make the ventricle stiffer) and therefore cause the pressure to increase out of proportion to the volume include myocardial ischemia and infarction, hemorrhagic and septic shock, pericardial effusions, right ventricular dilation and overload (causes the septum to shift to the left and impinge on the left ventricle), positive end-expiratory pressure (PEEP), and inotropic drugs (increase the strength of myocardial contraction). Factors that *increase ventricular compliance*[6,8] (make the ventricle less rigid) include relief of ischemia, vasodilator drugs (nitroprusside, nitroglycerin), and cardiomyopathies.

FACTORS THAT AFFECT VENOUS RETURN, PRELOAD, AND CARDIAC OUTPUT. The three main factors affecting the amount of blood returned to the heart are (1) changes in circulating blood volume, (2) changes in the distribution of the blood volume, and (3) atrial contraction.

Circulating Blood Volume. *Circulating blood volume* is obviously altered by bleeding but is also decreased by loss of other body fluids. Large amounts of urine output (as occurs with diuretics), wound drainage, diarrhea, perspiration, and gastric secretions can result in a large decrease in blood volume (hypovolemia). Fluid can also shift into the interstitial space. Sepsis, burns, and shock may result in tremendous amounts of fluid being moved into this so-called *third space.* On the other hand, fluids ingested or given

intravenously increase the circulating blood volume. Administration of colloids and dyes (large-molecular-weight solutions) pulls water from the interstitial space to "dilute out" the large molecules, resulting in an increase in blood volume. Small children can also have large increases in blood volume from respiratory care humidification, especially ultrasonic nebulizers.

Distribution of the Blood Volume. *Distribution of the blood volume* is altered not only by third-spacing but also by changes in *body position, venous tone, intrathoracic pressure,* and, rarely, by obstruction of the large veins returning to the heart. As the body changes position, blood tends to move to dependent areas. Standing decreases venous return; conversely, raising the legs of a patient who is lying down increases venous return. Venous tone also alters the distribution of blood in the body. Venous tone may increase (vasoconstriction) as a compensatory mechanism and shift more blood to the "core" (heart, lungs, and brain). Vasodilation therapy resulting from therapy with nitrates, nitroprusside (Nipride), isoproterenol (Isuprel), or furosemide (Lasix) relaxes vascular tone and may decrease venous return. Raised intrathoracic pressure decreases venous return. Pneumothorax (barotrauma), the Valsalva maneuver, breath-holding in children, prolonged bouts of coughing, and positive pressure ventilation increase intrathoracic pressure and thereby decrease venous return.

Blood or Fluid in the Pericardial Sac. Blood or fluid in the pericardial sac (cardiac tamponade), pericarditis (the pericardium becomes scarred and restrictive), or the mediastinum filling with blood after trauma or cardiac surgery will put pressure on the heart. Venous return meets resistance as the pressures around the heart increase. At first, pressure in the veins returning to the heart (central venous pressure) and heart rate increase, but arterial pressure remains fairly stable. However, if the tamponade continues, the pressure on the heart will exceed the pressure in the vessels returning blood to the heart, and blood will not be able to reenter the heart.

Atrial Contraction. *Atrial contraction* adds approximately 30% to cardiac output by loading the ventricle at the end of diastole. When a patient develops atrial fibrillation, atrioventricular dissociation, or third degree heart block, or is being paced by a ventricular pacemaker, this so-called *atrial kick* is lost, and cardiac output may fall.

CLINICAL APPLICATIONS OF VENTRICULAR FUNCTION CURVES. Preload is the major determinant of contractility, but ideal filling pressures vary greatly with compliance and the patient's condition. *Ventricular function curves* may be constructed to find a patient's ideal filling pressure at a given point in time and provide information about ventricular compliance. Cardiac output, stroke volume, or other measures of heart output are plotted on the vertical axis. Filling pressure (usually pulmonary artery diastolic or pulmonary capillary wedge pressure) is plotted on the horizontal axis. A baseline cardiac output reading is obtained, and the point corresponding to the cardiac output reading and simultaneous pressure reading is plotted (Fig. 13–5). A *fluid challenge* (discussed in Chapter 14) is administered, and another cardiac output and pressure reading is performed. Pressure is again plotted against cardiac output. As the plotting continues, a Starling (or ventricular function) curve is created. When a satisfactory cardiac output is achieved or the cardiac output begins to decline as the filling pressure increases, fluid challenges are stopped. The pressure that corresponds to the highest cardiac output reading obtained is used to indicate optimal preload. Volume can then be administered as needed to maintain the pressure at the point of maximal cardiac output.

USING HEMODYNAMIC SUBSETS TO ASSESS LEFT VENTRICULAR PERFORMANCE. In 1976 Forrester and others reported a comparison of clinical signs and hemodynamic values in patients following myocardial infarction. They defined pulmonary congestion clinically, based on the presence of dyspnea, crackles, and radiographic evidence of congestion, and found that pulmonary congestion correlated with a pulmonary capillary wedge pressure of greater than 18 mmHg. Clinical signs of peripheral hypoperfusion in-

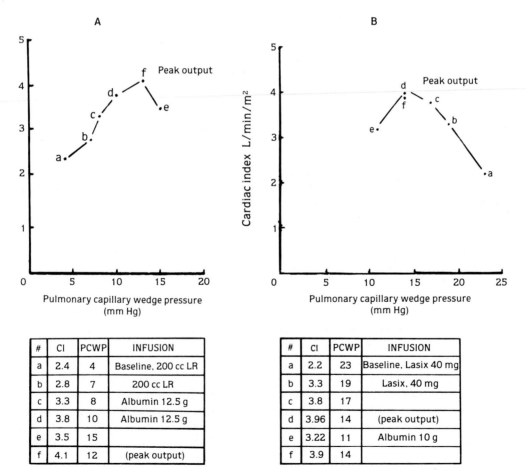

#	CI	PCWP	INFUSION
a	2.4	4	Baseline, 200 cc LR
b	2.8	7	200 cc LR
c	3.3	8	Albumin 12.5 g
d	3.8	10	Albumin 12.5 g
e	3.5	15	
f	4.1	12	(peak output)

#	CI	PCWP	INFUSION
a	2.2	23	Baseline, Lasix 40 mg
b	3.3	19	Lasix, 40 mg
c	3.8	17	
d	3.96	14	(peak output)
e	3.22	11	Albumin 10 g
f	3.9	14	

Fig. 13–5 *Ventricular function curves.* **A,** *Infusion curve of patient showing optimal myocardial performance level to be pulmonary capillary wedge pressure (PCWP) of 12 mmHg.* **B,** *Reverse curve of patient in cardiac failure. Diuresis occurred showing optimal PCWP of 14 mmHg.*

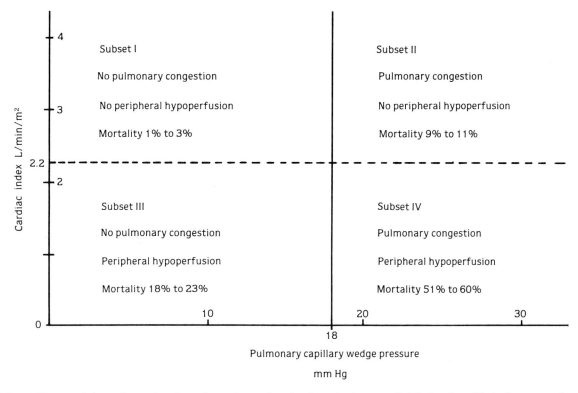

Fig. 13-6 *Forrester's hemodynamic subsets for patients after they have had myocardial infarction. Clinical status and mortality are given for each subset. Patient's position within subsets is determined by the intersection of the patient's pulmonary capillary wedge pressure and the cardiac index. (Data from Forrester JS and others: N Engl J Med 295:1356, 1404, 1976.)*

cluded obtundation, fatigue, reduced blood pressure, increased heart rate, cold skin, and oliguria (decreased urine output). Peripheral hypoperfusion was found to correlate with a cardiac index of less than 2.2 L/min/m². The patients were then grouped according to both the clinical signs and hemodynamics and were found to fall into four *hemodynamic subsets* (Fig. 13–6). Although it must be remembered that alterations in ventricular compliance may change the relationship of pressure and volume, construction of the patient's ventricular function curve over the graph for the hemodynamic subsets helps the novice understand what is happening to the patient. For example, if the patient's pulmonary capillary wedge pressure is 20 mmHg and the cardiac index is 2 L/min/m², the patient falls within subset IV. When the pulmonary capillary wedge pressure is high, the clinician can expect the patient to experience pulmonary congestion. When cardiac index is decreased, the patient can be expected to show clinical signs of decreased perfusion. Additionally, the combination of hypoperfusion and pulmonary congestion is accompanied by a high mortality if treatment does not move the patient back toward subset I (wedge pressure less than 18 mmHg, cardiac index greater than 2.2 L/min/m², and no clinical signs of hypoperfusion or pulmonary congestion).

EFFECTS OF MECHANICAL VENTILATION ON PRELOAD AND VENOUS RETURN.

Normal Spontaneous Breathing. During normal spontaneous *inspiration,* contraction of the dia-phragm and enlargement of the thoracic cage reduces the intrapleural pressure to approximately –6 cm H_2O. The decrease in intrapleural pressure enlarges the normally negative gradient between the intrathoracic and extrathoracic vessels, favors the movement of blood into the chest and heart, and increases venous return. These negative inspiratory pressures are also transferred to the heart. The resulting fall in intracardiac pressures pulls more blood into the heart, which augments preload. During spontaneous *expiration,* the reverse occurs. Recoil of the lung causes the intrathoracic pressure to rise augmenting output of the heart and creating the slight rise in arterial blood pressure that is normally seen with expiration. Thus spontaneous inspiration functions as a circulatory assist pump for the heart. During *labored breathing,* these pressure changes are increased and may result in a *paradoxical pulse*—a drop in blood pressure during inspiration of more than 10 mmHg.

Increased Intrapleural Pressure. Increased intrapleural pressure, as occurs during the Valsalva maneuver, decreases venous return, and cardiac output may be decreased.[9,10] Increased intrapleural pressure also occurs with loss of spontaneous breathing, disruption of the chest wall, collection of fluid or air in the pleural space, or positive pressure ventilation.

Positive Pressure Ventilation and Compliance. The effect positive breathing has on venous return depends on how much of the airway pressure is transferred to the pleural space.[8,9] When lung and thorax *compliances are equal,* only about half of the change in airway pressure is transmitted to the pleural space. If the lung becomes stiff (*decreased compliance*), as occurs with certain types of respiratory failure, less positive pressure is transmitted to the pleural space; thus these patients can better tolerate positive pressure ventilation with little effect on cardiovascular function.

When *chest wall compliance decreases,* more airway pressure is transmitted to the pleural space. This is commonly seen with abdominal distention or following surgery when the patients are splinting their chests and abdomens because of pain. If *chest wall compliance is decreased while lung compliance is increased* (e.g., chronic obstructive pulmonary disease, COPD), even more of the raised airway pressure is transmitted to the pleural space. These patients are more likely to develop problems of both decreased venous return and increased pulmonary vascular resistance resulting in decreased cardiac output during positive pressure ventilation.

PEEP and CPAP. Positive expiratory pressures including auto-PEEP not only exaggerate the inspiratory effects of positive pressure ventilation, they also maintain increased intrapleural pressure throughout expiration thus having an even greater potential of decreasing venous return. It has been shown that *venous return* is affected most by continuous mechanical ventilation (CMV) with PEEP, less by continuous positive airway pressure (CPAP), and least by spontaneous breathing ambient inspiratory pressure and PEEP.[8-12] *Cardiac output* is affected less by positive airway pressure (CMV, PEEP, CPAP) if intravascular volume is maintained or increased to offset the ventilator-induced fall in venous return.[13,14] In mechanically ventilated COPD patients with intrinsic (inadvertent) PEEP due to flow limitation, applied PEEP levels exceeding 85% of intrinsic PEEP caused further hyperinflation, decreased cardiac index and compromised hemodynamics and gas exchange.[15] The effect of mechanical ventilation on pulmonary artery pressure measurement is discussed in Chapter 14.

In summary, the heart, being inside the chest, is subject to the pressure changes occurring in the chest. Positive pressures around the heart "push" on the heart which makes it harder for blood to enter the heart (decrease venous return) but easier for blood to be ejected. On the other hand, negative pressures around the heart pull blood toward the heart (increase venous return and preload) but make it more difficult for blood to leave the heart.

Afterload

Afterload, the resistance or sum of the external factors that oppose ventricular ejection, has two components: tension in the ventricular wall and peripheral resistance (sometimes called impedance).

CARDIAC FACTORS. Cardiac factors that deter ventricular emptying include the following:
- Distention of the ventricle
- Increased intraventricular pressure
- Thin ventricular wall
- Negative intrathoracic pressure[16,17]

Resistance to ventricular emptying is even greater when both ventricle distention and intraventricular pressure are increased at the same time.

Increased Afterload. When the ventricle is distended from too much volume and pressure, tension in the muscle increases and more oxygen and energy are required for contraction: afterload is increased. Similarly, as intrathoracic pressure becomes more negative the vacuumlike effect favors the opening and filling of the ventricle but increases resistance to ventricular emptying.

Decreased Afterload. Positive intrathoracic pressure favors compression of the ventricle, decreases the pressure gradient across the ventricular wall, and decreases resistance to ventricular emptying, but opposes right ventricular filling.[18,19] Intermittent positive pressure breathing (IPPB) with PEEP has been shown to compress the heart during inspiration, "reducing the gradient for diastolic filling but at the same time enhancing systolic emptying, a perfect combination for many patients in congestive heart failure."[20,21] Afterload also decreases as the size of the ventricular muscles increases.

VASCULAR RESISTANCE. The peripheral component of afterload is determined by the following:
- The elasticity (compliance) of the vessels
- The size (radius) of the vessels
- The viscosity of the blood
- The changes in pressure from one end of the vessel to the other

Increased Vascular Resistance. The *radius* of the vessels is the greatest determinant of peripheral resistance to blood flow. When the vessels are constricted, the heart must exert more energy to eject the blood. Vasoconstriction increases afterload further because the constricted vessels are less compliant. As afterload is increased, the *myocardial oxygen demands* of the heart are also increased. When the heart is receiving an inadequate supply of oxygen (as occurs with coronary artery disease), it is not able to produce the amount of energy needed to eject efficiently against the afterload, and failure worsens. A downward cycle of cardiac failure ensures if the afterload is not decreased; inadequate cardiac output causes vasoconstriction, which causes increased work for the heart, which results in less cardiac output and more vasoconstriction, and so on. The cycle is broken by maximizing cardiac oxygenation and performance and decreasing the afterload, either by vasodilator therapy or with a cardiac assist device such as an intraaortic balloon pump.

Afterload is also increased as the *viscosity* of the blood increases. This is an important consideration in

Table 13-3 Normal Values and Formulas for Vascular Resistances*

Variable	Normal Range†	Formula
Pulmonary vascular resistance	<2 units 110–250 dynes/sec/cm⁵	PVR = (MPAP – PCWP)/CO PVR = (MPAP – PCWP)/CO × 80‡
Pulmonary vascular resistance index	225–315 dynes/sec/cm⁵/m²	PVRI = (MPAP – PCWP)/CI × 80‡
Systemic vascular resistance	15–20 units 900–1400 dynes/sec/cm⁵	SVR = (MAP – CVP)/CO SVR = (MAP – CVP)/CO × 80†
Systemic vascular resistance index	1970–2400 dynes/sec/cm⁵/m²	SVRI = (MAP – CVP)/CI × 80†

*Data from references 3–5.
†Normal values for adults. Sources vary in normal values reported, but values are within the same general ranges.
‡Conversion factors of 79.92 and 79.96 may also be used.[3,4]

patients with chronic pulmonary disease because the concentration of red cells in their blood is often abnormally high to increase their oxygen-carrying capacity. When hematocrits significantly exceed normal values, cardiac output decreases. Conversely, one of the causes of high cardiac output (hyperdynamic state) is anemia, low hematocrit.

Blood flows from high to low pressure. When the backpressure in the venous system increases, as occurs when the right heart is not able to pump blood efficiently, the pressure gradient across the capillary beds decreases. Flow from the arteries through the capillaries to the venous system is slowed. This damming effect causes the afterload to be increased.

Decreased Vascular Resistance. It is important to remember that although vasodilator therapy decreases afterload and therefore decreases the energy demands on the heart, it also increases the size of the "vascular container." If the container is made larger but the volume in the container stays the same, the amount of blood returning to the heart (venous return) is decreased, and preload is decreased. Conversely, when the volume in the ventricle is more than the ventricle can pump effectively, decreasing the preload can unload the ventricle and improve cardiac output. However, if the venous return is decreased too much, the stretch on the ventricle (preload) will be inadequate and cardiac output will fall. Additionally, if vasodilation causes the arterial diastolic pressure to fall below 50 mmHg or mean arterial pressure to fall below 60 mmHg, perfusion to the coronary arteries may be decreased, and cardiac output will be compromised even further.

CALCULATING SYSTEMIC AND PULMONARY VASCULAR RESISTANCE. Calculation of *systemic vascular resistance (SVR)* and *pulmonary vascular resistance (PVR)* provides numbers that can be used to evaluate the vascular component of afterload for each of the ventricles. As the numbers increase, afterload is increasing; decreasing numbers mean that afterload is decreasing. There are three sets of normal values for vascular resistance. They can be calculated in hybrid resistance units (mmHg/L/min), multiplied by 80 and

reported as absolute resistance units (dynes/sec/cm⁵) or divided by cardiac index and reported as an index. Formulas for calculating pulmonary and systemic vascular resistance and their normal values are listed in Table 13–3.

Elevated systemic vascular resistance can be caused by anything that causes vasoconstriction: cold, inadequate perfusion, hypertension, or drugs that vasoconstrict, such as norepinephrine (Levophed), methoxamine (Vasoxyl), or epinephrine (Adrenalin). Warming a hypothermic patient to normal temperature or administering vasodilators such as nitroprusside, isoproterenol, phentolamine (Regitine), or chlorpromazine (Thorazine) *decrease systemic vascular resistance.*

Pulmonary vascular resistance is increased by constriction, obstruction, or compression of the pulmonary vasculature or by backpressure from the left heart. Hypoxemia, acidosis, and release of histamine from an allergic response also cause vasoconstriction with an increase in pulmonary vascular resistance. Over time, increased pulmonary vascular resistance causes changes in the pulmonary vasculature, resulting in pulmonary hypertension and eventually cor pulmonale. Causes of pulmonary hypertension and cor pulmonale are listed in Table 13–4.

Contractility

The strength of a cardiac contraction is modified by two major influences:

1. Change in the initial muscle length caused by stretch of the cardiac muscle (preload)
2. Change in contractility or inotropic state of the heart at any given amount of muscle stretch[22]

For all practical purposes, contractility can be thought of as a change in the force and speed of shortening of the heart muscle that is independent of changes in preload or afterload.[22] Referring back to Fig. 13–3, it can be seen that an increase in contractility is associated with an increase in cardiac output despite no change in the preload. Conversely, heart failure is usually accompanied by decreased contractility with a

Table 13–4	Causes of Pulmonary Hypertension and Cor Pulmonale*
Mechanisms	**Related Disorders**
Loss of pulmonary vasculature and tissue (blockage, compression, destruction)	Primary pulmonary hypertension, multiple pulmonary emboli, pulmonary thrombosis
	Malignant metastasis, collagen-vascular diseases
	Inflammatory and fibrosing disease of the lung (diffuse interstitial pneumonia, sarcoidosis, the pneumonconioses)
Pulmonary vasoconstriction resulting from hypoxia and acidosis	COPD (emphysema, bronchitis, asthma)
	Neuromuscular disorders (e.g., myasthenia gravis, Guillain-Barré syndrome, poliomyelitis)
	Extreme obesity (pickwickian syndrome)
	Thoracic spine and chest wall deformities
Increased pulmonary venous pressure	Mitral valve stenosis, left atrial embolus or tumor, rheumatic heart disease
	Idiopathic veno-occlusive disease
Increased pulmonary blood flow (left-to-right shunt)	Ventricular septal defect, patent ductus arteriosus
Increased blood viscosity	Polycythemia

*Adapted from Margulies DM and Thaler MS: *The physician's book of lists.* New York, 1983, Churchill Livingstone.

downward shift of the ventricular function curve and a lowering of cardiac output for a given preload.

FACTORS RELATED TO CONTRACTILITY. Myocardial contractility is related to the following factors.

Sympathetic Nerve Stimulation. Sympathetic nerve stimulation with release of norepinephrine and other circulating catecholamines results in an increase in the strength and the rate of cardiac contraction: the "fight-or-flight" response. Conversely, inhibiting the sympathetic nervous system with a drug or by total spinal anesthesia depresses contractility. Parasympathetic stimulation (vagal stimulation) also decreases contractility.

Inotropic Drugs. Inotropic drugs are medications that affect the strength of contraction. A drug with a *positive inotropic effect* increases the force and velocity of contraction and myocardial oxygen consumption. Positive inotropic drugs include calcium, digitalis, epinephrine, norepinephrine, dopamine, dobutamine, amrinone, isoproterenol, and caffeine. If a positive inotropic drug is used to drive the heart when there is inadequate preload, myocardial oxygen supply and demand can become increasingly mismatched and even result in myocardial infarction. Therefore, preload must be maximized before driving the heart with these drugs.

Drugs with a *negative inotropic effect* decrease the strength of contraction but may also decrease the myocardial oxygen demand. Negative inotropic drugs include β blockers, barbiturates, and many of the antiarrhythmic agents such as procainamide and quinidine. In a patient with angina resulting from myocardial ischemia, negative inotropic agents such as β blockers may be used to enhance the relationship of myocardial oxygen supply to demand.

Physiologic Depressants. Physiologic depressants include hypoxia, hypercapnia, and acidosis. Decreased extravascular calcium and elevated potassium and sodium levels can severely depress contractility and cause the heart to become flaccid. An excess of calcium ions has the opposite effect, causing the heart

to go into spastic contraction. Low potassium and sodium levels are associated with cardiac fibrillation. Conduction disturbances and arrhythmia from any cause can decrease cardiac performance.

Damage to the Heart. Damage to the myocardium, valves, or conduction system reduces the pumping ability of the heart. Loss of ventricular substance results in decreased contractility because of the reduced effectiveness of muscle contraction, as in cardiomyopathy, myocardial ischemia, and myocarditis. The muscle in the area of a myocardial infarction may have no contraction or, over time, may even balloon out and develop into a ventricular aneurysm.

Chronic increase in the workload of the heart over time will result in enlargement of the chambers and hypertrophy of the muscle.

Coronary Blood Flow. Coronary blood flow is autoregulated within the range of mean aortic pressures of 60 to 180 mmHg.[23] Normal *coronary perfusion pressure (CPP)* is 60 to 80 mmHg and is calculated as follows[5]:

$$CPP = diastolic\ BP - PCWP$$

When mean arterial pressure or diastolic pressure falls, perfusion of the coronary sinus may be compromised resulting in decreased myocardial oxygen delivery and a subsequent fall in contractility.

VARIABLES USED TO ASSESS CONTRACTILITY. Unfortunately, it is not possible to directly conclude that the cause of low cardiac output is decreased contractility. Additionally, there is no absolute hemodynamic measure of contractility. *Stroke volume* is a good indicator of ventricular performance and is directly related to the degree of myocardial fiber shortening and circumferential ventricular size. Other variables used to describe ventricular performance and pumping efficiency include *ejection fraction, cardiac work, stroke work,* and their indices. These calculations

Table 13-5 Conditions Associated with Alteration in Hemodynamic Measurements Used to Evaluate Low Cardiac Output

Normal Hemodynamics*	Altered Hemodynamics	Conditions	Usual Correction
Preload Right heart 　CVP and RAP = 2–6 mmHg 　　or 4–12 cm H_2O Left heart 　LAP, PCWP, PADP = 　　6–15 mmHg 　EDV = 120–180 mL/beat Urine output 30 mL/hr	Low pressure or EDV ↓ CVP, ↓ PCWP, and ↓ urine output	1. Inadequate vascular volume 2. ↓ SVR (vasodilation) from drugs, spinal anesthetic, fever, sepsis 3. SVR may ↑ (vasoconstriction) to maintain MAP and CO if significant hypovolemia has developed	1. Volume expansion: IV solutions, blood, albumin 2. Stop vasodilators; volume expansion, vasoconstriction 3. Volume expansion; if SVR does not ↓, vasodilation and additional volume may be needed
	High pressure or EDV = poor pump/too much volume 1. ↑ CVP or PCWP	1. a. Cardiac failure 　b. Cardiac tamponade	1. a. Inotropic drugs, diuretics 　b. Volume expansion and isoproterenol until correction of tamponade
	2. ↓ CVP and ↑ PCWP	2. Left heart failure, intraoperative myocardial infarction, left heart valve malfunction	2. Inotropic drugs, vasodilate to ↓ SVR, surgical correction
	3. ↑ CVP and ↓ PCWP	3. a. Right heart failure/valve malfunction 　b. Chronic pulmonary disease 　c. Pulmonary embolism	3. a. Inotropic drugs, surgical correction 　b. ↓ PVR, watch for hypovolemia with low PCWP 　c. Heparin, inotropic drugs, vasopressors, surgical correction
Afterload SVR = <20 units or 　900–1400 dyne · sec/cm^5	1. ↑ SVR, ↓ CVP and PCWP	1. Vasoconstriction: body's natural response to maintain perfusion to vital organs when BP drops; ↓ temperature	1. Volume expansion; warm to normal temperature, watch for hypovolemia with vasodilation from warming
Urine output: 　Adult ≃ 30 mL/hr 　Pediatric ≥ 1 mL/Kg/hr	2. ↑ SVR and ↑ PCWP	2. ↑ SVR is compensation for failing pump; if uncorrected, will proceed to downward cycle of cardiac failure to cardiogenic shock	2. Vasodilators, diuretics, inotropic drugs
Extremities warm Capillary refill <3 sec	3. ↓ SVR	3. Vasodilation: spinal anesthetic, ↑ temperature, vasovagal response, sepsis	3. Stop vasodilators/diuretics; consider volume expansion; inotropic drugs, possible vasoconstrictors

*RAP = right atrial pressure; LAP = left atrial pressure; PADP = pulmonary artery diastolic pressure; CPP = cerebral perfusion pressure. For other abbreviations see text.

are used to describe the work the heart can do and thereby imply its contractile ability.

Rate-pressure product is a simplified approach to evaluating cardiac work. It is obtained by multiplying the easily obtained variables of heart rate and systolic blood pressure, based on the well-established fact that increases in heart rate and blood pressure result in increases in myocardial oxygen demand. Values that are greater than 12,000 are thought to indicate increased myocardial work and increased oxygen demand.

Echocardiography and radionuclide cardiac imaging, which are discussed later in this chapter, can provide for visual assessment of ventricular volumes and function. Transthoracic electrical bioimpedance, a noninvasive method of measuring cardiac performance variables, can also be used to assess the ventricular contractile state.

Table 13–5 lists the hemodynamic measurements most commonly used to evaluate each of the three determinants of cardiac output: preload, afterload, and contractility. It also lists changes in the variables that alter cardiac performance and gives some associated conditions and management.

Methods of Measuring Cardiac Output

The indicator-dilution method using optical dyes (dye-dilution), thermodilution, the estimated Fick method, echocardiography, transthoracic bioimpedence, and radionuclide imaging are the most common techniques for measurement of cardiac output in critical care units.

Invasive Methods

DYE-DILUTION CARDIAC OUTPUT. The *dye-dilution cardiac output* method requires insertion of a catheter into a central vein or pulmonary artery for

Table 13-5 Conditions Associated with Alteration in Hemodynamic Measurements Used to Evaluate Low Cardiac Output—*continued*

Normal Hemodynamics*	Altered Hemodynamics	Conditions	Usual Correction
Contractility CI = 2.5–4.0 L/min/m^2 SV = 60–130 mL SVI = 30–50 mL/m^2	Causes of decreased contractility: 1. ↓ Volume		1. Volume expansion; in some failing hearts, PCWP must be kept at 15–18 mmHg or higher to maintain contractility
RVSWI = 8.8 ± 0.9 g · min/m^2 LVSWI = 56 ± 6 g · min/m^2 MAP = 80–100 mmHg Diastolic BP = 60–80 mmHg CPP = 60–80 mmHg See Table 13–2 for formulas	2. Inadequate coronary perfusion/heart muscle	2. Inadequate diastolic pressure; Coronary stenosis, occlusion; Myocardial ischemia, infarction; Ventricular aneurysm, Congenital defects, Surgery	2. Maintain MAP > 60, diastolic pressure > 50 mmHg (watch for drop in diastolic pressure with vasodilators); Angioplasty, surgery Inotropic drugs when volume is adequate (driving heart when volume is low could lead to myocardial infarction) Low-dose inotropic support may be used continuously for 24–48 hr after surgery to support a weak myocardium
	3. HR >110 beats/min HR <60 beats/min		3. ↓ rate: assure adequate volume; β blockers, calcium antagonists ↑ rate: atropine; rarely, isoproterenol Pacemaker (CO may ↓ if loss of atrial kick)
	4. Arrhythmia	4. ↓ K$^+$, Ca^{2+}, O$_2$ Drug-induced Other	4. Replace K$^+$, Ca^{2+}, maintain adequate Pao$_2$ Withdraw/change medication Treat with antiarrhythmics, cardioversion, pacemaker
	5. Negative inotropic drugs, β blockers (propranolol), antiarrhythmics, barbiturates		5. ↓ or discontinue medication; inotropic drugs prn
	6. ↑ SVR (heart must work harder to pump against vasoconstriction)		6. Vasodilators with volume expansion if necessary; inotropic drugs
	7. ↓ Po$_2$, pH, K$^+$, Na$^+$, Ca^{2+}, ↑ Pco$_2$, K$^+$, Na$^+$		7. Correct oxygenation, electrolytes, acid-base balance

injection of the dye sample and an arterial catheter for withdrawal of blood. A bolus of dye (usually 5 mg of indocyanine green) is injected into the central venous catheter while arterial blood is withdrawn at a steady rate (usually 10 mL/min) through a densitometer cuvette by a syringe withdrawal pump. The densitometer is a device that sends a light beam through the blood to a photocell in the cuvette. When the bolus of dye crosses the light source, the amount of light that can pass through the blood decreases and a curve is produced on paper or in the computer (Fig. 13–7). As the concentration of dye in the blood increases, the light transmission decreases and the curve rises; then when the concentration of dye decreases, the curve falls. Cardiac output is inversely proportional to the area under the curve. If the cardiac output is low, the dye will spread over more blood and take longer to pass through the densitometer; therefore, there is more area under the curve. A high output generally produces a narrower curve (less area under the curve).

THERMODILUTION CARDIAC OUTPUT.

Thermodilution cardiac output measurement requires the placement of a thermodilution pulmonary artery catheter and the appropriate thermodilution cardiac computer for the type of catheter used. The indicator measured for this technique is change in blood temperature. Sterile dextrose in water or normal saline solution at least 2° C colder than blood temperature is injected into the proximal port (right atrium) of the pulmonary artery line. The temperature change (cooling, sometimes called *heat loss*) is detected by a thermistor bead located just behind the balloon of the catheter which is positioned in the pulmonary artery (Fig. 13–8). A temperature-time curve much like the dye-dilution curve is recorded by the computer. Thermodilution output measurements can be repeated as often as every 60 seconds because the blood rewarms in one pass through the system and there is no recirculation as with optical dyes.

Acceptable Variations in Thermodilution Injection Technique. Accurate thermodilution results can be achieved using iced, refrigerated, or room temperature injectant in most patients.[24-26] Injection can be via the proximal injectant lumen, proximal

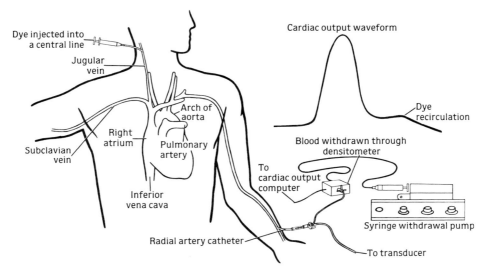

Fig. 13-7 *Dye-dilution cardiac output measurement.*

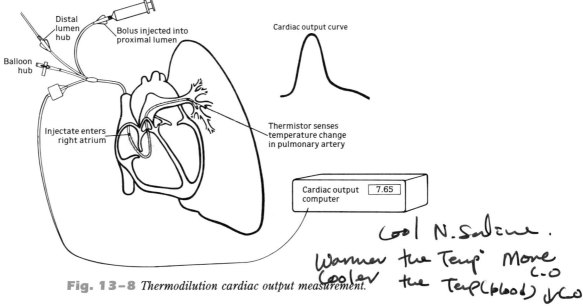

Fig. 13-8 *Thermodilution cardiac output measurement.*

infusion lumen, right atrial port, venous infusion port, or the side port of the introducer catheter.[27-29] An average of multiple determinations with *injections equally spaced throughout the respiratory cycle* has been shown to provide the best estimate of mean cardiac output.[30] Manual injection at end-exhalation may not accurately reflect the average cardiac output, especially in mechanically ventilated patients.[31] Use of an injection gun and a connecting system that measures the injectant temperature as it enters the catheter produces more consistent thermodilution cardiac output readings.[31,32]

Accuracy and reproducibility of results for both methods depend on extremely careful attention to detail and technique. Indicators must be measured precisely and injected as a bolus in less than 3 seconds. Computers must be calibrated, carefully maintained by biomedical engineers, and balanced before each measurement. Catheters must be properly located, patent,

and tips must be away from the wall of the vessel. The cardiac monitor should be watched during cardiac output measurements because arrhythmia may change the cardiac output. When a significant arrhythmia does occur, the cardiac output should be recorded separately (not averaged into the set) and noted to occur with the identified arrhythmia. Then another output measurement is obtained, averaged into the set, and recorded as cardiac output without the presence of arrhythmia.

FICK CARDIAC OUTPUT. The *Fick method of cardiac output* measurement is based on Adolph Fick's principle and can be calculated as follows.[1,2]

$$CO \text{ (L/min)} = \frac{O_2 \text{ absorbed by the lungs (mL/min)}}{\text{arteriovenous } O_2 \text{ difference (mL/L)}} = \frac{\dot{V}O_2}{C(a-v)O_2}$$

Accurate calculation of a Fick cardiac output reading requires the collection of inspired and expired gases as well as arterial and mixed venous blood samples while the patient is in a steady state. This method is usually considered the gold standard against which other forms of cardiac output measurement are validated, but it is rarely employed in the ICU. However, by using a normal or expected value of oxygen consumption and measuring the arteriovenous oxygen difference, an estimated Fick cardiac output reading can be obtained in the ICU setting. Three steps are required:

1. *Calculate the expected* oxygen consumption ($\dot{V}o_2$). The normal range of oxygen consumption[3] is 120 to 160 mL/min/m^2 with an average of 125 mL/min/m^2. For a patient with a body surface area of 2 m^2, oxygen consumption would be calculated as follows:

$$\dot{V}o_2 = 125 \text{ mL/min/m}^2 \times 2 \text{ m}^2 = 250 \text{ mL/min}$$

2. *Calculate the arterial and mixed venous oxygen contents and arteriovenous oxygen difference.* The following example is calculated for a hemoglobin of 14 g/100 mL, an arterial oxygen saturation (Sao_2) of 90%, and a mixed venous oxygen saturation ($S\bar{v}o_2$) of 60%.

O₂ Saturation	×	Hb	×	1.34 =	O₂ Content
Arterial	0.90 ×	14 ×	1.34 =	16.884	CaO_2
Mixed venous	0.60 ×	14 ×	1.34 =	11.256	$C\bar{v}O_2$
			$C(a-v)o_2 =$	5.628	

Arteriovenous oxygen difference, sometimes referred to verbally as the "a-v O$_2$ difference," is the difference between arterial and venous oxygen contents. The normal range for arteriovenous oxygen difference is 3.0 to 5.5 vol%.[33]

The *lower* the $C(a-v)o_2$, the smaller the amount of oxygen removed per 100 mL of blood passing through the capillaries. Low values are seen when:

- Well-oxygenated blood moves rapidly through the capillaries (high cardiac output)
- Cells extract less oxygen (septic shock)
- Oxygen is not released from hemoglobin (left-sided shift in the oxyhemoglobin dissociation curve)
- Anemia

Higher $C(a-v)o_2$ values indicate more oxygen was removed, as occurs when:

- Blood flow is slow (low cardiac output) *or*
- Tissue extraction of oxygen is high (increased oxygen consumption)

3. *Calculate the cardiac output. Remember to convert the mL/min/vol% to L/min:*

$$CO(L/min) = \frac{\dot{V}o_2}{C(a-v)o_2} = \frac{250 \text{ mL/min}}{5.628 \text{ vol}\%} = 44.8 \text{ mL/min/vol}\%$$

$$44.8 \times 100 = 4480 \text{ mL/min} = 4.48 \text{ L/min}$$

ESTIMATING CARDIAC OUTPUT. When patients do not have arterial or pulmonary artery lines in place, the following additional assumptions may be applied to obtain an estimated cardiac output; however, the chance of error is increased with each assumption used.

1. Arterial oxygen saturation is 95%.
2. Central venous blood is used for the blood sample rather than obtaining a true mixed venous sample from the pulmonary artery line.

The level of arteriovenous oxygen difference is linear and inversely proportional to CI as follows[34]:

C(a–v)o₂ (vol%)		Cardiac index (L/min/m²)
>6	≅	<2
>5	≅	<3
4	≅	3
>3	≅	<4
<3	≅	>5

CONTINUOUS CARDIAC OUTPUT MONITORING. Other invasive methods used successfully for continuous measurement of cardiac output include electromagnetic flow probes placed around the aorta; miniature ultrasound probes attached to the adventitia of the ascending aorta[35]; arterial pulse contour analysis; and transtracheal, transesophageal, and intravascular ultrasound. Modifications to the pulmonary artery catheter using fiberoptics, rapid response thermistors, Doppler ultrasound, electrode bands for measuring impedance, and electrodes for intracardiac electrocardiography (ECG) have made it possible to monitor cardiac output, Svo₂, right ventricular ejection fraction,[36-38] and other indices of right ventricular function at the bedside.[39] Methods for continuous cardiac output monitoring that have developed from this catheter technology include intracardiac impedance, "injectless" cold thermodilution, continuous thermodilution, and continuous Svo₂ monitoring. Their correlation with standard cardiac output methods is being evaluated. Whether these methods will prove to be reliable and accurate in multiple patient types remains to be seen.

Continuous Svo₂ Monitoring. Continuous Svo₂ monitoring has been suggested as an alternative to intermittent, serial cardiac output measurements. Based on the Fick equation, if total body oxygen consumption, hemoglobin, and Sao₂ remain constant, a change in cardiac output should be reflected by a parallel change in Svo₂. Although significant correlation between cardiac output and Svo₂ has been shown in critically ill patients who are in a steady state,[40-42] Svo₂ has not been found to be predictive of cardiac index in postoperative cardiac surgery patients[43] or mixed populations of critically ill patients.[44,45]

Pulse Contour Cardiac Output Monitoring.

The pulse contour method is an analysis of an arterial pressure waveform by an analog computer. It requires simultaneous measurement of the arterial pressure and cardiac output by another method such as thermodilution, dye-dilution, or the Fick method to obtain a baseline cardiac output reading. Thereafter, a continuous cardiac output reading may be obtained via the arterial catheter used for arterial blood pressure monitoring provided the patient does not have a change in peripheral vascular resistance. This technique has been shown to have moderate correlation with bolus thermodilution in pre- and postcardiopulmonary bypass patients.[46] Obtaining continuous cardiac output readings using a noninvasive finger blood pressure cuff is also being evaluated.[47]

Transtracheal, Transesophageal, and Intravascular Ultrasound.

Doppler ultrasonic transducers positioned on tubes or catheters measure the velocity of blood flow and the vessel diameter from which volumetric blood flow in liters per minute can be calculated. These transducers have been used in different body locations to obtain cardiac output measurements. The *transesophageal* transducer is positioned in the esophagus at the level of the fifth and sixth vertebrae (approximately 35 cm from the mouth) and pointed posteriorly to assess descending aortic blood flow. Signals can be obtained every 2 to 10 minutes. Transesophageal probes have been left in place for up to 4 days without significant complications.[48] *Transtracheal Doppler ultrasound*[49] is accomplished via a transducer which is attached to the end of an endotracheal tube so that it can be in continuous contact with the tracheal wall. Because these devices look at flow in the descending aorta, which does not contain total cardiac output, they cannot provide an actual cardiac output measurement. They can, however, provide measures of flow, including flow time, peak velocity, and stroke distance, which correlate with stroke volume. One-time calibration using transcutaneous Doppler ultrasound cardiac output measurements has been used in an attempt to find a proportionality factor which could be used to convert the flow measurements to actual cardiac output measurement. This technique has not proved to be reliable. However, these devices may find more use in situations where it is important to identify hemodynamic changes but where it is not necessary to know the actual cardiac output.

Continuous intravenous Doppler ultrasound cardiac output measurements[50] are obtained via a transducer which is mounted on the distal section of a pulmonary artery catheter and positioned in the main pulmonary artery proximal to the bifurcation. Cardiac outputs obtained by this method have a moderate correlation ($r = 0.73$) to bolus thermodilution.[51]

Continuous Thermodilution Cardiac Output.

Two methods for obtaining continuous cardiac output measurements using the thermodilution method are being used. They have the advantage of *not* requiring a calibration cardiac output measurement by another standard cardiac output technique. "Injectless" cold thermodilution uses a balloon on the proximal section of a pulmonary artery catheter. Iced solution is automatically injected into the balloon and withdrawn at intervals. The distal temperature changes are analyzed as they would be for a bolus thermodilution measurement. The practicality of using this automatic iced injector at the patient's bedside may be a limiting factor to the use of this technique.

Another continuous thermodilution technique measures volumetric flow using a specialized thermal filament located near the proximal injectant port of the pulmonary artery catheter. The filament, usually situated in the right ventricle, adds small amounts of heat to the blood in a specific, repetitive, on-off pattern which the computer can recognize as unique to the catheter and not caused by other physiologic or environmental events. These pulses serve as the indicator, which is then sensed by the distal thermistor in the same way it would be sensed using the standard bolus thermodilution technique. Computer analysis produces a curve much like the standard thermodilution curve and the cardiac output. Measurements are the average of data collected over the previous 3 to 5 minutes and are updated on the screen every 30 seconds. Heat production is minimal since the blood temperature sensed by the distal thermistor is typically less than $0.05°C$.

Noninvasive Methods for Measuring Cardiac Performance

Noninvasive methods for measuring cardiac performance include transthoracic electrical bioimpedance, echocardiography, radionuclide cardiac imaging, Doppler ultrasound, and estimates of cardiac index from pulse pressure.

CONTINUOUS MEASUREMENT OF CARDIAC PERFORMANCE USING TRANSTHORACIC ELECTRICAL BIOIMPEDANCE.

Transthoracic electrical bioimpedance provides continuous, real-time, noninvasive measurement of variables that describe global blood flow, left ventricular performance, pumping efficiency, and volume status.[52–59] Because blood is the most electrically conductive substance in the body and the thorax can act like a transducer, the electrical conductivity in the thorax can be translated into blood flow data. Eight ECG-type electrodes, two on either side of the neck and two on either side of the chest, form the interface between the patient and the computer terminal. Digitally displayed variables include cardiac output, stroke volume, heart rate, ejection velocity, ejection time, and thoracic fluid index. Additional variables include end-diastolic volume, peak flow, index of contractility, acceleration index, ejection ratio, and systolic time ratio.

PERIODIC NONINVASIVE MEASUREMENT OF CARDIAC PERFORMANCE.

Echocardiography. Echocardiography[60] provides a noninvasive method of obtaining periodic data on cardiac performance. The use of *Doppler color flow mapping* with *two-dimensional* and *M-mode echocardiography* allows assessment of global ventricular function, including left ventricular volume, ejection fraction, fractional shortening, and circumferential fiber shortening. Additionally, echocardiography can be used to describe intracardiac blood flow and the origin of intracardiac shunts, diagnose pathologic lesions in and around the heart and great vessels, evaluate regional wall motion and its relationship to coronary artery insufficiency and myocardial infarction, and suggest the possibility of rejection in the infant with a transplanted heart. Though echocardiography does not provide continuous assessment of cardiac function, the portability of the current machines allows quality studies to be performed at the patient's bedside in the ICU. However, bandages, obesity, inability to turn or maintain a desired position, and air trapping in the lungs (as occurs with emphysematous patients) may make it difficult to obtain an adequate study using transthoracic imaging.

When a quality image cannot be obtained using a chest transducer, *transesophageal imaging* can be performed. Esophageal imaging provides especially good images of the chambers and the mitral valve, because the transducer is positioned immediately behind the left ventricle or left atrium.

Radionuclide Cardiac Imaging. Radionuclide cardiac imaging[60] techniques can be used to provide periodic information about cardiac performance. Thallium 201 can be injected and myocardial perfusion scanning can be done with a gamma camera or single photon emission computed tomography (SPECT). Areas of decreased perfusion or scars pick up a reduced amount of thallium, creating "cold" spots on the image. Radionuclide angiography can be done by two techniques: *first pass* and *gated blood pool* (multiple gated acquisition, or MUGA). Technetium 99m is the radioisotope injected in both cases. The images obtained permit visualization of wall motion and calculation of ejection fraction.

Pulse Pressure. *Pulse pressure* (the difference between the systolic and diastolic arterial pressure) can be used as a rough estimate of stroke index (1 mmHg = 1 mL/m^2), because stroke volume is the major determinant of pulse pressure. This estimate does not take into account the effects of peripheral vascular resistance on cardiac output but may have some value for obtaining cardiac output trends when hemodynamics are changing rapidly and it is not possible to obtain cardiac outputs by any other method.

REVIEW QUESTIONS

1. Given a stroke volume of 62 mL and a heart rate of 88/min, what is the cardiac output?
   a. 5.5 L/min
   b. 6.2 L/min
   c. 7.0 L/min
   d. 11.0 L/min

2. What is the normal range for cardiac output in an adult?
   a. 2 - 4 L/min
   b. 4 - 8 L/min
   c. 6 - 10 L/min
   d. 10 - 13 L/min

3. T F Sympathetic nervous stimulation can cause the cardiac output to triple.

4. T F Organs with lower metabolic requirements need more oxygen to function optimally.

5. Which of the following are true regarding the distribution of blood flow and venous return?
   a. 30% of the total blood volume is in the venous system
   b. blood is shunted to vital organs during cardiac failure
   c. circulatory function and pressures can be maintained with a loss of 40% of the blood volume
   d. all of the above

6. What is the normal value of cardiac index?
   a. 0.2 - 1.3 L/min/m^2
   b. 1.5 - 2.6 L/min/m^2
   c. 2.5 - 4.0 L/min/m^2
   d. 4 - 8 L/min/m^2

7. Which of the following correlates best with the oxygen requirements of the heart?
   a. stroke volume
   b. ejection fraction
   c. end-diastolic volume
   d. cardiac work

8. T F An ejection fraction of 32% would result in a severe reduction in exercise tolerance.

9. The amount of precontraction stretch applied to the ventricles is a definition of which of the following?
   a. preload
   b. afterload

c. contractility

d. ejection fraction

10. Preload of the left ventricle is assessed by which of the following parameters?
    a. arterial diastolic blood pressure
    b. mean arterial pressure
    c. central venous pressure
    d. pulmonary capillary wedge pressure

11. Which of the following would cause the measurement of preload to be reduced?
    a. increased ventricular compliance
    b. increased venous return
    c. cardiac tamponade
    d. all of the above

12. T   F   Ventricular function curves are used to determine an optimal pressure/ volume relationship to maintain adequate preload.

13. Which of the following are possible hemodynamic effects of using mechanical ventilation?
    a. reduced preload
    b. reduced cardiac output
    c. decreased afterload
    d. all of the above

14. Which of the following would increase left ventricular afterload?
    a. pulmonic valve stenosis
    b. decreased blood viscosity
    c. positive end expiratory pressure
    d. none of the above

15. T   F   Systemic vascular resistance is a measure of right ventricular afterload.

16. Which of the following would increase pulmonary vascular resistance?
    a. hypoxemia
    b. acidosis
    c. pulmonary emboli
    d. all of the above

17. Which of the following is true regarding cardiac contractility?
    a. it cannot be directly measured
    b. it is increased by beta blocking drugs
    c. it is increased by hypercapnia
    d. is increased by parasympathetic neural stimulation

18. Which of the following invasive cardiac output techniques requires the measurement of inhaled and exhaled gas concentrations?
    a. dye dilution
    b. thermodilution
    c. Fick
    d. pulse contour

19. Which of the following invasive cardiac output techniques requires the placement of a pulmonary artery catheter?
    a. dye dilution
    b. thermodilution
    c. Fick
    d. pulse contour

20. Which of the following is a noninvasive technique for determining cardiac performance?
    a. echocardiography
    b. transthoracic electrical bioimpedance
    c. radionuclide cardiac imaging
    d. all of the above

REFERENCES

1. Guyton AC: *Textbook of medical physiology,* ed 7, Philadelphia, 1986, WB Saunders.
2. Guyton AC: *Human physiology and mechanisms of disease,* ed 4, Philadelphia, 1987, WB Saunders.
3. Shoemaker WC: Monitoring of the critically ill patient. In Shoemaker WC and others: *Textbook of critical care medicine,* ed 2, Philadelphia, 1989, WB Saunders.
4. Pollard E and Seliger E: *An implementation of bedside physiological calculations,* Waltham, Mass, 1985, Hewlett-Packard.
5. Daily EK and Schroeder JS: *Techniques in bedside hemodynamic monitoring,* ed 4, St Louis, 1989, Mosby.
6. Sibbald WJ and Driedger AA: Right and left ventricular preload and diastolic ventricular compliance: implications for therapy in critically ill patients. In Shoemaker WC and Thompson WL, editors: *Critical care state of the art,* vol 3, Fullerton, Calif, 1982, Society of Critical Care Medicine.
7. Tarnow J: Swan-Ganz catheterization: application, interpretation, and complications, *Thorac Cardiovasc Surg* 30:130, 1982.
8. Leasa DJ and Sibbald WJ: Respiratory monitoring in a critical care unit. In Simmons DH, editor: *Current pulmonology,* vol 9, St Louis, 1988, Mosby.
9. Douglas ME and Downs JB: Applied physiology and respiratory care. In Shoemaker WC and Thompson WL, editors: *Critical care state of the art,* vol 3, Fullerton, Calif, 1982, Society of Critical Care Medicine.
10. Slutsky RS, Dittrich H, Peck WW: Radionuclide analysis of sequential changes in central circulatory volumes: inspiration, expiration, and the Valsalva maneuver *Crit Care Med* 11:913, 1983.
11. Downs JB and others: Ventilatory pattern, intrapleural pressure and cardiac output, *Anesth Analg* 56:88, 1977.
12. Greenbaum DM: Positive end-expiratory pressure, constant positive airway pressure, and cardiac performance, *Chest* 76:248, 1979.
13. Walkinshaw M and Shoemaker WC: Use of volume loading to obtain preferred levels of PEEP: a preliminary study, *Crit Care Med* 8:81, 1980.
14. Jardin F and others: Influence of positive end-expiratory pressure on left ventricular performance, *N Engl J Med* 304:387, 1981.

15. Ranieri VM and others: Physiologic effects of positive end-expiratory pressure in patients with chronic obstructive lung disease during acute ventilatory failure and controlled mechanical ventilation, *Am Rev Respir Dis* 147:5, 1993.

16. Robotham JL and others: A re-evaluation of the hemodynamic consequences of intermittent positive pressure ventilation, *Crit Care Med* 11:783, 1983.

17. Robotham JL: Cardiovascular disturbances in chronic respiratory insufficiency, *Am J Cardiol* 47:941, 1981.

18. Weber KT: Contractile mechanics and interaction of the right and left ventricles, *Am J Cardiol* 47:686, 1981.

19. Wood LD and Prewitt RM: Cardiovascular management in acute hypoxemic respiratory failure, *Am J Cardiol* 47:963, 1981.

20. Pinksy MR: The influence of positive-pressure ventilation on cardiovascular function in the critically ill, *Crit Care Clin* 1:699, 1985.

21. Biondi JW, Schulman DS, and Matthay RA: Effects of mechanical ventilation on right and left ventricular function, *Clin Chest Med* 9:55, 1988.

22. Sonnenblick EH: Force-velocity relations in mammalian heart muscle, *Am J Physiol* 202:931, 1962.

23. Gilbert BW and Hew EM: Physiologic significance of hemodynamic measurements. In Armstrong PW and Baigrie RS: Hemodynamic monitoring in the critically ill. New York, 1980, Harper & Row.

24. Price P and Fowlow B: Thermodilution cardiac output determinations: a comparison of iced and refrigerated injectate temperatures in patients after cardiac surgery, *Heart Lung* 22:266, 1993.

25. Pesola GR, Ayala B, Plante L: Room-temperature thermodilution cardiac output: proximal injectate lumen vs proximal infusion lumen, *Am J Crit Care* 2:132, 1993.

26. Pesola GR and Carlon GC: Room temperature thermodilution cardiac output: central venous vs right ventricular port, *Crit Care Med* 19:563, 1992.

27. Medley RS, DeLapp TD, Fisher DG: Comparability of the thermodilution cardiac output method: proximal injectate versus proximal infusion lumens, *Heart Lung* 21:12, 1992.

28. Hunn D and others: Thermodilution cardiac output values obtained by using a centrally placed introducer sheath and right atrial port of a pulmonary artery catheter, *Crit Care Med* 18:438, 1990.

29. Vicari M and Ogle V: Comparison of thermodilution cardiac output measurements by injection of the proximal lumen versus side port of the Swan-Ganz catheter, *Heart Lung* 14:126, 1985.

30. Thrush DN and Varlotta D: Thermodilution cardiac output: comparison between automated and manual injection of indicator, *J Cardiothorac Vasc Anesth* 6:17, 1992.

31. Dixon CT and others: Hand-held thermodilution cardiac output injector, *Crit Care Med* 5:210, 1977.

32. Nelson LD and Houtchens BA: Automatic vs manual injections for thermodilution cardiac output determinations, *Crit Care Med* 10:190, 1982.

33. Nunn JF: *Applied respiratory physiology,* Boston, 1977, Butterworth.

34. Siegel JH: Acute post-traumatic pulmonary insufficiency and the adult respiratory distress syndrome. In Berk JL and Sampliner JE, editors: *Handbook of critical care,* ed 2, Boston, 1982, Little, Brown.

35. Keagy BA and others: Constant postoperative monitoring of cardiac output after correction of congenital heart defects, *J Thorac Cardiovasc Surg* 93:658, 1987.

36. Rafferty T and others: Thermodilution right ventricular ejection fraction measurement reproducibility study in patients undergoing coronary artery bypass graft surgery, *Crit Care Med* 20:1524, 1992.

37. Dorman G and others: Use of a combined right ventricular ejection fraction–oximetry catheter system for coronary bypass surgery, *Crit Care Med* 20:1650, 1992.

38. Diebel L and others: End-diastolic volume: a better indicator of preload in the critically ill, *Arch Surg* 127:817, 1992.

39. Guerroero JE and others: Right ventricular systolic time intervals determined by means of a pulmonary artery catheter, *Crit Care Med* 20:1529, 1992.

40. Lee J and others: Central venous oxygen saturation in shock: a study in man, *Anesthesiology* 36:472, 1972.

41. Waller JL and others: Clinical evaluation of a new fiberoptic catheter oximiter during cardiac surgery, *Anesth Analg* 61:676, 1982.

42. Krauss XH and others: On-line monitoring of mixed venous oxygen saturation after cardiothoracic surgery, *Thorax* 30:636, 1975.

43. Magilligan DR, Jr and others: Mixed venous oxygen saturation as a predictor of cardiac output in the postoperative cardiac surgical patient, *Ann Thorac Surg* 44:260, 1987.

44. Vaughn S and Puri VK: Cardiac output changes and continuous mixed venous oxygen saturation measurement in the critically ill, *Crit Care Med* 16:496, 1988.

45. Sommers MS and others: Mixed venous oxygen saturation and oxygen partial pressure as predictors of cardiac index after coronary artery bypass grafting, *Heart Lung* 22:112, 1993.

46. Stren H, Donovan JW, Hines RL: A new method for the measurement of continuous cardiac output: pulse contour method, *Crit Care Med*

47. Gratz I and others: Continuous noninvasive cardiac output as estimated from the pulse contour curve, *J Clin Monit* 8:20, 1992.

48. Huntsman LL and others: Noninvasive Doppler determination of cardiac output in man: clinical validation, *Circulation* 67:593, 1983.

49. Abrams JH, Weber RF, Holeman KD: Continuous cardiac output determinations using transtracheal Doppler: initial results in humans, *Anesthesiology* 7:11, 1989.

50. Allard MW, Robinson LM, Leone BJ: The continuous determination of cardiac output using a flow directed Doppler pulmonary artery catheters [abstract], presented at Society of Cardiovascular Anesthesiologists 12th Annual Meeting, Orlando, Fla, May 13–16, 1990, 207.

51. Segal J and others: *Instantaneous and continuous cardiac output using a Doppler pulmonary artery catheter.* Mountain View, Calif, 1989, Cardiometrics.

52. Itchiness CS: ANNA journal course: new technologies in anesthesia: update for nurse anesthetists—noninvasive, continuous, cardiac output monitoring by thoracic electrical bioimpedance, *ANNA J* 59:445, 1991.

53. Bernstein DP: Continuous noninvasive real-time monitoring of stroke volume and cardiac output by thoracic electrical bioimpedance, *Crit Care Med* 14:898, 1986.

54. Shoemaker WC and others: Multicomponent noninvasive physiologic monitoring of circulatory function, *Crit Care Med* 16:482, 1988.

55. Introna RP and others: Use of transthoracic bioimpedance to determine cardiac output in pediatric patients, *Crit Care Med* 16:1101, 1988.

56. Tibballs J: A comparative study of cardiac output in neonates supported by mechanical ventilation: measurement with thoracic electrical bioimpedance and pulsed Doppler ultrasound, *J Pediatr* 114:632, 1989.

57. Appel PL and others: Comparison of measurements of cardiac output by bioimpedance and thermodilution in severely ill surgical patients, *Crit Care Med* 14:933, 1986.

58. Spinale F, Reines HD, Crawford FA: Electrical bioimpedance as a method for continuous noninvasive estimation of cardiac output: experimental and clinical studies, *Crit Care Med* 15:364, 1987.

59. Kalkat GS and others: Reliability of bioimpedance cardiac output determinations in low and high flow states, *Crit Care Med* 16:430, 1988.

60. Clements FM and deBruijn NP: Noninvasive cardiac monitoring, *Crit Care Clin* 4:435, 1988.

BIBLIOGRAPHY

Armstrong PW and Baigrie RS, editors: *Hemodynamic monitoring in the critically ill.* New York, 1980, Harper & Row.

Ayres SM: Ventricular function. In Shoemaker WC and Thompson WL, editors: *Critical care state of the art,* vol 1, Fullerton, Calif, 1980, Society of Critical Care Medicine.

Bernstein DP: Noninvasive cardiac output measurement. In Shoemaker WC and others: *Textbook of critical care,* ed 2, Philadelphia, 1989, WB Saunders.

Bernstein DP: Continuous noninvasive real-time monitoring of stroke volume and cardiac output by thoracic electrical bioimpedance, *Crit Care Med* 14:898, 1986.

Biondi JW, Schulman DS, Matthay RA: Effects of mechanical ventilation on right and left ventricular function, *Clin Chest Med* 9:55, 1988.

Bone RC, George RB, Hudsom LD: Acute respiratory failure, New York, 1987, Churchill Livingstone.

Buda AJ and others: Effect of intrathoracic pressure on left ventricular performance, *N Engl J Med* 301:453, 1979.

Braunwald E Assessment of cardiac function. In Braunwald E, editor: *Heart disease,* ed 3, Philadelphia, 1988, WB Saunders.

Braunwald E and others: Mechanisms of cardiac contraction and relaxation. In Braunwald E, editor: *Heart disease,* ed 3, Philadelphia, 1988, WB Saunders.

Cain SM: Assessment of tissue oxygenation, *Crit Care Clin* 2:537, 1986.

Campbell S: Pharmacologic principles of cardiovascular drug administration to the critically ill, *Crit Care Clin* 1:471, 1985.

Cane RD and Shapiro BA: *Case studies in critical care medicine,* St Louis, 1985, Mosby.

Daily EK and Schroeder JS: *Techniques in bedside hemodynamic monitoring,* ed 4, St Louis, 1989, Mosby.

Darovic GO: *Hemodynamic monitoring: invasive and noninvasive clinical application.* Philadelphia, 1987, WB Saunders.

Finch CA and Lenfant C: Oxygen transport in man, *N Engl J Med* 286:407, 1972.

Gillman PA: Continuous measurement of cardiac output: a milestone in hemodynamic monitoring, *Am J Nurs* 199:55, 1992.

Goldbert HS and Rabson J: Control of cardiac output by systemic vessels: circulatory adjustments to acute and chronic respiratory failure and the effect of therapeutic interventions, *Am J Cardiol* 47:696, 1981.

Guyton AG, Jones CE, Coleman TG: *Circulatory physiology: cardiac output and its regulation,* ed 2, Philadelphia, 1973, WB Saunders.

Keagy BA and others: Constant postoperative monitoring of cardiac output after correction of congenital heart defects, *J Thorac Cardiovasc Surg* 93:658, 1987.

Kersten LD: *Comprehensive respiratory nursing care,* Philadelphia, 1989, WB Saunders.

Kreuzer F and Cain SM: Regulation of the peripheral vasculature and tissue oxygenation in health and disease, *Crit Care Clin* 1:453, 1985.

Magilligan DJ, Jr and others: Mixed venous oxygen saturation as a predictor of cardiac output in the postoperative cardiac surgical patient, *Ann Thorac Surg* 44:260, 1987.

Marini JJ: Monitoring during mechanical ventilation, *Clin Chest Med* 9:73, 1988.

Mark JB and others: Continuous noninvasive monitoring of cardiac output with esophageal Doppler ultrasound during cardiac surgery, *Anesth Analg* 65:1013, 1986.

Matthay RA and Wood LD: Seminar on cardiovascular function in respiratory failure: the functionally integrated cardiovascular-pulmonary unit, *Am J Cardiol* 47:683, 1981.

Mohr R and others: A method for continuous on-line monitoring of systemic vascular resistance (COMS) after open heart procedures, *J Cardiovasc Surg* 28:558, 1987.

Morganroth ML, editor: Mechanical ventilation, *Clin Chest Med* 9: March 1988.

Osgood CF and others: Hemodynamic monitoring in respiratory care, *Respir Care* 29:30, 1984.

Pinsky MR: The influence of positive-pressure ventilation on cardiovascular function in the critically ill, *Crit Care Clin* 1:699, 1985.

Price MS and Fox JD: *Hemodynamic monitoring in critical care,* Rockville, Md, 1987, Aspen Publishers.

Quaal SJ: *Comprehensive intra-aortic balloon pumping,* St Louis, 1984, Mosby.

Robotham JL: Seminar on cardiovascular function in respiratory failure: cardiovascular disturbances in chronic respiratory insufficiency, *Am J Cardiol* 47:941, 1981.

Robotham JL, Peters J, Takata M: Cardiorespiratory interactions. In Bone RC and others, editors: *Pulmonary and critical care medicine,* St Louis, 1993, Mosby.

Rubin LJ: Pulmonary hypertension and cor pulmonale. In Bone RC and others, editors: *Pulmonary and critical care medicine,* St Louis, 1993, Mosby.

Runciman WB, Ilsely AH, Rutten AJ: Monitoring other haemodynamic variables and oxygen consumption, *Anaesth Intensive Care* 16:58, 1988.

Sibbald WJ, editor: Cardiovascular crises in the critically ill, *Crit Care Clin* 1: Nov 1985.

Sprung CL, Drescher M, Schein RMH: Clinical investigation of the cardiovascular system in the critically ill: invasive techniques, *Crit Care Clin* 1:533, 1985.

Svennevig JL and others: Continuous monitoring of cardiac output postoperatively using an implantable Doppler probe, *Scand J Thorac Cardiovasc Surg* 20:145, 1986.

Teich S and Chernow B: Specific cardiovascular drugs utilized in the critically ill, *Crit Care Clin* 1:507, 1985.

Textbook of advanced cardiac life support, 1987. American Heart Association.

Thys DM and others: A comparison of hemodynamic indices derived by invasive monitoring and two-dimensional echocardiography, *Anesthesiology* 67:630, 1987.

Understanding hemodynamic measurements made with the Swan-Ganz catheter. Santa Ana, Calif, 1982, American Edwards Laboratories.

Vaughn S and Puri VK: Cardiac output changes and continuous mixed venous oxygen saturation measurement in the critically ill, *Crit Care Med* 16:495, 1988.

Vender JS, editor: Intensive care monitoring, *Crit Care Clin* 4: July 1988.

Williams GA and Ayres SM: Regulation of myocardial function in health and critical illness, *Crit Care Clin* 1:435, 1985.

Wood SE and Osguthorpe S: Cardiac output determination, *AACN Clin Issues Crit Care Nurs* 4:81, 1993.

Chapter 14

Invasively Monitored Hemodynamic Pressures

Susan Jones Krider

LEARNING OBJECTIVES

Upon completion of this chapter, the reader should be able to accomplish the following:

1. Recognize the following regarding arterial cannulation:
   a. indications
   b. cannulation sites
   c. possible complications
   d. normal pressures and their significance
   e. pressure waveforms
   f. significance of respiratory variation in the pressure waveform
   g. method of direct aortic pressure measurement and its significance

2. Identify the following regarding central venous pressure (CVP) monitoring:
   a. significance
   b. factors affecting measurement
   c. insertion sites
   d. types of catheters
   e. correct technique for pressure measurement
   f. parts of the CVP waveform
   g. effect of respiratory motion on the CVP waveform
   h. normal value for CVP
   i. relationship to left ventricular function

3. Recognize the following regarding pulmonary artery pressure monitoring:
   a. synonyms for the catheter
   b. indications and complications
   c. catheter description
   d. sizes used for adults and children
   e. position of distal and proximal catheter lumens
   f. average amount of air required to fill the catheter balloon
   g. procedure for placement of the catheter
   h. two synonyms for pulmonary capillary wedge pressure (PCWP) and the normal value for PCWP and pulmonary artery pressure (PAP)
   i. relationship between pulmonary artery diastolic pressure (PADP) and PCWP
   j. significance of pulmonary artery pressure (PAP) and PCWP measurements

Chapter Overview

Accurate and appropriate bedside hemodynamic monitoring of the critically ill is vital. It is performed to obtain information that will be pertinent to patient care, warn of impending problems, and guide decision making and therapeutic intervention toward the goal of improving patient outcome. Ideally, the information will be easily obtained, continuously available, reliable, and the process of obtaining the information will not harm the patient. Unfortunately, clinical assessment alone may inaccurately predict hemodynamics in some patients, while knowledge of invasively monitored measurements may result in changes to more appropriate therapy.[1,2] Noninvasive techniques for monitoring the critically ill are being developed and are the ideal tool, but they have not yet reached the capacity to *continuously* report information that *accurately* reflects the central hemodynamic status in all patients in all situations. Though the risk-benefit ratio of invasive monitoring as well as the cost-benefit ratio is questioned by some,[3-10] the bedside monitor and invasively measured values remain the cornerstones of today's critical care units.

    Bedside monitors acquire and calculate physiologic data with great speed and frequently transfer the data automatically to computers for trend analysis. But monitors do not always tell the truth.[11-13] Therefore, optimal invasive monitoring requires not only knowledge of the potential complications and appropriate clinical application of the acquired data but also understanding and control of the factors that alter the validity of the numbers. Therapeutic decision making based on the numbers alone is never appropriate and can be dangerous.

    This chapter provides an introduction to the hemodynamic pressures most frequently monitored invasively in critically ill patients: (1) arterial pressure, (2) central venous pressure (CVP), and (3) pulmonary artery pressure. Indications and complications of invasive monitoring, normal and abnormal pressure waveforms, and clinical applications are discussed. An invasive catheter-transducer-monitor system is described, with technical considerations for obtaining

Table 14-1 Normal Hemodynamic Pressure Values*

Pressure	Abbreviation	Normal Value
Arterial pressure	BP	120/80 mmHg (90/60 in teenage girls)
Mean arterial pressure	MAP	80–100 mmHg
Central venous pressure	CVP	<6 mmHg; <12 cm H_2O
Right atrial pressure	RAP	2–6 mmHg (mean pressure)
Right ventricular pressure	RVP	20–30/0–5 mmHg
Right ventricular end-diastolic pressure	RVEDP	2–6 mmHg
Pulmonary artery pressure	PAP	20–30/6–15 mmHg
Mean pulmonary artery pressure	MPAP or $\overline{PAP}$	10–20 mmHg
Pulmonary capillary wedge pressure	PCWP, PCWP, PAOP, PWP	4–12 mmHg
Left atrial pressure	LAP	4–12 mmHg (mean pressure)
Left ventricular pressure	LVP	100–140/0–5 mmHg
Left ventricular end-diastolic pressure	LVEDP	5–12 mmHg

*From Daily EK and Schroeder JS; *Hemodynamic waveforms: exercises in identification and analysis*, St Louis, 1983, Mosby.

optimal pressure readings. An in-depth presentation of hemodynamic monitoring is not within the scope of this text. The reader is encouraged to use the sources listed in the bibliography for more comprehensive study.

Table 14–1 summarizes the normal values and the most frequent abbreviations used for the pressures that are discussed. Although intracardiac pressures are essentially the same in adults and children, heart rate and blood pressure vary significantly by age. Table 14–2 lists normal heart rates and blood pressures for children from infancy through 16 years.[14] Remember that "normals" are obtained from studies on healthy people and may be neither normal nor desirable for a specific patient. Nevertheless, they serve well as reference ranges in the intensive care unit (ICU).

Arterial Pressure Monitoring

Arterial cannulation is indicated for (1) continuous arterial pressure monitoring; (2) to avoid arterial injury from multiple arterial punctures; and (3) for determining cardiac output using indocyanine green (Cardio-Green) dye. Although accurate mean blood pressure can be obtained automatically and noninvasively as often as every minute by automated oscillometry[15-18] (see Chapter 11), invasive arterial pressure monitoring continues to be recommended for patients receiving titrated vasoactive drugs and those experiencing extremes in blood pressure or increased systemic vascular resistance (SVR).

When SVR is elevated, as occurs in shock, diastolic runoff is slowed, decreasing the pressure gradient and therefore the jet flow heard when a cuff is deflated. Transmission of vibrations in the arterial wall may also decrease.[19] As a result, it may not be possible to obtain a cuff pressure measurement that reflects central arterial pressure.[20-24] Failure to recognize that a low peripheral arterial pressure does not necessarily indicate a low central arterial pressure may result in dangerous patient management.[25]

Table 14-2 Normal Heart Rates and Blood Pressures in Children*

Age	Blood Pressure Average for Males	Heart Rate† Average	Heart Rate† Range
Neonate	75/50	140	100–190
1–6 mo	80/50	145	110–190
6–12 mo	90/65	140	110–180
1–2 yr	95/65	125	100–160
2–6 yr	100/60	100	65–130
6–12 yr	110/60	80	55–110
12–16 yr	110/65	75	55–100
	Range: ±20%		
	Females 5% lower		

*Data from Rubenstein JS and Hageman JR: Monitoring of critically ill infants and children, *Crit Care Clin* 4:621, 1988.
†Heart rates rounded to nearest 5.

Disparities Between Direct and Indirect Arterial Pressures

Disparities between cuff and direct arterial pressure measurements of 5 to 20 mmHg may be considered normal as long as the direct pressure measurement is higher.[26] Disparities may exceed 30 mmHg in the face of severe vasoconstriction or when there is an overshoot in the direct arterial pressure trace.

When the indirect pressure is higher than the direct and there is no peripheral occlusive disease, the problem is usually technical. The monitoring system should be checked for leaks, air bubbles, or other causes of damped pressure as described at the end of this chapter. Additionally, the patient's position in relation to the transducer should be checked. If the vent port of the transducer is above the patient's right atrial level, the weight of the water in the tubing will pull away from the transducer and decrease the pressure. By moving the transducer up and down while the patient stays in one place, the numbers can be made to say anything.

Next time you are in the ICU, try this experiment. Look at a patient's pressure, then remove the transducer from its rack and raise it about a foot above the patient. The approximately 22 mmHg drop in displayed pressure is because the transducer was moved, not because the patient's pressure changed.

The example below shows the steps used to calculate exactly how much error an improperly positioned transducer would have on the pressure reading.

$$1 \text{ in.} = 2.540 \text{cm}$$
$$1 \text{ ft } (12 \text{ in.}) \times 2.540 = 30.48 \text{ cm H}_2\text{O}$$
$$\text{Since } 1.36 \text{ cm H}_2\text{O} = 1 \text{ mmHg}$$
$$\text{then } 30.48 \text{ cm H}_2\text{O}/1.36 = 22.4 \text{ mmHg}$$

If the transducer is placed about a foot below the patient, the displayed pressure will increase by about 22 mmHg.

Cannulation Sites

Arterial catheters are commonly placed in the radial artery, even in children, because of the excellent collateral circulation to the hand supplied by the ulnar artery. This site also permits easy access and care. The same precautions described in Chapter 6 for obtaining an arterial blood sample apply to assessment of the artery before catheter placement. Other arteries that may be used for invasive arterial monitoring include the brachial, axillary, femoral, dorsalis pedis, and, in the newborn, the umbilical artery.

Cannulation of the axillary, femoral, or umbilical arteries has the advantage of placing the catheter more centrally. This decreases errors caused by amplification in the waveform as the arteries narrow peripherally and possible underestimation of pressure in the severely vasoconstricted patient. A disadvantage of these sites is that a large amount of blood can leak into surrounding tissues before it is recognized.

Complications

ISCHEMIA. Ischemia secondary to embolism, thrombus, or arterial spasm is the major complication of direct arterial monitoring. It is evidenced by pallor distal to the insertion site and is usually accompanied by pain and paresthesias. Ischemia can proceed to tissue necrosis if the catheter is not repositioned or removed. Thrombosis is prevented by continuous irrigation with diluted heparinized solution. It must be remembered, however, that flushing can result in retrograde flow and cerebral embolization.[27]

HEMORRHAGE. Hemorrhage is possible if the line becomes disconnected or a stopcock is left open; therefore, the tubing should be kept on top of the bed sheets where it can be observed. Blood flow through an 18-gauge catheter is sufficient to allow a 500-mL blood loss per minute, and *exsanguination* can occur.[28] Bleeding and *hematoma* at the insertion site can occur, especially if the catheter was placed through a needle.

Sites should be assessed regularly while the catheter is in place and following removal.

INFECTION. As with all invasive lines, the presence of an arterial catheter increases the risk of infection. The degree of infection increases dramatically after 4 days of catheterization[29] and is directly related to care of the lines and transducers; frequency of dressing, tubing, and solution change; to-and-fro motion of the catheter; and altered host defenses. *Fever in any patient with invasive lines must trigger questions about the necessity of the lines and their implication in an infection process.*

Normal Pressures and Clinical Significance

NORMAL ARTERIAL PRESSURE. Normal arterial pressure in the adult is approximately 120/80 mm Hg and increases gradually with age. A rough estimate for the upper limit of normal systolic pressure can be obtained by adding 100 to the patient's age. Systolic pressures greater than 160 and diastolic pressures greater than 90 are considered hypertensive. A pressure of 90/60 is not uncommon in young females.

Although arterial pressure is one of the most frequently monitored vital signs, it reflects only the general circulatory status. Because neurovascular compensatory mechanisms can maintain blood pressure by vasoconstriction while flow is decreasing, low blood pressure is a late sign of deficits in blood volume or cardiac function.

ARTERIAL PRESSURE DECREASES. Arterial pressure decreases with hypovolemia from fluid or blood loss, during cardiac failure and shock, and with vasodilation. Diastolic pressure must be watched carefully during administration of vasodilators such as sodium nitroprusside, which may reduce diastolic pressure more rapidly than systolic or mean pressure. Since the coronary arteries receive most of their blood flow during diastole, diastolic pressure less than 50 mmHg and mean pressure less than 60 mmHg in the adult may result in compromised coronary perfusion.

ARTERIAL PRESSURE INCREASES. Arterial pressure increases with improvement in circulatory volume and function, sympathetic stimulation, vasoconstriction, and administration of vasopressors. Administration of inotropic agents may or may not increase blood pressure. If a positive inotropic drug drives the heart in the face of inadequate myocardial oxygenation or hypovolemia, the pressure may fall. Additionally, if the inotropic agent also causes vasodilation (e.g., isoproterenol [Isuprel]), the pressure may stay the same or fall as the medication is increased.

PULSE PRESSURE. The pulse pressure is the difference between the systolic and diastolic pressure. A decreasing pulse pressure is one of the first signs of inadequate volume. Conversely, an increasing pulse pressure is an early sign of volume restoration.[30]

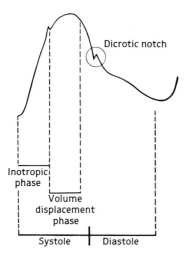

Fig. 14-1 *Arterial pressure waveform. Increase of circulating catecholamines can cause the inotropic phase to become steeper and form a point that may be higher than in the volume displacement phase. The circle marks the dicrotic notch that results from closure of the aortic valve. If the dicrotic notch cannot be visualized and the patient's systolic pressure is greater than 50 mmHg, it can be assumed that the plumbing system is damped. (See section on technical considerations later in this chapter.)*

Mean Arterial Pressure

Mean arterial pressure (MAP) is an average of pressures pushing blood through the systemic circulation; therefore, it is the more important of the arterial pressures and an indicator of tissue perfusion. However, MAP is not an arithmetic average of systolic and diastolic pressures, because the cardiac cycle spends about twice as long in diastole as in systole when the heart rate is in the normal range (50–100 beats per minute). Most monitors have a selector switch that computes MAP and displays it digitally. MAP can be estimated mathematically by either of the following formulas when it cannot be obtained from the monitor.

$$MAP = \frac{1}{3} \text{ pulse pressure} + \text{diastolic pressure}$$

or

$$\frac{\text{Systolic pressure} + (\text{diastolic pressure} \times 2)}{3}$$

Normal MAP

Normal MAP is considered to be 80 to 100 mmHg. Circulation to the vital organs (i.e., kidneys, coronary arteries) may be compromised when MAP falls below 60 mmHg. Following vascular surgery or in the presence of aneurysms, vasodilators and antihypertensive agents may be administered to keep the MAP below 100 mmHg.

MAP is used in calculating derived hemodynamic variables such as SVR, left ventricular stroke work, and cardiac work.

Arterial Pressure Waveforms

An arterial waveform should have a clear upstroke on the left with a dicrotic notch representing aortic valve closure on the downstroke on the right (Fig. 14–1). If the dicrotic notch is not visible, the pressure is probably inaccurate and the numbers will be lower than the patient's actual pressure. The dicrotic notch disappears in some patients when the systolic pressure drops below 50 or 60 mmHg, but this is usually associated with difficulty hearing and palpating a cuff pressure.

Arterial pressure waves take on many different configurations in patients in the ICU (Fig. 14–2). The left side of the pressure wave becomes straight and even pointed on the top when there is an increase in circulating catecholamines that causes an increased inotropic response. A tall narrow pressure wave is also seen in patients with stiff aortas (hypertension). In these patients the diastolic pressure may also fall, producing an exaggerated tall and narrow complex. As mentioned earlier, increases in stroke volume increase the pulse pressure (increase systolic and decrease diastolic pressure); however, the visual appearance of the waveform stays approximately the same. Increases in heart rate and peripheral vascular resistance (PVR) increase diastolic pressure. On the other hand, vasodilation that decreases PVR can cause the diastolic pressure to drop rapidly. Because approximately 70% of coronary artery perfusion occurs during the diastolic phase, coronary artery perfusion may be compromised if the diastolic pressure falls below 50 mmHg.

Respiratory Variation in the Arterial Pressure Waveform

Respiratory variation in the arterial pressure waveform normally goes unnoticed because arterial pressure is so high relative to the magnitude of usual respiratory pressure changes. Additionally, the sensitivity of the monitor is usually set so that the screen covers a pressure range of 0 to 300 mmHg, making changes of 10 mmHg barely visible. When respiratory variation is seen, the possibility of cardiac tamponade or other causes of *paradoxical pulse* (pressure decreasing with inspiration) must be considered (Fig. 14–3). Increases in arterial pressure during inspiration (*reverse pulsus paradoxus*) are seen in patients following heart surgery and patients with left ventricular failure who are mechanically ventilated with positive end-expiratory pressure (PEEP) (see also Chapter 11). Dysrhythmias and pulsus alternans also cause variations in the height and shapes of the waveforms.

Direct Aortic Pressure Measurement

Aortic pressures are occasionally measured and can be used to obtain continuous cardiac output readings by the pulse contour method. Direct aortic pressure mea-

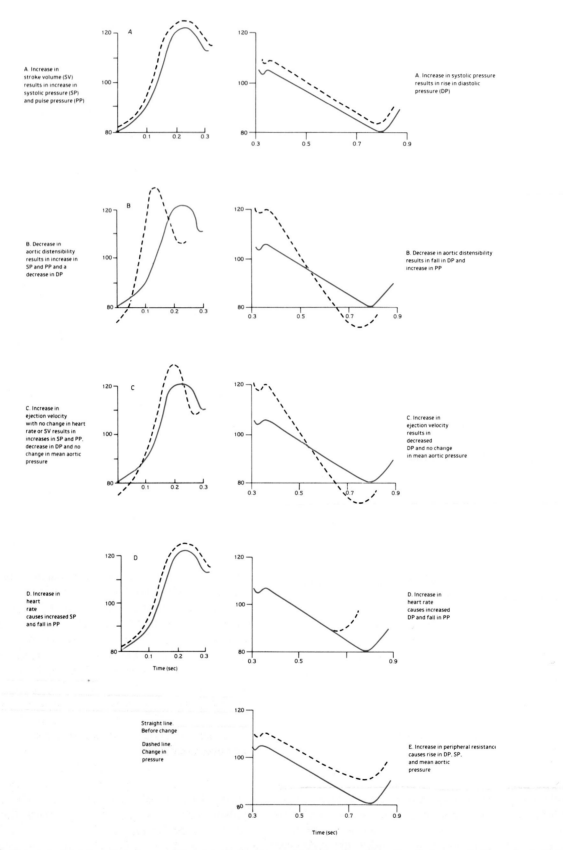

Fig. 14-2 *Determinants of aortic pressures. Diagrams indicate general tendencies when other factors are held constant. (Adapted from Smith JJ and Kampine JP: Circulatory physiology—the essentials, Baltimore, 1980, Williams & Wilkins. By permission.)*

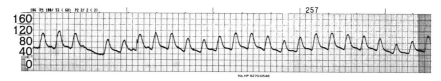

Fig. 14–3 *Arterial pressure waveform showing respiratory-induced changes in pressure.*

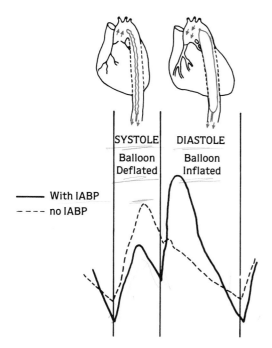

Fig. 14–4 *Intraaortic balloon positioned just below the aortic arch. Note deflation of the balloon at the beginning of systole decreases the systolic pressure, thereby unloading the ventricle and enhancing ejection. Inflation during diastole increases the aortic pressure and displaces the blood in the aorta, augmenting coronary blood flow and forward perfusion. Elevation of the diastolic portion of the waveform during intraaortic balloon pumping (IABP) produces an arterial pressure waveform that resembles a two-humped camel, with the diastolic segment as high as or higher than the systolic segment.*

surement is most commonly seen in patients undergoing intraaortic balloon pumping (IABP). A lumen extends the length of the intraaortic balloon catheter, opening at the tip of the catheter. The balloon is classically inserted via the femoral artery until the tip is in the descending aorta just below the aortic arch (Fig. 14–4). When the lumen is filled with fluid and connected to a transducer, aortic pressure can be measured continuously and is used to time the balloon pump.

The aortic and arterial pressure waveforms are altered during balloon pumping. *Inflation of the balloon occurs during diastole* and displaces blood back toward the coronary arteries, enhancing coronary perfusion. This increase in aortic pressure during diastole (diastolic augmentation) causes the pressure waveform to rise during diastole, resulting in pressure complexes resembling a two-humped camel (Fig. 14–4). The *balloon deflates almost instantly at the beginning of systole,* creating a "vacuum" in the aorta and "unloading" the ventricle, thereby decreasing systolic pressure and left ventricular afterload and increasing blood flow toward the periphery. Because of this increase in diastolic pressure and decrease in systolic pressure, IABP is often referred to as *counterpulsation.* A discussion of IABP is beyond the scope of this text, but it has been presented in detail in other texts.[31]

Central Venous Pressure Monitoring

Central venous pressure (CVP) is the pressure of the blood in the right atrium or the vena cava, where the blood is returned to the heart from the venous system. Since the tricuspid valve is opened between the right atrium and ventricle during diastole (ventricular filling), right atrial pressure or CVP also represents the end-diastolic pressure in the right ventricle (RVEDP) and is a reflection of preload for the right ventricle.

Normal CVP and Clinical Significance of Changing CVP

Central venous pressure is regulated by a balance between the ability of the heart to pump blood out of the right atrium and the amount of blood being returned to the heart by the venous system (venous return). In general, any peripheral factor that decreases the amount of blood returning to the heart decreases CVP, and any factor that increases venous return increases CVP. When the pumping capacity of the right heart is increased, more blood is moved out of the right ventricle and CVP decreases. Conversely, decreased pumping ability of the heart or increased pulmonary vascular resistance results in an increase in CVP, sometimes as high as the 20 to 30 mmHg range. *Normal CVP is less than 6 mmHg or less than 12 cm H_2O.*

Elevations of CVP measurements occur under the following conditions:

1. Volume overload or fluids being given more rapidly than the heart can tolerate
2. Increased intrathoracic pressure (CVP increases with positive pressure breath or pneumothorax)
3. Compressions around the heart: constrictive pericarditis, cardiac tamponade
4. Pulmonary hypertension (primary or secondary) (see Chapter 13, Table 13–4)
5. Right ventricular failure (e.g., myocardial infarction, cardiomyopathy)

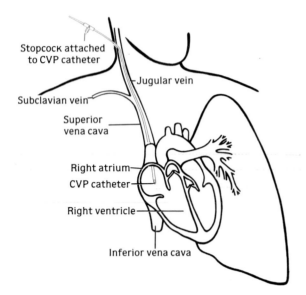

Fig. 14-5 *Central venous pressure (CVP) catheter inserted through the jugular vein with the tip positioned in the right atrium.*

6. Left heart failure
7. Pulmonary valvular stenosis
8. Tricuspid valvular stenosis or regurgitation
9. Pulmonary embolism
10. Increased large vessel tone throughout the body resulting in venoconstriction
11. Arteriolar vasodilation that increases the blood supply to the venous system[32]
12. Infusion of solution into the CVP line (especially by infusion pumps)

Causes of *decreased CVP* measurements include the following:

1. Vasodilation (by drug or increase in body temperature)
2. Inadequate circulating blood volume (hypovolemia) caused by dehydration; actual blood loss; or large amounts of gastrointestinal loss, wound drainage, perspiration, urine output (diuresis), insensible losses (high temperature, low humidity), and losses to the interstitial space (edema, "third spacing")
3. Spontaneous inspiration
4. Placement of the transducer or zero level of the water manometer *above* the patient's right atrial level
5. Air bubbles or leaks in the pressure line

When a patient is hypovolemic but has pulmonary hypertension with a resulting decrease in right ventricular function, the CVP reflects the elevated pressure from the loss of ventricular function and does not fall to levels that would be expected with hypovolemia.

CVP Catheters and Insertion Sites

Central venous pressure catheters are positioned so that their tips are in the vena cava or the right atrium (Fig. 14-5). CVP may also be obtained from the proximal port of a pulmonary artery line, described later in this chapter.

The most common sites for introduction of the catheter (either percutaneously or by cutdown) are the external and internal jugular, subclavian, or antecubital veins and rarely the femoral veins. The internal jugular vein has become the most popular site because of the ease of insertion (it is nearly a straight line from the right internal jugular vein to the right atrium), decreased risk of pneumothorax from pleural puncture, and good visibility if hematomas form in the neck. However, the subclavian route is usually preferred by ICU nurses (even though the risk of pneumothorax during insertion is greater) because the catheter, tubing, and connections are easier to stabilize and less subject to kinking, separation, and breakage when the patient is awake and actively moving the head and neck. Placement in the antecubital and femoral veins is least preferred because it is necessary to immobilize the extremity to protect the catheter. Following placement of the catheter, a chest x-ray film is performed to verify the position of the catheter tip and to rule out pneumothorax.

CVP catheters are now available with multiple lumina (Fig. 14-6). The multiple-lumen catheter allows infusion of blood and various medications and solutions through different ports and permits aspiration of blood samples or injections for cardiac output measurements without interrupting the infusion of medication. The catheter should not be confused with the pulmonary artery catheter (see pulmonary artery catheter discussion). There is no balloon on a CVP catheter: *air is never injected into any port of a CVP line.*

Once the CVP catheter is in place, it can be used for administration of fluids, blood, and drugs, including vasoactive substances and hypertonic solutions that cannot be given in the peripheral veins. It also provides a site for aspiration of blood for laboratory work. However, it is preferable to aspirate samples for mixed venous oxygen measurements from the pulmonary artery catheter rather than from the CVP catheter. Significant differences in the extraction of oxygen occur in the upper and lower halves of the body and therefore in the oxygen content of blood being returned to the right atrium. The blood is not "mixed" until it passes through the ventricle and is ejected into the pulmonary artery.[33,34]

CVP Using a Water Manometer

Central venous pressure can be obtained using a transducer system or a water manometer (Fig. 14-7). The advantage of the water manometer is that it is inexpensive, readily available, and relatively easy to use. The manometer is filled with intravenous fluid to a point above the expected CVP measurement. With the patient in the supine position, the zero level of the manometer is placed at the patient's right atrial level

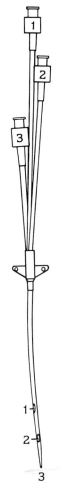

Fig. 14-6 *Triple-lumen central venous pressure catheter designed for placement through the internal or external jugular vein. The tip ends in the right atrium. The catheter does not have a balloon; air is never injected into ports.*

and the stopcock is turned so that the manometer is opened to the patient. The fluid level in the stopcock is turned so that the manometer should fall rapidly until the level of the patient's CVP is reached, and then it should oscillate with respiration. The CVP is ideally read at the end of expiration, since spontaneous inspiration causes the pressure to fall and mechanical ventilation causes the pressure to rise. The pressure obtained is in centimeters of water and must be converted to millimeters of mercury for use in calculating SVR. This is accomplished by dividing the centimeters of water by 1.36, since 1.36 cm H_2O equals 1 mmHg.

$$8 \text{ cm } H_2O = \frac{8 \text{ cm } H_2O}{1.36} = 5.9 \text{ mmHg}$$

The criteria for interpretation of CVP by a water manometer include the following:

1. X-ray verification that the tip of the catheter is in central venous position
2. Free-flowing intravenous fluid
3. Ability to easily aspirate a blood sample from the CVP catheter

4. A rapidly falling water column when the pressure is obtained
5. Small oscillations at the top of the water column indicating the changes in the CVP throughout a cardiac cycle
6. Larger oscillations occurring with respiration

Unfortunately, comparison of water manometer methods with transducer methods has demonstrated that the water manometer readings usually overestimate transducer-determined mean right atrial pressure (CVP).[34] This is because the water only falls to the highest pressure in each cardiac cycle and not to the mean pressure. Additionally, the location of the catheter tip cannot be verified, since wide fluctuations of the water column do not occur even when the catheter is located in the right ventricle and changes in the individual waves (a and v) cannot be seen.

Transduced CVP

When CVP is measured using a transducer system, careful attention must be given to technique before obtaining a pressure reading. The catheter must be patent, the waveform clear and nondamped, the patient in the supine position, the transducer zero-balanced to the patient's right atrial level, and the pressure recorded at end-expiration (see Technical Considerations for Invasive Hemodynamic Monitoring at the end of this chapter).

As with most hemodynamic measurements, the trend of the CVP changes is more important than any single number.[35,36] Since the position of the tricuspid valve cannot be identified precisely, patients become their own control for pressure regulation. It is imperative that the right atrial position selected for the patient be marked with indelible ink and the transducer or water manometer be zero-balanced to that point before each pressure measurement is obtained (Fig. 14–8). For example, a CVP reading of 6 mmHg by itself may have little significance, but a drop of 1 mmHg/hr over a 4-hour period would be highly suggestive of volume loss, especially if combined with tachycardia and increasing PVR. However, if someone decides the original zero-reference point on the patient was incorrect and elects to move it 4 cm higher on the patient's side, an approximately 3 mmHg decrease (4/1.36) in the displayed pressure will result. The apparent decrease in the pressure is due to the change in the zero-reference point and not to an actual decrease in the patient's pressure. Readjustment of the zero-reference point has the same effect on pulmonary pressures readings.

CVP Waveform

Central venous pressure waveforms (like left atrial pressure [LAP] and pulmonary capillary wedge pressure [PCWP] waveforms) have three waves for each cardiac cycle: *a, c, v* (Fig. 14–9). The *a wave* results

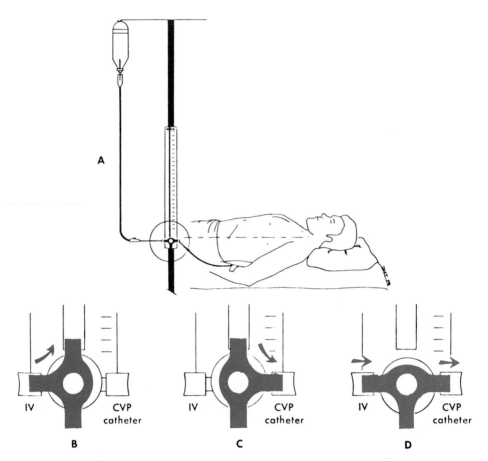

Fig. 14-7 *Procedure for measuring central venous pressure (CVP) with manometer.* **A,** Manometer and intravenous (IV) tubing in place. **B,** *Turn stopcock so that manometer fills with fluid above level of expected pressure.* **C,** *Turn stopcock so that IV flow is off and fluid in manometer flows to patient. Obtain reading after fluid level stabilizes.* **D,** *Turn stopcock to resume IV flow to patient.* *(From Daily EK and Schroeder JS:* Techniques in bedside hemodynamic monitoring, *ed 4, St Louis, 1989, Mosby.)*

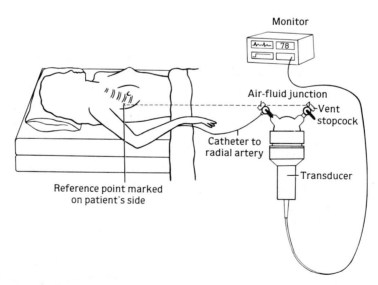

Fig. 14-8 *Zero-referencing the transducer to the patient's atrial level. The air-fluid junction of the transducer (vent port of stopcock) is leveled with the atrial position marker placed on the patient's side.*

from atrial contraction and occurs during ventricular diastole. When there is no atrial contraction (atrial fibrillation), there is no a wave. Conversely, when the atrium contracts against a closed valve, as occurs dur-

ing atrioventricular (AV) dissociation or with some junctional or ventricular pacemaker rhythms, large a waves called *cannon waves* occur. The downslope of the wave, called the *x descent,* results from the decrease in

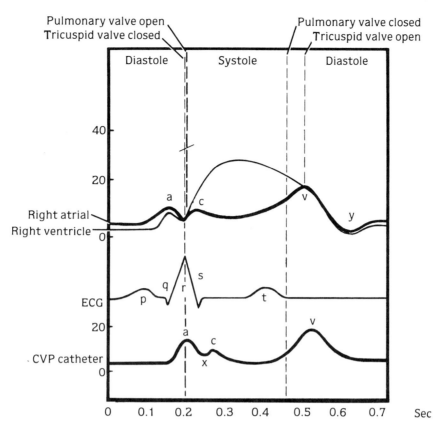

Fig. 14-9 *Central venous (CVP) and right atrial pressure traces with a, c, and v waves shown in relation to the electrocardiogram (ECG) and ventricular pressure waves. When traces are recorded from long catheters, especially pulmonary artery catheters, there is usually a time delay in visualizing the pressure waveform so that the a wave coincides with the QRS complex rather than preceding it slightly as occurs with the right atrial pressure trace.*

atrial pressure as the blood fills the ventricle and ends with the closure of the AV valve (tricuspid on right, mitral on left).

The *c wave* occurs when the ventricle begins to contract, causing the AV valves to bulge backward toward the atrium because of the increasing pressure in the ventricle.

The *v wave* is a gradual ascent resulting from the filling of the right atrium while the tricuspid valve is closed during ventricular contraction. The downslope of the v wave, called the *y descent,* occurs when the tricuspid and mitral valves open and the ventricle begins to fill with blood. When an AV valve does not close all the way (*incompetent or leaky valve*), some of the blood is ejected backward into the atrium during systole (tricuspid *regurgitation*), creating exaggerated v waves and an elevated CVP measurement.

Respiratory Variations in the CVP Waveform

Respiratory-induced pressure changes are normal on CVP waveforms. If no respiratory artifact is seen on the trace and the patient is not holding his or her breath, the pressure must be assumed to be inaccurate. The most likely cause would be a kink or air in the tubing, a stopcock turned in the wrong direction, or a small clot

or kink in the catheter. Rarely, when a hypovolemic patient is breathing spontaneously with a small tidal volume, no respiratory artifact or a, c, and v waves will be seen. If the patient is asked to take a deep breath, the waveform should fall below baseline as intrathoracic pressure falls with inspiration. The catheter and tubing should still be checked carefully for air and other causes of damped pressure traces (see the section on technical considerations later in this chapter).

CVP decreases with spontaneous inspiration and increases with mechanical ventilation. When a patient is on intermittent mandatory ventilation (IMV), the pressure decreases with the spontaneous breaths. When the patient triggers a mechanical breath, the pressure decreases and then immediately rises above baseline levels when the ventilator breath is initiated (Fig. 14–10).

The patient who is awake and alert can be asked to suspend breathing for several cardiac cycles until a mean venous pressure without respiratory artifact can be obtained. When the patient cannot assist and is *not on PEEP,* the ventilator can be disconnected for several cardiac cycles to obtain a pressure reading. When a patient is mechanically ventilated with PEEP, the pressures should be recorded on paper, and the average end-expiratory pressure over several respiratory cycles should be used for both CVP and pulmonary artery pressure measurements. Routine measurements are

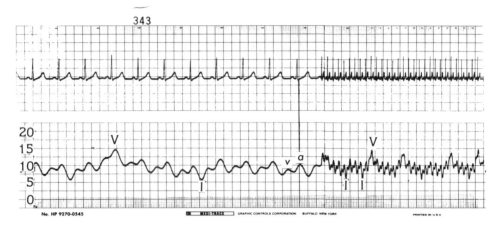

Fig. 14–10 *Right atrial pressure trace from proximal port of pulmonary artery catheter. Note a and v waves; c wave is not visible. The first portion of the trace was recorded at a paper speed of 25 mm/sec; the later portion was at a speed of 10 mm/sec so that the effects of the ventilator on the central venous pressure waveform are more clearly identified. Patient was on intermittent mandatory ventilation, 12; positive end-expiratory pressure, 5 cm H_2O; tidal volume, 850 mL; fraction of inspired oxygen, 40%. Central venous pressure reading on the monitor varied between 6 and 15 mmHg. Mean end-expiratory pressure measured on the recording varied consistently between 8 and 9 mmHg. I, spontaneous breaths; V, intermittent ventilator breath.*

done without interrupting the PEEP.[37,38] Unless these precautions are taken, numbers obtained from the monitor represent the extremes of the patient's respiratory efforts and not the mean CVP.

CVP as a Reflection of Left Ventricular Function

Can CVP be used to estimate left ventricular filling pressures and performance? In patients with an ejection fraction of more than 0.50 (50% of the LVEDV) and no left ventricular dyssynergia, excellent correlation has been found between CVP and PCWP.[39] CVP is a less invasive option for management of intraoperative, postoperative, or volume replacement[40,41] in the young patient with no history of heart disease or hypertension. The patient should have normal physical examination of the heart, normal cardiac size and configuration, absence of pulmonary vascular redistribution or congestion on chest x-ray films, and nonthoracic illness or injury. However, in patients with valvular heart disease[42] or coronary artery disease[43] and in critically ill patients,[44,45] CVP may not correlate well with wedge pressure readings.

In the patient with pulmonary disease, the left heart pressures remain normal or may even be decreased, whereas the pulmonary artery pressure and therefore right heart pressures are significantly elevated. Therefore, in the patient with pulmonary hypertensive disease, both the left and right heart pressures must be monitored.[46]

Left Atrial Pressure Monitoring

Left atrial pressure is directly measured in some patients during and following cardiac surgery; however, its use has become more limited since many patients have a pulmonary artery catheter placed at the time of induction of anesthesia. Additionally, LAP monitoring increases the risk of clot or air embolus to the coronary or cerebral arteries. An air embolus can occur if as little as 0.05 mL of air enters the plumbing system and the heart and then flows to the brain or coronary artery. To prevent complications, LAP lines are rarely used for blood sampling or infusions. Irrigation of the catheter is done minimally and with great care if it is permitted at all. The LAP waveform is the same as the CVP waveform (see Fig. 14–9). Normal LAP is 4 to 12 mmHg, the same as normal PCWP.

Transthoracic Intracardiac Catheters

The percutaneous approach is used for most catheter placements. However, in children and occasionally in adults, transthoracic intracardiac catheters may be placed to monitor right atrial, pulmonary artery, or left atrial pressures. This approach is most commonly seen in infants and children following repairs of congenital heart defects when it is feared that even a small catheter placed percutaneously might impede blood flow in an infant's tiny vessels. Catheters with one lumen are usually used for this approach; however, if a wedge pressure is wanted, a small pulmonary artery catheter may be used.

The catheter is placed through the wall of the right atrium while the chest is open during surgery. The other end of the catheter is pushed through the anterior chest wall so the tissue seals around the catheter. A pursestring suture is placed in the tissue around the atrial insertion point and connected to the catheter. When the catheter is removed, the suture should tighten and seal the insertion site. To permit assessment of bleeding secondary to removal of transthoracic catheters, mediastinal chest tubes are usually left in place until the transthoracic intracardiac catheters have been successfully removed.

Complications of transthoracic intracardiac monitoring include (1) migration of the catheter tip into the atrial appendage or pulmonary vein[47] resulting in erroneous pressure readings; (2) kinking of the catheter and inability to obtain a correct (if any) pressure reading; (3) breakage and retention of the catheter; and (4) intrathoracic bleeding when the catheter is removed. Studies of transthoracic catheter use in pediatric patients undergoing cardiac surgeries have shown a low incidence of bleeding and catheter retention for left atrial, right atrial, and pulmonary artery catheters placed through the wall of the atrium.[48]

Pulmonary Artery Pressure Monitoring

The development of the pulmonary artery catheter by Swan and Ganz in the late 1960s[49] began a new era in assessment of left ventricular and pulmonary performance. Placement of a flow-directed pulmonary artery catheter into the patient's pulmonary artery allows assessment of the following:

1. Left ventricular preload via measurement of pulmonary artery diastolic pressure (PADP) and PCWP
2. Pulmonary vascular resistance via continuous monitoring of pulmonary systolic and pulmonary mean pressures
3. Cardiac output by bolus, continuous thermodilution, or Doppler ultrasound (see Chapter 13)
4. Arteriovenous oxygen difference $(C[a-v]O_2)$, oxygen consumption $(\dot{V}o_2)$,[50] and venoarterial admixture $(\dot{Q}s/\dot{Q}t)$ from aspiration of mixed venous blood sample
5. Right ventricular function including preload, ejection fraction,[51,52] stroke work, and right ventricular infarction
6. Pulmonary edema: separating cardiogenic from noncardiogenic pulmonary edema, and effects of PEEP on oxygen delivery (Do_2) in adult respiratory distress syndrome (ARDS)[53]
7. Afterload reduction of left ventricle with vasodilator therapy[54]
8. Patient's response to therapy, position within hemodynamic subsets,[55] and construction of left ventricular function curves
9. Acute rupture of intraventricular septum[56] or mitral valve regurgitation[55]
10. Continuous monitoring of mixed venous blood saturation with oxygen $(S\bar{v}o_2)$[57–59] (see Chapters 12 and 13)
11. Atrial, ventricular, and AV sequential pacing by either bipolar pacemaker bands or insertion of pacing leads through the catheter lumen[60–62]
12. Estimation of the oxygen utilization coefficient by pulmonary artery oximetry or dual oximetry (combined pulse and pulmonary artery oximetry)[63,64] (see Chapter 12)

Description of Balloon Flotation Catheters

Pulmonary artery catheters, also called *Swan-Ganz catheters,* are made of radiopaque polyvinylchloride and are approximately 400 cm long and marked in 10-cm increments. The balloon at the tip of the catheter is used both to float the catheter into position and to obtain wedge pressure measurements. The catheter is also called a *balloon-tipped, flow-directed* catheter (Fig. 14–11). The size, configuration, and thermodilution computer requirements vary according to manufacturer and specific application. Four- and 5F catheters with two or three lumina are available for use in children. Five- to 8F catheters with four to six lumina are more commonly used for adults. The *distal lumen* terminates at the tip of the catheter and is positioned in the pulmonary artery for measuring pulmonary artery pressures, aspirating mixed venous blood samples, and injecting medications. The fiberoptic filaments used for $S\bar{v}o_2$ monitoring also exit at the tip of the catheter (see Chapter 12).

The *balloon lumen* exits inside of the balloon just behind the tip of the catheter. Most balloons hold approximately 1.5 mL of air and extend beyond the tip of the catheter when fully inflated. The balloon is fully inflated during insertion to provide a cushion around the tip of the catheter. The inflated balloon helps the catheter float into the pulmonary artery and helps to prevent premature ventricular contractions (PVCs) when the catheter is passed through the ventricle. *Once the catheter is in place, only the amount of air necessary to obtain a wedge pressure reading is placed in the balloon.*

The *proximal lumen* ends approximately 30 cm back from the tip of the catheter and rests in the right atrium when the catheter is properly placed. The proximal port is used for aspirating blood samples, measuring CVP, injecting drugs, and injection of the thermal bolus used for thermal dilution cardiac output measurements. Some catheters have two lumina ending in the right atrium: one for routine infusion of drugs or continuous pressure monitoring, the other for infusion of thermodilution materials and other periodic injections.

Thermodilution cardiac output catheters have a *thermistor bead* located approximately 1½ in. from the tip of the catheter. The thermistor senses temperature changes in the blood and is used for obtaining body core temperature as well as thermodilution cardiac output measurements.

Pulmonary artery catheters with bands for atrial, ventricular, or AV sequential cardiac pacing are also

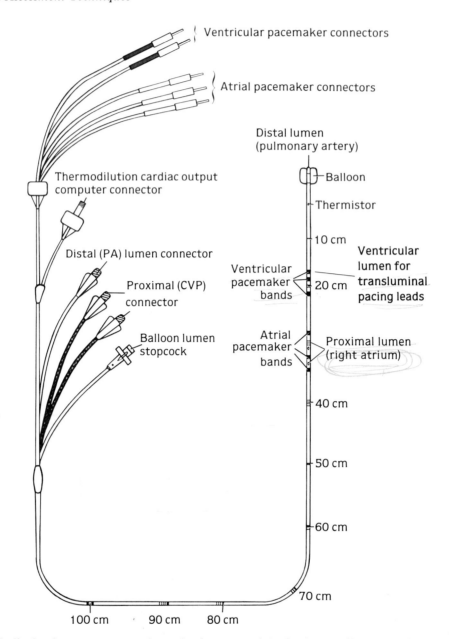

Fig. 14-11 *Idealized pulmonary artery catheter showing many of the features available on pulmonary artery catheters—no catheters have all the features shown. Distal lumen opens into the pulmonary artery (PA). Fiberoptic filaments used for $S\bar{v}o_2$ monitoring (see Fig. 12–9) and the balloon are also located at the tip. The thermistor bead is located 1½ in. from the tip and is connected by a wire through the catheter to the connector for the thermodilution cardiac output computer. The proximal lumina located 30 cm back from the tip open into the right atrium. Catheters are available for ventricular, atrial, or atrioventricular sequential pacing using either pacemaker bands positioned on the catheter or pacing leads, which are passed through the lumen. Ventricular bands or lumina are located 20 cm from the tip; atrial, 30 cm from the tip.*

available. The pacemaker bands must stay in contact with the wall of the atrium or ventricle to work effectively. Another type of <u>pulmonary artery pacing catheter has a ventricular lumen 20 cm back from the tip</u> in addition to the proximal (atrial) lumen. Specially designed pacing leads may be passed through the lumen and positioned more securely against the wall of the chamber.[60] The pacer leads are then connected directly to the pacemaker. If cardiac pacing is not required, the lumen can be used for infusions and blood sampling. A pulmonary artery catheter, which will allow continuous cardiac output readings by constant measurement of the diameter of the pulmonary artery and velocity of blood flow, is currently in clinical trials.

Assessing the Response of Cardiopulmonary Drugs Infused Through a Pulmonary Artery Catheter

When a cardiopulmonary drug infusion is started through a pulmonary catheter, as much as 6 minutes can elapse before the drug reaches the patient's blood. The

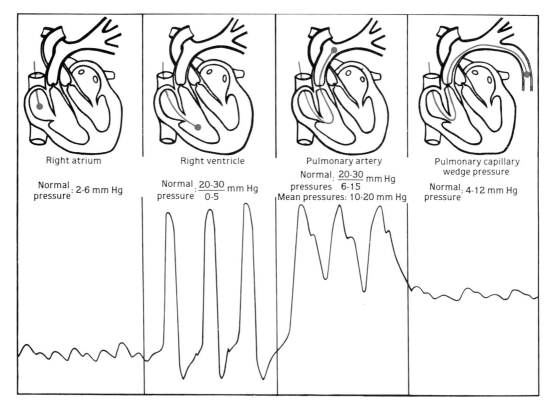

Fig. 14-12 *Schematic of waveforms and normal pressures visualized as the pulmonary artery catheter is floated into position.*

time delay varies with the size of the lumen selected for drug administration and the speed of the IV infusion pump. It has been recommended that the rate of infusion should begin at 99 drops/min until the drug reaches the central circulation: 37 seconds for the distal lumen, 28 seconds for the proximal lumen, and 16 seconds for infusion through the introducer.[64] Alternately, the internal volume of each lumen can be measured using a 1-mL syringe to slowly aspirate the lumen until a flush of blood is seen at the hub of the syringe. The amount of fluid in the syringe is equal to the internal volume of the catheter lumen. The catheter lumen can then be loaded with a volume of drug solution equal to the internal volume of the lumen. Connecting the filled catheter lumen to an intravenous tubing system that has been flushed with the cardiopulmonary drug solution allows infusion to reach the patient's blood without a time delay.

Placement of the Pulmonary Artery Catheter

The catheter may be positioned using fluoroscopy but is more often floated into place using the pressure waveforms to indicate the catheter's position. The distal lumen of the catheter is connected to a transducer-monitor system; both the distal and proximal lumina are flushed until they are free of air bubbles, and then the catheter is placed through an introducer in one of the same vessels used for placement of CVP catheters.

RIGHT ATRIUM. When the tip of the catheter reaches the great vessels, a CVP waveform appears on the monitor (Fig. 14-12). The balloon is fully inflated while the catheter is still in the *atrium* to decrease the risk of PVCs occurring while the catheter is in the ventricle.

RIGHT VENTRICLE. A rapid increase in the height of the pressure waveform is seen when the catheter passes through the tricuspid valve into the *right ventricle.* The ventricular waveform is easily distinguished from the pulmonary artery waveform because the right side of the waveform (downstroke) drops straight down to just below zero as the ventricle relaxes during diastole. As soon as the ventricle relaxes, the tricuspid valve opens and blood begins to flow into the ventricle causing the pressure wave to increase gradually. *End-diastolic pressure* occurs just prior to the upstroke created by ventricular isovolumetric contraction (see Fig. 14-12).

The catheter is supposed to float from the right ventricle into the pulmonary artery; however, achieving catheter placement in the pulmonary artery can take from minutes to more than an hour. Insertion is even more difficult in patients with altered pulmonary circulation secondary to longstanding or chronic pulmonary disease. In most adults, catheters inserted through the subclavian or jugular vein are positioned in the pulmonary artery when approximately 50 cm of catheter is inserted into the patient. When more than that amount has been inserted and no pulmonary waveform is

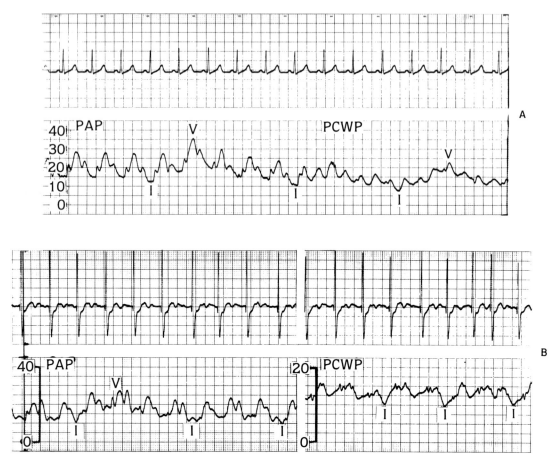

Fig. 14-13 *Pulmonary artery pressure (PAP) trace converting to wedge pressure.* **A,** *Patient is on intermittent mandatory ventilation of 12 and positive end-expiratory pressure of 5 cm* H_2O. *Note respiratory swing in pressure wave. I, spontaneous inspiration; V, intermittent ventilator breath. Heart rate, 98 beats/min, normal sinus rhythm; PAP, 27/15 mmHg; pulmonary capillary wedge pressure (PCWP), 13 mmHg.* **B,** *Note difference in appearance of waveforms in patient with atrial fibrillation. Heart rate, 87–102, PAP, 23/14 mmHg, PCWP, 13 mmHg.*

obtained, it is generally assumed that the catheter is curling in the atrium or ventricle. The balloon is deflated and the catheter is withdrawn until the tip is in the atrium, and then reinserted.

PULMONARY ARTERY. Entry into the *pulmonary artery* is recognized by a change in the diastolic portion of the waveform. The pulmonary artery waveform is a miniature of the peripheral arterial waveform having a dicrotic notch and a gradual diastolic runoff that does not drop to zero level.

Normal pulmonary artery *systolic pressure* is between 20 and 30 mmHg; *diastolic* is 6 to 15 mmHg; and the *mean* is between 10 and 20 mmHg. Pressures in excess of 45 mmHg are occasionally seen in patients with severe left heart disease and chronic obstructive pulmonary disease (COPD). These pressure waves may have a steep appearance on both sides and may be easily confused with the ventricular pressure waves. However, close examination of the diastolic portion of the waveform shows that ventricular waves fall to below baseline before leveling off in diastole, whereas the pulmonary artery waveforms do have a dicrotic notch and diastolic runoff (see Fig. 14–12).

WEDGE POSITION. When the catheter *wedges* in a smaller branch of the pulmonary artery, the forward flow of the pulmonary arterial blood is occluded. With pulsatile arterial blood flow stopped, the tip of the catheter "sees" the backpressure from the pulmonary venous system and left atrium and the waveform takes on the appearance of an atrial pressure (CVP) waveform with a, c, and v waves (Figs. 14–12 and 14–13). The pulmonary artery waveform should return when the balloon is deflated.

WEDGE PRESSURE. *Normal pulmonary artery wedge pressure (PAWP)* is 4 to 12 mmHg. Wedge pressure is lower than mean pulmonary artery pressure and is usually about 2 mmHg lower than PADP. These normal pressure relationships are easy to remember by keeping in mind that blood flows from higher pressure to lower pressure. Wedge pressure is also called *pulmonary capillary wedge pressure (PCWP)* and *pulmonary artery occlusion pressure (PAOP)*. (See other sources for a more complete discussion of pulmonary artery pressure monitoring,[65,66] of catheter placement, and of waveform analysis.[67])

Complications of Pulmonary Artery Catheterization

Pulmonary artery catheterization has been associated with multiple complications.[4,5,68–72] During cannulation of a central vein, it is possible for pneumothorax, hydrothorax, air embolism, and damage to the vein, nearby arteries, or nerves to occur. Movement of the catheter inside the heart can trigger bundle-branch block and supraventricular or ventricular dysrhythmia. Hypoxemia, acidosis, hypokalemia, hypocalcemia, and hypomagnesemia increase the likelihood of dysrhythmia. Additionally, *perforation* of the heart or pulmonary artery is possible.

The pulmonary artery catheter, like all other invasive lines, is a source of *embolus, thrombosis, bleeding, hematoma, site infection,* and *sepsis.* The constant movement of the catheter with heartbeat, breathing, and patient movement can result in catheter migration. It should be remembered that a balloon left inflated or a catheter that migrates into wedge position acts like a pulmonary embolus. *Pulmonary infarction* and even *pulmonary rupture* can occur from overfilling the balloon while obtaining a wedge pressure as well as from *catheter migration.* Pulmonary infarction should be suspected and assessed whenever a patient with a pulmonary catheter coughs up blood-tinged sputum. An overfilled balloon can rupture causing possible fragment or *air embolism.*

Catheter movement and catheter removal can trigger dysrhythmia as well as *looping of the catheter* in the ventricle with possible knotting and valve damage. Lidocaine and emergency resuscitation equipment should be immediately available at both insertion and removal. Blood gases and serum electrolytes should be optimized to decrease the risk of dysrhythmia. Catheter resistance during removal is not normal and is an indication for chest radiography to assess the cause.

Interpretation of Pulmonary Artery Pressures

PULMONARY ARTERY SYSTOLIC PRESSURE.
Pulmonary artery systolic pressure is the highest pressure created when the right ventricle ejects blood through the pulmonary valve and into the pulmonary artery and lungs. Like systemic arterial pressure, pulmonary artery pressure is a product of the volume of blood ejected by the ventricle and the resistance of the pulmonary circulation. Pulmonary artery pressures *decrease* when the volume of blood ejected by the right ventricle decreases or when the pulmonary vasculature relaxes or dilates (decreased pulmonary vascular resistance). Conversely, pulmonary artery pressures *increase* when pulmonary blood flow increases or when pulmonary vascular resistance increases.

The right ventricle pumps increased amounts of blood into the lungs with volume overload or when it receives excess blood from left-to-right intracardiac shunts (e.g., atrial or ventricular septal defects or patent ductus arteriosus). Resistance to pulmonary flow (*increased pulmonary vascular resistance*) can be caused by constriction, obstruction, or compression of the pulmonary vasculature or by backpressure from the left heart. For example, emboli obstruct flow, and acute or chronic pulmonary parenchymal disease compresses and destroys vascular pathways. Cardiac tamponade or increased intrathoracic pressure compresses the vasculature and impedes forward flow. Left heart failure and mitral valve stenosis (narrowing) cause backpressure from the left heart into the lungs. Hypoxia, acidosis, hypoxemia, and vasoactive drugs cause vasoconstriction and increased pulmonary vascular resistance (see Table 13–4).

Pulmonary arterial pressures average about 22/8 mmHg with a mean pressure of about 13 mmHg.[73] However, in advanced pulmonary disease it is not uncommon for the systolic pressure to exceed 45 mm Hg and the mean pulmonary pressure to exceed 35 mm Hg. Such severe pulmonary hypertension may depress right ventricular function and thereby decrease left ventricular preload. Subsequently, left ventricular stroke volume and systemic oxygen transport may also decrease.[44,74,75]

PULMONARY ARTERY DIASTOLIC PRESSURE.
Pulmonary artery diastolic pressure, under normal conditions, is dependent on the downstream pressures: pulmonary venous, left atrial, and because the mitral valve is open during diastole, LVEDP. Additionally, pulmonary capillary resistance and impedance to flow are normally minimal.[76] Therefore, in the absence of severe pulmonary vascular changes, marked tachycardia, or pulmonary embolism, pulmonary artery diastolic pressure can be used to monitor left heart function without risk of problems induced by inadvertent wedging of the catheter.[76,77] In some institutions, when a normal comparison of pulmonary artery diastolic and wedge pressure is identified, the catheter is withdrawn into a larger section of the pulmonary artery where it cannot be wedged. Positioning the catheter in a large arterial segment and using the PADP to reflect LAP decreases the chances of complications from catheter migration and accidental wedging.

Relationship between PADP and PCWP

Normally, PADP is approximately 2 mmHg higher than wedge pressure, but elevated pulmonary vascular resistance increases the gradient. Factors such as clot, hypoxia, acidosis, sepsis, fibrosis, and drugs that increase pulmonary vascular resistance will cause the PADP to exceed the PCWP. In fact, a PADP-PCWP gradient that is greater than 5 mmHg is characteristic of ARDS, sepsis, excessive PEEP, or other conditions that increase pulmonary vascular resistance. In contrast, pulmonary hypertension due to increased LAP is

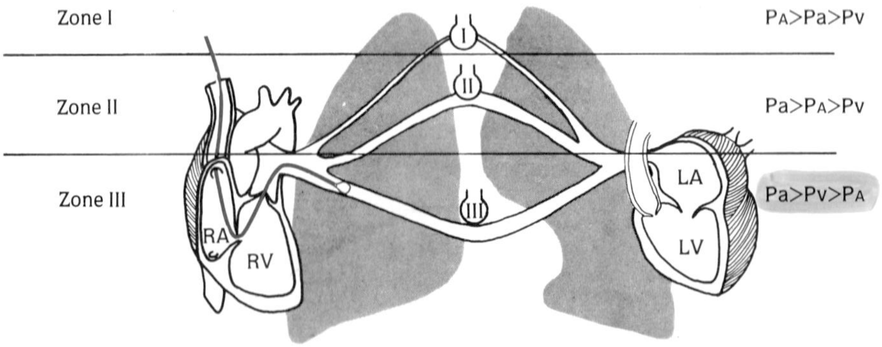

Fig. 14–14 *Pulmonary artery catheter wedged in zone III, where both pulmonary arterial and venous pressures are greater than alveolar pressure, resulting in uninterrupted blood flow to the left heart and a pulmonary capillary wedge pressure that reflects pulmonary venous and left heart pressures. Relationship of pressures is shown at the right. See text for explanation of West's zones I, II, III, Pₐ, alveolar pressure, Pa, pulmonary arterial pressure, Pv, pulmonary venous pressure, RA, right atrium, RV, right ventricle, LA, left atrium, LV, left ventricle.*

characterized by a normal PADP-PCWP gradient (<5 mmHg).

With heart rates greater than 120 beats per minute, the time for diastolic runoff is shortened and PADP increases.[78] Therefore, in the presence of tachyarrhythmias, vasoconstriction, pulmonary emboli, or increased or fluctuating pulmonary vascular resistance, PADP significantly overestimates PCWP and should not be used to reflect left heart pressures.[76–80] On the other hand, when the tip of the catheter is in a vessel above the level of the heart (zone I or II), the vessel may become occluded by airway pressure, causing the pulmonary diastolic pressure to fall below the wedge and left-sided pressures (Fig. 14–14).

Relationship of Wedge Pressure to Pulmonary Venous and Left Atrial Pressures

Under normal conditions, pulmonary wedge pressure can be used to represent pulmonary venous, left atrial, and left ventricular end-diastolic pressure because, when the mitral valve is open, there are no barriers between the tip of the catheter and the left heart. Additionally, inflation and wedging of the balloon closes off forward flow from the right heart so the catheter only "sees" a backward reflection of pressure from the left heart. However, when obstructions or alterations in blood flow exist, PCWP will overestimate LVEDP. Conditions in which PCWP *overestimates* left heart filling pressure include mitral valve stenosis, mitral valve regurgitation, wedge pressures greater than 25 mm Hg,[81] pulmonary venous obstruction,[82] or pulmonary venoconstriction.[83] Additionally, if compliance of the ventricle is decreased[78,84,85] or intrathoracic pressure is increased[82,87] (as discussed in Chapter 13), PCWP may represent end-diastolic pressure but will not be an accurate measure of end-diastolic volume and preload. Table 14–3 summarizes situations in which PCWP overestimates left heart filling.

Obtaining an Accurate PCWP

Studies have indicated that approximately one third of the wedge pressure readings have some type of error.[13,88,89] Table 14–4 summarizes the technical criteria used to ensure that the pressure measured is wedge pressure. The technical aspects of setting up a pressure monitoring system include calibrating the monitor and transducer, positioning the transducer and patient, verifying and maximizing frequency response and damping characteristics, and recording the pressures at end-expiration. Attention to proper management of the technical steps is vital to obtaining accurate pulmonary artery and wedge pressure measurements. The criteria are discussed at the end of this chapter.

CATHETER POSITIONED IN ZONE III. For PCWP to reflect pulmonary venous and therefore left atrial pressure, blood flow must be uninterrupted between the catheter tip and the left heart. This condition only exists in what West has called *zone III*,[91,92] an area of the lung where both pulmonary arterial and venous pressures exceed alveolar pressure. As depicted in Fig. 14–14, zone I theoretically has no blood flow, because alveolar pressure exceeds both pulmonary venous and MAP. In zone II, alveolar pressure exceeds venous pressure but is less than MAP. Because breathing (inspiration and expiration) and pulmonary artery pressure (systolic and diastolic) are phasic, flow is intermittent. Hence, a catheter located in zone II measures pulmonary arterial pressure with the balloon deflated but reflects *alveolar* pressure when it is wedged.

The lung zones are not anatomically fixed zones but rather functional, gravity-dependent zones, which are altered by position, blood flow and pressure, and ventilatory status (CPAP, PEEP, air trapping). Zone II conditions dominate in supine patients. However, because the catheters are flow-directed, they tend to advance to areas of continuous blood flow. Nevertheless, the location of the catheter tip at or below left atrial level should be verified by a lateral chest film.[93] *To measure left heart pressure accurately, the catheter 'ip*

Table 14-3 Recognizing When PCWP Overestimates Left Ventricular Filling*†

Catheter Tip in Zone I or II[88] During PEEP or CPAP	Technical Problems	Physiologic Conditions
PADP < PCWP	Overinflation	Pulmonary venous obstruction/compression
Smooth trace: no a or v waves	Incomplete wedge	(e.g., lung or mediastinal tumors, left atrial
With changes in Peep:	Catheter fling	myxoma)
PCWP increase >50% PEEP increase	Underdamped trace	Mitral valve stenosis or occlusion
PCWP decrease >50% PEEP reduction	Occluded catheter tip: clot, vessel wall,	Mitral valve insufficiency—large v waves
With catheter wedged:	embolism, eccentric inflation	Decreased left ventricular compliance[84,85]
Inability to withdraw blood	Transducer below left atrial level	Inotropic drugs, hypertension
Mixed venous blood rather than "arterialized"	Not end-expiratory reading	Acute cardiac dilation
blood	Tubing or patient movement	Myocardial ischemia, hypertrophy, injury,
Catheter tip above left atrial level on lateral	Cough or Valsalva maneuver during wedge	infarction, infiltrate
chest film		Pericardial disease or tamponade
		Increased intrathoracic pressure:
		PEEP or CPAP > 10 cm H_2O

*Data from references 78, 82.
†PCWP = pulmonary capillary wedge pressure; PEEP = positive end-expiratory pressure; PADP = pulmonary artery diastolic pressure; CPAP = continuous positive airway pressure.

Table 14-4 Criteria for PCWP That Represents Left Heart Filling Pressure*

Criteria	Characteristics
Distinct and valid pulmonary artery pressure trace before inflation	Frequency response not over- or underdamped
	Transducer calibrated at left atrial level
	Patient supine, head of bed ≤ 45 degrees
Catheter tip in zone III	At or below left atrial level with lateral x-ray film
PADP > PCWP	If PAPD < PCWP, consider non-zone III, tachycardia > 120 beats/min
	and increased pulmonary vascular resistance
Distinct PCWP trace immediately on wedge	a and c waves clearly visible
	Elevated v waves suggest mitral regurgitation; may also be seen
	with MI and mitral stenosis
Free flow with catheter wedged[88,89]	No overinflation (climbing wave)
	Easy withdrawal of blood
	Nondamped trace
Change in PCWP < ½ change in airway pressure	Applies to both increase and decrease of PEEP or CPAP
Aspiration of "arterialized" blood from distal port while catheter is	$Pwo_2 - Pao_2 ≥ 19$ mmHg
wedged[90]	$Paco_2 - Pwco_2 ≥ 11$ mmHg
	pHw – pHa ≥ 0.08
Pressure reading using the a wave at end-expiration	Obtained from paper if IMV or labored breathing
	If monitor has algorithm to find end-expiration and verification
	between paper recording and digital agree[82]:
	Use systolic pressure for spontaneous breathing
	Use diastolic pressure for continuous mechanical ventilation

*PADP = pulmonary artery diastolic pressure; PCWP = pulmonary capillary wedge pressure; MI = myocardial infarction; PEEP = positive end-expiratory pressure; CPAP = continuous positive airway pressure; PWo_2 = wedge pressure, oxygen; Pao_2 = arterial oxygen tension; $Paco_2$ = arterial carbon dioxide tension; $Pwco_2$ = wedge pressure, carbon dioxide; pHw = wedge pH; pHa = arterial pH.

must be in zone III.[88] When intravascular volume decreases (diuresis, hypovolemia, hemorrhage) or alveolar pressure increases (PEEP), zone III areas can convert to zone I or II. Catheters located at or below the left atrial level are less likely to be affected by these changes. Characteristics of non-zone III catheters[94] are listed in Table 14-3.

WEDGING THE BALLOON. Ideally, the catheter ends up in a portion of the pulmonary artery that is at or below left atrial level, where a wedge trace with very clear a and v waves is obtained using 0.8 to 1.5 mL of air.[95] Locating the catheter tip in a slightly larger segment of the artery reduces the risk associated with catheter migration and decreases the likelihood of overinflation and eccentric balloon inflation. Subse-

quently, the balloon should be inflated with the *minimum* amount of air necessary to obtain a clear wedge reading.

Placing too much air in the balloon (*overwedging*) results in a pressure waveform without clearly distinguishable a and v waves that gradually climbs upward across the screen. Rarely, overwedging may produce a waveform that gradually declines, again without clearly distinguishable a and v waves.

The balloon should be left inflated only long enough to obtain the wedge trace; however, it must be remembered that it may take from 5 to 20 seconds for equilibration of the left heart and pulmonary pressures following balloon inflation.[82] Integrity of the balloon is extended if it is permitted to empty on its own rather

Table 14-5	Obtaining Blood Samples from a Pulmonary Artery (PA) Catheter*
Obtaining a Mixed Venous Blood Sample*	**Obtaining a Wedge ("Capillary") Blood Sample**
Verify or obtain a clear PA trace.	Verify or obtain a clear PCWP trace with a and v waves PADP > PCWP
Balloon deflated	Balloon inflated
Slowly withdraw to clear PA port (3–6 mL); *discard*	Withdraw 15–20 mL; *discard*
Using a heparinized syringe, *slowly* withdraw 2–3 mL	Using a heparinized syringe, withdraw 2–3 mL
Mark syringe *mixed venous.*	Mark syringe *wedge sample*
Simultaneously draw arterial blood; mark syringe *arterial*	Draw arterial blood; mark syringe *arterial*
Criteria for mixed venous sample compared to *arterial* blood:	Criteria for wedged (arterialized or capillary) blood[90]:
$P\bar{v}co_2 - Paco_2 \geq 2$ mmHg	$Pwo_2 - Pao_2 \geq 19$ mmHg
	$Paco_2 - Pwco_2 \geq 11$ mmHg
	$pHw - pHa \geq 0.08$

*$P\bar{v}co_2$ = mixed venous carbon dioxide pressure. For other abbreviations, see footnote to Table 14–4.

than by aspiration. Deflation of the balloon is confirmed by a clear pulmonary artery trace.

VERIFYING WEDGE POSITION. The wedge position is verified first by the waveform. Prior to balloon inflation, the pulmonary artery trace should be very clear, with systolic, dicrotic notch, and diastolic segments. On inflation the waveform should immediately convert to a clear atrial pressure trace with no systolic segment or dicrotic notch. On balloon deflation, the waveform should convert immediately to a crisp pulmonary artery trace.

It is possible to obtain a *partial wedge,* in which the systolic pressure is high enough to push blood around the inflated balloon but the artery is occluded during diastole. The trace is recognized by a systolic wave that converts to a wedge trace during diastole: half pulmonary artery trace and half wedge trace. This waveform produces a pressure that is higher than true wedge pressure.

Wedge pressure readings are normally about 2 mm Hg lower than pulmonary artery pressure readings[82,88] because blood flows from high pressure to low pressure. If the wedge pressure were higher, blood would be flowing backward. In fact, that does occur with mitral valve regurgitation where the valve does not close completely during systole and blood is ejected backward into the left atrium. This problem can be recognized by giant v waves, which are more than 10 mmHg higher than the a waves. Recording the waveform on paper and using the a wave[96,97] (atrial systole) at the end of expiration will result in a more consistent and accurate reflection of left ventricular end-diastolic volume.

CONFIRMING WEDGE POSITION BY BLOOD GAS ANALYSIS. *Wedge blood* is obtained by aspirating blood backward from the pulmonary capillaries while the inflated balloon prevents aspiration of mixed venous blood from the pulmonary artery. Because gas exchange will have already taken place in blood that has passed the capillaries, the sample is referred to as "arterialized." In fact, wedge blood should have a higher oxygen pressure (Po_2) and lower carbon dioxide pressure (Pco_2) than arterial blood.[82,90]

Obtaining arterialized blood confirms that the vascular channel is open between the catheter tip and left heart (zone III) condition, and that the pressure obtained should be representative of left heart pressure.[90]

Table 14–5 summarizes the difference in technique and outcome for obtaining mixed venous and wedge blood samples. A *mixed venous sample is obtained with the balloon deflated and is withdrawn slowly* to prevent accidental withdrawal of arterialized blood. The catheter is cleared using the same "slow draw" technique.

A *wedge sample is drawn at normal to rapid speed with the balloon inflated.* Note that the PADP should be higher than the wedge pressure and that the PCWP waveform should have clearly visible a and v waves. The catheter should be cleared by aspirating and discarding 15 to 20 mL after balloon inflation to ensure that capillary blood is obtained.

MEASURING THE PRESSURE AT END-EXPIRATION. Alterations in ventilatory patterns cause fluctuations in intrapleural pressure. End-expiration minimizes the influence of the pressure swings for both spontaneous and mechanical ventilation, provided the patient is not exhaling against positive pressure. Ideally, the pressure will be recorded from a calibrated paper trace that also records the ventilatory pattern so that the end-expiratory pressures are clearly identified over several respiratory cycles.[98-110]

Digital displays are less accurate because they report an average of several beats and may even average artifact.[11,13] When the digital display is used, the cooperative patient can be asked to suspend breathing on exhalation for several cardiac cycles. Adjusting the systolic or diastolic pressure switch on the monitor according to the patient's mode of ventilation will help to improve the accuracy of digitally displayed pressures. Using the *systolic* pressure setting during spontaneous ventilation gives the most reliable reading because intrapleural pressure is highest on expiration. On the other hand, the *diastolic* pressure setting provides the most accurate reading for the patient on continuous mechanical ventilation[105] where intrapleural pressure is lowest at end-expiration.[82] For patients with labored or shallow breathing, the mean setting probably gives the best result.

Even monitors with respiratory algorithms[110] cannot accurately track the pressures of patients on IMV who have both negative and positive inspiratory changes. For continuous monitoring of pulmonary pressures, the mean pressure setting should be used; however, a paper trace should be used for pressures that are to be recorded, trended, or used for specific therapeutic interventions. The technique for reading a paper trace is discussed in the technical section at the end of this chapter.

RELATIONSHIP BETWEEN TRANSMURAL PRESSURE AND PCWP. Transmural pressure is the net distending pressure within the ventricle. It provides a true estimation of left ventricular end-diastolic filling because the effect of pressure around the heart is considered. Transmural pressure cannot be measured directly but is calculated by *subtracting* the pressure around the heart (juxtacardiac pressure) from the measured filling pressure in the heart. Wedge pressure is used to estimate left ventricular filling pressure. Intrapleural or esophageal pressure is used to approximate juxtacardiac pressure.

During spontaneous breathing, intrapleural pressure is nearly zero at end-expiration. Therefore, as shown in the example below, end-diastolic pressure and transmural pressure are approximately equal and wedge pressure is a good estimator of left ventricular filling pressure in the patient with normal spontaneous breathing.[78,82] However, positive pressure ventilation, labored respiratory effort, coughing, and the Valsalva maneuver cause large swings in the intrapleural pressure. These pressure fluctuations can cause wedge pressure to over- or underestimate left ventricular filling pressure.

The following example shows how a PCWP of 12 mmHg can occur with very different transmural pressures. Remember that left ventricular filling pressure (PCWP) minus pressure around the heart (pleural pressure) equals pressure distending the left ventricle (transmural pressure).

	PCWP – Pleural pressure	=	Transmural pressure
Spontaneous breathing	12 – 0	=	12 mmHg
20 cm PEEP	12 – 10	=	–2 mmHg
Partial airway obstruction	12 – -10	=	22 mmHg

The relationship between PCWP and transmural pressure must be kept in mind when interpreting the numbers. The example "20 cm PEEP" shows how transmission of positive pleural pressure can cause the PCWP to appear normal (12) while, in fact, the patient is really hypovolemic with a transmural pressure of – 2 mmHg.

The example of "partial airway obstruction" shows how filling pressure can appear to be normal (12) when in fact, the true filling pressure would be high (22).

TRANSMURAL PRESSURE AND THE EFFECTS OF PEEP. Clinically, PEEP levels less than 10 cm H_2O have a limited effect on intrapleural pressure. However, when PEEP exceeds 15 cm H_2O, the effect of PEEP on transmural pressure is uncertain and is altered by lung compliance and changing venous return. As lung compliance decreases, less of the positive pressure is passed to the pleural space. This has led to the practice of estimating the effect of PEEP on PCWP by converting the PEEP to millimeters of mercury (1.36 cm H_2O = 1 mmHg) and subtracting part of the PEEP from the PCWP as follows[111]:

$$\text{Compliant lungs: subtract} \frac{1}{2} \text{ of PEEP from PCWP}$$
$$\text{Noncompliant lungs: subtract} \frac{1}{4} \text{ of PEEP from PCWP}$$

The effects of PEEP on transmural pressure can also be assessed by measuring pleural pressure. In practice, *esophageal pressure*[112] is measured with a fluid-filled tube while the patient is in the lateral decubitus position. The esophageal pressure, which is essentially the same as pleural pressure, is then subtracted from the wedge pressure.

PRESSURE MEASUREMENTS ON AND OFF PEEP. Removing the patient from PEEP while the wedge pressures are obtained has been suggested.[113] However, this maneuver alters the pressure gradient for venous return to the thorax and may result in sudden "autotransfusion."[114,115] Additionally, sudden removal of PEEP has been reported to cause deterioration in gas exchange that is not readily corrected.[116] In patients with left ventricular dysfunction, removal from mechanical ventilation with PEEP may be associated with increased pulmonary artery pressure, hypoxemia, and deterioration in cardiac function.[117] Removal of patients from mechanical ventilation with PEEP to obtain pressure readings is not recommended.

Clinical Applications

Clinical Interpretation Using Both CVP and PCWP

In the absence of impaired left heart function, changes in CVP parallel those of wedge pressure and LVEDP. Therefore, the CVP can be used to monitor the heart's response to fluid challenges[118] without the attendant risks of pulmonary artery catheterization (see Tables 14–10 and 14–11). It is important to note however, that this *does not apply* to the patient with impaired left ventricular function, especially following acute myocardial infarction (MI).[44] As shown in Table 14–6, CVP remains normal or only slightly elevated even in pa-

Table 14-6   Hemodynamic Changes in Clinical Conditions Associated with Low Cardiac Output*†

	CO	CVP	PAP	PCWP
Mild left ventricular (LV) failure	↓	—	↑	↑↑
Severe LV failure	↓↓	—↑	↑↑	↑↑
Mitral regurgitation	↓	—↑	↑↑	↑↑ (v wave)
Ventricular septal defect	↓↑	—↑	—	—↑
Right ventricular infarction	↓	↑↑	↓↑	↓↑
Pulmonary hypertension	↓	↑↑	↑↑	—
Tamponade	↓	↑↑	↑	↑
Pulmonary embolism	↓	↑↑	↑↑	—↓
Shock states‡				
Obstructive shock	↓	↑↑	↑↑	—↓
Cardiogenic shock	↓	↑↓	↑↑	↑↑
Hypovolemic shock	↓	↓↓	↓↓	↓↓
Distributive shock	↓↑	—	—	—

*From Weil MH, vonPlanta M, and Rackow EC: Acute circulatory failure (shock). In Braunwald E, editor, *Heart disease*, ed 3, Philadelphia, 1988, WB Saunders.
†↓, decreased; ↓↓, greatly decreased; ↑, increased; ↑↑, greatly increased; —, normal or little or no change; ↓↑ = increase or decrease.
‡*Obstructive shock:* Blood flow is obstructed in the heart or great veins: pericardial tamponade, ball-valve thrombi, pulmonary embolism, or aortic dissection. *Distributive shock:* Major alterations in the distribution of blood flow without critical decreases in intravascular volume, cardiac function, or obstruction of blood flow. Two types are described: *Low-resistance* (low systemic vascular resistance [SVR]) occurs with inflammatory vasodilation or arteriovenous shunting, as in gram-negative sepsis (hyperdynamic shock), pneumonia, peritonitis, abscess, reactive hyperemia. *High or normal* SVR occurs with increase in venous capacitance, which results in decreased venous return: advanced (hypodynamic) septic shock, autonomic blockade, spinal shock, and tranquilizer, sedative, and narcotic overdose.

Table 14-7   Clinical Decision Making Using Wedge Pressure (PCWP), Cardiac Output (CO), and Oxygen Delivery (Do₂)*

PCWP	CO	Do₂	Therapeutic Course
Low	Normal	Normal	Continue monitoring
Low	Low	Low	Administer fluid to increase LVEDV and SV
High	Normal	Normal	Consider diuretic
High	Low	Low	Assess for decreased left ventricular compliance or increased LVEDV; if blood pressure is normal, consider vasodilator to improve compliance, with additional volume to augment LVEDV and SV

*Data from Leasa DJ and Sibbald WJ: Respiratory monitoring in a critical care unit. In Simmons DH, editor: *Current pulmonology*, vol 9, St Louis, 1988, Mosby.
†LVEDV = left ventricular end-diastolic volume; SV = stroke volume.

tients with cardiogenic shock following acute MI unless cardiac tamponade, right heart disease, or lung disorders are also present. Nevertheless, it is important to monitor the right heart filling pressure routinely.

CVP rises as the efficiency of the right heart to move blood through the lungs decreases. When the CVP is elevated and accurately measured while pulmonary pressures are normal or low, the cause of the problem resides in the right heart; e.g., right ventricular infarction or right heart valvular disease. If, however, both the CVP and pulmonary artery pressures are elevated while the left-sided filling pressures are normal, the problem most likely resides in the lung: pulmonary embolism, ARDS, or pulmonary hypertension induced by hypoxemia or preexisting pulmonary heart disease.[119] Table 14-6 summarizes the relationships of hemodynamic pressures in clinical problems often associated with low cardiac output.

Clinical Interpretation Using Wedge Pressure and Other Measures

Table 14-7 shows how the combination of wedge pressure, cardiac output, and oxygen delivery can suggest the clinical problem and therapeutic course.

In 1976, Forrester and others[120] reported a comparison of clinical signs, hemodynamic values, and medical therapy using hemodynamic subsets in patients following MI. As shown in Fig. 14-15 and 13-6, these hemodynamic subsets are constructed by comparing PCWP and cardiac index. A PCWP greater than 18 mm Hg is considered elevated and is usually associated with pulmonary vascular congestion secondary to decreased left ventricular function. A cardiac index less than 2.2 L/min/m² is considered low and is associated with peripheral hypoperfusion. Low cardiac output is most commonly caused by the loss of ventricular muscle function but may also occur because of inadequate volume (preload). Although further research is indicated before

Subset I PCWP low to normal, adequate CI **Goal:** "Fine tune" patient's clinical status prevent pulmonary congestion or fall in CI **Treatment Options:** treat tachycardia and dysrhythmia ↓ myocardial O_2 demand: nitroglycerin & beta blockade fluid administration to "optimal PCWP"	Subset II PCWP elevated, adequate CI **Goal:** Reverse/prevent pulmonary congestion without jeopardizing preload, contractility, CO **Treatment Options:** IV vasodilators ACE inhibitors diuretics
Subset III PCWP low to normal, low CI *consider hypovolemia, third spacing, right MI* **Goal:** Correct hypovolemia with appropriate fluid optimize preload & afterload, treat bradycardia **Treatment Options:** aggressive fluid therapy to "optimal PCWP" inotropes/vasopressors if ↓ contractility after volume use chronotropic drugs with caution to avoid ↑ myocardial O_2 demand	Subset IV PCWP elevated, low CI *consider cardiogenic shock, pulmonary embolus* **Goal:** Reduce afterload, improve contractility & CI, reverse pulmonary congestion but optimize preload **Treatment Options:** vasodilators vasopressors diuretics IABP thrombolytic therapy

Cardiac Index 2.2 L/min/m² — 0 — 18 mm Hg — **Pulmonary Capillary Wedge Pressure**

Fig. 14–15 *Forrester's hemodynamic subsets and treatment considerations for patients following myocardial infarction.*[120] *The patient's position within the subsets is determined by the intersection of a PCWP of 18 mmHg and a cardiac index of 2.2 L/min/m². See also Fig. 13–6. IABP, intraaortic balloon pump; see Fig. 14–4 and related text. PCWP, pulmonary capillary wedge pressure.*

these subsets can be generalized to all critically ill patient populations, the subsets can be used as a framework for integrating hemodynamic measurements with clinical assessment[121] and understanding clinical decision making. The most common therapeutic goals and treatment options for each subset are listed in Fig. 14–15. The overall therapeutic goal is to maintain or obtain adequate perfusion (cardiac index >2.2 L/min/m²) and preload while avoiding volume overload and pulmonary congestion (PCWP >18 mmHg). The balance of myocardial oxygen supply and demand is enhanced by assuring adequate volume (preload) before medications such as pressors, inotropic agents, or chronotropic drugs are initiated to "drive" myocardial performance. Additionally, the use of vasodilators and IABP increase pump efficiency by decreasing the resistance to ventricular emptying (afterload).

Fig. 14–16 shows two logic trees that use a three-factor approach for interpreting these hemodynamic data in patients with and without pulmonary vascular disease. Patients are sorted into one of the two logic trees based on their pulmonary vascular resistance. A normal pulmonary vascular resistance indicates no pulmonary vascular disease. Patients with elevated pulmonary vascular resistance are considered

to have pulmonary vascular disease. Once the appropriate logic tree has been selected, PCWP is used as an estimate of left ventricular end-diastolic volume and function. Cardiac output is used for the final decision toward choosing a diagnostic pathway.

Relationship of PCWP to Pulmonary Edema

Pulmonary edema is an abnormal accumulation of fluid within the parenchyma (functioning tissue) of the lung. Pulmonary edema occurs with increased hydrostatic pressure (PCWP), decreased oncotic pressure, or increased permeability of the pulmonary capillaries.

The gas exchange units of the lung (*acini*) resemble clusters of grapes composed of bronchioles branching to alveolar ducts, alveolar sacs, and finally alveoli (Fig. 14–17). Each of the estimated 8,000 alveoli within an acinus is surrounded by a meshwork of capillaries. Microscopic *alveolar-capillary membranes* (across which the gases diffuse to oxygenate and remove excess carbon dioxide from the blood) separate the air space within an alveolus from the blood in the capillaries (see insert of Fig. 14–17). Type I alveolar epithelial cells form the lining of the alveoli and are

A No pulmonary vascular disease

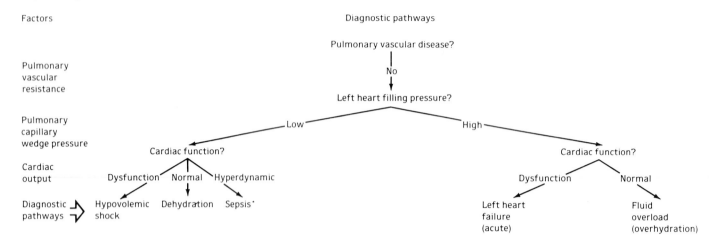

*Sepsis may be associated with normal left heart filling pressures.

Pulmonary vascular disease

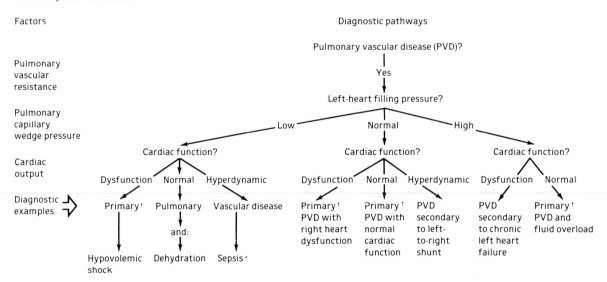

* Sepsis may be associated with normal left heart filling pressures.
† Primary PVD may be caused by pulmonary emboli, pulmonary artery disease (vasculitis, "primary" pulmonary hypertension), respiratory distress syndromes, hypoxic vasoconstriction, or drugs.

Fig. 14-16 *Three-factor approach to interpreting hemodynamic data. Pulmonary vascular resistance reflects the presence or absence of pulmonary vascular disease. Pulmonary capillary wedge pressure reflects the filling pressure of the left heart. Cardiac output reflects myocardial function.* **A,** *Patterns with no pulmonary vascular disease,* **B,** *Patterns with pulmonary vascular disease. Examples of common diagnoses associated with various abnormal patterns. (From Osgood CF and others:* Respir Care 29:30, 1984.)

relatively impermeable to fluids and solutes. A potential space called the *interstitial space* exists between the wall of the alveoli and the highly permeable endothelial wall of the capillaries. Fluid filtering from the pulmonary capillaries normally moves into the interstitial space, comes to the almost impermeable alveolar epithelium, and is channeled to the peribronchial and perivascular interstitium where it can flow into the lymphatics.[122] When the amount of fluid filtered from the capillaries exceeds the removal capacity of the lymph system, pulmonary edema develops.

Pulmonary edema has two stages: interstitial and alveolar.[123] In the interstitial phase, excessive amounts of fluids filtered from the capillaries engorge the interstitial space, but fluid does not enter the alveoli. A significant amount of fluid can collect with no apparent clinical signs other than possible subtle changes in pulmonary wedge pressure, compliance, and chest x-ray films. If the cause of pulmonary edema continues, fluid begins to move into the air spaces of some alveoli and eventually floods the alveoli, leaving no available air space. The rate of gas transfer across the alveolar-

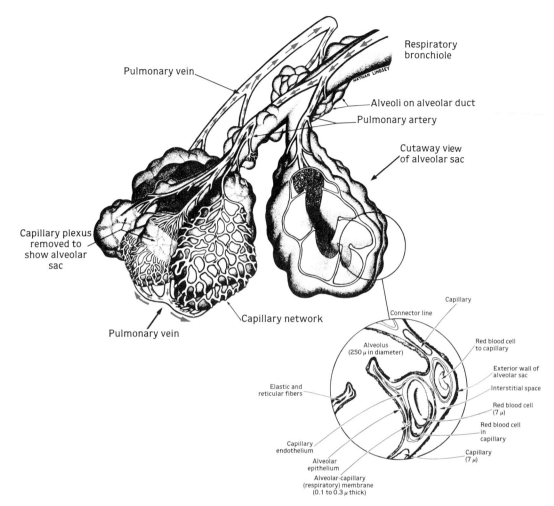

Fig. 14-17 *Respiratory unit or lobule (acinus) made up of respiratory bronchioles branching into alveolar ducts budding with alveoli, alveolar ducts, and alveoli (0.25 mm in diameter). Alveoli are encased by a meshwork of interconnecting capillaries averaging 8 μm in diameter. Red blood cells also average approximately 8 μm in diameter so that their membrane is usually in contact with the capillary wall, decreasing the amount of plasma respiratory gases that must pass between the red blood cell and alveolus. Insert, alveolor-capillary membrane (respiratory membrane) is made up of multiple layers: capillary endothelium, capillary basement membrane, interstitial space, epithelial basement membrane, alveolar epithelium, and surfactant and other substances lining the alveolus. Despite the number of layers, the overall thickness of the microscopic alveolar-capillary membrane is only 0.1 to 0.3 μm.*

capillary membranes is decreased (diffusion defect); ventilation becomes unevenly distributed throughout the lung (ventilation-perfusion [V̇/Q̇] mismatching and shunt); the lungs become stiff; and the patient develops hypoxemia and dyspnea. If alveolar fluid moves up into the airway, it is rapidly mixed with air and is coughed up as characteristically pink, frothy sputum.

Pulmonary edema can vary from mild (apparent only on x-ray films) to fulminating (an acute emergency situation in which massive amounts of fluid block the exchange of oxygen at the alveolar-capillary membrane and obstruct the airways). Pulmonary edema is most commonly associated with left heart failure and valvular disease. The inefficient left ventricle causes blood to "dam up" in the pulmonary circulation, increasing hydrostatic pressure in the capillaries (PCWP) and causing excessive extravasation of fluid. Neurogenic and high altitude pulmonary edema also result from in-

creased pulmonary blood flow and elevated pulmonary artery pressures. Pulmonary edema resulting from increased capillary membrane permeability (ARDS) is usually not associated with elevations in PCWP.

Studies have shown a relationship between PCWP and pulmonary edema. The results of two studies are summarized in Tables 14-8 and 14-9. One study[124] showed that wedge pressures less than 18 mmHg were not associated with chest radiographic indications of congestion and pulmonary edema, whereas pressures in excess of 25 mmHg are associated with severe congestion and classic findings of pulmonary edema. Another study[125] looked at colloid osmotic pressure and pulmonary artery pressure in patients with and without pulmonary edema. It was found that the difference between the colloid oncotic pressure (pressure drawing fluid back into the capillary) and the PCWP was the most significant. Patients without pulmonary

Table 14–8	Comparison of Pulmonary Capillary Wedge Pressure (PCWP) and Chest Radiographic Indication of Pulmonary Edema*

PCWP (mmHg)	Radiographic Findings
<18	No signs of pulmonary edema
18–20	Onset of pulmonary congestion
20–25	Mild to moderate pulmonary congestion
25–30	Moderate to severe pulmonary congestion
>30	Classic findings of pulmonary edema

*Data from Forrester JS and Swan HJC: Acute myocardial infarction: a physiological basis for therapy, *Crit Care Med* 2: 2283, 1974.

edema had gradients of approximately 9.7 mmHg compared to less than 3 mmHg in patients with pulmonary edema.

PCWP as an Indicator of Adequate Left Ventricular Preload: Optimal PCWP

As described earlier in this chapter, PCWP can be used to estimate LVEDP when there is neither mitral valve obstruction nor very high filling pressures which would cause the PCWP to overestimate LVEDP. However, because the relationship of PCWP, LVEDP, left ventricular preload, and cardiac output can be drastically affected by conditions such as myocardial ischemia or hypertrophy, shock, high doses of pressors, and changes in ventricular compliance, optimal PCWP must be determined individually for each patient. *Optimal PCWP* is defined as the PCWP above which further increases in pressure result in little or no increase in cardiac output, stroke volume, or left ventricular stroke work (LVSW or LVSWI). In healthy persons, LVSW plateaus at a PCWP of 10 to 12 mmHg. After acute MI or at high levels of PEEP, a PCWP of 18 mmHg may produce the optimal cardiac output. On the other hand, in patients undergoing volume resuscitation for hypovolemic shock, a PCWP of 14 to 18 mmHg may actually represent relative hypovolemia because of reduced left ventricular compliance. Therefore, the optimal PCWP must be determined for each patient. Maintaining a PCWP higher than necessary may be detrimental to a patient at risk for pulmonary edema or ARDS. Conversely, the patient with hypovolemia, hypotension, or shock should receive volume infusion until optimal PCWP and cardiac output are obtained. Construction of individual left ventricular function curves to identify the patient's optimal filling pressure was discussed in Chapter 13.

Use of Right and Left Heart Filling Pressures for Fluid Challenges

Although the veins and venous reservoirs are capable of redistributing volume and maintaining cardiac performance when up to 15% of the blood volume has been lost, an acute reduction in plasma volume to less than 70% of normal is life-threatening. The obvious cause of such a volume reduction is hemorrhage; however, the critically ill patient may become severely hypovolemic without actual blood loss. Large losses of body fluids such as urine, wound drainage, gastric fluid, diarrhea, or perspiration may result in significant hypovolemia. Additionally, altered hydrostatic and oncotic pressures and increased capillary membrane permeability allow fluid to be lost to the interstitial space, resulting in hypovolemia. Since preload is the single largest contributor to cardiac output, volume replacement represents one of the most important therapeutic interventions performed in the ICU. However, overzealous fluid administration, especially with decreased cardiac performance, may result in further decompensation and pulmonary edema. PCWP and CVP reflect both vascular volume and ability of the ventricle to pump its volume. Therefore, these pressures can be used to guide fluid challenge. Table 14–10 outlines how the 2-5 rule is used when CVP governs the fluid challenge; the 3-7 rule is used for PCWP.[40]

The filling pressure (CVP or PCWP) is observed for 10 minutes, and a decision is made about the volume of fluid to administer. The volume selected is given as a fluid challenge over a 10-minute period. The filling pressure is observed throughout the 10-minute infusion; if at any time during the infusion the CVP rises more than 5 cm H_2O or the PCWP rises more than 7 mmHg, the infusion is stopped. Following the infusion, if the increase in CVP is less than 2 cm H_2O (PCWP < 3 mmHg), the challenge is repeated. If the pressure increases between 2 and 5 cm H_2O for the CVP (3–7 mmHg for the PCWP), the patient is observed for 10 minutes. Following the 10-minute wait, if CVP does not fall to within 2 cm H_2O of the starting pressure (3 mm Hg for PCWP), the challenge is stopped; if the pressure continues to fall, the challenge is repeated. Fluid challenges are repeated using the immediately preceding pressure as the new reference point until the 2-5 or 3-7 rule is violated. Table 14–11 shows how a modification of Weil's 3-7 rule is used for fluid challenges in children.[14,126]

Technical Considerations for Invasive Hemodynamic Monitoring

Values obtained through invasive monitoring are only meaningful when they reflect the actual pressures occurring in the patient. Despite the fact that intravascular pressures can be measured, errors in the monitoring system or the observer's selection of values to record can result in nearly meaningless data and possible erroneous assessment and intervention.[11–13,127] When patients are ill enough to warrant invasive moni-

Table 14-9 Relationship of Pulmonary Edema to Colloid Oncotic Pressure (COP), Pulmonary Capillary Wedge Pressure (PCWP), and COP-PCWP Gradient*

	COP (mmHg)	PCWP (mmHg)	COP-PCWP gradient
No pulmonary edema	20.8 ± 1.0	11.0 ± 1.2	9.7 ± 1.7 mmHg
Pulmonary edema	16.9 ± 1.1	15.7 ± 1.5	1.2 ± 1.3 mmHg
			>3.0 in only 3/14 patients with pulmonary edema

*Data from DaLuz PL: The relationship of pulmonary edema to hydrostatic and colloid osmotic pressure in man. In Weil MH and DaLuz PL: *Critical care medicine manual*, New York, 1978, Springer-Verlag.

Table 14-10 Guidelines for Fluid Challenge in Adults: Weil's 2-5 and 3-7 Rules*†

Assessment	2-5 Rule (CVP in cm H₂O)	3-7 Rule (PCWP in mmHg)	Action
Observe pressure for 10 min and determine action.	<8	<12	200 mL × 10 min
	8-14	12-16	100 mL × 10 min
	≤14	≤16	50 mL × 10 min
Infuse challenge over 10 min; continuously monitor pressure			
During challenge, if pressure rise is:	>5	>7	STOP; monitor
Immediately following infusion, if pressure rise is:	≤2	≤3	Repeat challenge
	2-5	3-7	Wait 10 min
After 10 min, if pressure rise is:	>2	>3	STOP; monitor
	≤2	≤3	Repeat challenge

*Data from Weil MH: Patient evaluation, "vital signs," and initial care. In Shoemaker WC and Thompson WL, editors: *Critical care state of the art*, vol 1, Fullerton, Calif, 1980, Society of Critical Care Medicine. †CVP = central venous pressure; PCWP = pulmonary capillary wedge pressure.

Table 14-11 Guidelines for Fluid Challenge in Children: A Modification of Weil's 3-7 Rules*†

Assessment	2-4 Rule (CVP in mmHg)	3-7 Rule (PCWP in mmHg)	Action
Observe pressure for 10 min and determine action	<10	<15	Give 4 mL/Kg
	≥10	≥15	Give 2 mL/Kg
Infuse challenge over 10 min; continuously monitor pressure			
During challenge, if pressure rise is:	>4	>7	STOP; monitor
Immediately following infusion, if pressure rise is:	≤2	≤3	Repeat challenge
	2-4	3-7	Wait 10 min
After 10 min, if pressure rise is:	>2	>3	STOP; monitor
	≤2	≤3	Repeat challenge

toring with its attendant risks, every attempt should be made to obtain accurate and reliable data.

It is beyond the scope of this book to discuss all the technical aspects of monitoring. (To develop technical expertise, see the sources listed in the references.) This section discusses sources of error that can be readily controlled in the clinical setting before recording and using hemodynamic pressures in the development of a comprehensive pulmonary assessment.

Invasive Monitoring Systems

An invasive monitoring system consists of a vascular catheter connected to a transducer and amplifier by a fluid-filled tubing system. The transducer converts the water pressure received from the catheter and tubing to an electric signal displayed on the monitor as a waveform and either a digital or analog display of the patient's pressure (Fig. 14–18). From the amplifier the signal can be sent to other monitors and recording devices as required for continuous observation and documentation. The catheter is kept patent by continuous irrigation with heparinized intravenous solution. There are several continuous irrigation devices on the market that deliver 3 to 6 mL/hr of irrigating solution when the bag of solution is maintained at 300 mmHg pressure with a blood infusion bag. Alternatively, when it is necessary to irrigate with a smaller volume of fluid, a continuous infusion syringe pump can be connected to the line; however, extremely close observation of the catheter is required to prevent clotting.

Amplifier

The pressure amplifiers in most monitors have built-in electric calibration signals that yield predetermined pressure values. Calibrating the monitor ensures that the amplifier is set to the correct sensitivity and should

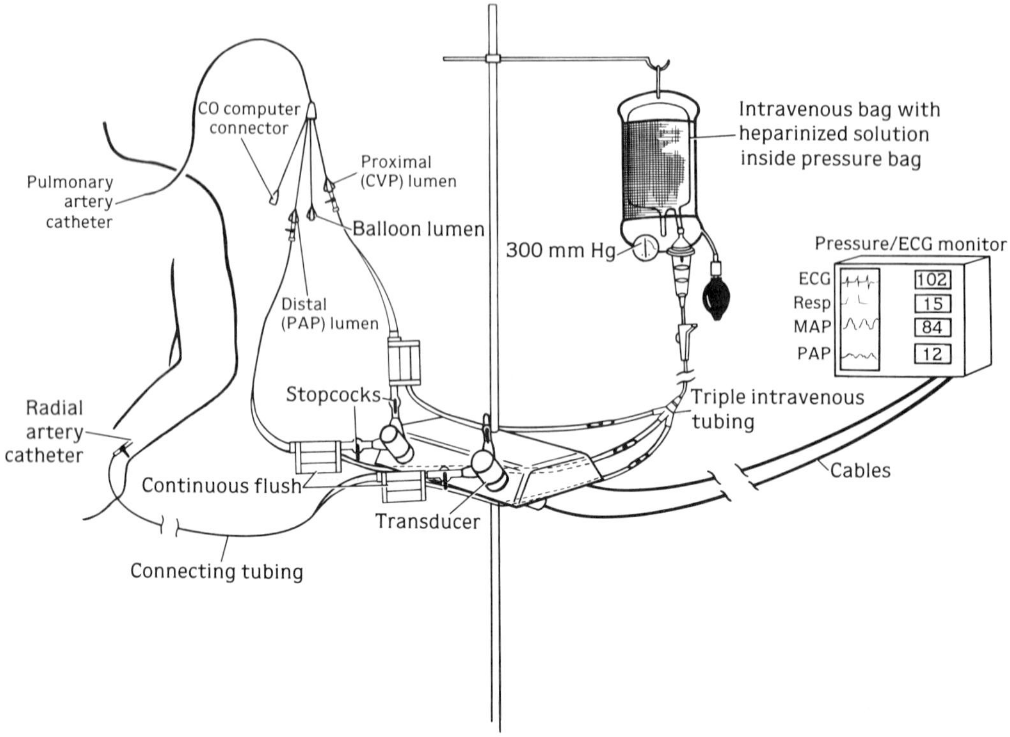

Fig. 14-18 *Two-transducer invasive monitoring setup designed for continuous monitoring of radial and pulmonary artery pressures (PAP) and intermittent monitoring of central venous pressure (CVP). Lines are continuously irrigated by flush devices connected to pressurized bags of heparinized saline solution. To obtain CVP reading, the stopcock between the transducer and the proximal lumen of the pulmonary artery catheter is turned off to the transducer; then the opposite stopcock is opened to the proximal port of the pulmonary artery catheter. After the CVP reading has been obtained, stopcocks are repositioned and the PAP is again monitored continuously. MAP, mean arterial pressure.*

be done when monitoring is initiated, at shift changes, and whenever there is a discrepancy between the clinical picture and the pressures. With the transducer vented to air, the monitor is adjusted to read zero; then the calibration (test) button is depressed to obtain the calibration signal. Some amplifiers have a gain or sensitivity control that can be adjusted if the reading does not exactly match the predetermined pressure value. In monitors without this capability, the use of a transducer-amplifier combination that does not read out the predetermined value results in inaccurate pressure readings when the system is connected to the patient. Calibrating the monitor does not ensure that the transducer is calibrated. The transducer's accuracy must be confirmed by the application of known pressure *following* warming of the transducer and monitor and calibration of the monitor.

Transducer

Transducers should be calibrated using a mercury manometer before each use, whenever transducer damage is suspected, and whenever there is a question regarding the accuracy of the numbers obtained. Calibration is accomplished by connecting the transducer to the monitor and the manometer (Fig. 14–19). The

transducer is vented to air and the monitor zero-balanced and then pressurized by introducing air into the dome via a syringe or pressure bulb. To ensure that the transducer is calibrated in low, middle, and high ranges and is functioning linearly, the pressure on the monitor and manometer should agree at the following points: 200, 100, and 50 mmHg. If pressures do not agree within ± 3 mmHg, the transducer must be assumed to be inaccurate and a new transducer obtained.

When the transducer dome and plumbing system are sterile and in use on a patient, they must be protected from contamination by the nonsterile manometer. This may be accomplished by inserting a sterile component such as a 0.2 μm bacteria filter or a 6-ft length of tubing between the transducer dome and the manometer connection. Extreme care must be taken to prevent inadvertent introduction of air into the patient, resulting in an air embolus. The advantages and disadvantages of several alternative in-use calibration techniques have been reported.[128]

The transducer dome must be connected in accordance with the manufacturer's directions and screwed on tightly enough to ensure a snug contact between the membrane of the dome and the diaphragm of the transducer. A sudden decline in pressure, especially in conjunction with moving the patient or with activity of

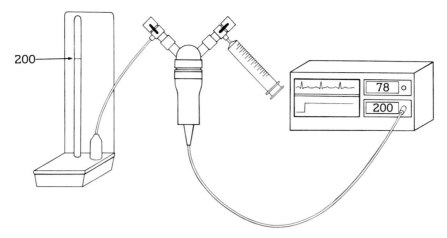

Fig. 14-19 *Transducer calibration against mercury column.*

Zero Reference

Zero reference (sometimes called *zero-balancing* or *zeroing*) is a technique used to cancel the effects of atmospheric and hydrostatic pressure on the ultimate pressure reading. With the air-fluid junction of the transducer (vent port of the stopcock) placed at the same level as the patient's heart (see Fig. 14-18) and opened to atmosphere, the monitor is adjusted to read zero. This procedure tells the monitor to consider atmospheric pressure to be zero so that only the pressure within the vessel or heart chamber is measured when the vent port is closed and the transducer is opened to the patient. Positioning the vent port and the heart at the same level prevents alterations in pressure resulting from effects of hydrostatic pressure within the plumbing system. Since fluid has weight, a pressure proportional to the height of the fluid column is added to the pressure reading if the transducer is placed lower than the atrial level of the heart. Conversely, positioning the transducer above the heart can result in erroneously low pressure readings.[129]

ATRIAL LEVEL. The level of the atria is considered the zero reference point for hemodynamic monitoring transducers: the right atrium for CVP monitoring and the left atrium for pulmonary artery and PCWP measurements. Various landmarks have been suggested for locating the atrial level: (1) measuring the distance from the anterior to posterior chest wall and marking the halfway point on the lateral chest wall, the *midchest level*; (2) selecting a point 10 cm up from the top of the mattress[65]; (3) selecting a point at the fourth intercostal space and anterior axillary line; (4) selecting a point at the fourth intercostal space and midaxillary line[130]; or (5) identifying the phlebostatic axis. The *phlebostatic axis* is defined as "the junction between the transverse plane of the body passing through the fourth intercostal space at the lateral margin of the sternum and a frontal plane of the body passing through the midpoint of a line from the outermost point of the sternum to the outermost point of the posterior chest,"[25,131,132] or, more simply stated, the midchest level at the fourth intercostal space (Fig. 14-20). Echocardiography has shown that this midanteroposterior phlebostatic axis is a valid external reference point for both the right and left atrium when the patient is supine.[133]

The atrial reference point should be marked on the patient's side and used consistently to zero-reference the transducer (also see Fig. 14-8). When the patient's position is changed, the transducer(s) must be repositioned and zero-referenced (Fig. 14-21). As long as the transducer is consistently zero-referenced to the same point, there should be no significant difference in pressure when the patient is in the supine position with the head of the bed elevated between 0 and 60 degrees.[133-135] There is a slight decrease in pressure when the patient is upright (90 degrees) with legs dangling over the edge of the bed.[132,133]

A uniform atrial reference point has not been identified for prone and lateral positions; therefore, it is recommended that the patient be supine with the head of the bed elevated to 60 degrees or less when intracardiac pressures are recorded.[132-135] A limited study showed that reliable pulmonary artery and wedge pressures can be obtained using a reference point at the fourth intercostal space and the midsternal line or midline of the spinal column when the patient is in the *lateral decubitus position*[130] (Fig. 14-22). However, the small sample size and specific characteristics of the population (pleural effusion) make it difficult to generalize the findings to other patients and various lateral positions.

Plumbing System

The dynamic response characteristics of a plumbing system significantly affect the accuracy of the pressure readings.[136-138] An overdamped system reduces the

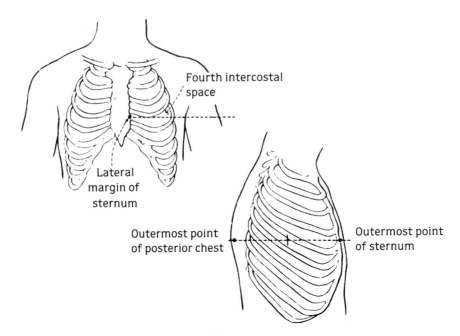

Fig. 14-20 *The phlebostatic axis is the junction between the transverse plane of the body passing through the fourth intercostal space at the lateral margin of the sternum and the frontal plane of the body passing through the midpoint of a line from the outermost point of the sternum to the outermost point of the posterior chest. (From Shinn JA, Woods SL, and Huseby JS: Heart Lung 8:324, 1979.)*

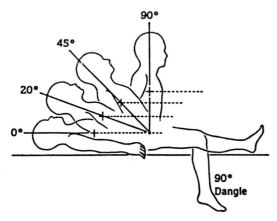

Fig. 14-21 *Phlebostatic (atrial) levels for five positions used for pressure measurements. (From Woods SL and Mansfield L: Heart Lung 5:84, 1976.)*

amplitude of the major components of the waveform resulting in erroneously low systolic and high diastolic pressure readings. An underdamped system with a low resonant frequency accentuates artifact and amplitude resulting in an overestimation of systolic pressure. Since most monitors look only at the highest and lowest points on a waveform to determine systolic and diastolic pressures respectively, alterations in response characteristics and artifacts in the pressure trace can result in clinically significant error.

The dynamic response of a catheter tubing system should be assessed at the beginning of each shift and each time the system is opened and the pressure is questioned. A "snap test" can be performed by rapidly pulling and releasing the "pigtail" of a Sorenson Intraflo or by creating a "fast flash"[127,137-139] with other continuous irri-

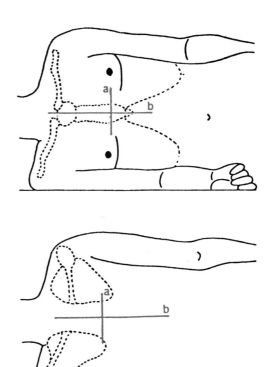

Fig. 14-22 *Determination of anterior and posterior measuring points for lateral decubitus positions. Top: line a, fourth intercostal space; line b, midsternal line. Bottom: line a, fourth intercostal space (T4-6 level); line b, midline of spinal column. (From Kennedy GT, Bryant A, and Crawford M: Heart Lung 13:155, 1984.)*

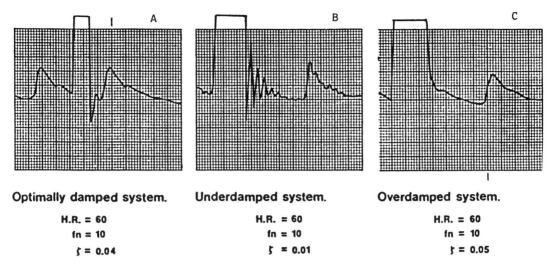

Fig. 14-23 *Using the fast flush square wave test (snap test) to test dynamic characteristics of the monitoring system.* **A,** *Optimally damped system can be verified when the square wave ends with a slight undershoot, followed by an even smaller overshoot (before the next patient trace begins).* **B,** *Underdamped system: typical monitoring system. It is free of air and compliant components, but it has such low natural frequency and damping coefficient that the pulse pressure is exaggerated, and the apparent systolic pressure is higher than the actual. "Ringing" or oscillating can be seen in the waveform following the square wave. Accudynamic placed anywhere in line near the transducer can be adjusted until the response shows that the system is optimally damped.* **C,** *Overdamped system. System is overdamped when fast flush square wave returns slowly to baseline and the patient trace resumes without any hint of oscillation. The most likely cause is air trapped in the system or a compliant or loose component. Pressure produces a systolic pressure that is lower than the actual pressure until the problem is isolated and corrected. (From How to "optimize" a monitoring line with Accudynamic (5/83-S3101), Salt Lake City, 1983, Sorenson Research Co., Inc.)*

gating devices connected to high pressure sources. When the flush device is opened and rapidly released (snapped), a rapidly falling pressure wave occurs. The resulting oscillations show how the hydraulic system is working. A snap test should be timed so that the downstroke of the square wave occurs during diastole to prevent superimposing the pressure waveform on the flush results. Several flushes may need to be performed to obtain a properly positioned waveform.[127,137,138] When radial artery pressures are being obtained, a blood pressure cuff may be applied to the arm above the catheter and inflated momentarily to eliminate the patient waveform while the snap test is performed.

Fig. 14-23, *A* shows the flush results desired to obtain optimal waveforms that reflect the patient's true pressure: one undershoot followed by a small overshoot and then settling to the patient's waveform or back to baseline (if a cuff is used). When the system is overdamped, the overshoot and undershoot may be lost completely (Fig. 14-23, *C*), resulting in artificially low pressure readings. Underdamped systems produce oscillations ("ringing"[129]) following the downstroke before settling back to the baseline or the patient's waveform (Fig. 14-23, *B*). These oscillations are added to the patient's pressure waveforms resulting in elevated pressure readings. "Simple visualization of the waveforms is not sufficient to determine the adequacy of dynamic response due to the large physiologic variation in waveforms between patients and dynamic characteristics of each system."[137,138]

Implementing the following suggestions optimizes dynamic response characteristics and decreases the chance of obtaining erroneous pressures.[65,127,129,136,138]

1. Keep the system as short as possible, preferably not more than 3 to 4 ft.
2. Keep the system simple, with the fewest connections possible.
3. Use only transparent, low-compliance (stiff) tubing, stopcocks, and connections.
4. Keep all connections and the dome tight.
5. Remove all air bubbles. Large air bubbles, clots, loose connections, and soft tubing act like pillows that absorb pressure and decrease or damp the pressure reading. Small bubbles often trapped in stopcocks, domes, and connections can accentuate an underdamped system. These bubbles are most easily removed by aspirating the plumbing system with a syringe and then slowly flushing the blood or air from the line without introducing new bubbles from the irrigating system.
6. If the system is still underdamped, a damping device (such as Sorenson's Accudynamic) may be inserted near the transducer and adjusted until an optimal snap test is obtained.[137]

Respiratory Changes in Pressures

During spontaneous breathing, central venous and pulmonary artery pressures follow intrathoracic pressure fluctuations. Respiratory-induced variation in intravascular pressures is especially marked when the mechanical breath is induced by a spontaneous respiratory effort, as occurs when the patient receives mechanical ventilation in the assist mode or with synchronized IMV (Fig. 14-24). Since most monitors are only capable of

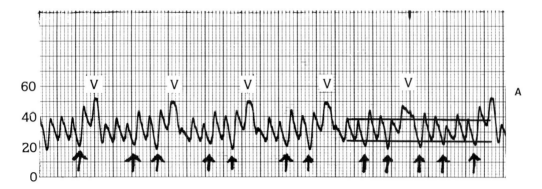

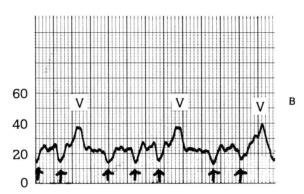

Fig. 14-24 *Analog recording of pulmonary artery pressures in a patient on synchronized intermittent mandatory ventilation (SIMV) of 14/min with a spontaneous respiratory rate of 31/min. Sweep speed is 10 mm/sec.* **A,** *Pulmonary artery pressure recording. Horizontal lines drawn on the right side of the trace indicate end-expiratory pressures of 38/22 mmHg. (Digital readout was 49/18 mmHg.)* **B,** *Pulmonary capillary wedge pressure with end-expiratory pressure of 24 mmHg.* ↑, *spontaneous breath; V, ventilator breath.*

registering the highest point on each waveform as systolic pressure and the lowest point as diastolic pressure, large variations in both pressures are observed on the digital readout. To avoid this significant source of error, pressure should be recorded at end-expiration in all patients whether they are breathing spontaneously or receiving mechanical ventilation.[25,98-110,140-142]

Obtaining an end-expiratory pressure from the digital readout may be accomplished only if the monitor updates pressure immediately with each beat (most do not) or is connected to a computer programmed to analyze the respiratory cycles and display the end-expiratory pressures. Additionally, the digital signal should not be used unless it has been compared with analog data and found to be similar.[98]

Recording the pressure on an analog (strip chart) recorder allows the graphic data to be correlated to changes in intrathoracic pressure. The end-expiratory point is most easily identified when a simultaneous recording of vascular and airway pressure is available. As alternatives, the vascular pressure recording may be marked at the points of inspiration by an observer, or a cooperative patient may be asked to suspend breathing during exhalation for several cardiac cycles. Once the end-expiratory points have been located, pressures are obtained by averaging the corresponding systolic, diastolic, and mean pressures over several respiratory cycles.[25,100-103,127]

Summary

In summary, the following steps ensure that pressures obtained by invasive hemodynamic monitoring are suitable for use in developing a comprehensive pulmonary assessment of the critically ill patient[143]:

1. Before initiating monitoring and whenever pressures are inconsistent with the clinical picture:
   a. Verify that the amplifier and transducer have been warmed for 15 minutes to decrease electronic drift.
   b. Verify the calibration of the transducer.
   c. Verify the calibration of the amplifier (monitor).
2. At the beginning of each shift and whenever the line is opened, the patient's position is changed, or the pressures change significantly:
   a. Zero-balance with the air-fluid junction of the transducer's referencing stopcock at the patient's right atrial level.
   b. Perform a snap test and correct over-damping or underdamping.
3. Determine CVP and pulmonary vascular pressures-at end-expiration from a calibrated paper recording obtained while the patient is in the supine position with the head of the bed elevated between 0 and 45 degrees.

REVIEW QUESTIONS

1. T   F   *Continuous measurement of blood pressure can be performed via arterial cannulation.*

2. Which of the following is not a site used for arterial cannulation?
   a. umbilical artery
   b. radial artery
   c. femoral artery
   d. carotid artery

3. Which of the following are possible complications of arterial cannulation?
   a. infection
   b. arterial spasm
   c. thromboembolism
   d. all of the above

4. Which of the following is true regarding mean arterial pressure?
   a. it is normally 80 - 100 mmHg
   b. it is the arithmetic average of the systolic and diastolic pressures
   c. organ perfusion will be reduced if MAP is less than 80 mmHg
   d. all of the above

5. The dichrotic notch on the arterial pressure waveform represents which of the following?
   a. pulmonic valve closure
   b. aortic valve closure
   c. tricuspid valve closure
   d. mitral valve closure

6. T   F   *The presence of a dichrotic notch in the arterial pressure waveform indicates an accurate pressure measurement.*

7. T   F   *Respiratory variation in the arterial pressure waveform may indicate cardiac tamponade.*

8. Which of the following is not true regarding the use of an intraaortic balloon pump?
   a. direct aortic pressure measurements can be taken
   b. its action increases left ventricular afterload
   c. it deflates at the beginning of systole and inflates during diastole
   d. it is also called counterpulsation

9. Central venous pressure (CVP) is a reflection of which of the following?
   a. right ventricular preload
   b. right atrial pressure
   c. right ventricular end-diastolic pressure
   d. all of the above

10. Which of the following would cause the CVP to increase?
    a. vasodilator therapy
    b. spontaneous inspiration
    c. fluid overload
    d. air in the pressure sensing line

11. Which of the following is (are) true regarding the CVP catheter?
    a. it is commonly inserted via the subclavian vein
    b. the catheter can have multiple lumina
    c. a balloon is located on the distal end
    d. a and b only

12. T   F   *A CVP catheter can be used to administer intravascular drugs.*

13. Which of the following is the correct method of measuring CVP in a patient on mechanical ventilation with PEEP?
    a. at end-inspiration on the ventilator
    b. at end-inspiration off the ventilator
    c. at end-exhalation on the ventilator
    d. at end-exhalation off the ventilator

14. The c wave of a CVP waveform represents which of the following?
    a. atrial contraction
    b. ventricular contraction
    c. right atrial filling
    d. none of the above

15. T   F   *Respiratory variation in the CVP waveform is an abnormal finding.*

16. What is the normal value for CVP?
    a. less than 6 mmHg
    b. 6 - 8 mmHg
    c. 8 - 12 mmHg
    d. 12 - 18 mmHg

17. T   F   *In certain situations CVP can be a good indicator of left ventricular function.*

18. Pulmonary artery pressure monitoring can be accomplished via the use of which of the following?
    a. pulmonary artery catheter
    b. Swan-Ganz catheter
    c. balloon-tipped flow-directed catheter
    d. all of the above

19. What size catheter is typically used for adults to monitor pulmonary artery pressures?
    a. 4 - 5 French
    b. 5 - 8 French
    c. 8 - 10 French
    d. 10 - 15 French

20. T F The distal catheter lumen is located approximately 30 cm from the tip of the catheter.

21. What is the approximate amount of air required to fill the balloon on a PA catheter?
    a. 0.5 cc
    b. 1.0 cc
    c. 1.5 cc
    d. 2.0 cc

22. During insertion of the PA catheter when is the balloon inflated?
    a. immediately after the catheter is inserted into the venous site
    b. when the catheter enters the right atrium
    c. when the catheter enters the right ventricle
    d. when the catheter enters the left atrium

23. Which of the following is true regarding pulmonary capillary wedge pressure (PCWP)?
    a. it is normally 4 - 12 mmHg
    b. it is normally higher than pulmonary artery diastolic pressure (PADP)
    c. it reflects left ventricular afterload
    d. all of the above

24. What would be considered a normal value for pulmonary artery pressure (PAP)?
    a. 15/4 mmHg
    b. 18/10 mmHg
    c. 25/10 mmHg
    d. 36/22 mmHg

25. Which of the following would increase PAP?
    a. severe hypoxemia
    b. thromboemboli
    c. acidosis
    d. all of the above

26. T F A PADP of 14 mmHg and a PCWP of 12 mmHg indicate Zone III catheter placement.

27. Which of the following could cause PCWP to be artificially elevated?
    a. PEEP or CPAP greater than 10 cm H_2O
    b. mitral valve stenosis
    c. reduced left ventricular compliance
    d. all of the above

28. Which of the following can cause pulmonary edema?
    a. increased hydrostatic pressure
    b. increased oncotic pressure
    c. decreased pulmonary capillary permeability
    d. all of the above

29. T F Fluid challenges are done to assess the adequacy of intravascular volume and can be monitored via the use of CVP and PCWP.

30. Zero referencing the transducer involves maintaining the transducer at the level of the
    a. pressure monitor
    b. amplifier
    c. patient's heart
    d. patient's head

REFERENCES

1. Eisenberg PR, Jaffe AS, Schuster DP: Clinical evaluation compared to pulmonary artery catheterization in the hemodynamic assessment of critically ill patients, *Crit Care Med* 12:549, 1984.
2. Tuchschmidt J and Sharma OMP: Impact of hemodynamic monitoring in a medical intensive care unit, *Crit Care Med* 15:840, 1987.
3. Ayers SM and others: NIH consensus conference—critical care medicine, *JAMA* 250:798, 1983.
4. Gore JM and others: A community-wide assessment of the use of pulmonary artery catheters in patients with acute myocardial infarction, *Chest* 92:721, 1987.
5. Robin ED: Death by pulmonary artery flow-directed catheter, *Chest* 92:727, 1987.
6. Shoemaker WC: Use and abuse of the balloon tip pulmonary artery (Swan-Ganz) catheter: are patients getting their money's worth?, *Crit Care Med* 18:1294, 1990.
7. Shoemaker WC and others: The efficacy of central venous and pulmonary artery catheters and therapy based upon them in reducing mortality and morbidity, *Arch Surg* 125:1332, 1990.
8. Pearson KS and others: A cost/benefit analysis of randomized invasive monitoring for patients undergoing surgery, *Anesth Analg* 69:338, 1989.
9. Isaacson IJ and others: The value of pulmonary artery and central venous monitoring in patients undergoing abdominal aortic reconstructive surgery: a comparative study of two selected, randomized groups, *J Vasc Surg* 12:754, 1990.
10. Naylor CD and others: Pulmonary artery catheterization: can there be an integrated strategy for guideline development and research promotion?, *JAMA* 269:2407, 1993.
11. Maloy L and Gardner RM: Monitoring systemic arterial blood pressure: strip recording versus digital display, *Heart Lung* 15:627, 1986.
12. Morris AH, Chapman RH, Gardner RM: Frequency of technical problems encountered in measurement of pulmonary artery wedge pressure, *Crit Care Med* 12:164, 1984.
13. Morris AH, Chapman RH, Gardner RH: Frequency of wedge pressure errors in the ICU, *Crit Care Med* 13:705, 1985.
14. Rubenstein JS and Hageman JR: Monitoring of critically ill infants and children, *Crit Care Clin* 4:621, 1988.
15. Colan SD and others: Noninvasive determination of systolic, diastolic and end-systolic blood pressure in neonates, infants and young children: comparison with central aortic pressure measurements, *Am J Cardiol* 52:869, 1983.
16. Borow KM and Newburger JW: Noninvasive estimation of central aortic pressure using the oscillometric method: a comparative study of brachial artery pressure with simultaneous central aortic pressure measurements, *Am Heart J* 103:879, 1982.
17. Venus B and others: Direct versus indirect blood pressure measurements in critically ill patients, *Heart Lung* 14:228, 1985.

18. Manolio TA and others: Evaluation of the Dinamap continuous blood pressure monitor, *Am J Hypertens* 1(3, Pt 3):161S, 1988.

19. Cohn JN: Blood pressure measurement in shock: mechanism of inaccuracy in auscultatory and palpatory methods. *JAMA* 199:118, 1967.

20. Stern DH and others: Can we trust the direct radial artery pressure immediately following cardiopulmonary bypass?, *Anesthesiology* 62:557, 1985.

21. Mohr R, Lavee J, Goor DA: Inaccuracy of radial artery pressure measurement after cardiac operations, *J Thorac Cardiovasc Surg* 94:286, 1990.

22. Keckeisen M and Monsein S: Techniques for measuring arterial pressure in the postoperative cardiac surgery patient, *Crit Care Nurs Clin North Am* 3:699, 1991.

23. Henneman E and Hennenan PL: Intricacies of blood pressure measurement: reexamining the rituals, *Heart Lung* 18:263 1989.

24. Hand HL: Direct or indirect blood pressure measurement for open heart surgery patients: an algorithm, *Crit Care Nurs* 12:52, 1992.

25. Kaye W: Invasive monitoring techniques. In McIntyre KM, and Lewis AJ, editors: *Textbook of advanced cardiac life support,* ed 2, Dallas, 1987, American Heart Association.

26. Harrington DP: Disparities between direct and indirect arterial systolic blood pressure managements, *Cardiovasc Pulmonary Techniques* 6:40, 1978.

27. Johnson FE, Sumner DS, Strandness DE: Extremity necrosis caused by indwelling arterial catheters, *Am J Surg* 131:375, 1976.

28. Lantiegne KC and Civetta JM: A system for maintaining invasive pressure monitoring, *Heart Lung* 7:610, 1978.

29. Kaye W: Catheter and infusion-related sepsis: the nature of the problem and its prevention. In McIntyre KM and Lewis AJ, editors: *Textbook of advanced cardiac life support,* ed. 2, Dallas, American Heart Association.

30. Shoemaker WC: Monitoring of the critically ill patient. In Shoemaker WC, Thompson WL, Holbrook PR: *Textbook of critical care,* ed 2, Philadelphia, 1988, WB Saunders.

31. Quaal SJ: *Comprehensive intra-aortic balloon pumping,* St Louis, 1984, Mosby.

32. Guyton AC: *Textbook of medical physiology,* ed 7, Philadelphia, 1986, WB Saunders.

33. Lee J and others: Central venous oxygen saturation in shock: a study in man, *Anesthesiology* 36:473, 1972.

34. Civetta JM: Invasive catheterization. In Shoemaker WC and Thompson WL, editors: *Critical care state of the art,* vol 1, Fullerton, Calif, 1980, Society of Critical Care Medicine.

35. Weil MH, Shubin H, Rosoff L: Fluid repletion in circulatory shock: central venous pressure and other practical guides, *JAMA* 192:668, 1965.

36. Brisman R, Parks LC, Benson DW: Pitfalls in the clinical use of central venous pressure, *Arch Surg* 95:902, 1967.

37. Davidson R, Parker M, Harrison RA: The validity of determinations of pulmonary wedge pressure during mechanical ventilation, *Chest* 73:352, 1978.

38. Rajacich N and others: Central venous pressure and pulmonary capillary wedge pressure as estimates of left atrial pressure: effects of positive end-expiratory pressure and catheter tip malposition, *Crit Care Med* 17:7, 1989.

39. Mangano DT: Monitoring pulmonary arterial pressure in coronary disease, *Anesthesiology* 53:364, 1980.

40. Weil MH: Patient evaluation, "vital signs," and initial care. In Shoemaker WC and Thompson WL, editors: *Critical care state of the art,* vol 1, Fullerton, Calif, 1980, Society of Critical Care Medicine.

41. Hanashiro PK and Weil MH: Reliability of central venous pressure as a measure of changes in left sided intracardiac pressure, *Chest* 62:479, 1972.

42. Bell H, Stubbs D, Pugh D: Reliability of central venous pressure as an indicator of left atrial pressure: a study in patients with mitral valve disease, *Chest* 59:169, 1971.

43. Civetta JM and Gabel JC: Flow directed pulmonary artery catheterization in surgical patients: indications and modifications of technique, *Ann Surg* 176:753, 1972.

44. Forrester JS and others: Filling pressures in right and left sides of the heart in acute myocardial infarction, *N Engl J Med* 285:190, 1971.

45. Delaurentis DA and others: Does central venous pressure accurately reflect hemodynamic and fluid volume patterns in the critical surgical patient?, *Am J Surg* 126:415, 1973.

46. DelGuercia LRM and Cohn JD: Monitoring: methods and significance, *Surg Clin North Am* 56:977, 1976.

47. Molajo AO and others: Clinical implication of inadvertent monitoring of pulmonary artery pressure via a "left atrial" catheter. *Cathet Cardiovasc Diagn* 13:42, 1987.

48. Gold JP and others: Transthoracic intracardiac monitoring lines in pediatric surgical patients: a ten year experience, *Ann Thorac Surg* 42:185, 1986.

49. Swan HJC and others: Catheterization of the heart in man with use of a flow-directed balloon-tipped catheter, *N Engl J Med* 283:447, 1970.

50. Bodai BI and Halcroft IW: Use of the pulmonary artery catheter in the critically ill patient, *Heart Lung* 11:406, 1982.

51. Rafferty T and others: Thermodilution right ventricular ejection fraction measurement reproducibility study in patients undergoing coronary artery bypass graft surgery, *Crit Care Med* 20:1524, 1992.

52. Dorman G and others: Use of combined right ventricular ejection fraction-oximetry catheter system for coronary bypass surgery, *Crit Care Med* 20:1650, 1992.

53. Leatherman JW and Marini J: Clinical use of the pulmonary artery catheter. In Hall JB, Schmidt GA, Wood LDH: *Principles of critical care,* New York, 1992, McGraw-Hill.

54. Tarnow J: Swan-Ganz catheterization: application, interpretation and complications, *Thorac Cardiovasc Surg* 30:120, 1983.

55. Forrester JS and others: Medical therapy of acute myocardial infarction by application of hemodynamic subsets, *N Engl J Med* 295:1356, 1976.

56. Meister SG and Helfant RH: Rapid bedside differentiation of ruptured interventricular septum from acute mitral insufficiency, *N Engl J Med* 295:1024, 1975.

57. Jaquith S: Continuous measurement of $S\bar{v}o_2$: clinical applications and advantages for critical care nursing, *Crit Care Nurse* 5(2):1985.

58. Birman H and others: Continuous monitoring of mixed venous oxygen saturation in hemodynamically unstable patients, *Chest* 85:753, 1985.

59. *Understanding continuous mixed venous oxygen saturation ($S\bar{v}o_2$) monitoring with the Swan-Ganz oximetry TD system,* Santa Ana, Calif, 1986, American Edwards Laboratories.

60. Product descriptions, Santa Ana, Calif, March 1989, American Edwards Laboratory.

61. Trankina MF and White RD: Perioperative cardiac pacing using an atrioventricular pacing pulmonary artery catheter, *J Cardiothorac Anesth* 3:154, 1989.

62. Lumb PD: Atrioventricular sequential pacing with transluminal atrial and ventricular pacing probes inserted via a pulmonary artery catheter: a preliminary comparison with epicardial wires, *J Clin Anesth* 1:292, 1989.

63. Rasanen J and others: Estimation of oxygen utilization by dual oximetry, *Ann Surg* 206:621, 1987.

64. Kahn JK and Kirsh MD: The infusion delivery time of the flow-directed pulmonary artery catheter: clinical implications, *Heart Lung* 12:630, 1983.

65. Daily EK and Schroeder JS: *Techniques in bedside hemodynamic monitoring,* ed 4, St Louis, 1989, Mosby.

66. Sprung CL, editor: *The pulmonary artery catheter: methodology and clinical application,* Baltimore, 1983, University Park Press.

67. Daily EK and Schroeder JS: *Hemodynamic waveforms: exercises in identification and analysis,* St Louis, 1983, Mosby.

68. Boyd K and others: A prospective study of complications of pulmonary artery catheterizations in 500 consecutive patients, *Chest* 84:245, 1983.

69. Keefer J and Barash P: Pulmonary artery catheterization—a decade of clinical progress? *Chest* 84:241, 1983.

70. Sladen A: Complications of invasive hemodynamic monitoring in the intensive care unit, *Curr Probl Surg* 25:69, 1988.

71. Matthay MA and Chatterjee K: Bedside catheterization of the pulmonary artery: risks compared with benefits, *Ann Intern Med* 109:826, 1988.

72. Damen J and Wever JE: The use of balloon-tipped pulmonary artery catheters in children undergoing cardiac surgery, *Intensive Care Med* 13:266, 1987.

73. Rushmer RF: *Cardiovascular dynamics*, ed 3, Philadelphia, 1970, WB Saunders.

74. Civetta JM, Gabel JC, Laver MG: Disparate ventricular function in surgical patients, *Surg Forum* 22:136, 1971.

75. McIntyre K and Sasahara AA: Determinants of right ventricular function and hemodynamics after pulmonary embolism, *Chest* 84:126, 1974.

76. Falicov RE and Resnekov L: Relationship of the pulmonary artery end-diastolic pressure to the left ventricular end-diastolic and mean filling pressures in patients with and without left ventricular dysfunction, *Circulation* 42:65, 1970.

77. Gabriel S: The difference between pulmonary artery diastolic pressure and the pulmonary wedge pressure in chronic lung disease, *Acta Med Scand* 190:555, 1971.

78. Vender JS: Invasive cardiac monitoring, *Crit Care Clin* 4:455, 1988.

79. Bouchard RJ, Gault JH, and Ross JR, Jr: Evaluation of pulmonary arterial end-diastolic pressure as an estimate of left ventricular end-diastolic pressure in patients with normal and abnormal left ventricular performance, *Circulation* 44:1072, 1971.

80. Lappas D and others: Indirect measurement of left atrial pressure in surgical patients: pulmonary-capillary wedge pressure and pulmonary-artery diastolic pressures compared with left-atrial pressure, *Anesthesiology* 38:394, 1973.

81. Walston A and Kendall ME: Comparison of pulmonary artery wedge pressure with left atrial pressure in man, *Am Heart J* 86:159, 1973.

82. O'Quinn R and Marini JJ: Pulmonary artery occlusion pressure: clinical physiology, measurement, and interpretation, *Am Rev Respir Dis* 128:319, 1983.

83. Marini JJ: Hemodynamic monitoring with the pulmonary artery catheter, *Crit Care Clin* 2:551, 1986.

84. Sibbald WJ and others: Concepts in the pharmacological and nonpharmacological support of cardiovascular function in critically ill surgical patients, *Surg Clin North Am* 63:445, 1983.

85. Leasa DJ and Sibbald WJ: Respiratory monitoring in a critical care unit. In Simmons DH, editor: *Current pulmonology*, vol 9, St Louis, 1988 Mosby.

86. Pinksy MR: The influence of positive-pressure ventilation on cardiovascular function in the critically ill, *Crit Care Clin* 1:699, 1985.

87. Biondi JW, Schulman DS, Matthay RA: Effects of mechanical ventilation on right and left ventricular function, *Clin Chest Med* 9:55, 1988.

88. Kane PB and others: Artifacts in the measurement of pulmonary artery wedge pressure, *Crit Care Med* 6:36, 1978.

89. Morris AH and others: Frequency of technical problems encountered in measurement of pulmonary artery wedge pressure, *Crit Care Med* 12:164, 1987.

90. Morris AH and Chapman RH: Wedge pressure confirmation by aspiration of pulmonary capillary blood, *Crit Care Med* 13:756, 1985.

91. West JB and Dollery CT: Distribution of blood flow and pressure volume-relationships of the whole lung, *J Appl Physiol* 20:175, 1965.

92. West JB: *Respiratory physiology: the essentials*, ed 2, Baltimore, 1979, Williams & Wilkins.

93. Shasby DM and others: Swan-Ganz catheter location and left atrial pressure determine the accuracy of the wedge pressure when positive end-expiratory pressure is used, *Chest* 80:666, 1981.

94. Marini JJ: Obtaining meaningful data from the Swan-Ganz catheter, *Respir Care* 30:572, 1988.

95. Culver BH: Hemodynamic monitoring: physiologic problems in interpretation. In Fallat RJ and Luce JM, editors: *Critical care clinics: cardiopulmonary critical care management*, New York, 1988, Churchill Livingstone.

96. Rehimtoola SH and others: Relationship of pulmonary artery to left ventricular diastolic pressures in acute myocardial infarction, *Circulation* 46:283, 1972.

97. Fisher ML, DeFelice CE, Parisi AF: Assessing left ventricular filling pressure with flow-directed (Swan-Ganz) catheters, *Chest* 68:542, 1975.

98. Gershan JA: Effect of positive end-expiratory pressure on pulmonary capillary wedge pressure, *Heart Lung* 12:143, 1983.

99. Shinn JA, Woods SL, Huseby JS: Effect of intermittent positive pressure ventilation upon pulmonary artery and pulmonary capillary wedge pressures in acutely ill patients, *Heart Lung* 8:322, 1979.

100. Wild LR and Woods SL: Comparison of three methods for interpreting pulmonary wedge pressure waveforms with respiratory variation, *Heart Lung* 14:308, 1985.

101. Campbell ML and Breenberg CA: Reading pulmonary artery wedge pressure at end-expiration, *Focus Crit Care* 15:60, 1988.

102. Riedinger MS, Shellock FG, Swan HJC: Reading pulmonary artery and pulmonary capillary wedge pressure waveforms with respiratory variations, *Heart Lung* 10:675, 1981.

103. Cengiz M, Crapo RO, Gardner RM: The effect of ventilation on the accuracy of pulmonary artery and wedge pressure measurements, *Crit Care Med* 11:502, 1983.

104. McGrath RB: Invasive bedside hemodynamic monitoring, *Prog Cardiovasc Dis* 29:129, 1986.

105. Silverman H and others: Measurement of pulmonary capillary wedge pressure from graphic and digital recorders, *Chest* 86:335, 1984.

106. Booker KJ and Arnold JS: Respiratory-induced changes on the pulmonary capillary wedge pressure tracing, *Crit Care Nurse* 13:80, 1993.

107. Bridges EJ and Woods SL: Pulmonary artery pressure measurement: state of the art, *Heart Lung* 22:99, 1993.

108. Ahrens TS: Effects of mechanical ventilation on hemodynamic waveforms, *Crit Care Nurs Clin North Am* 3:629, 1991.

109. Gardner PE: Pulmonary artery pressure monitoring, *AACN Clin Issues Crit Care Nurs* 4:98, 1993.

110. Ellis D: *An algorithm for reduction of respiratory artifact in pulmonary artery pressure measurement*, Waltham, Mass, 1983, Hewlett-Packard.

111. Chapin JC and others: Lung expansion, airway pressure transmission and positive end expiratory pressure, *Arch Surg* 114:1193, 1979.

112. Rajacich N and others: Esophageal pressure monitoring: a practical adjuvant to hemodynamic monitoring with positive end-expiratory pressure, *Heart Lung* 17:483, 1988.

113. Iberti TJ and Fisher LJ: A prospective study on the use of the pulmonary artery catheter in a medical intensive care unit, its effect on diagnosis and therapy, *Crit Care Med* 11:238, 1983.

114. Qvist J and others: Hemodynamic responses to mechanical ventilation with PEEP: the effect of hypervolemia, *Anesthesiology* 42:45, 1975.

115. Zarins C and others: The effect of vascular volume on positive and expiratory pressure-induced cardiac output depression and wedge left atrial discrepancy, *J Surg Res* 23:348, 1977.

116. DeCampo T and Civetta JM: The effect of short-term discontinuation of high level PEEP in patients with acute respiratory failure, *Crit Care Med* 7:47, 1979.

117. Lookinland S: Comparison of pulmonary vascular pressure based upon blood volume and ventilator status, *Nurs Res* 38:68, 1989.

118. Weil MH and Henning RJ: New concepts in the diagnosis and fluid treatment of circulatory shock, *Anesth Analg* 58:124, 1979.

119. Hanashiro PK and Weil MH: Reliability of central venous pressure as a measure of changes in left sided intracardiac pressures, *Chest* 62:479, 1972.

120. Forrester JS and others: Medical therapy of acute myocardial infarction by application of hemodynamic subsets, parts I and II, *N Engl J Med* 295:1356, 1404, 1976.

121. Urban N: Integrating the hemodynamic profile with clinical assessment, *AACN Clin Issues Crit Care Nurs* 4:161, 1993.

122. Robin ED, Cross CE, Zelis R: Pulmonary edema, *N Engl J Med* 288:239, 1973.

123. Modell JH and Boysen PG: Respiratory crisis. In Shoemaker WC and Thompson WL, editors: *Critical care state of the art,* vol 1, Fullerton, Calif, 1980, Society of Critical Care Medicine.

124. Forrester JS and Swan HJC: Acute myocardial infarction: a physiological basis for therapy, *Crit Care Med* 2:2283, 1974.

125. DaLuz PL: The relationship of pulmonary edema to hydrostatic and colloid osmotic pressure in man. In Weil MH and DaLuz PL: *Critical care medicine manual,* New York, 1978, Springer-Verlag.

126. Raphaely RC and Browning RA: The role of preload in the manipulation of the failing circulation. In Swenlow DB and Raphaely RC, editors: *Cardiovascular problems in pediatric critical care,* New York, 1986, Churchill Livingstone.

127. Gardner RM and Chapman RH: Trouble-shooting pressure monitoring systems: when do the numbers lie? In Fallat RJ and Luce JM, editors: *Clinics in critical care medicine: cardiopulmonary critical care management,* New York, 1988, Churchill Livingstone.

128. Air embolism during calibration of invasive blood pressure monitoring systems and alternative in-use calibration techniques, *Health Devices,* November 1982, p. 22.

129. *Guide to physiological pressure monitoring,* Waltham, Mass, 1977, Hewlett-Packard Co.

130. Kennedy GT, Bryant A, Crawford MH: The effects of lateral body positioning on measurements of pulmonary artery and pulmonary artery wedge pressure, *Heart Lung* 13:155, 1984.

131. Winsor R and Burch GE: Use of the phlebomanometer: normal venous pressure values and a study of certain clinical aspects of venous hypertension in man, *Am Heart J* 31:387, 1946.

132. Woods SL and Mansfield LW: Effect of body position upon pulmonary artery and pulmonary capillary wedge pressures in non-critically ill patients, *Heart Lung* 5:83, 1976.

133. Kee LL and others: Echocardiographic determination of valid zero reference levels in supine and lateral positions, *Am J Crit Care* 2:72, 1993.

134. Doering LV: The effect of positioning on hemodynamics and gas exchange in the critically ill: a review, *Am J Crit Care* 2:208, 1993.

135. Laulive JL: Pulmonary artery pressures and position changes in critically ill adult, *Dimens Crit Care Nurs* 1:28, 1982.

136. Brunner JMR: *Handbook of blood pressure monitoring,* Littleton, Mass, 1978, PSG Publishing.

137. Gardner RM: Direct blood pressure measurement: dynamic response requirements, *Anesthesiology* 54:227, 1981.

138. Gibbs NC and Gardner RM: Dynamics of invasive pressure monitoring systems: clinical and laboratory evaluation, *Heart Lung* 17:43, 1988.

139. Nursing 80 Books: *Nursing photobook: using monitors,* Horsham, Pa. 1980, Intermed Communications.

140. Maran AG: Variables in pulmonary capillary wedge pressure: variation with intrathoracic pressure, graphic and digital recorders, *Crit Care Med* 8:102, 1980.

141. Berryhill RE, Benumof JL, Raushcer LA: Pulmonary vascular pressure reading at the end of exhalation, *Anesthesiology* 49:365, 1978.

142. Pace NL: A critique of flow-directed pulmonary arterial catheterization, *Anesthesiology* 47:455, 1977.

143. Gardner RM and Hollingsworth KW: Optimizing the electrocardiogram and pressure monitoring, *Crit Care Med* 14:651, 1986.

BIBLIOGRAPHY

Armstrong PW and Baigrie RS, editors: *Hemodynamic monitoring in the critically ill,* New York, 1980, Harper & Row.

Biondi JW, Schulman DS, Matthay RA: Effects of mechanical ventilation on right and left ventricular function, *Clin Chest Med* 9:55, 1988.

Bone RC, George RB, Hudsom LD: *Acute respiratory failure,* New York, 1987, Churchill Livingstone.

Cain SM: Assessment of tissue oxygenation, *Crit Care Clin* 2:537, 1986.

Daily EK and Schroeder JS: *Hemodynamic waveforms: exercises in identification and analysis,* St Louis, 1983, Mosby.

Daily EK and Schroeder JS: *Techniques in bedside hemodynamic monitoring,* ed 4, St Louis, 1989, Mosby.

Damen J: The microbiological risk of invasive hemodynamic monitoring in adults undergoing cardiac valve replacement, *J Clin Monit* 2:87, 1986.

Damen J and Wever JE: The use of balloon-tipped pulmonary artery catheters in children undergoing cardiac surgery, *Intensive Care Med* 13:266, 1987.

Darovic GO: *Hemodynamic monitoring: invasive and noninvasive clinical application,* Philadelphia, 1987, WB Saunders.

Ellis D: *An algorithm for reduction of respiratory artifact in pulmonary artery pressure measurement,* Waltham, Mass, 1983, Hewlett-Packard Co.

Fields AI: Invasive hemodynamic monitoring in children, *Clin Chest Med* 8:611, 1987.

Gardner RM: Hemodynamic monitoring: from catheter to display, *Acute Care* 12:3, 1986.

Halfman-Franeya M: Current trends in hemodynamic monitoring of patients in shock, *Crit Care Nurs Q* 11:9, 1988.

Kahn JK and Kirsh MM: The infusion delivery time of the flow-directed pulmonary artery catheter: clinical implications, *Heart Lung* 12:630, 1983.

Kennedy GT, Bryant A, Crawford M: The effects of lateral body positioning on measurements of pulmonary artery and pulmonary wedge pressure, *Heart Lung* 13:155, 1984.

Kersten LD: *Comprehensive respiratory nursing care,* Philadelphia, 1989, WB Saunders.

Lazar NM and Luce JM: Hemodynamic assessment and management of patients with the adult respiratory distress syndrome, *Crit Care Clin* 2:601, 1986.

Leasa DJ and Sibbald WJ: Respiratory monitoring in a critical care unit. In Simmons DH, editor: *Current pulmonology,* vol 9, St Louis, 1988, Mosby.

Loach J and Thompson MR, Jr: Hemodynamic assessment and management of patients with the adult respiratory distress syndrome, *Crit Care Clin* 2:610, 1986.

Lough ME: Introduction to hemodynamic monitoring, *Nurs Clin North Am* 22:89, 1987.

Luce JM and Pierson DJ: *Critical care medicine,* Philadelphia, 1988, WB Saunders.

McGrath RB: Invasive bedside hemodynamic monitoring, *Prog Cardiovasc Dis* 29:129, 1986.

Marini JJ: Hemodynamic monitoring with the pulmonary artery catheter, *Crit Care Clin* 2:551, 1986.

Marini JJ: Monitoring during mechanical ventilation, *Clin Chest Med* 9:73, 1988.

Murray JF and Nadel JA: *Textbook of respiratory medicine,* Philadelphia, 1988, WB Saunders.

Norris D and Klein LA: What all those pressure readings mean . . . and why, *RN* 44:43, Oct 1981.

Osgood CF and others: Hemodynamic monitoring in respiratory care, *Respir Care* 29:30, 1984.

Parrillo JE: *Current therapy in critical care medicine,* Philadelphia, 1987, BC Decker.

Pinsky MR: The influence of positive-pressure ventilation on cardiovascular function in the critically ill, *Crit Care Clin* 1:699, 1985.

Pollard D and Seliger E: *An implementation of bedside physiological calculations,* Waltham, Mass, 1985, Hewlett-Packard Co.

Price MS and Fox JD: *Hemodynamic monitoring in critical care,* Rockville, Md, 1987, Aspen.

Rajacich N and others: Esophageal pressure monitoring: a practical adjuvant to hemodynamic monitoring with positive end-expiratory pressure, *Heart Lung* 17:483, 1988.

Robotham JL, Peters J, Takata M: Cardiorespiratory interactions. In Bone RC and others, editors: *Pulmonary and critical care medicine,* St Louis, 1993, Mosby.

Rubin LJ: Pulmonary hypertension and cor pulmonale. In Bone RC and others, editors: *Pulmonary and critical care medicine,* St Louis, 1993, Mosby.

Runciman WB, Ilsely AH, Rutten AJ: Monitoring other haemodynamic variables and oxygen consumption, *Anaesth Intensive Care* 16:58, 1988.

Sasahara AA and others: The clinical and hemodynamic features of acute pulmonary embolism. In Simmons DH, editor: *Current pulmonology,* vol 9, St Louis, 1988, Mosby.

Shinn JA, Woods SL, Huseby JS: IPPV effect on wedge pressures in the acutely ill, *Heart Lung* 8:324, 1979.

Shoemaker WC and others: *Textbook of critical care,* ed 2, Philadelphia, 1989, WB Saunders.

Sibbald WJ, editor: Cardiovascular crises in the critically ill, *Crit Care Clin* 1:1985.

Sivak ED and Wiedemann HP: Clinical measurement of extravascular lung water, *Crit Care Clin* 2:511, 1986.

Sprung CL, Drescher M, Schein RMH: Clinical investigation of the cardiovascular system in the critically ill: invasive techniques, *Crit Care Clin* 1:533, 1985.

Taylor T: Monitoring left atrial pressures in the open-heart surgical patient, *Crit Care Nurse* 6:62, 1986.

Textbook of advanced cardiac life support, Dallas, 1987, American Heart Association.

Tuchschmidt J and Sharma OP: Impact of hemodynamic monitoring in a medical intensive care unit, *Crit Care Med* 15:840, 1987.

Understanding hemodynamic measurements made with the Swan-Ganz catheters, Santa Ana, Calif, 1982, American Edwards Laboratories.

Vender JS, editor: Intensive care monitoring, *Crit Care Clin* 4:1988.

Wiedemann HP, Matthay MA, Matthay RA: Cardiovascular pulmonary monitoring in the intensive care unit, part I, *Chest* 85:537, 1984.

Woods SL, Growe BL, Laurent-Bopp D: Effect of backrest position on pulmonary artery pressures in critically ill patients, *Cardiovasc Nurs* 18:19, 1982.

Woods SL and Mansfield L: Effects of body position upon pulmonary artery and pulmonary capillary wedge pressures in noncritically ill patients, *Heart Lung* 5:83, 1976.

Yang SC and Puri VK: Role of preoperative hemodynamic monitoring in intraoperative fluid management, *Am Surg* 52:536, 1986.

Chapter 15

Nutritional Assessment of Patients with Respiratory Disease

James A. Peters and Kenneth I. Burke

LEARNING OBJECTIVES

1. *Recognize how nutrition and respiration are interrelated.*

2. *Recognize the functional importance of oxygen in nutrition.*

3. *Identify the nutritional significance of measuring oxygen uptake ($\dot{V}O_2$).*

4. *Identify the value of determining the basal metabolic rate (BMR) and basal energy expenditure (BEE).*

5. *Recognize how starvation affects the following:*
   a. *body weight*
   b. *muscle mass (diaphragm and other respiratory musculature)*
   c. *FVC, FEV_1, and D_LCO*
   d. *surfactant production*

6. *Recognize how some respiratory treatment modalities may inhibit the nutritional status of patients.*

7. *Identify the by-products of anaerobic (without oxygen) metabolism.*

8. *Identify oxygen's importance in terms of ATP production.*

9. *Recognize how fat, carbohydrate, and protein metabolism affect the respiratory quotient (RQ).*

10. *Recognize the daily nutritional requirements for carbohydrate, protein, and fat.*

11. *Identify the protein requirements for normal and severely catabolic patients.*

12. *Recognize the significance of measuring nitrogen balance.*

13. *Recognize the problems associated with a low protein diet.*

14. *Recognize the advantages and disadvantages of a high carbohydrate diet in regards to the pulmonary system.*

15. *Identify the importance of vitamins and minerals in respiratory function.*

LEARNING OBJECTIVES — cont'd

16. *Recognize the methods available for meeting nutritional requirements and their advantages and disadvantages.*
17. *Recognize the methods for assessing nutritional status.*
18. *Identify the role of the respiratory care practitioner in nutritional assessment in relation to inspection, auscultation, and laboratory findings.*

Chapter Outline

Interdependence of Respiration and Nutrition

Respiration and nutrition are interdependent (Fig. 15–1). Air and food share common pathways during ingestion and then separate only briefly during "digestion," with air going to the lungs and food to the stomach. Oxygen and nutrients soon blend together in the blood and are distributed to the tissues of the body. The use of food for energy at the cellular level requires oxygen to support a controlled combustion process that produces energy molecules of adenosine triphosphate (ATP), which are used in a multitude of body processes (Fig. 15–2).

Titrating in the proper amount of oxygen and eliminating carbon dioxide, the metabolic "smoke" of the combustion process, is the job of the respiratory system coupled closely with the cardiovascular system. The respiratory system must be sensitive to the metabolic needs of the whole body. To accomplish this requires an integration of several organ systems. The respiratory system consists of neurologic components, cardiovascular components, respiratory muscles, and lungs (Fig. 15–3).

The metabolic rates of the tissues dictate the amount of oxygen to be picked up in the lungs. Oxygen uptake ($\dot{V}O_2$) is a respiratory factor that can be measured in the laboratory or at the bedside.[1–3] Nutritionally speaking, it is this measure that indicates the energy requirement of the patient. If $\dot{V}O_2$ is measured while a person is in a resting, nonstressed state, one can then calculate the basal metabolic rate (BMR) or basal energy expenditure (BEE). The Harris-Benedict equation, which follows, is commonly used for estimating BEE.[4,5] It can be adjusted for energy expenditures above the basal level by applying certain correction factors that account for the patient's metabolic condition.

1. Basal energy expenditure (BEE)

Men:

$$BEE = 66 + (13.7 \times W) + (5 \times H) - (6.8 \times A)$$

Women:

$$BEE = 655 + (9.6 \times W) + (1.7 \times H) - (4.7 \times A)$$

where

W = weight in kilograms
H = height in centimeters
A = age in years

2. Energy requirements

Type of Therapy	Kilocalories Required (per 24 hr)
Parenteral anabolic	1.75 × BEE
Oral anabolic	1.50 × BEE
Oral maintenance	1.20 × BEE

Although BEE is commonly estimated, whenever possible the metabolic rate should be measured to obtain the most accurate assessment of the patient's status. Following is a summary of the energy measurement procedure.

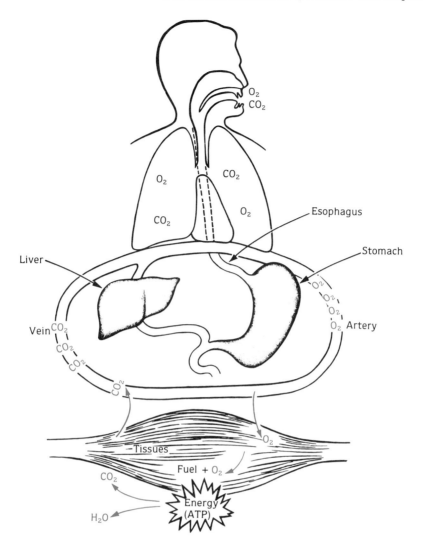

Fig. 15–1 *Nutrition and breathing are interrelated. Food and air share common ports of entry into the body, separate briefly in lungs or stomach, and then travel together in the circulation. At the tissue level, food energy is released in the presence of oxygen. Final nutrient-air interaction results in production of adenosine triphosphate (ATP), CO_2, and H_2O.*

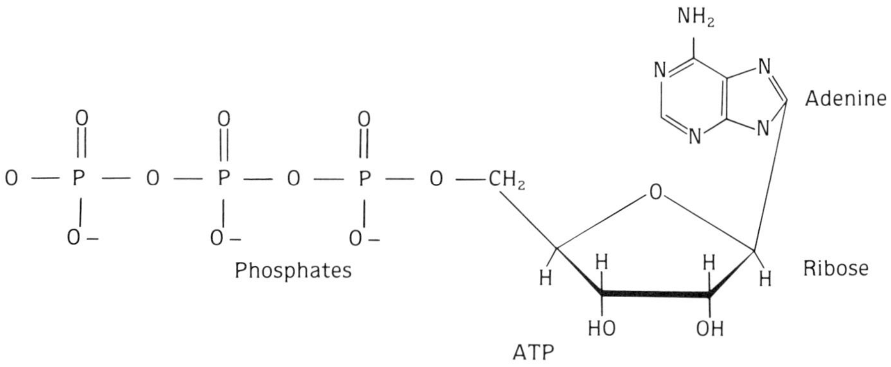

Fig. 15–2 *Functions of adenosine triphosphate (ATP) are as follows: (1) muscle contraction and relaxation, (2) active transport of substances across membranes, (3) substrate for cyclic adenosine monophosphate (cAMP), (4) energy for synthesis of various chemical compounds, and (5) energy storage.*

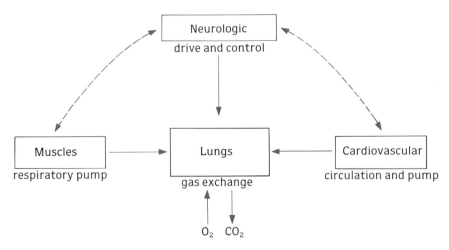

Fig. 15-3 *Block diagram illustrating components of the respiratory system. The neurologic component drives and controls respiration at the lungs via the respiratory muscles. It also affects the cardiovascular system by altering heart function and circulatory resistance. All components are necessary to achieve respiration. Nutritional quality and quantity directly affect the functioning of each system.*

1. Collect expired gas in a bag or Tissot spirometer for several minutes.
2. Analyze for carbon dioxide and oxygen (or oxygen and nitrogen).
3. Measure the volume of the gas collected in the bag.
4. Calculate:
   a. If oxygen and carbon dioxide are measured:

$$\dot{V}_{O_2 STPD} =$$

$$\left[\frac{\dot{V}_{E_{ATPS}} \times (P_B - H_2O) \times 21.55}{\text{collection time} \times (273 + \text{temp} °C)} \right]$$

$$\times \frac{1 - F_{EO_2} - F_{ECO_2} - \left(\dfrac{P_{H_2O}}{P_B}\right)}{\dfrac{1 - F_{IO_2}}{F_{IO_2}}} - (F_{EO_2})$$

$$\text{note:} \left(\frac{273° \text{ K} \times 60 \text{ sec}}{760 \text{ mmHg}} \right) = 21.55$$

If gas is analyzed with desiccant in line, then

$$\left(\frac{P_{H_2O}}{P_B} \right) = 0$$

where

$\dot{V}_{O_2 STPD}$ = oxygen uptake, standard conditions
$\dot{V}_{E_{ATPD}}$ = minute volume; ambient temperature and pressure, dry
F_{EO_2} = fraction of expired oxygen
F_{ECO_2} = fraction of expired carbon dioxide
$P_{H_2}O$ = water vapor pressure
P_B = barometric pressure
F_{IO_2} = fraction of inspired oxygen

   b. $\dot{V}_{CO_2} = \dot{V}_{E_{STPD}} \times (F_{ECO_2} - 0.0003)$

where $\dot{V}_{CO_2}$ = carbon dioxide production

   c. $RQ = \dfrac{\dot{V}_{CO_2}}{\dot{V}_{O_2}}$

where RQ = respiratory quotient

   d. If only oxygen and nitrogen are measured:

$$\dot{V}_{O_2} = \dot{V}_E \times \left(\frac{F_{EN_2}}{F_{IN_2}} \right) \times F_{IO_2} - (\dot{V}_E \times F_{EO_2})$$

where

F_{EN_2} = fraction of expired nitrogen
F_{IN_2} = fraction of inspired nitrogen

For patients confined to a hospital bed, portable equipment must be used. For patients that are not intubated and whose condition does not allow them to cooperate with the procedure using a nose clip and mouthpiece, a special hood or tent apparatus becomes necessary. A method for continuously measuring the $\dot{V}_{O_2}$ using a plastic tent hood has been described.[6-8] Metabolic measurements are more commonly determined with a metabolic cart that is composed of a volume or flow measuring device, oxygen and carbon dioxide analyzers, and a computer that calculates and displays the results. The respiratory care practitioner's interactions with the nutritional support team for metabolic measurements are most helpful, since respiratory therapy departments are usually equipped and therapists trained for such measurements.

In nutrition, energy is quantified in terms of kilocalories (kcal); 1 kcal is the amount of energy it takes to raise the temperature of 1 kg of water 1° C. (Although kilocalories have been used most frequently in clinical nutrition, the kilojoule (kJ) is often used in research. To convert kilocalories to kilojoules multiply: kcal × 4.184.) For approximately every 5 kcal burned, 1 L of oxygen is used by the tissues. Therefore if a patient's $\dot{V}_{O_2}$ is measured as 300 mL oxygen/min, then 300 mL oxygen × 60 minutes × 24 hours equals 432 L of oxygen required per day. And 5 kcal × 432 L oxygen/day equals 2,160 kcal/day that should be given to the patient. If less than this amount of energy is given, the patient is forced to use body energy stores, which often are depleted. The Weir or Lusk equation is used for more precise conversion of $\dot{V}o_2$ to kilocalories.[9,10]

The Weir equation is as follows:

$$kcal/min = 3.94 \times \dot{V}o_2 + 1.11 \times \dot{V}co_2$$
$$BEE = kcal/min \times 1{,}440 \text{ min}$$

Nutritional Depletion and Respiration

A patient who is not ingesting food enterally (via the gastrointestinal tract) and yet is only receiving 2 to 3 L/day of 5% dextrose is receiving at most about 600 kcal/day ($0.05 \times 3{,}000$ mL × 3.41 kcal/g glucose). (Glucose when given in hydrated form [intravenous D5/W, etc.] yields 3.41 kcal/g; otherwise the yield is about 4 kcal/g.) This is far from sufficient to meet a person's energy needs, much less protein, vitamin, and mineral needs. Liver glycogen stores (from which blood glucose levels are maintained in a fasting state) can be depleted in less than a day when there is inadequate carbohydrate intake.[11] This results in blood glucose levels being maintained by gluconeogenesis (production of glucose primarily from amino acids). Since there are no protein stores in the body, the amino acids for this process come from muscle and enzyme systems, with subsequent loss of functional tissue. The diaphragm and other respiratory muscles are not spared from this wasting, and they, along with other skeletal muscles, lose muscle mass.[12-14] In starvation or semistarvation states, respiratory muscle strength can diminish, producing a decrease in forced vital capacity (FVC)[15] and forced expiratory volume in 1 second (FEV_1).[16-18] Also occurring in starvation is a decrease in carbon monoxide diffusing capacity. (DL_{CO}). The decline in FEV_1 also correlates with a decreased creatinine-height index (CHI) indicative of loss of muscle mass.

If the calorie intake is less than needed, there will be a decrease in weight, as is commonly seen in patients with chronic obstructive pulmonary disease (COPD).[19-22] Patients with emphysema are more commonly underweight than those with chronic bronchitis.[16,22-27] Emphysema produces a catabolic state that results in weight loss even when a normal quantity of food is consumed. (If an increased amount of food is consumed, weight can begin to normalize, but emphysematous patients are not comfortable eating larger quantities of foods. If not continuously encouraged to do so they return typically to eating their "normal" amount which is insufficient to maintain a normal weight.)[25] Patients with chronic protein energy malnutrition (PEM; also known as protein-calorie malnutrition [PCM]) experience higher morbidity and mortality than

comparable patients who maintain normal weight.[29] With loss of body protein there is a subsequent loss not only of muscle and various enzyme systems but also of immunoglobulins, i.e., IgA, IgG, and IgM. Thus susceptibility to respiratory infections is increased because of decreased immunocompetence.[30-34]

Therapeutic Interactions of Respiration and Nutrition

Nutritional repletion in respiratory patients is often hindered by some of the necessary therapeutic actions. Bronchodilators may produce nausea; oxygen by nasal cannula disturbs the sense of smell—and therefore taste; other medications may interact with nutrients and render them less available for absorption or inhibit specific metabolic enzymes[35-38]; and intubation complicates the process of eating. Furthermore, since large meals may hamper function in an already less functional diaphragm, frequent small meals may be necessary, requiring greater effort in food preparation. These factors, along with shortness of breath, increased work of breathing, and a greater prevalence of peptic ulcers,[39-41] increase the risk of malnutrition. Being knowledgeable about these facts can help to improve both nutritional status and respiratory function.

The respiratory response to the body's need for oxygen and carbon dioxide elimination is usually regulated by the carbon dioxide produced ($\dot{V}_{CO_2}$). Sometimes increased hydrogen ion (H^+) concentration in addition to carbon dioxide will drive ventilation; this can occur when the amount of oxygen present is insufficient with respect to metabolic need, resulting in lactic acidosis. Oxygen itself or the lack thereof can become an important stimulus for breathing when it drops to levels in the body that are low enough, either through decreased exchange across the lungs or through scarcity in the atmosphere. Additionally, a semistarved state can decrease hypoxic drive, rendering a patient less sensitive to the need for more oxygen.[42,43]

Oxygen uptake and carbon dioxide excretion are as much a part of nutrition as are eating and the elimination of food by-products via the gastrointestinal tract and kidneys. Usually respiration is not thought of in this way because of the abundance of air and the minimal effort involved in its continuous "ingestion" (breathing). However, patients with respiratory disease often find themselves needing higher levels of the "nutrient" oxygen, or assistance in getting rid of the metabolic waste, carbon dioxide. Under these conditions, breathing becomes a more conscious and deliberate effort. Often in critical care patients, both feeding and breathing require continuous assistance. Just as patients require intubation when the ventilatory status is compromised sufficiently, they may require nasogastric (NG) or enteral tubes or parenteral (outside of the gastrointestinal tract) intravenous (IV) feeding when nutritional status warrants it. Matching a patient's energy and nutritional needs with ventilatory needs can become a challenge.

Respiratory System and Nutritional Needs

For optimal ventilatory function, proper nutrition is needed for all components of the respiratory system (see Fig. 15–3).

Neurologic Component

The neurologic component drives and controls ventilation. The higher the $\dot{V}co_2$ level (through increased metabolism or increased buffering of fixed acid), the greater the blood carbon dioxide concentration will be and therefore the greater the stimulus to the chemoreceptors. This in turn increases the electrical activity in the respiratory centers of the central nervous system (CNS), resulting in increased minute ventilation. The nervous system's fundamental requirement is for glucose. The energy derived from glucose is used to maintain an electrical charge across the nerve cell membrane, allowing for depolarization (action potential) and subsequent repolarization. The neurotransmitters at the synaptic ends are amino acids themselves or derivatives of them, and their presence is necessary for the relay of information from one neuron to another and from nerve to muscle. Apparently the sensitivity of the respiratory centers (either peripheral or central chemoreceptors) is affected by the amount and quality of protein ingested. The respiratory response to carbon dioxide or low levels of oxygen is increased with large amounts of protein intake.[44] However, too much protein may make some patients too sensitive to gas partial pressure changes, thus increasing the work of breathing. Giving the optimal amount of protein is the task of the nutritional support team.

Respiratory Muscle Component

The respiratory muscles make up the pump that drives the lungs. They receive the final stimulus from the CNS and produce the appropriate breathing rate and tidal volume as dictated by the CNS and local feedback pathways. The muscles require energy for contraction and relaxation. This energy is derived from blood glucose, free fatty acids from fat stores, and muscle glycogen. The muscle glycogen stores are the most readily available source of energy for the muscles; however, the amount of glycogen stored depends on the level of carbohydrate in the diet as well as on the previous exercise history of the muscle.[45] An exercised muscle can store more glycogen after exercise and subsequent nutritional repletion than it can after adequate nutrition alone.[45,46] In any case, for the body to store muscle glycogen there must be an adequate amount of carbohydrate in the diet.

Cardiovascular Component

The requirements of the cardiovascular system for food energy for the heart muscle are similar to those of the respiratory muscles. Protein is needed for buffering actions, clotting factors, transport of lipids and iron, and maintenance of oncotic pressure; carbohydrate is needed as fuel for heart muscle, 2,3-diphosphoglycerate (2,3-DPG), and various other cell components; fat is needed for cell membranes and as fuel for heart muscle; vitamins and minerals are needed for maintenance of the metabolic pathways and integrity of cell membranes, including iron for oxygen transport. Thus the quality and functional value of the heart and blood depend on fluid and nutrient intake.

Gas Exchange Component (Lungs)

The lungs, which interface air from the atmosphere with the circulatory system, require a delicate balance of various systems to achieve gas exchange efficiently. Alveolar ventilation must be matched with alveolar circulation to allow the efficient transfer of gases between blood and air. To prevent alveolar collapse, surfactant is needed to lessen the surface-active forces that promote collapse of the lung. Starvation leads to decreased surfactant synthesis as well as emphysematous changes in the lung.[47-49] Humidity and mucociliary performance in the lung require adequate hydration. Smooth muscle function, macrophage activity, and secretion of immunoglobulins (e.g., IgA) into mucus all depend on good nutrition.

Metabolism

Since basic requirements for both oxygen and nutrients are determined by the cellular metabolic rate, an understanding of metabolism is essential for both respiratory and nutritional assessment.

Metabolism is the body's way of transferring energy from food to the body's energy currency molecules—ATP. The metabolic process can be divided into two pathways: those that break molecules down as energy is released (catabolism) and those that build up new molecules (anabolism) to be used in either a structural or a functional role. The catabolic pathways produce ATP, which is used in the anabolic pathways for growth and maintenance of the organism or simply for the organism's movement in the environment. Therefore energy is the fundamental need of the body. If sufficient food is eaten, the body can maintain its equilibrium and satisfy the demands placed on it by changes in the environment. However, if too little food is ingested, the body must rely on energy previously stored. If the stored energy—fat and carbohydrate (glycogen)—is not sufficient, the body will break down protein to produce ATP. As mentioned previously, this condition is undesirable, since the protein comes from functioning tissue and therefore lessens the functional capability of the organism.

If too much food energy is taken in, the body must use some of its energy to store the excess in the form of fat. As the level of body fat increases, the metabolic cost of moving and breathing increases along with the risk of various diseases. Again the functional capability of the organism is decreased.

A basic understanding of the metabolic pathways is essential when planning nutritional and ventilatory support. Fig. 15–4 illustrates schematically the major energy-producing pathways used by almost every cell of the body. The reader is encouraged to refer to biochemistry or physiology texts for a more complete discussion of metabolism.

The metabolic process can be viewed as having four major phases (see Fig. 15–4). The first is the digestive phase, in which the food materials are broken down to the basic components: fat (fatty acids), carbohydrates (sugars), and protein (amino acids). The food components are then absorbed from the gastrointestinal tract into the blood, where they eventually travel to every cell in the body.

The second phase involves the catabolism of the food components, within the cell, down to a common molecule, acetylcoenzyme A (acetyl CoA). A small amount of the food energy is used directly to produce a few ATP molecules or transferred to molecular energy shuttles (energy intermediates) in this phase, but acetyl CoA still contains the bulk of the food energy. It is also possible for the metabolic pathways in this phase to go in the opposite direction, from acetyl CoA to form the basic food components again. However, molecules only move in this anabolic direction when the cell has plenty of energy currency (ATP) available. Also note that anaerobic metabolism (energy—ATP—being formed without the presence of oxygen) can occur only in this second phase of metabolism, in the pathway labeled *glycolysis*. In anaerobic metabolism, pyruvate produces lactate (lactic acid) rather than acetyl CoA. The greater the energy production without sufficient oxygen, the more lactic acid produced. This can result in *lactic acidosis*. If this occurs, then the acid must be buffered with bicarbonate (HCO_3), and carbon dioxide is produced in the process. This requires increased minute ventilation to breathe off the carbon dioxide that is generated.

Whereas the phases just described have different pathways for each of the food components, the third phase uses the same tricarboxylic acid (TCA) pathway (also referred to as the Krebs or citric acid cycle), regardless of the origin of the acetyl CoA. The rest of the food energy is removed in the TCA phase, again transferring the energy to molecular energy shuttles. It is here that most of the energy-depleted carbon "skeletons" are discarded as carbon dioxide. For the TCA cycle to be active, the energy shuttles NAD (nicotinamide-adenine dinucleotide) and FAD (flavoprotein adenine dinucleotide) have to be able to unload their energy-rich hydrogen and electrons into the respiratory transport chain (oxidative phosphorylation). This requires the presence of oxygen. Without it, the TCA cycle grinds to a halt.

The fourth phase is the final destination of the molecular energy shuttles, where they "dump" their energy-rich loads of hydrogen and electrons into the oxidative phosphorylation system, where ATP molecules are mass-produced. This is also the final destination of the oxygen that was breathed in. Here the energy is extracted from the hydrogen and electrons; in the energy-depleted form, the hydrogen and electrons combine with oxygen to form water.

It is in the metabolic pathways outlined above where the body's oxygen is used and carbon dioxide is produced. The oxygen used can be measured and is expressed as the oxygen uptake per minute, $\dot{V}_{O_2}$. The measured carbon dioxide produced per minute is expressed as the $\dot{V}_{CO_2}$. The ratio of $\dot{V}_{CO_2}$ to $\dot{V}_{O_2}$ is the respiratory quotient (RQ). (What is actually measured at the mouth is referred to as the respiratory exchange ratio, or REE.) The RQ is determined simply by the amount of fat, carbohydrate, or protein that one has eaten or is metabolizing. Pure fat metabolism has an RQ of 0.7; protein has a value of 0.85; and carbohydrate has a value of 1.0. A mixture of the three different types of foods used for energy at the same time results in an RQ of around 0.8. (This is the R value used most often in the alveolar air equation.)

Nutritional Requirements

The basic nutritional requirements include carbohydrate, protein, fat, vitamins, minerals, and water.[50] In light of the present discussion it would not be wrong to include oxygen as a nutrient since food is of no value unless oxygen is present, although traditionally it is not included in discussions of nutritional requirements. Carbohydrate, protein, and fat provide the energy the body needs as well as the basic chemical skeletons on which structural and functional body systems are built. Vitamins, being part of coenzymes, work along with enzymes in various metabolic pathways and allow specific reactions to occur. Minerals are often elements of specific molecules; for example, hemoglobin, cytochromes, and thyroxin. Water is the medium in which the various chemical reactions take place within cells. It

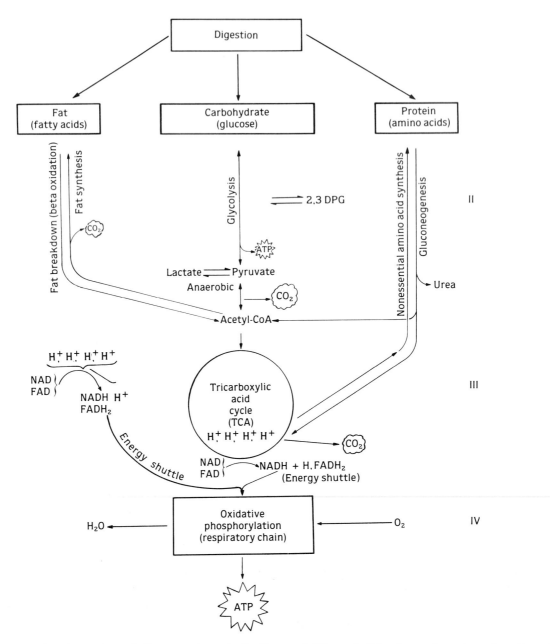

Fig. 15-4 *Four major phases of metabolism are schematically illustrated.* **Phase I,** *Digestion and nutrient absorption of fat, carbohydrate, and protein.* **Phase II,** *Breakdown of fatty acids, glucose, and amino acids to acetyl-CoA, which can either go on to synthesize, directly or indirectly, fat, carbohydrate, or amino acids, as need be, or have more energy extracted from it in phases III and IV.* **Phase III,** *Tricarboxylic acid cycle, where most of the body's CO_2 is produced and where most of the molecular energy shuttles (NAD, FAD) receive their energy supply in the form of hydrogen atoms. Shuttles transport energy to the respiratory chain.* **Phase IV,** *Inner mitochondrial membrane where oxidative phosphorylation (production of ATP in the presence of oxygen) occurs. Oxygen is the final acceptor of the now energy-depleted electrons and hydrogen ions.*

is also responsible for the fluidity of the blood, which allows blood to circulate.

The optimal amount of each of the nutritional elements has not been precisely determined, especially for those required in trace amounts. There is agreement that a minimum nutrient level should be high enough so that deficiency symptoms cannot be detected and low enough to prevent toxicity. Within this range there is much discussion as to what is the right amount, since nutritional requirements can vary from person to person. Greater or lesser amounts of specific nutrients may be needed because of genetically induced enzyme defects, various disease states, varying amounts of energy expenditure, and various drug-nutrient interactions. Because of the complexity of nurturing the body, a careful nutritional assessment by a nutritional support team, composed of at least a physician, dietitian, and nurse, is essential. A clinical pharmacologist, for diets that are given parenterally, and a respiratory therapist, for assessing $\dot{V}o_2$ and $\dot{V}co_2$, are important additions to the team.

Carbohydrate

The single element that should compose the largest amount of the dietary intake is carbohydrate. Carbohydrate can be broadly classified as complex or simple. The complex carbohydrates are starches (sugar molecules linked together in long branching chains) and are readily found in a variety of foods, the best sources being grains, vegetables, and fruits. Foods high in complex carbohydrates usually contain the vitamins required in the metabolic pathways for catabolism. In addition, these foods provide water, fiber, protein, and chemical components that may inhibit disease processes. Simple carbohydrates are free sugars and, of the natural foods, are found in the largest amounts in fruits. However, the majority of sugar consumed comes from processed, refined foods. Ingestion of simple carbohydrates should be held to a minimum, since their nutritional value is quite low but their metabolic demand is quite high (i.e., they travel down the glucose metabolic pathway or go to fat synthesis, but do not "pay any taxes" in the form of vitamins and protein for the maintenance of the metabolic machinery). They can provide a quick form of energy, but when ingested alone they can stimulate an exaggerated insulin response because of their rapid absorption from the intestinal tract. Complex carbohydrates tend not to trigger this response because they have to be broken down to free sugars—which takes time—before they are absorbed.[51] Various complex carbohydrate foods may differ from one another in their effects on blood sugar levels.[52,53]

Carbohydrate has often been contrasted with fat. Since the $\dot{V}_{CO_2}$ with fat metabolism is lower than that with carbohydrate, it has been suggested by some that minimizing the dietary intake of carbohydrate is to the respiratory patient's advantage.[26] A patient's response to carbohydrate should be evaluated so that adverse effects can be avoided. It appears, however, that when high levels of carbohydrate are given enterally to patients with COPD who retain carbon dioxide, elevated arterial carbon dioxide tension (Pa_{CO_2}) levels do not always occur.[54-57] In fact, there are even some advantages. A load of ingested carbohydrate can elevate the arterial blood oxygen level (Pa_{O_2}) by a modest amount of 7 to 9 mmHg.[54,58,59] This is of definite benefit to patients with low oxygen saturations. When the oxygen saturation is low, small increases in Pa_{O_2} can produce significant increases in oxygen content. Additionally, a high carbohydrate diet can significantly increase endurance[60] as well as allow a given amount of work to be performed with less oxygen when compared to low carbohydrate diets.[11,61] Possibly the low $\dot{V}_{CO_2}$ advantages of a high fat diet are offset in some patients by the increased oxygen requirement for a given work rate. The major problem that has arisen with carbohydrate intake in patients with respiratory disorders occurs when glucose has been given in excess. The increased $\dot{V}_{CO_2}$ (a result of both the high RQ of glucose metabolism and its conversion to fat) has induced respiratory difficulty in patients being weaned from mechanical ventilators.[62-66] This has been observed primarily when glucose has been administered by the parenteral (IV) route.

Clearly the problem with glucose lies not in its use but in its abuse. It is recommended that with the use of parenteral nutrition in critically ill patients, fat be infused along with the glucose.[64] The infused fat not only helps provide energy but inhibits the fat synthesis pathway, thereby preventing excessive carbon dioxide production.

Generally, carbohydrates should make up 60% or more of the caloric intake of enterally fed patients. Follow-up assessment of the patients will allow for adjustments of the carbohydrate intake to match individual needs.

Protein

Protein should make up 12% to 15% of the caloric intake. The recommended dietary allowance (RDA) of protein for a healthy person has been set at 0.8 g/Kg of body weight each day.[67] Thus a 70-Kg person should obtain about 56 g of protein each day. Typically a person who ingests an adequate number of calories each day, from a variety of foods, will get sufficient protein. Following are two methods for estimating protein needs in healthy or sick people.

1. Caloric-nitrogen ratio
   150:1 for the average hospitalized patient
   100:1 for extreme hypermetabolism
   450:1 for renal insufficiency (without dialysis)
   300:1 for the normal healthy adult
2. Grams of protein per kilograms of body weight
   0.8 g/Kg for the normal healthy adult
   1.2 to 1.5 g/Kg for the average hospitalized patient
   2.0 to 2.5 g/Kg for severe catabolic problems

Nitrogen values are often referred to when discussing protein requirements because every amino acid (all proteins are made up of various kinds and amounts of amino acids) contains an acid group, COOH, and an amino group, NH_2, that contain nitrogen. Specific laboratory methods are used to measure nitrogen in the blood (blood urea nitrogen [BUN]) or in the urine (urinary urea nitrogen [UUN]). Since every 100 g of many proteins contains 6.25 g of nitrogen, one can readily convert grams of nitrogen to grams of protein by multiplying by 6.25. Conversely, to find how much nitrogen there is in a given amount of protein, in grams, one simply divides by 6.25 (or the appropriate factor for the specific protein).

When considering adequacy of protein intake, both quantity and quality of the protein must be considered. The quality of a protein is determined by the amount of essential amino acids it contains. Essential amino acids cannot be synthesized by the body in sufficient quantities to meet body needs—or cannot be synthesized at all. Of the 20 amino acids, 9 are considered essential for the healthy adult: histidine, isoleucine, leucine, lysine, methionine, phenylalanine, threonine, tryptophan, and valine. The greater the number of essential amino acids in a protein, the higher its quality.

As with anything else, the extremes of protein intake, either too little or too much, can have detrimental effects. Too little protein compromises the immune system, promotes edema and ascites, produces generalized wasting of muscle tissue, and retards growth and proper development in children. Too much protein, although not as harmful, increases the requirements for some other nutrients, notably calcium[68] and water.[69] In addition, there may be an increase in the work of breathing,[40] as noted previously, and increased stress on the liver and kidneys (mostly of concern in patients with liver or renal failure). The final consideration involves the body's acid-base balance. Protein is the major source of fixed acids that are ingested (fixed acids have to be cleared by the kidney; volatile acids, like carbon dioxide, can be cleared by the lungs). Patients with COPD that are in a state of respiratory acidosis may experience more difficulty if an increased fixed acid load—large quantity of protein—is ingested.

To establish the optimal amount of protein that a patient needs requires the measurement of protein intake (nitrogen intake) and nitrogen excretion. A patient whose intake of nitrogen equals excretion of nitrogen is said to be in *nitrogen balance*. If more nitrogen is excreted than ingested, then *negative* nitrogen balance exists. Conversely, *positive* nitrogen balance exists when the nitrogen intake is greater than the nitrogen excretion. Patients who are severely ill or who are simply not getting enough calories will often be in negative nitrogen balance. This is undesirable, since it indicates that body protein is being used for energy. Patients who are nutritionally depleted need to be in positive nitrogen balance to build up body tissues. In the well-nourished patient, the clinical goal is to maintain nitrogen balance.

Fat

Dietary fat is important for several reasons: (1) it can carry the fat-soluble vitamins (A, D, E, K) and allow for their absorption; (2) it is energy-dense so that a given quantity ingested yields more energy than carbohydrate or protein; (3) it gives flavor and adds the satiation aspect to food; (4) it can prolong the digestion process, giving rise to fewer hunger feelings between meals; and (5) it contains two essential fatty acids the body must have but cannot synthesize, linolenic and linoleic acids (used for prostaglandin synthesis).

Within the body, fat is involved in many different functions. Notably, fat is a component of all cell membranes, provides energy storage and organ protection, and is the major component of surfactant (dipalmityl lecithin). To accomplish these tasks, however, does not require much fat to be eaten. The typical American diet takes more than 30% of calories from fat. This is too much. With excess dietary fat comes increased risk of heart disease, breast cancer, colon cancer, and recently, a reported increased risk of lung cancer in women.[70] Fat may also decrease oxygenation of the tissues,[71-73] impair pulmonary D_{LCO},[74] and hinder capillary circulation by the clumping of red blood cells.[75-78] However, other studies have shown no changes in blood gas values or D_{LCO}.[65,79,80]

The main concern of nutritionists is to determine the optimal percentage of calories that should come from carbohydrate and protein. With that established, the remaining amount of calories required can come from fat.

With the quantity of fat determined, one must be concerned with the quality of fat. Fat can be either saturated (no double bonds present in the fatty acid chain) or unsaturated (some of the fatty acid carbons contain double bonds). Most of the fat eaten should be unsaturated. Good-quality fat or oils will have a polyunsaturated to saturated ratio (P/S ratio) greater than 1. Diets that contain higher P/S ratios tend to decrease the blood cholesterol level and are associated with a lower risk of heart disease.[81] A specific type of polyunsaturated fat may also play a role.[82,83] It should be noted that even fat of good quality (high P/S ratio) does not negate the effects of too much fat.

Despite all the information available about the advantages and disadvantages of given foods and optimal combinations of carbohydrate, fat, and protein, dietary patterns established early in life are difficult to change in later years. Patients should be encouraged to eat foods that provide good nutrition and at the same time do not aggravate a compromised respiratory condition. However, some patients will not adapt to a change in diet, and in these cases any nutrition is better than no nutrition.

Vitamins and Minerals

Vitamins can be classified into two main categories: water-soluble and fat-soluble. Water-soluble vitamins are those of the B group and vitamin C. The fat-soluble vitamins are A, D, E, and K. The minerals can be divided into either macronutrient elements or micronutrient (trace) elements.

For most people who eat a variety of food each day, ingesting the recommended amounts of vitamins and minerals is not difficult. But when physiologic functioning has been altered by a disease process, an increased need for specific nutrients may arise. Furthermore, various medications can interact with the absorption, function, or excretion of some nutrients, thereby altering the required amount.[84]

A few nutrients deserve special mention because of their importance in patients with lung disease. Iron's role in oxygen transport and use in hemoglobin, myoglobin, and within the respiratory transport chain makes it necessary for iron to be maintained at normal levels. Vitamin A promotes optimal functioning of mucous membranes and helps in promoting resistance to respiratory tract infections.[85] β-Carotene, a vitamin A precursor, and vitamin C have been found to be associated with a decreased risk of certain types of lung cancers.[86,87] Vitamins E and C and selenium, which are antioxidants, appear to help lessen the effects of oxygen toxicity and ozone on lung tissue.[88-92] Any chronically ill patient may have altered eating habits that are insufficient to meet nutrient requirements. The severity of nutritional depletion appears to be related to the severity of COPD despite an adequate caloric intake.[93] This may result in a need for supplementation of some or all of the vitamins and minerals. For further information the reader is referred to any of the many nutrition texts.

Fluids and Electrolytes

Adequate fluid intake is extremely important for patients with respiratory disorders. Proper function of the lung's mucociliary clearance mechanism requires good hydration. Although the body is composed of about 60% water by weight, it is constantly losing water via urine, feces, sweat, breathing, and, in patients with respiratory problems, expectoration. This requires continual fluid replacement.[94-98]

Patients with respiratory problems often develop heart failure (right or left or eventually both), which complicates the fluid replacement process. The need for fluids must be carefully balanced with the need to restrict fluids because of the fluid retention secondary to the heart problem. When dealing with a patient who has a heart problem, both fluid and sodium intake must be monitored. Sodium levels determine how much water the body will retain; therefore dietary sodium must often be limited.

Water is the best fluid to replace water. However, fruit or vegetable juices add some variety as well as some nutrition. Low-sodium juices can be obtained. Drinks containing caffeine promote bronchodilation to some extent because caffeine is in the same family as theophylline, both being xanthines.[99] But if a patient is using theophylline-type bronchodilators and is also a heavy user of drinks containing caffeine, there is a greater chance of side effects. Because the ingestion of alcohol has been correlated with decreased FVC and FEV_1,[100,101] bronchoconstriction,[102,103] impairment of lung defenses,[104] and increased likelihood of sleep apnea,[105] its use is contraindicated. Good nutrition for the respiratory system involves not only getting enough of that which is essential but also avoiding that which is harmful.

Patients receiving fluids IV must have the input and output amounts monitored continually so that neither too much nor too little is given. Fluid overload frequently results in pulmonary congestion or edema, further complicating a poorly functioning lung.

In addition to serum sodium levels, potassium and chloride values should be checked. All of these electrolytes play an important role in acid-base balance. Potassium also plays an important role in heart, muscle, and nerve function, as well as in stimulation of aldosterone secretion (along with angiotensin II) from the adrenal cortex.

One must not forget that fluid and sodium intake can occur with medication and normal saline nebulization. Nebulized fluid retention is most critical when dealing with small children and infants—especially when an ultrasonic nebulizer is used.[106]

Methods of Meeting Nutritional Requirements

Nutritional requirements can only be met once the food has entered the body. This is obvious; however, it is not always easily achieved. Nutritionists often work against such patient factors as loss of appetite, dyspnea that is increased with eating, inability to eat normal amounts of solid food, fluid restrictions, inability to take food by mouth, and a comatose state. Careful evaluation of a patient's nutritional needs, food preferences, educational and economic status, cooking facilities, and self-help level is necessary. All factors influence a patient's ability to reach the nutritional goals set.

The routes of nutritional administration can be either enteral or parenteral. The preferred route is enteral. If a patient is intubated and cannot take food by mouth, then tube feeding will be instituted via an NG tube. The last resort, when all other attempts at feeding are unsuccessful, is total parenteral nutrition (TPN). TPN is the feeding of patients by direct infusion of nutrients into either a peripheral or a central vein. There is a reluctance to feed patients by TPN because it is not as efficient as the enteral route, it is expensive, and there are increased risks of complications such as infection, but since nutrition is so important, it is used. Nutritionally depleted or hypermetabolic patients should never go without nutritional support for more than a day.

Patients with emphysema are often underweight and need to gain, while those with chronic bronchitis are likely to be overweight and need to lose.[16,25-28] Patients with COPD may find it uncomfortable to eat a large meal because a flattened diaphragm along with a full stomach makes it even more difficult to function. To avoid this problem, frequent small meals may be helpful. The goal for a patient with emphysema is a positive nitrogen balance and an increase in caloric intake since respiratory muscle function improves with an increase in weight (muscle mass). The goal for an overweight patient with bronchitis is maintenance of nitrogen balance with decreased caloric intake since respiratory muscle function improves with a loss of weight (fat).

Patients being assisted by continuous mechanical ventilation provide an additional nutritional challenge. Studies in dogs suggest that positive pressure breathing can affect splanchnic (internal organs of the abdomen) circulation[107] as well as increased resistance to portal blood flow,[108] increased resistance to bile flow down the bile duct,[109] and decreased blood flow to the kidneys.[110] These effects are increased as the pressure is increased and are most pronounced with the use of continuous positive airway pressure (CPAP) or positive end-expiratory pressure (PEEP). These effects, however, may only reach significance for a minority of patients. Yet any alteration in blood flow in the gastrointestinal tract, liver, or kidneys can have an impact on the nutritional status of the patient, thus making it more difficult to meet the nutritional requirements set.

Nutritional Assessment

The respiratory care practitioner is not responsible for the nutritional assessment of the patient, but should be familiar with the process and may actually participate in it. Since the respiratory therapist and the nurse usually spend the most time with a patient, their observations are valuable. A complete nutritional assessment is performed by the dietitian, with some factors being assessed by other members of the nutritional support team. The components of nutritional assessment consist of medical and diet histories, anthropometric (weight and various body) measurements, biochemical evaluations, and immunologic evaluations. The areas to be assessed in determining the patient's nutritional profile are summarized in the accompanying box.

Data Gathering and Interpretation

HISTORY. Following is a list of some conditions to be sought in the medical history.

> Multiple surgical or nonsurgical trauma
> Fever
> Infection
> Burns
> Long bone fractures
> Hyperthyroidism
> Prolonged corticosteroid therapy

These conditions increase a patient's metabolic rate or caloric and other nutrient requirements, or all of these. Such metabolic challenges pose a serious threat to the homeostatic maintenance of a marginally nourished patient with COPD. A patient with one of these conditions should be further evaluated with a metabolic rate assessment (BEE).

AREAS REQUIRING ASSESSMENT TO DETERMINE PATIENT'S NUTRITIONAL PROFILE

Physiologic
Type(s) of disease(s) present
Severity of illness
Metabolic stress of disease
Medications being used
Genetic deficiencies
Activity level
Resting metabolic rate
Food allergies
Present nutritional status
  Anthropometric
  Biochemical
  Immunologic

Psychosocial
Mental state (mood, alertness)

Culture
Food preparation skills
Appetite
Learned eating behaviors/habits (food preferences)
Motivation
Habits: alcohol, smoking
Education
Income

Environmental
Mechanical hinderances to eating (continuous mechanical ventilation and tracheostomy)
Food availability
Temperature
Humidity

During the patient interview, information in the following important areas is sought.

> Occupation and usual daily activity
> Use of supplemental oxygen
> Usual energy and nutrient intake via 24-hour recall, food frequency pattern, etc.
> Special diet at home
> Food aversions, intolerances, and allergies
> Medications and nutritional supplements
> Mechanical feeding problems (chewing, swallowing, etc.)
> Changes in appetite
> Changes in food intake or food patterns
> Gastrointestinal problems (nausea, vomiting, heartburn, etc.)
> Elimination pattern and consistency of stool
> Maximum weight attained and how long ago it was attained
> Usual weight
> Alcohol intake
> Smoking or other tobacco habits

This information is usually obtained from the patient or family members during the initial workup.

PHYSICAL EXAMINATION. The physical examination often yields clues to the patient's nutritional status; however, many signs of nutritional deficiency

Table 15–1   Height and Weight (16)*

	Men				Women		
Height	Small Frame	Medium Frame	Large Frame	Height	Small Frame	Medium Frame	Large Frame
5'2"	128–134	131–141	138–150	4'10"	102–111	109–121	118–131
5'3"	130–136	133–143	140–153	4'11"	103–113	111–123	120–134
5'4"	132–138	135–145	142–156	5'0"	104–115	113–126	122–137
5'5"	134–140	137–148	144–160	5'1"	106–118	115–129	125–140
5'6"	136–142	139–151	146–164	5'2"	108–121	118–132	128–143
5'7"	138–145	142–154	149–168	5'3"	111–124	121–135	131–147
5'8"	140–148	145–157	152–172	5'4"	114–127	124–138	134–151
5'9"	142–151	148–160	155–176	5'5"	117–130	127–141	137–155
5'10"	144–154	151–163	158–180	5'6"	120–133	130–144	140–159
5'11"	146–157	154–166	161–184	5'7"	123–136	133–147	143–163
6'0"	149–160	157–170	164–188	5'8"	126–139	136–150	146–167
6'1"	152–164	160–174	168–192	5'9"	129–142	139–153	149–170
6'2"	155–168	164–178	172–197	5'10"	132–145	142–156	152–173
6'3"	158–172	167–182	176–202	5'11"	135–148	145–159	155–176
6'4"	162–176	171–187	181–207	6'0"	138–151	148–162	158–179
Weight at ages 25 to 59 in shoes and 5 lb of indoor clothing.				Weight at ages 29 to 59 in shoes and 3 lb of indoor clothing.			

*From 1979 Build Study. Society of Actuaries and Association of Life Insurance Medical Directors of America, 1980; courtesy Metropolitan Life Insurance Co.

can be missed by the inexperienced practitioner. Look at the health of the patient's hair and check for sparseness, dyspigmentation, or easy "pluckability." Does the patient's skin show areas of drying, cracking, or pigment change? Are there swollen parotid glands or an enlarged liver? Is there weight loss or muscle wasting, edema, mental apathy or confusion? These are some of the points to look for in assessing nutritional status, realizing, of course, that other factors may be causing some of the changes. These signs are rather nonspecific and therefore only suggestive of malnutrition.[111–113] When these signs are present in a patient, more sensitive and objective methods of assessment should be used to confirm or rule out compromised nutritional status.

Following is a summary of some basic anthropometric measurements and their nutritional assessment value.

Measurement	Indication
Skinfold thickness	Amount of body fat
Skinfold + arm circumference = arm, muscle circumference, muscle and fat area	Body protein reserves, an indicator of protein-energy nutrition Body fat stores, an indicator of energy reserves
Weight for height	Result of long-term nutritional status

The assessment most commonly used and easiest to perform during the physical examination involves weighing and measuring. Measurements of weight, height, and arm circumference require little effort or time yet give important information. Since height and weight can vary with the time of day and the amount of clothing or shoe heel height, the measurements should be performed in the same way each time and the pertinent information recorded so that serial measurements are meaningful. Bed scales can be used for weighing ventilator-dependent patients. The weight of any ventilator tubing should be subtracted from the total. A weight of less than 80% of the weight for height from standard tables (Table 15–1), or a loss of 5% of the usual body weight, or an unintentional weight loss of 10 lb or more indicates increased nutritional risk. Although body weight has limited value in detecting malnutrition,[114] values less than 85% of the weight-for-height standards of the Metropolitan Life Insurance Company correlate with poor medical outcome.[115] The clinical team should make certain that water retention is not masking a weight loss and that water loss is not interpreted as nutritional depletion. If a fluctuation or change in weight of several pounds is observed during a 24-hour period, one can be quite sure that it is caused by water retention or loss.

A quick estimate of ideal body weight can be determined from the following rule of thumb: allow 105 pounds for the first 5 feet of height and 5 pounds for each additional inch. This does not account for variations in frame size but is useful for rapid estimation as to appropriateness of a patient's weight. The ideal body weight can also be used for estimating a patient's anatomic dead space (1 mL/lb ideal body weight) or for determining a starting tidal volume for a ventilator-dependent patient (5–7 mL/lb ideal body weight). The term *ideal body weight* simply refers to the weight the patient probably *should* weigh. Body weight is often divided into two types: fat weight and lean body weight (lean body weight = total weight – fat weight). The problem is never simply a weight problem. A patient only weighs too much when the percentage of total body weight made up of fat exceeds about 14% for males and 24% for females. A method for estimating the percent of body fat is the skinfold *measurement*.

Triceps Skinfold Thickness. Measurement of skinfold thickness with the use of calipers is a fairly simple procedure (proper technique is important) that

Table 15-2 Current Laboratory Biochemical Tests and Guidelines for Interpretation

Measurement or Index	Deficient	Normal	Sensitivity
Creatinine-height index (CHI) (%)	40	60	Poor
Serum albumin level (g/dL)	2.5	3.5–5.0	Limited because of long half-life (20 days)
Serum transferrin level (mg/dL)	100	200–400	Poor; unpredictable response to refeeding
Total iron-binding capacity (TIBC) (mg/dL)	<250	250–350	Poor; increased in pregnancy, iron deficiency, oral contraceptive use; iron may bind to proteins other than serum transferrin
Nitrogen balance	Negative balance	Equilibrium	Poor; nitrogen excretion often underestimated
Thyroxin-binding prealbumin (TBPA) (mg/dL)	<10	10–20	Very good; half-life short (2 days)
Retinol-binding protein (RBP) (μg/dL)	<3	3–6	Very good; half-life short (12 hr)
Total lymphocyte count (cells/mm^3)	<1,200	2,000–3,500	Limited; decreased in injury, chemotherapy, radiotherapy, surgery; increased in infection
Differential count for lymphocytes (%)		20–45	Limited
Skin antigen testing	Negative	Positive	Good

yields data on the fat and protein reserves in the body. The triceps skinfold is the most common place of measurement; however, several other sites can be used, usually in addition to the triceps area. Skinfold thickness coupled with measurements of the upper arm circumference, arm muscle circumference, and arm muscle area provide accepted estimates of protein energy malnutrition.[116,117] The arm fat area may also be calculated and, when used along with triceps skinfold measurements, improves the body fat weight estimate.[118] These measurements are all compared with standard normal values to assess the degree of malnutrition. As with other tests, the exact value obtained with any one measurement may not be as important as the trend seen with serial measurements. It is important to establish baseline data for a patient when first admitted. Then the first signs of malnutrition can be detected and appropriate treatment implemented before serious deficiency symptoms occur.

Other, more accurate methods for assessment of body fat include underwater weighing,[119] body volume displacement,[120] and electrical bioimpedance measurements.[121,122] Only the last has a role to play in the hospital setting.

LABORATORY BIOCHEMICAL TESTS. Laboratory biochemical tests tend to reflect body changes more quickly and be more accurate than anthropometric tests. Table 15–2 summarizes their relative sensitivities to body nutritional change and suggests guidelines for interpretation.

Creatine phosphate is used in muscle as an energy reserve molecule. When there is an increased demand for ATP, creatine will donate a phosphate to ADP, making ATP. The more muscle mass there is in the body, the more creatine there will be. Creatine is metabolized to creatinine, the form in which it is largely excreted. The clearance of creatinine from the blood by the kidneys is a good indicator of renal function. Measurement of 24-hour urinary excretion of creatinine correlates with the patient's lean body weight (muscle mass): the greater the muscle mass, the higher the urinary excretion of creatinine. When expressed in terms of height, a measure relatively unaffected by malnutrition, urinary excretion of creatinine can be used as a general measure of malnutrition. The creatinine-height index (CHI) reportedly does not correlate with arm muscle circumference,[123–125] probably because of the many factors that govern the excretion of creatinine. A recent study found it to be of limited value as a predictor of muscle mass in malnourished young females but a good predictor of muscle mass in malnourished young males. In young females and elderly males, if the creatinine excretion is related to the total arm length, the ability to predict malnutrition is improved.[114]

Levels of serum albumin, the major protein fraction of blood, correlate well with body protein reserves of muscle mass. The measurement of serum albumin levels provides a useful screening tool for detecting protein energy undernutrition.[125,126] However, since the turnover of serum albumin is relatively slow (half-life is 20 days), a change in nutritional status is not soon reflected by this measurement. The time lag of 1 to 2 weeks for the serum albumin level to show a change after a nutritional alteration has occurred is too long to effectively manage the nutrition of most critically ill patients.

Prealbumin, also called thyroxin-binding prealbumin (TBPA) because it carries about one third of the body's thyroxin (thyroid hormone), also carries retinol-binding protein (RBP). These two proteins quickly reflect nutritional deprivation or refeeding treatment because of their short half-lives (TBPA, 2 days; RBP, 12 hours).[127–131] Either one or both can be used for assessing nutritional repletion in critically ill patients, since the response time for these values is 3 days or less.[132]

Serum transferrin, the protein that transports iron in the body, has a half-life of 4 to 8 days. However, because of its wide range of normal values and its unpredictable response to refeeding in depleted patients, it has limited clinical use in nutritional assessment.[132–134] The total iron-binding capacity (TIBC) of transferrin may also be used. However, it may overestimate transferrin levels since iron can also bind to other proteins in the blood to a certain extent. Transferrin levels may be elevated during iron deficiency anemia, the second and third trimesters of pregnancy, estrogen therapy, or oral contraceptive use.[135,136] Other hormones and disease states have a variable effect on serum transferrin levels and TIBC.[136,137]

Nitrogen balance measurements, using 24-hour urine specimens, are essential for protein assessment and are commonly performed in acute care settings. However, an underestimation of nitrogen excretion can occur in patients with burns, diarrhea, vomiting, or other nitrogen-losing conditions.[138] A commonly used clinical estimation is: nitrogen balance = grams of nitrogen intake − (24-hour grams of urine urea nitrogen + 4 g).

Immunocompetence, being dependent on globulin proteins, as mentioned previously, can also be used to help assess PEM. Either total lymphocyte count (lymphocytes make the immunoglobulins) or their function can be measured. An easy test of their function (which requires them to have ample protein to make their antibodies) is to challenge them with skin antigen testing. Antigens used are those to which a patient is most likely to have been previously exposed. With these, a quick antigen-antibody reaction should be seen at the skin testing site (much like a positive tuberculin skin test reaction). However, if the patient is protein-deficient, the skin test reaction will be greatly diminished or absent.[139] It should be noted that an iron deficiency can also diminish the response.[140]

• • •

As can be seen, no one test constitutes a perfect assessment of a patient's nutritional status. But with the appropriate use of selected anthropometric and biochemical measurements, along with astute observations by respiratory care practitioners, an adequate nutritional profile can be developed. Other sources should be consulted for further discussion of nutritional assessment.[141–144]

Role of Respiratory Care Practitioners in Nutritional Assessment

The members of the health team not involved in direct nutritional assessment, if alert to the information discussed so far, can contribute significantly to achieving good nutrition for patients with respiratory disorders. Signs or symptoms of potential nutritional problems should be sought while dealing with the routine of patient care.

In examining a patient with respiratory problems, the first step is to observe. Although malnutrition can never be diagnosed by simple inspection, except in extreme cases, much information can be learned by simply looking. It is during this time that various differential diagnoses can be formulated, which subsequent findings will confirm or disprove.

INSPECTION FINDINGS. One should note the effects of body mass on breathing efficiency. Cachectic (nutritionally depleted) patients will have readily outlined bony structures with depression of the intercostal spaces. Accessory muscles of respiration are often visible in these patients. Since severe muscle wasting can decrease lung function in those *without* lung disease, malnourished patients with COPD have compounded breathing difficulties. Patients who are obese will have difficulty breathing in direct proportion to their excess fat weight. Obesity imposes a restrictive condition on top of whatever lung condition already exists. Fig. 15–5 illustrates the effects of excess fat weight on the mechanics of breathing. Note the increased energy that must be expended during inspiration. Pregnancy can produce similar interference with the mechanics of breathing.

During inspection of the patient, the amount of effort that can be generated during coughing should be observed. Muscle weakness accompanies poor nutrition. Also, the viscosity of the sputum should be noted. This, along with jugular venous pressure (JVP) estimation, can give clues to fluid balance. Of course, in patients with right ventricular heart failure the JVP will be elevated by factors other than simple fluid overload. Additionally, a distended abdomen, as with ascites (fluid retention), may cause fluid balance as well as breathing problems. Edema of the extremities should also be noted; when present, it may require alterations in the patient's fluid and sodium intake.

AUSCULTATION FINDINGS. Hearing moist crackles (rales) in the lung bases on auscultation can indicate either fluid overload or a loss of blood protein (oncotic pressure). Wheezing may be associated with some food intolerances or foods that contain yellow food coloring.[145] As previously mentioned, alcohol can produce wheezing in some people. Misplaced nutrition can produce wheezing as a result of aspirated food. The fine, late inspiratory crackles of atelectasis may be from decreased surfactant production secondary to malnutrition. Hearing the S_3 heart sound of congestive failure could suggest that fluid problems may occur. An S_4 heart sound can be associated with severe anemia.

LABORATORY FINDINGS. Decreases in pulmonary function measures such as FVC or FEV_1 may indicate protein energy deficiency or severe malnutrition. Decreased FVC can also occur with excess fat weight because of fat's restrictive effects. Decreases in peak expiratory pressure (PEP) and peak inspiratory pressure (PIP) are also associated with poor nutrition. Altered lung compliance, as measured in the laboratory, or effective compliance, as measured when taking ventilator parameters, can result from fluid and serum albumin changes acutely or from chronic malnutrition.

Arterial blood gas (ABG) values can be altered with nutrition, as mentioned before. Increased Pa_{CO_2} levels can result from excess parenteral infusion of

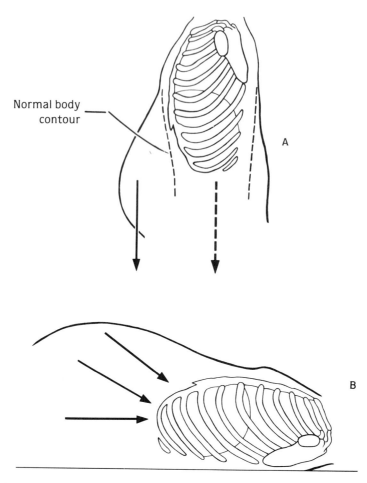

Normal body
contour

A

B

Fig. 15–5 *Effects of obesity on mechanics of breathing.* **A,** *In normal-weight persons, the weight of viscera is borne by the pelvic area, and the net weight force is in the direction of the dotted arrow. However, in obese people the net force of the weight (solid arrow) is not being supported by the pelvic area, and weight pulls directly down on the ribs. This favors the expiratory phase, making inspiration more difficult.* **B,** *In the supine position, the weight of viscera pushes up on the diaphragm, again making inspiration difficult.*

glucose or simply from insufficient muscle energy to achieve adequate ventilation. The chemoreceptor "set point" can also be altered by changes in protein (amino acid) intake, thereby altering sensitivity to $Paco_2$ levels. Oxygenation parameters (oxygen saturation, oxygen content, hemoglobin) are all affected by nutritional status. Anemias can result from deficiencies in iron, folic acid, or vitamin B_{12}. Some patients may not be able to tolerate high intakes of fat or lipid infusions because of the resulting lowered Pao_2.

Changes in pH can indicate changes in dietary intake of potassium, sodium, or foods that leave an alkaline or acidic residue. Low Pao_2 levels, with subsequent lactate production, can lower pH as well. As alluded to earlier, any change in the $Paco_2$ set point can alter acid-base balance.

The respiratory care practitioner can become directly involved in the nutritional assessment of patients by measuring $\dot{V}o_2$ in determining energy needs. In addition, the eating environment and conditions that may affect the eating process should be assessed. An effort should be made to have clean equipment in the

patient's room, to empty suction bottles, and to remove or hide sputum cups during mealtimes. A prerequisite to good nutrition is a good appetite, and a good appetite is hard to invoke unless the surroundings are pleasant. The respiratory care practitioner can further assist by helping patients receive adequate oxygen therapy during and after meals and by scheduling breathing treatments so as not to interfere with mealtimes. Patients who are using oxygen masks should have an order for oxygen via cannula while eating. Attending to the oxygenation of the patient is of great nutritional importance. A decrease in oxygen saturation while eating can occur in patients with severe COPD.[146] A patient who is short of breath may not eat, and if the patient does eat, food metabolism may be compromised.

Rarely is a respiratory problem caused by nutrition alone; however, the respiratory care practitioner will often see nutritional deficiencies complicating an existing lung problem. Being alert to the impact nutrition has on respiratory function may help stabilize the condition of a patient with lung disease that was previously deteriorating because of nutritional neglect.

REVIEW QUESTIONS

1. T F *Oxygen is required for the optimal production of ATP.*

2. T F *Oxygen uptake ($\dot{V}O_2$) is a nutritional indicator of the energy needs of the patient.*

3. Which of the following is (are) true regarding the basal energy expenditure?
   a. requires a $\dot{V}O_2$ measurement in order to calculate
   b. gives an estimation of the nutritional needs of the patient
   c. if not met, use of body energy stores is required
   d. all of the above

4. Which of the following are pulmonary effects of starvation?
   a. increased D_{LCO}
   b. increased FEV_1
   c. decreased surfactant production
   d. none of the above

5. Which of the following might hinder attempts at nutritional repletion in patients with respiratory disease?
   a. the use of bronchodilators
   b. simple oxygen therapy
   c. intubation
   d. all of the above

6. Which of the following is (are) true regarding anaerobic metabolism?
   a. can cause a metabolic acidosis
   b. results in excess lactate production
   c. reduces the amount of ATP produced
   d. all of the above

7. What is the RQ value of a patient on a pure carbohydrate diet?
   a. 0.60
   b. 0.70
   c. 0.85
   d. 1.00

8. Which of the following should the majority of dietary intake be comprised of?
   a. fat
   b. carbohydrate
   c. protein
   d. none of the above

9. What is nitrogen balance useful in determining?
   a. the adequacy of protein intake
   b. the adequacy of carbohydrate intake
   c. the need for vitamin supplementation
   d. fluid and electrolyte balance

10. Which of the following is (are) associated with a diet that is low in protein?
    a. increased work of breathing
    b. increased fixed acid load
    c. immune compromise
    d. increased stress on the kidneys

11. Which of the following is (are) associated with a high carbohydrate diet?
    a. increased $\dot{V}CO_2$
    b. increased PaO_2
    c. difficulty in weaning from mechanical ventilation
    d. all of the above

12. What mineral plays a very important role in oxygen transport?
    a. calcium
    b. iron
    c. zinc
    d. magnesium

13. T F *Total parenteral nutrition (TPN) is the first choice for nutritional supplementation.*

14. Which of the following might indicate poor nutritional status?
    a. body weight less than ideal
    b. negative nitrogen balance
    c. negative response to skin antigen testing
    d. all of the above

15. T F *Malnutrition may cause crackles to be heard upon auscultation.*

16. T F *Aiding a patient's nutritional status may be as simple as helping to relieve their dyspnea.*

REFERENCES

1. Hunker FD and others: Metabolic and nutritional evaluation of patients supported with mechanical ventilation, *Crit Care Med* 8:628, 1980.
2. Bursztein PS and others: Determination of energy metabolism from respiratory functions alone, *J Appl Physiol* 42:117, 1977.
3. Prakash O and Meij S: Use of mass spectrometry and infrared CO_2 analyzer for bedside measurement of cardiopulmonary function during anesthesia and intensive care, *Crit Care Med* 5:180, 1977.
4. Harris JA and Benedict FG: A biometric study of basal metabolism in man, Washington, DC, 1919, Carnegie Institute of Washington, publication no. 279.
5. Roza AM and Shizgal HM: The Harris Benedict equation reevaluated: resting energy requirements and the body cell mass, *Am J Clin Nutr* 40:168, 1984.
6. Neuhof H and Wolf H: Method for continuously measured oxygen consumption and cardiac output for use in critically ill patients, *Crit Care Med* 6:155, 1978.

7. Webb P and Troutman SJ, Jr.: An instrument for continuous measurement of oxygen consumption, *J Appl Physiol* 28:867, 1970.

8. Lister G, Hoffman JIE, Rudolph AM: Oxygen uptake in infants and children: a simple method for measurement, *Pediatrics* 53:656, 1974.

9. Wier JB and De V: New methods for calculating metabolic rate with special reference to protein metabolism, *J Physiol* 109:1, 1949.

10. Lusk G: *The elements of sciences of nutrition,* Philadelphia, 1928, WB Saunders.

11. Hultman E: Liver as a glucose supplying source during rest and exercise, with special reference to diet. In Parizkova J and Rogozkin VA, editors: *Nutrition, physical fitness, and health,* Baltimore, 1978, University Park Press.

12. Arora NS and Rochester DF: Effect of general nutritional and muscular states on the human diaphragm, *Am Rev Respir Dis* 115:84, 1977.

13. Aguilaniu B and others: Muscle protein degradation in severely malnourished patients with chronic obstructive pulmonary disease subject to short-term total parenteral nutrition, *JPEN J Parenter Enteral Nutr* 16:248–254, 1992.

14. Rochester DF: Respiratory muscles and ventilatory failure: 1993 perspective, *Am J Med Sci* 305:394–402, 1993.

15. Keys A and others: *Biology of human starvation,* Minneapolis, 1950, University of Minnesota Press.

16. Openbrier DR and others: Nutritional status and lung function in patients with emphysema and chronic bronchitis, *Chest* 83:17, 1983.

17. Schols AM and others: Energy balance in chronic obstructive pulmonary disease, *Am Rev Respir Dis* 143:1248–1252, 1991.

18. Schols AM and others: Prevalence and characteristics of nutritional depletion in patients with stable COPD eligible for pulmonary rehabilitation, *Am Rev Respir Dis* 147:1151–1156, 1993.

19. Hunter AMB, Carey MA, Larsh HW: The nutritional status of patients with chronic obstructive pulmonary disease, *Am Rev Respir Dis* 124:376, 1981.

20. Mitchel RS and Filley GF: Chronic obstructive bronchopulmonary disease: clinical features, *Am Rev Respir Dis* 89:360, 1964.

21. Burrows BA and others: Chronic obstructive lung disease: relationship of clinical and physiologic findings to the severity of airway obstruction, *Am Rev Respir Dis* 91:665, 1964.

22. Wilson NL, Wilson RH, Farber SM: Nutrition in pulmonary emphysema, *J Am Diet Assoc* 45:530, 1964.

23. Sahebjami H and others: Anthropometric and pulmonary function test profiles of outpatients with stable chronic obstructive pulmonary disease, *Am J Med* 94:469–474, 1993.

24. Hofford JM and others: The nutritional status in advanced emphysema associated with chronic bronchitis. A study of amino acid and catecholamine levels, *Am Rev Respir Dis* 141:902–908, 1990.

25. Otte KE and others: Nutritional repletion in malnourished patients with emphysema, *JPN J Parenter Enteral Nutr* 13:152–156, 1989.

26. Brandstetter DE and Brandstetter RD: Guidelines to good nutrition in COPD patients, *J Respir Dis* 4:25, 1983.

27. Efthimiou J and others: The effect of supplementary oral nutrition in poorly nourished patients with chronic obstructive pulmonary disease, *Am Rev Respir Dis* 137:1075–1082, 1988.

28. Rogers RM, Donahoe M, Costantino J: Physiologic effects of oral supplemental feeding in malnourished patients with chronic obstructive pulmonary disease. A randomized controlled study, *Am Rev Respir Dis* 146:1511–1517, 1992.

29. Vandenberg E, van de Woestijne KP, Gyselen A: Weight changes in the terminal stages of chronic obstructive pulmonary disease; relation to respiratory function and prognosis, *Am Rev Respir Dis* 95:556, 1967.

30. Bistrian BR and others: Cellular immunity in semi-starved states in hospitalized adults, *Am J Clin Nutr* 28:1148, 1975.

31. Law DK, Durick SJ, Abdou NI: Immunocompetence of patients with protein calorie malnutrition, *Ann Intern Med* 79:545, 1973.

32. Axton JHM and Gile HM: Lung aspirate and blood culture taken immediately after death in malnourished children, *S Afr Med J* 46:563, 1972.

33. Green GM and Kass EH: Factors influencing the clearance of bacteria by the lung, *J Clin Invest* 43:769, 1964.

34. James JW: Longitudinal study of the morbidity of diarrhea and respiratory infections in malnourished children, *Am J Clin Nutr* 25:690, 1972.

35. Ubbink JB and others: Evidence of a theophylline-induced vitamin B_6 deficiency caused by noncompetitive inhibition of pyridoxal kinase, *J Lab Clin Med* 113:15–22, 1989.

36. Ubbink JB and others: Relationship between vitamin B-6 status and elevated pyridoxal kinase levels induced by theophylline therapy in humans, *J Nutr* 120:1352–1359, 1990.

37. Vaz Fragoso CA and Miller MA: Review of the clinical efficacy of theophylline in the treatment of chronic obstructive pulmonary disease, *Am Rev Respir Dis* 147:540–547, 1993.

38. Weir MR and others: Depression of vitamin B_6 levels due to theophylline, *Ann Allergy* 65:59–62, 1990.

39. Cohen AC and Jenney FS: The frequency of peptic ulcer in patients with chronic pulmonary emphysema, *Am Rev Respir Dis* 85:130, 1962.

40. Zasly L, Baum GL, Rumball JM: The incidence of peptic ulceration in chronic obstructive pulmonary emphysema: a statistical study, *Dis Chest* 37:400, 1960.

41. West WO and others: The syndrome of chronic pulmonary disease and gastroduodenal ulceration, *Arch Intern Med* 103:897, 1959.

42. Doekel RC and others: Clinical semi-starvation: depression of hypoxic ventilatory response, *N Engl J Med* 295:358, 1976.

43. Gorini M and others: Neural respiratory drive and neuromuscular coupling in patients with chronic obstructive pulmonary disease (COPD), *Chest* 98:1179–1186, 1990.

44. Weissman C and Askanazi J: Nutrition and respiration, *Clin Consult Nutr* 2(Suppl):5, 1982.

45. Bergstrom J and Hultman E: Muscle glycogen synthesis after exercise: an enhancing factor localized to the muscle cells in man, *Nature* 210:309, 1966.

46. Gertz I and others: Muscle metabolism in patients with chronic obstructive lung disease and acute respiratory failure, *Clin Sci Mol Med* 52:396, 1977.

47. Sahebjami H and Wirman JA: Emphysema-like changes in the lungs of starved rats, *Am Rev Respir Dis* 124:619, 1981.

48. Gail DB, Massaro GD, Massaro D: Influence of fasting on the lung, *J Appl Physiol* 42:88, 1977.

49. Sahebjami H, Vassallo CL, Wirman JA: Lung mechanics and ultrastructure in prolonged starvation, *Am Rev Respir Dis* 117:77, 1978.

50. Harper HA, Rodwell VW, Mayes PA: *Review of physiological chemistry,* ed 16, Los Altos, Calif, 1977, Lange Medical Publications.

51. Normand S and others: 13C appearance in plasma glucose and breath CO_2 during feeding with naturally 13C-enriched starchy food in normal humans, *Am J Clin Nutr* 55:430–435, 1992.

52. Guezennec CY and others: Oxidation of corn starch, glucose, and fructose ingested before exercise, *Med Sci Sports Exerc* 1989. 21:45–50, 1989.

53. Hiele M and others: $13CO_2$ breath test to measure the hydrolysis of various starch formulations in healthy subjects, *Gut* 31:175–178, 1990.

54. Gieseke T, Gurushanthaiah G, Glauser FL: Effects of carbohydrates on carbon dioxide excretion in patients with airway disease, *Chest* 71:55, 1977.

55. Prusaczyk WK and others: Differential effects of dietary carbohydrate on RPE at the lactate and ventilatory thresholds, *Med Sci Sports Exerc* 24:568–575, 1992.

56. Sue CY and others: Effect of altering the proportion of dietary fat and carbohydrate on exercise gas exchange in normal subjects, *Am Rev Respir Dis* 139:1430–1434, 1989.

57. Talpers SS and others: Nutritionally associated increased carbon dioxide production. Excess total calories vs high proportion of carbohydrate calories, *Chest* 102:551–555, 1992.
58. Saltzman HA and Salzano JV: Effects of carbohydrate metabolism upon respiratory gas exchange in normal men, *J Appl Physiol* 30:228, 1971.
59. Hansen JE, Hartley H, Hogan RP: Arterial oxygen increase by high-carbohydrate diet at altitude, *J Appl Physiol* 33:441, 1972.
60. Astrand PO: Something old and something new ... very new, *Nutr Today* 1968, p 9.
61. Saltin B: Fluid, electrolyte, and energy losses and their replenishment in prolonged exercise. In Parizkova J and Rogozkin VA, editors: *Nutrition, physical fitness, and health,* Baltimore, 1978, University Park Press.
62. Askanazi J and others: Respiratory changes induced by the large glucose loads of total parenteral nutrition, *JAMA* 243:1444, 1980.
63. Askanazi J and others: Influence of total parenteral nutrition on fuel utilization in injury and sepsis, *Ann Surg* 191:40, 1980.
64. Askanazi J and others: Nutrition for the patient with respiratory failure: glucose versus fat, *Anesthesiology* 54:373, 1981.
65. Efthimiou J and others: Effect of carbohydrate rich versus fat rich loads on gas exchange and walking performance in patients with chronic obstructive lung disease, *Thorax* 47:451–456, 1992.
66. De Meo MT, Mobarhan S, Van De Graaff W: The hazards of hypercaloric nutritional support in respiratory disease, *Nutr Rev* 49:112–115, 1991.
67. *Recommended dietary allowances,* ed 9, Washington, DC, 1980, The National Research Council–National Academy of Sciences.
68. Anand CR and Linkswiler HM: Effect of protein intake on calcium balance of young men given 500 mg calcium daily, *J Nutr* 104:695, 1974.
69. Albanese AA and Orto LA: The proteins and amino acids. In Goodhart RS and Shils ME, editors: *Modern nutrition in health and disease,* ed 5, Philadelphia, 1973, Lea & Febiger.
70. Select Committee on Nutrition and Human Needs, United States Senate: *Diet and killer diseases with press reaction and additional information,* Washington, DC, 1977, US Government Printing Office.
71. Kuo PT and Joyner CR: Angina pectoris induced by fat ingestion in patients with coronary artery disease, *JAMA* 158:1008, 1955.
72. Swank RL and Nakamura H: Oxygen availability in brain tissues after lipid meals, *Am J Physiol* 198:217, 1960.
73. Talbott GD and Frayser R: Hyperlipidemia, a cause of decreased oxygen saturation, *Nature* 200:684, 1963.
74. Greene HL, Hazlett D, Demaree R: Relationship between intralipid-induced hyperlipemia and pulmonary function, *Am J Clin Nutr* 29:127, 1976.
75. Friedman M, Byers SO, Rosenman RH: Effect of unsaturated fats upon lipemia and conjunctival circulation: a study of coronary-prone (pattern A) men, *JAMA* 193:110, 1965.
76. Swank RL: Changes in blood produced by fat meal and by intravenous heparin, *Am J Physiol* 164:798, 1951.
77. Cullen CF and Swank RL: Intravascular aggregation and adhesiveness of blood elements associated with alimentary lipemia and injections of large molecular substances; effect of blood-brain barrier, *Circulation* 9:335, 1954.
78. Williams, AV, Higginbotham AC, Knisel MH: Increased blood cell agglutination following ingestion of fat, a factor contributing to cardiac ischemia, coronary insufficiency, and anginal pain, *Angiology* 8:29, 1957.
79. Cain SM: Effects of fat emulsion on O_2 transport and alveolar-arterial gas tensions, *J Appl Physiol* 17:263, 1962.
80. Jarnberg P, Lindholm M, Eklund J: Lipid infusion in critically ill patients: acute effects on hemodynamics and pulmonary gas exchange, *Crit Care Med* 9:27, 1981.
81. Stamler J: Diet-related risk factors for human atherosclerosis: hyperlipidemia, hypertension, hyperglycemia—current status. In Sirtori C, Ricci G, Gorini S, editors: *Diet and atherosclerosis,* New York, 1973, Plenum.
82. Fraser G and others: A possible protective effect of nut consumption on risk of coronary heart disease: the Adventist health study, *Arch Intern Med* 152:1416–1424, 1992.
83. Sabate J and others: Effects of walnuts on serum lipid levels and blood pressure in normal men, *N Engl J Med* 328:603–607, 1993.
84. Hartshorn EA: Food and drug interactions, *J Am Diet Assoc* 70:15, 1977.
85. Goodman DS: Vitamin A and retinoids in health and disease, *N Engl J Med* 310:1023, 1984.
86. David S and others: The risk of cancer and serum vitamins A and E and carotenoids, *N Engl J Med* 311:121, 1984.
87. Willett WC and others: Relation of serum vitamins A and E and carotenoids to the risk of cancer, *N Engl J Med* 310:430, 1984.
88. Jam J and Roberts RJ: Pharmacological alteration of oxygen-induced lung toxicity, *Toxicol Appl Pharmacol* 47:367, 1979.
89. Kann HE, Jr. and others: Oxygen toxicity and vitamin E, *Aerospace Med* 35:840, 1964.
90. Cross CE and others: Enhanced lung toxicity of O_2: in selenium-deficient rats, *Res Commun Chem Pathol Pharmacol* 16:695, 1977.
91. Richard C and others: Vitamin E deficiency and lipoperoxidation during adult respiratory distress syndrome, *Crit Care Med* 18:4–9, 1990.
92. Frank L: Antioxidants, nutrition, and bronchopulmonary dysplasia, *Clin Perinatol* 19:541–562, 1992.
93. Fiaccadori E and others: Hypercapnic-hypoxemic chronic obstructive pulmonary disease (COPD): influence of severity of COPD on nutritional status, *Am J Clin Nutr* 48:680, 1988.
94. Barr SI, Costill DL, Fink WJ: Fluid replacement during prolonged exercise: effects of water, saline, or no fluid [see comments], *Med Sci Sports Exerc* 23:811–817, 1991.
95. Brem AS: Electrolyte disorders associated with respiratory distress syndrome and bronchopulmonary dysplasia, *Clin Perinatol* 19:223–232, 1992.
96. Cavaliere F and others: Airway secretion electrolytes: reflection of water and salt states of the body, *Crit Care Med* 17:891–894, 1989.
97. Coyle EF and Montain SJ: Benefits of fluid replacement with carbohydrate during exercise, *Med Sci Sports Exerc* 24(Suppl 9):S324–S330, 1992.
98. Rubin BK and others: Respiratory mucus from asymptomatic smokers is better hydrated and more easily cleared by mucociliary action, *Am Rev Respir Dis* 145:545–547, 1992.
99. Becker AB and others: The bronchodilator effects and pharmacokinetics of caffeine in asthma, *N Engl J Med* 310:743, 1984.
100. Chan-Yeung M and others: Respiratory survey of workers in a pulp and paper mill in Powell River, British Columbia, *Am Rev Respir Dis* 2:122, 1980.
101. Lebowitz MD: Respiratory symptoms and disease related to alcohol consumption, *Am Rev Respir Dis* 123:16, 1981.
102. Beslin ABX, Hendrick DJ, Pepys J: Effect of disodium cromoglycate on asthmatic reactions to alcoholic beverages, *Clin Allergy* 3:71, 1973.
103. Geppert EF and Boushey HA: Case report: an investigation of the mechanism of ethanol-induced bronchoconstriction, *Am Rev Respir Dis* 118:135, 1978.
104. Heinemann HO: Alcohol and the lung: a brief review, *Am J Med* 63:81, 1977.
105. Dolly FR and Block JA: Increased ventricular ectopy and sleep apnea following ethanol ingestion in COPD patients, *Chest* 83:469, 1983.
106. Shapiro BA, Harrison RA, Trout CA: *Clinical application of respiratory care,* ed 2, St Louis, 1979, Mosby.
107. Johnson EE: Splanchnic hemodynamic response to passive hyperventilation, *J Appl Physiol* 38:156, 1975.
108. Johnson EE and Hedley-Whyte J: Continuous positive-pressure ventilation and portal flow in dogs with pulmonary edema, *J Appl Physiol* 33:385, 1972.
109. Johnson EE and Hedley-Whyte J: Continuous positive-pressure ventilation and choledochoduodenal flow resistance, *J Appl Physiol* 39:937, 1975.

110. Drury DR, Henry JP, Goodman J: The effects of continuous pressure breathing on kidney function, *J Clin Invest* 26:945, 1947.

111. Cristakis G: *Nutritional assessment in health programs,* Washington, DC, 1974, American Public Health Association.

112. Dudrick SJ, Jensen TG, Rowlands RJ: Nutritional support: assessment and indication. In Deital M, editor: *Nutrition in clinical surgery,* Baltimore, 1980, Williams & Wilkins.

113. Vandenberg E, van de Woestijne KP, Gyselen A: Weight changes in the terminal stages of chronic obstructive pulmonary disease: relation to respiratory function prognosis, *Am Rev Respir Dis* 95:556, 1967.

114. Mitchell CO and Lipschitz DA: The effect of age and sex on the routinely used measurements to assess the nutritional status of hospitalized patients, *Am J Clin Nutr* 36:340, 1982.

115. Harvey KB and others: Hospital morbidity-mortality risk factors using nutritional assessment (abstract), *Clin Res* 26:581, 1978.

116. Frisancho AR: Triceps skinfold and upper arm muscle size norms for evaluation of nutritional status, *Am J Clin Nutr* 27:1052, 1974.

117. Jensen TG, Durick SJ, Johnson D: A comparison of triceps skinfold and arm circumference values measured in standard and supine positions, *JPEN J Parenter Enteral Nutr* 3:513, 1979.

118. Frisancho AR: New norms of upper limb fat and muscle areas for assessment of nutritional status, *Am J Clin Nutr* 34:2540, 1981.

119. Katch FI, Michael ED, Horvath SM: Estimation of body volume by underwater weighing: description of a simple method, *J Appl Physiol* 23:811, 1967.

120. Brozek J and Henschel A, editors: *Techniques for measuring body composition,* Washington, DC, 1961, National Academy of Sciences–National Research Council.

121. Segal KR and others: Lean body mass estimation by bioelectrical impedance analysis: a four-site cross-validation study, *Am J Clin Nutr* 47:7, 1988.

122. Schols AM and others: Body composition by bioelectrical-impedance analysis compared with deuterium dilution and skinfold anthropometry in patients with chronic obstructive pulmonary disease, *Am J Clin Nutr* 53:421–424, 1991.

123. Jelliffe DB: *The assessment of nutritional status of the community,* monograph 53, Geneva, 1966, World Health Organization.

124. Standard KL, Wills VG, Waterlow JC: Indirect indicators of muscle mass in malnourished infants, *Am J Clin Nutr* 7:271, 1959.

125. Reindorp S and Whitehead RG: Changes in serum creatinine kinase and other biological measurements associated with musculature in children recovering from kwashiorkor, *Br J Nutr* 25:273, 1971.

126. Viteri FE and Alvardo J: The creatinine-height index: its use in the estimation of protein depletion and repletion in protein-calorie malnourished children, *Pediatrics* 46:696, 1970.

127. Ingenbleek Y, DeVisscher M, DeNayer P: Measurement of prealbumin as an index of protein-calorie malnutrition, *Lancet* 2:106, 1972.

128. Ingenbleek Y and others: The role of retinol-binding protein in protein-calorie malnutrition, *Metabolism* 24:633, 1975.

129. Ingenbleek Y, Van Den Schrieck HG, DeNayer P: Albumin, transferrin and thyroxin-binding prealbumin/retinol-binding protein (TBPA-RBP) complex in assessment of malnutrition, *Clin Chem Acta* 63:61, 1975.

130. Smith FR and others: Serum vitamin A, retinol-binding protein, and prealbumin concentrations in protein-calorie malnutrition. I. A functional defect in hepatic retinol release, *Am J Clin Nutr* 63:973, 1973.

131. Gofferje H: Prealbumin and retinol-binding protein highly sensitive parameters for the nutritional state in respect to protein, *Med Lab* 5:38, 1979.

132. Shetty PS and others: Rapid turnover transport proteins: an index of subclinical protein-energy malnutrition, *Lancet* 2:230, 1979.

133. Reeds PJ and Ladita AA: Serum albumin and transferrin in protein-energy malnutrition, *Br J Nutr* 36:255, 1976.

134. Young GA, Chem C, Hill GL: Assessment of protein-calorie malnutrition in surgical patients from plasma proteins and anthropometric measurements, *Am J Clin Nutr* 31:429, 1978.

135. Law DK, Dudrick SJ, Abdou NI: Immunocompetence of patients with protein-calorie malnutrition: the effects of nutritional repletion, *Ann Intern Med* 79:545, 1973.

136. Sher PP: Drug interference with laboratory tests: serum iron: iron binding capacity, *Drug Ther (Hosp)* 7:63, 1977.

137. Wallach J: *Interpretation of diagnostic tests: a handbook synopsis of laboratory medicine,* ed 3, Boston, 1970, Little, Brown.

138. Blackburn GL and others: Nutritional and metabolic assessment of the hospitalized patient, *JPEN J Parenter Enteral Nutr* 1:11, 1977.

139. Vitale J: Impact of nutrition on immune function. In *Nutrition in disease series,* Columbus, Ohio, 1979, Ross Laboratories.

140. Strauss RG: Iron deficiency infections and immune function: a reassessment, *Am J Clin Nutr* 31:660, 1978.

141. Peters JA, Burke K, White D: Nutrition in the pulmonary patient. In Hodgkin JE, Zorn E, Connors G: *Pulmonary rehabilitation: guidelines to success,* Woburn, Mass, 1984, Butterworth.

142. Schneider HA, Anderson CE, Coursin DB: *Nutritional support of medical practice,* New York, 1977, Harper & Row.

143. Bashir Y and others: Nutritional state of patients with lung cancer undergoing thoracotomy, *Thorax* 45:183–186, 1990.

144. De Meo MT and others: Nutrition in acute pulmonary disease, *Nutr Rev* 50:320–328, 1992.

145. Buswell RS and Lefkowitz MS: Oral bronchodilators containing tartrazine, *JAMA* 235:1111, 1976.

146. Brown SE, Casciari RJ, Light RW: Arterial oxygen desaturation during eating in patients with severe chronic obstructive pulmonary disease (COPD) (abstract), *Chest* 3:346, 1979.

Chapter 16

Assessment of Sleep and Breathing

Ralph Downey III and James R. Dexter

LEARNING OBJECTIVES

Upon completion of this chapter, the reader should be able to accomplish the following:

1. *Identify the percent of adult males believed to have problems related to sleep apnea.*

2. *Identify the characteristics of NREM and REM sleep.*

3. *Identify the physiologic effect of the different types and stages of sleep on the cardiovascular and respiratory systems in the healthy adult.*

4. *Recognize a definition of central, obstructive, and mixed sleep apnea.*

5. *Identify the factors believed to be responsible for the pathophysiology of obstructive sleep apnea.*

6. *Identify the clinical features of patients with obstrucive sleep apnea.*

7. *Identify the sleep characteristics that may be useful in screening the patient for obstructive sleep apnea.*

8. *Identify the parameters typically monitored during a polysomnogram.*

9. *Identify the criteria for mild, moderate, and severe sleep apnea.*

10. *Identify the age at which the peak incidence of sudden infant death occurs.*

11. *Identify the abnormalities associated with obstructive sleep apea in infants and children.*

12. *Recognize the importance of identifying sleep-related breathing disorders in patients with preexisting lung disease.*

Sleep and Patients with Lung Disease

Role of the Respiratory Care Practitioner in the Sleep Disorders Center

Chapter Overview

For most people, sleep is a time to relax and recover from the day's efforts. For those with sleep disorders, however, sleep may not provide refreshment and recovery. Additionally, when a sleep-related breathing disorder is present, sleep can precipitate life-threatening problems.

Sleep-related breathing problems occur in 5% of adult men, with this figure being somewhat lower in women.[1] In adults over 60 years of age, the incidence of sleep-related breathing abnormalities increases significantly, one report identifying a 37% incidence in this age group.[2] Breathing difficulty in sleep can lead to a variety of consequences, some of which can be deadly.

Sleep disorders centers (SDCs) exist to evaluate and diagnose sleep-related breathing problems and a host of other sleep disorders. The recognition of sleep apnea problems and their clinical importance has caused a dramatic increase in the number of SDCs. Respiratory care practitioners (RCPs) serve as technicians for the SDCs because of their expertise in respiratory problems. In this setting, the RCP may be employed as a sleep technician to evaluate patients with sleep disorders. In the hospital setting, RCPs have many opportunities to observe patients with sleep disorders. In order to understand disturbed sleep it is helpful to understand the basics of normal sleep.

Normal Sleep Stages

Everyone sleeps. Most humans sleep about 8 hours a night. Until recently, sleep was thought to be a homogeneous state of dormancy; however, sleep is a heterogeneous physiologic state of activity. The normal sleeper progresses through a relatively standard sequence of sleep during the night. Two basic types of sleep exist: nonrapid eye movement (NREM) and rapid eye movement (REM) sleep. The sleep stages of NREM and REM cycle every 60 to 90 minutes.

NREM Sleep

Healthy sleepers first enter NREM sleep. NREM sleep has four different stages: sleep stage 1, 2, 3, and 4 (Fig. 16–1). Normal sleepers enter sleep stage 1 first. This stage is characterized by large eye rolls and low-amplitude waves on the electroencephalogram (EEG). During this transitional stage between sleep and wakefulness the sleeper experiences drowsiness.

Within minutes of entering sleep stage 1, most sleepers progress to sleep stage 2. Sleep stage 2 is characterized by sleep spindles on the EEG recording (a quick burst of waveforms at 12 to 14 Hz), along with

K complexes (large 75-μV waves) (see Fig. 16–1). Sleep stage 2 is a "deeper sleep state" than sleep stage 1 and is the predominant stage of NREM sleep. Approximately 10 to 20 minutes after entering sleep stage 2, the sleeper moves into sleep stages 3 and 4, which reflect increased depth of sleep. During sleep stages 3 and 4, commonly referred to as slow wave sleep, the sleeper may be difficult to rouse. Slow wave sleep is characterized by the presence of extremely high-amplitude waves (in excess of 75 μV) (see Fig. 16–1). The amount of time the sleeper stays in slow wave sleep decreases with age and pathologic states.

Respiratory rate slows during NREM sleep.[3] The decrease in ventilation that results often causes a rise in arterial carbon dioxide pressure ($Paco_2$) in the early stages of sleep. Also during the beginning moments of sleep, respiration tends to be irregular in most persons.[3–5] However, once deeper stages of NREM sleep are reached, ventilation generally becomes rhythmic and continues to be so until the person wakens or enters REM sleep. Blood pressure decreases during NREM sleep about 5% to 10% during stages 1 and 2 and 8% to 14% in delta sleep.[6]

REM Sleep (Dreaming)

REM sleep begins in normal sleepers after 60 to 90 minutes of sleep. REM sleep is characterized by dreaming and by many profound physiologic changes, described later. Sleepers awakened from REM sleep almost always report dreaming, whereas those awakened from slow wave sleep rarely report dreamlike experiences.

The normal sleeper will experience four or five REM episodes each night. REM episodes increase progressively in length and intensity throughout the night. The initial REM episode may last only 5 minutes whereas the later episodes occurring toward morning may last 30 to 60 minutes. REM sleep accounts for about 20% to 25% of total sleep time over the human life span.

Since dreaming takes place in REM sleep, it may be regarded by the sleeper as a time of pleasure, but to the sleeper with breathing difficulties, REM sleep poses an increased hazard. During REM sleep, muscle tone, as measured by the electromyogram (EMG), is at a minimum. Thus during REM sleep the sleeper is partially paralyzed. In addition, respiratory efforts are relatively chaotic, even in healthy persons.[1,4] REM sleep, unlike slow wave sleep, is associated with a diminished response to hypercapnia and hypoxemia.[5] This effect, coupled with a decrease in upper airway muscle tone, increases vulnerability to upper airway obstruction and hypoxemia during sleep. This is particularly true when respiration is compromised by pulmonary disease or small upper airway dimensions (e.g., excessive upper airway tissue). Furthermore, the heart rate is variable during REM sleep, and cardiac dysrhythmias are more common. Blood pressure often increases slightly over its NREM level.

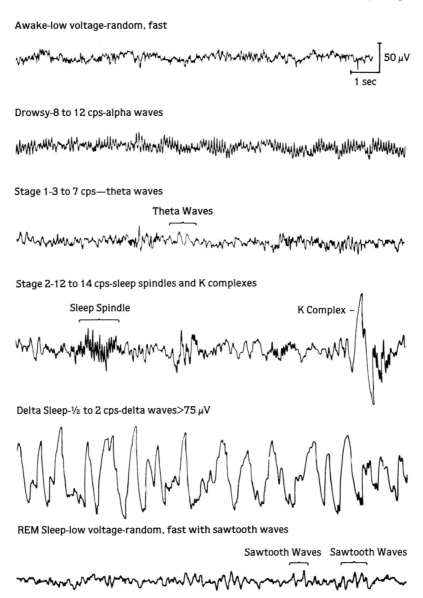

Fig. 16–1 *Human sleep stages. (From Hauri P:* The sleep disorders: current concepts, *ed 2, Kalamazoo, Mich, 1982, Upjohn.)*

Sleep Disorders

People with sleep disorders can exhibit a diverse spectrum of sleep difficulties, from sleeplessness (insomnia) to excessive daytime sleepiness. Sleep disorders may be present at birth but are much more common in adulthood and old age.

Millions of people have difficulty falling asleep or staying asleep. Chronic insomnia may be related to an underlying psychiatric condition, to associated stresses, alcohol or drug withdrawal or usage, periodic movements of the legs in sleep, or unknown causes. Insomnia may also stem from sleep-related breathing disorders such as sleep apnea.

Most sleepers recognize sleep as occurring somewhere between 4 and 10 minutes after EEG evidence of sleep appears.[7,8] Patients who are awakened near the beginning of sleep may not perceive that they were asleep. Thus, patients may complain of insomnia because of the early fragmentation of their sleep. Some patients with sleep-related breathing disorders may experience this early fragmentation of sleep and complain of sleep-onset insomnia. When a person wakens many times during the night, so that he or she receives less than 10 minutes of sleep per sleep period, that person is likely to experience a significant increase in daytime sleepiness.[9,10] This is often the case in patients with moderate to severe levels of sleep apnea.

Sleep Apnea

Sleep apnea is defined as a cessation of airflow for at least 10 seconds, which occurs during sleep. Three types of apnea have been identified: *obstructive, central,* and *mixed.* Obstructive apnea occurs when respiratory effort is present but the upper airway is so occluded that no air enters the lungs. Central apnea is characterized by the absence of respiratory effort. Mixed apnea consists of periods of both obstructive and central apnea during sleep.

Obstructive Sleep Apnea

Obstructive sleep apnea (OSA) is the most common form of sleep apnea. OSA is thought to occur because of an upper airway occlusion during sleep. This occlusion may be caused by several factors, including micrognathia (small lower jaw), large tongue, large tonsils, retrognathia (underdevelopment of the mandible), and deviated septum. While the exact mechanism remains unclear, it is clear that the site of the obstruction is in the pharynx.

PATHOPHYSIOLOGY. During sleep, the tissues in the upper airway relax to levels not seen during the waking state. As the airway becomes occluded there is a tremendous increase in upper airway resistance. In response to the occlusion, the inspiratory muscles contract more forcefully and cause an increased negative intrathoracic pressure (-70 to -80 cm H_2O) to overcome the obstruction. This is analogous to breathing through a wet soda straw. As you try to pull air through the straw, it actually closes more tightly. The upper airway obstruction may cause apnea, hypercarbia, and hypoxemia. The events eventually rouse the patient to a lighter stage of sleep or wakefulness, and muscle tone returns to the upper airway. Breathing resumes and the patient's blood gases return to baseline levels. As the patient returns to a deeper stage of sleep the process starts again. Thus, the patient with OSA may cycle between deeper and lighter stages of sleep several hundred times each night.

CLINICAL FEATURES OF OBSTRUCTIVE SLEEP APNEA. Persons with OSA suffer a number of consequences from their disorder (see box). Excessive daytime sleepiness is experienced by most persons with OSA. Such excessive sleepiness is thought to result from fragmentation of sleep as noted by EEG records.[9-13] Excessive daytime sleepiness may lead to impaired cognitive and psychomotor function. As a result, patients with OSA are more likely than others to be involved in auto accidents.[14] Drivers who fall asleep tend to be involved in more serious collisions.[15-16]

The general appearance of the patient with OSA is often positive for obesity. The patient often has a short, thick neck and may have a large tongue. Inspection of the upper airway for skeletal and soft tissue abnormalities is needed. Daytime vital signs are often normal at rest, although about 50% of patients with OSA are hypertensive during waking hours.[6] Breathing pattern and chest auscultation are normal during waking hours unless an underlying cardiopulmonary illness, such as chronic obstructive pulmonary disease (COPD), is present.

CLINICAL FEATURES OF OBSTRUCTIVE SLEEP APNEA

Snoring
Excessive daytime sleepiness
Morning headaches
Sleep fragmentation
Memory loss
Confusional awakenings
Personality changes
Impotence
Night sweats
Cardiac dysrhythmias
Pulmonary and systemic hypertension
Congestive heart failure
Enuresis

Another common clinical feature of OSA is snoring. While almost all persons with OSA snore, not all snorers have sleep apnea. It is estimated that about 25% of men and 15% of women habitually snore,[17-19] but the incidence of OSA is not this high.

Persons with OSA generally regard themselves as "good sleepers." Frequently the spouse is the one most conscious of the sleeping problem. Persons with OSA may regard themselves as good sleepers because (1) sleepers generally rate sleep as better when conscious awakenings do not occur; (2) research subjects typically underestimate the number of times they wake up during a night in the sleep laboratory; (3) as sleep becomes more fragmented, the depth of sleep increases[20]; and (4) as sleep becomes deeper, conscious awakenings are less likely to occur. Ironically, the more severe the sleep fragmentation, the less likely the person with OSA is to report being a poor sleeper.

Changes in the heart rate and cardiac dysrhythmias are frequent during episodes of OSA. Bradycardia often occurs during the apneic period and is followed by tachycardia immediately after the apnea.[21] Premature ventricular contractions occur in approximately 20% of patients with OSA and represent the most frequent dysrhythmia.[22] Asystole occurs in about 10% of cases and usually lasts for a few seconds.

These patients may also experience hypertension, periodic leg movements of the anterior tibialis muscle causing disruption of sleep, nocturnal confusion upon awakening, enuresis (bed wetting), impotence, morning headaches (possibly secondary to their hypoxia), automatic behavior (acting with little conscious recognition of what they are doing), memory loss, and personality changes.

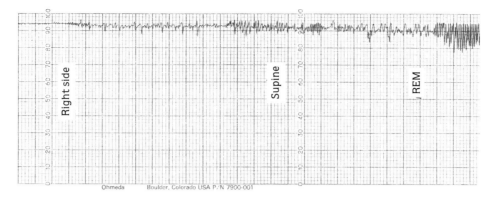

Fig. 16–2 *Continuous ear oximetry from a patient with severe sleep apnea demonstrating intermittent but significant arterial oxygen desaturation. Note that the patient's sleeping position is written periodically on the recording and that the SaO_2 drops below 80% with the patient in the supine position during REM sleep.*

Central Sleep Apnea

Central sleep apnea is seen less frequently than OSA in SDCs. Documented cases of central apnea make up less than 10% of all cases of sleep apnea.[23] This may be true because there are fewer of these patients in the general population or because fewer of these patients are studied in the sleep laboratory. Since persons with central sleep apneas appear to have fewer noticeable symptoms than those with OSA, the latter explanation seems reasonable.

PATHOPHYSIOLOGY. Central sleep apnea occurs when there is a cessation of airflow secondary to lack of movement of the diaphragm; thus, central apnea represents a loss of ventilatory drive or rhythmicity. During sleep, behavioral control of ventilation may be absent, placing ventilation under the control of the metabolic system. Ventilation is governed by afferent input from chemoreceptors and vagal intrapulmonary receptors during sleep. The development of sleep-induced apnea represents instability of these control mechanisms that serve to maintain normal blood gas homeostasis.[24] This may be because sleep serves to depress both hypoxic and hypercapnic ventilatory response.

CLINICAL FEATURES OF CENTRAL SLEEP APNEA. Many patients with central sleep apnea experience little daytime effect from their disorder; in fact, most do not recognize that a problem exists. The most common complaint of those with symptoms is insomnia.

Clinical differences are typically present between those with OSA and those with central sleep apnea. Although pure central apnea is rare, those with predominantly central sleep apnea often have a normal body habitus and only mild or no snoring compared to those with OSA. Since most persons with sleep apnea have components of both central and obstructive apnea, many of the clinical features of each type are common to most patients with sleep apnea. The reason most sleepers have a mixed component of apnea is not known.

Assessment of Sleep-Related Breathing Disorders

Observation of the hospitalized patient during sleep may provide the opportunity to evaluate the patient's gross sleeping characteristics. The evaluator should identify whether the patient snores and should pay strict attention to whether or not the patient has pauses in respiration. If pauses are present, they should be timed. As part of this observation, the sleeping position, presence or absence of cyanosis, and breathing effort should be noted. If the patient is hospitalized for several days or nights, a series of observations may coalesce into a broad evaluation of the patient's sleeping pattern. If the patient is noted to have pauses in breathing with sleep, a referral to a sleep center for the appropriate diagnosis is in order.

Finger or ear pulse oximetry is a useful tool on the ward to evaluate the patient for sleep apnea or hypoventilation. Run continuously with a paper strip recorder, pulse oximetry monitoring of arterial oxygen saturation (SaO_2) can provide a clear representation of the desaturation profile of the patient. A gradual decrease of the saturation may be evidence of nocturnal hypoventilation and is not typical of sleep apnea. A pattern in which there are sharp declines in saturation followed by sharp increases in saturation back to baseline levels is more indicative of sleep apnea (Fig. 16–2). While the exact type of sleep apnea is not detectable by oximetry, this method is very helpful for apnea screening and the identifying degree of arterial oxygen desaturation associated with the apnea. More advanced PCO_2 monitoring may be helpful or midsternum esophageal balloon monitoring to measure the actual work of breathing.

Laboratory Assessment, Techniques, and Procedures

A two-channel EEG, a two-channel electro-oculogram (EOG) to measure eye movements, and a chin EMG

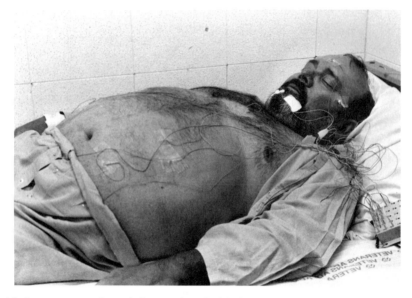

Fig. 16–3 *Patient with sleep apnea syndrome being monitored with electrodes to detect chest and abdominal movement. EEG lead placement includes C3-A2, OZ-A1, and electrodes to detect eye movements. Chin EMG detects muscle tension.*

recording are used to record sleep[25] (Fig. 16–3). All of these measurements are used to identify when the patient is asleep and what stage of sleep is occurring. Recordings are made on a polygraph machine and the recording is called a *polysomnogram* (PSG).

The typical clinical PSG also includes a one-lead ECG and a leg EMG (electrodes placed over the anterior tibialis muscles of both legs to determine if the patient experiences leg jerks during sleep). To record respirations, electrodes are placed on the upper and lower chest or abdomen to detect movement in these regions, and a dual bead thermistor is used to detect oral and nasal airflow (Fig. 16–4).

Abdominal leads are often more sensitive than chest leads in detecting the efforts of breathing. For this reason, many sleep laboratories use one chest lead and one abdominal lead. Oximetry, PCO_2, and esophageal pressure monitoring have been discussed.

How Sleep Apnea Is Quantified

The severity of sleep apnea is quantified based upon the number of apneas per hour of total sleep time. This number is commonly referred to as the *apnea index* or *respiratory disturbance index*. Normal levels of sleep apnea are said to be present when patients have fewer than 5 apneas per hour of sleep. Those who experience between 5 and 20 apneas per hour of sleep are considered to have mild levels of sleep apnea; those who experience between 20 and 40 apneas per hour of sleep are considered to have moderate levels of sleep apnea; and those who experience more than 40 apneas per hour of sleep are considered to have severe sleep apnea. These categories of apnea severity were rather arbitrarily defined. The aggressiveness of the treatment will depend upon such factors as the

degree of desaturation associated with the apneas, the presence of cardiac dysrhythmias associated with the apneas, and the presence and severity of other symptoms as determined by the patient history. Patient compliance is an important factor in determining treatment.

Treatment

Apnea is more likely to be experienced if the patient is supine during sleep rather than lying on one side. In some cases, apnea may be eliminated by sleeping on the side. This simple change in position may obviate the need for more aggressive treatment. The sleep laboratory may be instrumental in documenting the effect of changes in position on the patient's sleep. Many patients, however, have difficulty learning to sleep in a different position.

For moderate to severe cases, most sleep clinicians recommend continuous positive airway pressure (CPAP) (Fig. 16–5). CPAP effectively eliminates obstructive or central apneas in nearly all patients who tolerate it. CPAP is thought to work for patients with OSA because it acts as a "pneumatic splint" and thus increases the patency of the upper airway during inspiration.[26]

If CPAP is indicated from the initial PSG, a repeat PSG with the patient receiving CPAP is needed to determine the appropriate level. The key is to identify the minimum CPAP level effective in completely eliminating the sleep apnea and snoring. The sleep study begins by having the patient sleep without CPAP for approximately 1 hour to document the existence of the predetermined obstructive apnea. This is done to assure that the patient's condition has not changed since the original study. After about 1 hour, the CPAP trial is initiated at 5 cm H_2O, and the number of apneas is noted.

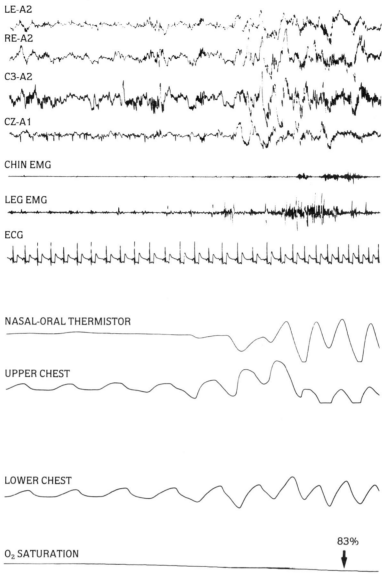

LE-A2

RE-A2

C3-A2

CZ-A1

CHIN EMG

LEG EMG

ECG

NASAL-ORAL THERMISTOR

UPPER CHEST

LOWER CHEST

83%

O_2 SATURATION

Fig. 16–4 *Sleep recording from a patient undergoing clinical polysomnography (sleep study):*
Channel 1—electro-oculogram (EOG); left eye (LE) electrode referenced to right ear electrode (A2)
Channel 2—EOG; right eye (RE) electrode referenced to (A2)
Channel 3—electroencephalogram (EEG): C3 placement referenced to A2; note that patient is in stage 2 sleep
Channel 4—EEG: CZ placement referenced to A1
Channel 5—chin EMG
Channel 6—leg EMG
Channel 7—electrocardiogram (ECG)
Channel 8—nasal-oral thermistor measures airflow through the mouth and nose
Channel 9—upper chest movement
Channel 10—lower chest movement (abdomen)
Channel 11—oxygen saturation reading from oximeter

If loud snoring or obstructive apneas are present after a 30-minute trial, the CPAP is increased 2.5 cm H_2O. This process is repeated until both apneas and snoring are eliminated (see accompanying box). The maximum level of CPAP attained by most current CPAP systems is 20 cm H_2O, but this is rarely needed (Fig. 16–6).

OXYGEN THERAPY. In some patients, apnea elimination may unmask nocturnal hypoventilation, a con-dition characterized by low oxygen saturation and elevated carbon dioxide levels, which are unrelated to apneas but may be due, for example, to COPD. In our center, oxygen therapy is initiated in these patients when oxygen saturation is below 85% for more than 30 minutes. The fraction of inspired oxygen (FIO_2) is increased in small increments until saturation is generally maintained above 90% in both REM and NREM sleep.

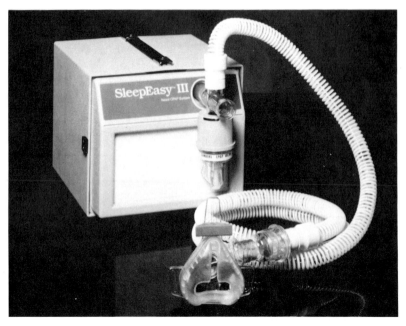

Fig. 16-5 *Continuous positive airway pressure device. (Courtesy of Respironics Inc and John Bensimon C&L Medical Inc.)*

CRITERIA USED FOR ASSURING CORRECT LEVEL OF CPAP FOR PATIENTS WITH OBSTRUCTIVE SLEEP APNEA

---

1. Elimination of obstructive apneas and hypopneas. (Central sleep apneas may be present for several hours or days following successful elimination of obstructive apneas by CPAP.)
2. Elimination of snoring.

CORRECTIVE SURGERY. When CPAP is not tolerated, patients may elect corrective surgery. A uvulopalatopharyngoplasty (UPPP) can be done to remove redundant tissue from the upper airway. The surgery leads to an alleviation of snoring in most cases but is only effective in eliminating the sleep apnea in less than one half of the cases.[27] There is no single test that can predict with a high degree of certainty that UPPP will be successful in any one patient with OSA.[28]

Several weeks after UPPP, it is recommended that the patient have a repeat sleep study to determine if the apnea was eliminated by the procedure. If the UPPP patient has a tracheostomy tube in place after surgery, a sleep study is conducted with the tube open initially and then with the tube closed. If, while the tube is closed, the patient no longer experiences sleep apnea or experiences only mild levels of sleep apnea, removing the tube and closure of the stoma is reasonable. If the patient still has significant levels of sleep apnea and desires that the tube be removed and

the tracheostomy closed, a trial of nasal CPAP is recommended.

It is important to note that moderate to severe levels of OSA probably should be treated. A recent 7-year study found that patients with an apnea index greater than 20 that did not receive either CPAP or a tracheostomy had a higher incidence of mortality than patients that received CPAP or tracheostomy.[29] More studies are needed in this area to determine if the apnea level is related to mortality and whether reversal of sleep apnea results in increased longevity.

Sleep-Disordered Breathing In Children

Breathing problems during sleep are not limited to adults. They can occur in infants and children of all ages. In many cases, sleep disorders in children are more problematic because they affect children more quickly and may result in dramatic changes in their daily functioning. Academic and social function performance can suffer significantly when sleep disorders are occurring.

Sudden Infant Death Syndrome

Most people associate breathing problems in infants with sudden infant death syndrome (SIDS); however, SIDS is only one of many potential sleep-related breathing disorders in children. SIDS, by definition, has no known cause. It is a leading cause of death in children under the age of 1 year. SIDS has a peak incidence between 2 and 4 months of age and the majority of cases occur in the first 6 months of life.[30]

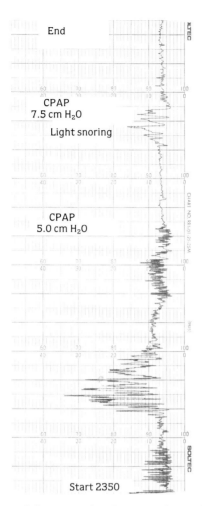

End

CPAP
7.5 cm H₂O

Light snoring

CPAP
5.0 cm H₂O

Start 2350

Fig. 16–6 *Oximetry tracing from a patient using continuous positive airway pressure (CPAP). Note the severe desaturation that occurs prior to initiation of 5 cm H₂O of CPAP.*

Obstructive Sleep Apnea in Infants and Children

Any child with a narrowed upper airway or abnormal airway reflexes is prone to airway occlusion during sleep. Certain groups, however, are more prone to have upper airway occlusion during sleep. This is generally seen in patients with craniofacial abnormalities such as Pierre Robin syndrome, Treacher-Collins syndrome, cleft palate, or when the mid-face is not fully developed as in mid-face hypoplasia. Frequently, children with enlarged tonsils and adenoids are victims of OSA.

In general, children with OSA suffer similar symptoms as adults. Rather than snoring, some children exhibit the inspiratory stridor type of sounds during sleep. Retractions may also be seen during sleep. Cardiopulmonary abnormalities during the daytime are rare in children with OSA. OSA may be a SIDS risk factor.

Upper Airway Resistance in Infancy and Childhood

Upper airway resistance syndrome (UARS) was first witnessed by Guilleminault and colleagues in 1982.[31] The discovery came when children developed symptoms (e.g., excessive daytime sleepiness) similar to OSA patients and were studied in the sleep laboratory. The classic PSG findings associated with OSA were not seen, although sleep fragmentation was noted. An esophageal balloon was placed in the children to measure intrathoracic pressure changes during sleep. The children demonstrated similar large swings in pleural pressure with breathing during sleep, as do OSA patients. This finding suggests that the UARS children have significant increased work of breathing during sleep. The excessive work of breathing may cause the sleep fragmentation in these children. These patients respond to treatment like their OSA counterparts.

Sleep and Patients with Lung Disease

Up to two thirds of asthma patients have increased bronchospasms at night.[32] Nocturnal bronchospasm may not be related to sleep itself and does not appear to be related to particular sleep stages.[33] Potential causes of nocturnal bronchospasm include aspiration of gastric contents, which are allowed into the esophagus by a relaxed esophageal sphincter during sleep, and, in older patients, accumulation of fluid in the lungs during prolonged recumbency (cardiac asthma). Some patients are allergic to down pillows and wheeze during sleep. Sleep disruption will continue until the offending pillow is removed.

Although asthma is not a sleep disorder per se, patients with asthma often complain about their sleep. The nocturnal breathlessness of asthmatic persons is most likely to be related to circadian changes in cortisol and catecholamine levels (which are at their lowest at night).[34] As a result, the sleep of asthmatic persons is often fragmented. Unfortunately, while some bronchodilators (theophylline-based) help with asthma, they can also contribute to fragmented sleep.

In patients with chronic lung diseases such as COPD, pulmonary fibrosis, or cystic fibrosis, nocturnal changes in breathing can be particularly troublesome. The normal oxygen desaturation associated with sleep (drop in arterial oxygen tension [Pao₂] of 10–20 mm Hg) can result in significant nocturnal hypoxemia in these patients since they are already hypoxemic in many cases. Hypoventilation is a major cause of hypoxemia during REM sleep in patients with COPD.[35] In a minority of patients, the problem of nocturnal hypoxemia can be further complicated by the existence of sleep apnea. Because these patients may be hypoxemic before the apneas, they may be more prone to the hypoxic complications of the sleep apnea syndrome.[36]

Role of the Respiratory Care Practitioner in the Sleep Disorders Center

The RCP may work in a SDC as a PSG technician. In this position, the RCP is responsible for patient hook-ups and close monitoring of the patient during the night. This may include making accurate notes of the patient's sleep position, the level of snoring (if any), and other factors such as movements of the body in sleep, all of which help determine the correct diagnosis and treatment plan.

The RCP is also likely to attend weekly meetings with the medical staff to discuss the history of the patient and the completed sleep study. In this regard, the RCP is often the only person on the staff who has monitored the patient sleeping and is thus a valuable source of information.

As a sleep technician the RCP may also score sleep recordings using standard scoring techniques.[36] The scoring of sleep recordings is a skill that may require many months of training. This input is crucial to the sleep laboratory, as the diagnosis depends upon accurate recording and interpretation of sleep stages and other measurements. The RCP is the backbone of a successful sleep center.

Case Study 1

D.B. is a 40-year-old man who presents to his attending physician in the outpatient clinic with complaints of severe fatigue and daytime sleepiness. D.B. is accompanied by his wife who states that her husband snores loudly throughout the night with occasional pauses in breathing followed by gasping for air. D.B.'s wife indicates that D.B. is a restless sleeper. D.B. smokes two packs of cigarettes per day and has been smoking for the past 22 years.

Physical examination: *D.B. is 68 in. in height and weighs 240 lb. He appears lethargic but is oriented to time, place, and person. His vital signs at rest are blood pressure, 140/85 mmHg; respiratory rate, 26 breaths per minute; and heart rate, 110 beats per minute. D.B. has a short, thick neck with enlarged tonsils and a hypopharynx that is narrowed by excessive fatty tissue. D.B. is a mouth breather with nasal-sounding speech. His breath sounds are diminished bilaterally. A loud P_2 was noted during auscultation over the precordium.*

Laboratory data: *A routine ECG revealed right axis deviation and was consistent with cor pulmonale. The complete blood count was normal except for polycythemia. A chest film revealed mild cardiomegaly. The patient was*

referred to the sleep center for a PSG. The PSG study revealed:

Apnea index	50
Central apnea index	0
Minimum SaO$_2$	75%
No. of desaturation events	137
Arousals per hour of sleep	50
Stage 1 sleep	50% (normal = 1%–5%)
Stage 2 sleep	25% (normal = 45%–55%)
Stage 3 and 4 sleep	0% (normal = 0%–5%)
REM sleep	20% (normal = 15%–25%)
Technician comments	Loud snoring in all sleep positions; restlessness observed throughout the night

Impression: *Severe OSA is present since the apnea index is greater than 40. Frequent arousals occur, which probably explains D.B.'s excessive daytime sleepiness. The frequent episodes of desaturation may be contributing to the cor pulmonale since the hypoxemia triggers significant increases in pulmonary vascular resistance. The distribution of sleep is abnormal and consistent with frequent nocturnal arousals. The patient is experiencing no delta sleep (stages 3 and 4), less than normal amounts of stage 2 sleep, and an increased amount of stage 1 sleep. Fig. 16–7 provides a sample of the PSG demonstrating the obstructive apnea in this case.*

Recommendations:
1. *Ear, nose, and throat consultation for evaluation of the upper airway problems.*
2. *Consider medical management, which may include CPAP trial.*
3. *Orthodontic appliance evaluation.*
4. *Dietary consultation and endocrinology evaluation for obesity.*
5. *Follow-up sleep study to evaluate effects of treatment.*

REVIEW QUESTIONS

1. *What percent of adult males are thought to have a sleep-related breathing disorder?*
   a. *1%*
   b. *5%*
   c. *7.5%*
   d. *10%*

2. *What is the predominant stage of NREM sleep?*
   a. *stage 1*
   b. *stage 2*
   c. *stage 3*
   d. *stage 4*

3. T F *Breathing tends to be irregular during the early stages of NREM sleep.*

4. T F *Blood pressure tends to increase during the initial stages of sleep.*

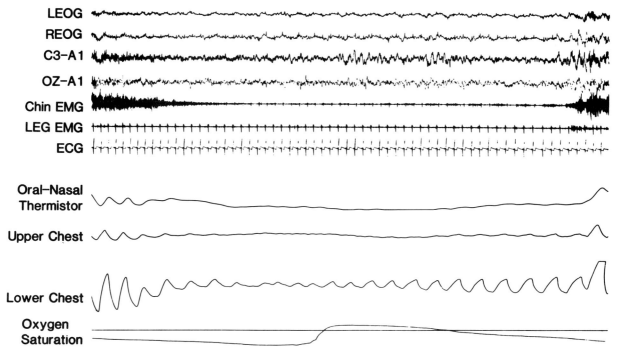

LEOG
REOG
C3–A1
OZ–A1
Chin EMG
LEG EMG
ECG

Oral–Nasal Thermistor

Upper Chest

Lower Chest

Oxygen Saturation

Fig. 16-7 *Polysomnogram demonstrating obstructive sleep apnea. Note the lack of flow noted by the oral-nasal thermistor lead with simultaneous effort of breathing as noted by the lower chest movements. The oxygen saturation is reduced at the beginning of the tracing from a previous period of apnea. The oxygen saturation tracing lags behind the changes in the patient's breathing pattern.*

5. T F *During REM sleep the sleeper is partially paralyzed.*

6. T F *Breathing is very regular during REM sleep in most sleepers.*

7. *Which of the following is the key concept related to the definition of central sleep apnea?*
    a. *intermittent absence of respiratory effort*
    b. *intermittent upper airway obstruction*
    c. *intermittent central airway obstruction*
    d. *intermittent reductions in tidal volume*

8. *Which of the following is not believed to be responsible for the onset of obstructive sleep apnea?*
    a. *relaxation of the upper airway muscles*
    b. *tremendous increase in upper airway resistance*
    c. *more forceful contraction of the inspiratory muscles*
    d. *significant decrease in static lung compliance*

9. *Which of the following clinical features is not typical for adult patients with obstructive sleep apnea?*
    a. *excessive daytime sleepiness*
    b. *inspiratory stridor during daytime examination*
    c. *loud snoring during sleep*
    d. *impaired cognitive function*

10. *Which of the following sleep characteristics is most helpful in screening the patient for obstructive sleep apnea?*
    a. *total sleep time per night*
    b. *length of time it takes to fall asleep*
    c. *snoring during sleep*
    d. *sleep position*

11. *Which of the following parameters is not typically monitored during a polysomnogram?*
    a. *EEG*
    b. *ECG*
    c. *leg EMG*
    d. *minute volume*

12. *What is the criteria for severe sleep apnea?*
    a. *more than 20 apneas per hour of sleep*
    b. *more than 30 apneas per hour of sleep*
    c. *more than 40 apneas per hour of sleep*
    d. *more than 50 apneas per hour of sleep*

13. *What is the peak age of onset for sudden infant death syndrome?*
    a. *birth to 2 months*
    b. *2 to 4 months*
    c. *3 to 8 months*
    d. *6 to 10 months*

14. *Which of the following is most likely to cause obstructive sleep apnea in children?*
    a. *enlarged tonsils and adenoids*
    b. *diffuse bronchospasm*

c. *upper airway infection*

d. *encephalitis*

15. *Why are sleep-related breathing disorders particularly of concern in patients with preexisting lung disease?*

   a. *because they are very sensitive to hypercarbia*

   b. *because they often have daytime hypoxemia*

   c. *because they already have sleep problems*

   d. *all of the above*

REFERENCES

1. White DP: Disorders of breathing during sleep: introduction, epidemiology and incidence, *Semin Respir Med* 9:529, 1988.
2. Carskadon M and Dement W: Respiration during sleep in the aged human, *J Gerontol* 36:420, 1981.
3. Douglas NJ, White DP, Weil JV: Respiration during sleep in normal man, *Thorax* 37:840, 1982.
4. Kreiger J: Breathing during sleep in normal subjects, *Clin Chest Med* 6:577, 1985.
5. Naifeh KH and Kamiya J: The nature of respiratory changes associated with sleep onset, *Sleep* 4:49, 1981.
6. Shepard JW and Bradley TD: Hypertension, cardiac arrhythmias, myocardial infarction, and stroke in relation to obstructive sleep apnea, *Clin Chest Med* 13:437, 1992.
7. Bonnet MH and Moore SE: The threshold of sleep: perception of sleep as a function of time asleep and auditory threshold, *Sleep* 5:267, 1982.
8. Rechtshaffen A: Polygraphic aspects of insomnia. In Gastaut and others, editors: *The abnormalities of sleep in man,* Bologna, 1968, Gaggi.
9. Bonnet MH: Effect of sleep disruption on sleep, performance, and mood, *Sleep* 8:11, 1985.
10. Bonnet MH: Performance and sleepiness as a function of frequency and placement of sleep disruption, *Psychophysiology* 23:263, 1986.
11. Bonnet MH: Performance and sleepiness following moderate sleep disruption and slow wave sleep deprivation, *Physiol Behav* 37:915, 1986.
12. Downey R and Bonnet MH: Performance during frequent sleep disruption, *Sleep* 10:354, 1987.
13. Colt HG, Helmut H, Rich GB: Hypoxemia vs sleep fragmentation as cause of excessive daytime sleepiness in obstructive sleep apnea, *Chest* 100:1542–1548, 1991.
14. Findley LJ, Unverzagt ME, Suratt PM: Automobile accidents involving patients with obstructive sleep apnea, *Am Rev Respir Dis* 138:337, 1988.
15. Findley LJ, Weiss J, Jabour E: Serious automobile crashes caused by undetected sleep apnea, *Arch Intern Med* 151:1451–1452, 1991.
16. Findley LJ, Levinson MP, Bonnie RJ: Driving performance and auto accidents in patients with sleep apnea, *Clin Chest Med* 13:427, 1992.
17. Lugaresi E and others: Some epidemiological data on snoring and cardiocirculatory disturbances, *Sleep* 3:221, 1980.
18. Lugaresi E, Coccagna G, Cirinotta F: Snoring and its clinical implications. In Guilleminault C and Dement WC, editors: *Sleep apnea syndromes,* New York, 1978, Alan R Liss.
19. Lugaresi E, Coccagna G, Mantovani M: Hypersomnia with periodic apneas. In Weitzman ED, editor: *Advances in sleep research,* vol 4, New York, 1978, Spectrum.
20. Schneider LM and others: Awakening thresholds as a function of schedule of sleep disruption, *Sleep Res* 16:210, 1987.
21. Zwillich CW and others: Bradycardia during sleep apnea: its characteristics and mechanisms, *Am Rev Respir Dis* 125:234, 1982.
22. Romaker AM and Ancoli-Israel S: The diagnosis of sleep-related breathing disorders, *Clin Chest Med* 8: 1987.
23. Guilleminault C, van den Hoed J, Mitler M: Clinical overview of the sleep apnea syndromes. In Guilleminault C and Dement W, editors: *Sleep apnea syndromes,* New York, 1978, Alan R Liss.
24. Onal E: Central sleep apnea, *Semin Respir Med* 9:547, 1988.
25. Rechtschaffen A and Kales A, editors: A manual of standardized terminology: techniques and scoring system for sleep stages of human subjects, Los Angeles, 1968, UCLA Brain Information Service/Brain Research Institute.
26. Sullivan CE and Grunstein RR: Continuous positive airways pressure in sleep-disordered breathing. In Kryger MH, Roth T, Dement W, editors: *Principles and practice of medicine,* Philadelphia, 1989, WB Saunders.
27. Silvestri R, Guilleminault C, Simmons FB: Palatopharyngoplasty in the treatment of obstructive sleep apnea. In Guilleminault C and Lugaresi E, editors: *Long term evaluation and natural history of sleep disorders,* New York, 1983, Raven Press.
28. Kryger MH: Management of obstructive sleep apnea, *Clin Chest Med* 13:481, 1992.
29. He J and others: Mortality and apnea index in obstructive sleep apnea: experience in 385 male patients, *Chest* 94:9, 1988.
30. Brooks JG: Sudden infant death syndrome and apparent life-threatening events. In Levin DL and Morriss FC, editors: *Essentials of pediatric intensive care,* St Louis, 1990, Quality Medical.
31. Guilleminault C et al: Children and nocturnal snoring—evaluation of the effects of sleep related respiratory resistive load and daytime functioning, *Eur J Pediatr* 139:165–171, 1982.
32. Connolly CK: Diurnal rhythms in airway obstruction, *Br J Dis Chest* 73:357, 1979.
33. Kales A and others: Sleep studies in asthmatic adults: relationship of attacks to sleep stage and time of night, *J Allergy* 41:164, 1968.
34. Douglas NJ: Asthma. In Kryger MH, Roth T, Dement W: *Principles and practice of sleep medicine,* Philadelphia, 1989, WB Saunders.
35. Douglas NJ: Nocturnal hypoxemia in patients with COPD, *Clin Chest Med* 13:437, 1992.
36. Douglas NJ: Breathing during sleep in patients with respiratory disease, *Semin Respir Med* 9:586, 1988.

BIBLIOGRAPHY

Barnes C and Orem J, editors: *Physiology in sleep,* New York, 1980, Academic Press.

Fletcher E, editor: *Abnormalities of respiration during sleep,* Orlando, Fla, 1986, Grune & Stratton.

Guilleminault C, editor: *Sleeping and waking: indications and techniques,* Menlo Park, Calif, 1982, Addison-Wesley Publishing.

Guilleminault C and Ariagno R: Apnea during sleep in infants and children. In Kryger MH, Roth T, Dement W: *Principles and practice of sleep medicine,* Philadelphia, 1989, WB Saunders.

Hauri P: *Current concepts: the sleep disorders,* ed 2, Kalamazoo, Mich, 1982, Upjohn.

Kryger MH, Roth T, Dement WC, editors: *Principles and practice of sleep medicine,* Philadelphia, 1989, WB Saunders.

Lydic R and Biebuyck JF, editors: *Clinical physiology of sleep,* New York, 1988, Oxford University Press.

Phillipson EA and Bradley TD, editors: Breathing disorders in sleep, *Clin Chest Med* 13(2):1992.

Tyner F, Knott JR, Mayer WB: *Fundamentals of EEG technology,* vol 1, *Basic concepts and methods,* New York, 1983, Raven Press.

Chapter 17

Assessment of the Home Care Patient

Susan L. McInturff and Patrick J. Dunne

LEARNING OBJECTIVES

Upon completion of this chapter, the reader should be able to accomplish the following:

1. *Identify the importance and benefits of respiratory home care.*

2. *Identify the type of patients that receive home respiratory care.*

3. *Recognize the key elements involved in home respiratory care assessment.*

4. *Recognize the role of the respiratory care practitioner in home care.*

5. *Recognize how accreditation by the JCAHO has affected respiratory home care.*

6. *Identify the components involved in the initial home care evaluation.*

7. *Recognize the purpose and the procedure for performing a plan of care for a patient.*

8. *Recognize the purpose of performing follow-up care.*

Chapter Overview

Although home care has been performed for many years, it is only now receiving recognition as a specialty area of clinical practice. Respiratory care practitioners (RCPs) who were interested in the field of home care were often considered either "burnt out" or unable to practice in the highly technical acute care facilities. Furthermore, the home care industry was conspicuous for its lack of standards of practice.

These perceptions are changing, however. The specialty practice of home care is emerging as an essential component of the short-term and long-term treatment of the patient with pulmonary impairment. It is also a highly technical field filled with highly skilled practitioners who frequently have left the critical care arena in search of a new challenge.

The Importance of Home Care

Soaring costs for acute medical care and changes in third-party reimbursement have modified the focus of care toward reducing the length of a patient's hospital stay.[1,2] At the same time, expanding technology has provided the health care industry with the ability to manage patients at home whose medical conditions may previously have kept them in the hospital. Procedures such as intravenous (IV) therapy, tracheostomy tube changes, and ventilator care, once performed only in an intensive care unit (ICU), are now common in the home. The availability of such services coupled with the personnel to perform them enables physicians to discharge their patients earlier. Patients now go home who otherwise might have had to spend the remainder of their life in an acute or long-term care facility.[3]

The major benefits of home care are obvious: it can decrease total hospital days; it can decrease the total of medical dollars spent; it can allow patients to go home who otherwise would not be able to do so; and it can help reduce the number and length of future hospitalizations.[4,5]

Types of Patients Receiving Home Care

A wide array of patients can benefit from home care services. Patients who have suffered an acute exacerbation of their chronic obstructive pulmonary disease (COPD) may need home care services designed to instruct and evaluate them on the use of home oxygen equipment, compressor nebulizer therapy, or a new medication schedule. Assessments would be done on this patient to determine need, response to therapy, compliance, and to identify emergent problems that could lead to a rebound hospitalization.

Conversely, a patient requiring mechanical ventilation for life support would require home care services for as long as he or she remains at home. The highly technical nature of home ventilators and the necessary ancillary equipment requires frequent evaluation and maintenance to ensure proper and continued function. These patients will also require frequent physical assessments, again to determine response to therapy, compliance, and to identify emergent problems. The patient's caregivers will also be assessed to ensure that they too are managing the equipment and home care

procedures properly and that they continue to remain satisfactory caregivers.

In the middle of the spectrum are patients who may require home care for days, weeks, or even months for such conditions as the treatment of infections, management of a tracheostomy, or perhaps stabilization on a program of noninvasive ventilation. Patients whose needs or diagnoses have changed, or who have had a change in resources such as environment, caregivers, or reimbursement, may need to reactivate home care services that were previously terminated.

Hospital vs. Home Care Assessment

Assessment of the patient at home utilizes many of the same methods used in the acute care setting. The techniques of physical examination described in this book are performed in the same manner. The primary differences in home care assessment are the parameters assessed and the types of diagnostic tools used. Table 17–1 outlines the key aspects of home care assessment, including the patient, and his or her environment and resources.

The primary tools used to conduct home care assessments are very basic and may be considered rudimentary by the critical care practitioner. Stethoscopes, sphygmomanometers, and oximeters are the most common devices used. Peak flowmeters and respirometers may be used for basic spirometry. End-tidal carbon dioxide monitors and portable diagnostic sleep recorders are used with increasing frequency but are less commonly available.

Arterial blood sampling and analysis can be performed in the home, frequently by mobile blood gas laboratories. Sputum and blood samples are often collected, and even electrocardiograms (ECGs) can be obtained in the home. Results of these tests are given to the physician who orders treatment, if indicated, thus helping the patient avoid hospitalization in many instances.

Respiratory therapy is certainly not the only discipline that is involved in the assessment and treatment of the pulmonary patient at home. Frequently, the home care setting requires a team of professionals comprised of nurses, speech therapists, and physical and occupational therapists, nutritionists, and social workers, along with the RCP. As a team they gather vital information about the patient that will be useful in developing or revising the patient's comprehensive plan of care.

Qualifications and the Role of the Home Care Therapist

The role of the RCP in home care is to select, set up, and train the patient in the use of respiratory equipment and to monitor and assess patients for continued

Table 17–1	Key Aspects of Home Care Assessment
Patient	**Environment**
History	Electricity
Symptom profile	Heating, cooling
Nutritional status	Space
Functional limitations	Stairways
Psychosocial evaluation	Cleaning, storage space
Medications	Emergency access
Physical examination	Telephone
Caregiver	

Table 17–2 Respiratory Equipment That Commonly Receives RCP Home Follow-up*

Ventilators	Percussors
Oxygen therapy equipment	Portable diagnostic devices
Compressor nebulizers	Suction machines
IPPB	Oximeters
Large-volume nebulizer therapy	Apnea monitors
CPAP/bilevel pressure devices	Tracheostomy tubes

*IPPB-intermittent positive pressure breathing; CPAP continuous positive airway pressure.

safe use of that equipment.[6] RCPs who choose home care must be highly competent and extremely versatile. Their job requires well-honed skills including the abilities to: (1) teach a patient to use a complex piece of equipment with confidence; (2) evaluate a patient using the most basic tools in an uncontrolled environment; and (3) make good decisions regarding the patient's plan of treatment. It is very common for home care RCPs to have a background in acute care because home medical equipment (HME) providers frequently hire practitioners who have had several years of hospital patient care experience.

The RCP may be the only skilled professional the home care provider employs. Therefore, home care RCPs must also be extremely versatile. They may be called upon to set up and troubleshoot many types of equipment that they have never worked with in the hospital. For example, it is not uncommon for the RCP to have to set up, instruct, and maintain a patient on enteral feeding or IV pump equipment.

The field of home care presents a continual challenge to the RCP owing to the extremely dynamic state of technology and third-party reimbursement. New devices are frequently invented and current equipment modified to treat medical problems never treated before at home. Furthermore, changes in reimbursement, particularly Medicare, occur so rapidly that it is difficult to remain current with the regulations. Yet the RCP is expected to keep abreast of the changes and to know what items and services are covered by third-party payers.

JCAHO and the Home Care Industry

Within the last few years accreditation by the Joint Commission on Accreditation of Healthcare Organizations (JCAHO) has been available to the HME industry. In the past, many home care providers did not employ licensed RCPs to instruct patients on respiratory and related equipment, but would instead use laypersons to perform these technical services. Patients were not being assessed, and there was no plan of treatment or goals. There were no standards in effect, and as a result quality of care suffered.

The advent of JCAHO accreditation for home care providers required that certain standards of care be practiced. This accreditation has validated the role of the RCP in home care.[7] Therapists are now able to use their assessment and decision-making skills during a home visit and patients are no longer using equipment for prolonged periods of time that is either unsuitable or unnecessary. The RCP employed by a company that is accredited for clinical respiratory services is actively involved in evaluating the patient and developing an ongoing plan of care in order to meet the goals of therapy the physician has prescribed.

Patient Assessment

One of the most important aspects of home care is patient assessment. The results of the assessment will affect all other aspects of the patient's care, such as the type of equipment required, instruction of the patient and caregivers, whether ancillary services such as nursing are necessary, and the type of monitoring and follow-up the patient will need. The RCP is generally notified about a new patient when certain types of HME need to be placed in the patient's home. Table 17–2 outlines the types of prescribed medical equipment for which a patient may need instruction, assessment, and follow-up by the home care RCP. Assessment of the patient, his or her physical environment, and the caregivers is done as part of the initial evaluation.

Initial Evaluation

During the first home visit, the RCP will interview the patient and caregivers and examine the patient. The patient interview is conducted to establish a "symptom profile," pulmonary risk factors, and any previous medical history.[5,8–10] Identification of the patient's pulmonary and nonpulmonary symptoms, as well as the ability to self-manage his or her symptoms, is extremely important. Assessment of the patients' and caregivers' cognitive abilities and of their functional limitations is essential to determine whether they will understand instruction and be able to manage the medical equipment and therapy regimen that have been prescribed.

Psychosocial factors are also evaluated at the initial interview. Family dynamics can play a distinct role in the success or failure of a patient being cared for at home. It will be important to ascertain during the initial interview which family members are going to be participating in the patient's care. Home care patients may be depressed over their state of health and may feel that they are a burden to their family. They may also have difficulty coping with being dependent on others (role reversal), which often takes place in a family when illness occurs. Other patients may be hostile, may deny that they are ill, or have no intention of following their physician's orders. Cultural, ethnic, and religious beliefs may also affect the home care program.

Nutritional status is also evaluated. Patients may need instruction on energy conservation techniques in order to prepare food as well as eat it; it is common for patients to decline food rather than suffer the dyspnea associated with preparation and consumption. Patients using continuous oxygen will frequently remove their oxygen during a meal and need to be instructed against this. Choreworkers or aides may need to be hired to assist the patient with meal preparation. Patients who have difficulty swallowing may need to have a feeding tube placed in order to receive adequate nutrition. Careful questioning and observation can identify areas of need.

An evaluation of the patient's medication use is also done. Identification of all prescription and nonprescription medications is vital, particularly when the patient with pulmonary disease is on a complicated medication regimen. The RCP questions the patient to determine his or her level of understanding about how to take the medications and to determine compliance with the regimen prescribed.

Another important issue discussed during the initial interview is the patient's desire for advanced directives about emergency medical care. The patient may or may not have considered whether he or she wants to receive cardiopulmonary resuscitation (CPR) or other advanced life-support measures. For some patients, even antibiotic therapy may be considered life support. It is important to determine and document what the patient wishes in order to avoid emergency medical treatments they do not want.

During the initial home visit and evaluation, a physical assessment is usually performed. Age, height, weight, and general appearance should be recorded. Vital signs, including blood pressure, pulse rate, and respiratory rate and their quality, should be taken. Auscultation, palpation of the chest, and observation for cyanosis, clubbing, and peripheral edema are also indicated. Chapters 3 and 4 of this book review the techniques of physical examination that may be used.

Some aspects of the physical evaluation may need to be altered to protect the privacy of the patient. The home care RCP may be the only person in the home with the patient when the evaluation is being done.

Therefore, it may be considered improper to ask patients to disrobe in order to auscultate their lungs, particularly in the case of the male RCP evaluating the female patient. In such a case, auscultation is usually done over a shirt or nightclothes. Keep in mind that extraneous sounds may occur when the patient's clothing rubs against the chest piece of the stethoscope. There are also patients who might not wish to have their feet and legs examined for edema by a therapist of the opposite sex. Requesting the patient's permission prior to performing assessment procedures is always helpful in making the encounter comfortable for both the patient and the examiner.

Part of the physical examination may include some form of diagnostic testing. Pulse oximetry and measurement of spontaneous tidal volume and forced vital capacity are commonly done during the initial evaluation.[10]

HME providers that are JCAHO-accredited for clinical respiratory services can perform an initial physical assessment without a physician's request; however, the RCP can only perform ongoing physical assessments under a physician's written order for such. Physician orders should likewise be obtained whenever pulse oximetry is performed.[11]

Environmental Assessment

The environmental assessment is done to determine if problems exist within the home environment that would prove to be a detriment to the patient's care. Evaluation of the home, the caregivers, and the patient's equipment needs are performed during this assessment.

The Home

The home is inspected to identify any health, fire, and safety hazards that may exist.[12] Electrical outlets are inspected for proper grounding and to determine if enough amperage exists to service the patient's medical equipment in addition to the appliances that are already on the electrical circuit. Patients requiring multiple pieces of medical equipment may need to have modifications in or additions to their home's wiring. Patients who do not have grounded electrical outlets will need to be advised of the potential for electric shock if the outlets are left ungrounded.

The home is also inspected for adequate storage space for the equipment and supplies that may be needed, particularly when hospital beds and patient lifts are ordered. Equipment powered by compressors, such as oxygen concentrators, nebulizers, and ventilators, must have enough free space around them to allow for adequate airflow and cooling. Hallways and door openings must be wide enough for the patient to pass through with ambulatory aids such as walkers or wheelchairs. Floors must be free of anything that could present a hazard to the patient who has a gait problem.

Patients with pulmonary impairment may not tolerate wide fluctuations in ambient temperature. The home may be inspected for heating and cooling needs. Emergency exit routes need to be identified, and a plan for the quick removal of the patient from the home should be familiar to all caregivers, particularly in the case of the bedbound patient whose only access to the outside may be by stairs.

The home should also have adequate facilities for cleaning equipment. Many types of medical equipment have parts that must be cleaned and disinfected on a periodic basis. This should be done in an area that can be kept clean, preferably not a bathroom.

The Caregivers

The patient and his or her caregivers are evaluated to determine their ability and willingness to care for the equipment and perform the procedures required. A patient's spouse who has severe arthritis may not be able to disassemble tubings and other parts for cleaning, or to turn an oxygen tank on and off. The caregiver with a language barrier may not receive instruction well and may require an interpreter as well as materials written in a language he or she can read. The person who is in poor health or has functional limitations may not be able to provide care to the patient.

Some family members may be resistant to learning many of the procedures required for the patient's care, such as suctioning or tracheostomy care. Even patients themselves who are physically capable may be resistant to learning how to perform these procedures.

Other caregivers may simply be incapable of learning the techniques or may not be able to manage the highly technical nature of some types of medical equipment. Managing life-support devices such as mechanical ventilators may prove to be too daunting a task for some. Careful observation and requesting return demonstrations will help identify any areas of deficiency in caregiver ability.[14]

Equipment

The nature of the patient's illness will usually dictate the type of medical equipment that is required. However, the environmental assessment will indicate the suitability of that equipment and the adaptations that may be necessary. The patient who lives in the older home with poor electrical wiring or frequent power outages may require a liquid or compressed oxygen system rather than an oxygen concentrator. The home ventilator patient may need backup equipment, or a ventilator mounted on a wheelchair to allow for portability. The patient who lives in a small mobile home may not have room for a hospital bed, and if that patient

were unable to lie flat when sleeping it would be necessary to find other ways to elevate the head during sleep or facilitate frequent change of position.

Stairways, carpeting, and sharp turns can create difficulties for the patient who ambulates in the home while using equipment like portable oxygen or IV poles. It may be necessary to place oxygen equipment on each floor of a multilevel home, or move the patient to a room on the ground floor in order to avoid stairs. Patients who are ambulatory outside the home may require battery-powered equipment like suction machines and compressor nebulizers. Careful observation of where and how the equipment will be used is essential.

Plan of Care

The objective of all the assessments done during the initial evaluation is to provide vital pieces of information the practitioner will use to develop an individualized plan of care.[15] The JCAHO defines a plan of care as "a systematic process or method of planning for the delivery of patient/client services."[12] HME providers that are JCAHO-accredited for clinical respiratory services are expected to follow standards that put this process into action and that supply a method of documenting the plan.

The physician orders home care services for a patient because that patient has specific medical needs. The type of service the physician orders is the *plan of treatment*. This is essentially a prescription which includes the type of therapy, dose, frequency, and method of administration, as well as physical parameters the physician wants assessed, such as oxygen saturation or vital capacity. For example, the plan of treatment for the home oxygen patient might state: "Oxygen at 1 L/min via nasal cannula at rest and 2 L/min with activity by oxygen concentrator and pulse oximetry spot check monthly and prn." During the initial visit the RCP will assess the patient, provide treatment, instruct the patient and caregivers in the use of the equipment and the treatment ordered, and evaluate the patient's environment.

During the initial evaluation the RCP will also identify specific problems or needs the patient may have in conjunction with the treatment he or she is to receive. The patient whose spouse cannot turn on the oxygen tank owing to the functional limitations imposed by arthritis will have the problem of being unable to use the equipment as prescribed. The ventilator patient who wants to leave the home has a need for battery-powered equipment. The patient who cannot remember how to use the medication in the compressor nebulizer has a problem with competency that may require assistance with the treatments. It is common to identify multiple problems during the initial evaluation.

Table 17-3 Interpretation of Signs and Symptoms in the Home Care Patient

Finding	Possible Cause	Action
Dyspnea, cyanosis	Malfunction of equipment; poor compliance with treatment; change in physical status	Check oxygen equipment; assess patient; review energy conservation techniques, pursed lips breathing; contact physician
Wheezing	Bronchospasm; congestive heart failure; pulmonary infection	Examine patient; verify compliance with medication regimen; review medication nebulizer procedures; contact physician
Increased sputum or change in sputum color	Lung or airway infection	Assess patient; check temperature; check compliance with therapy and cleaning of equipment; contact physician
Pedal edema	Heart failure; fluid overload	Assess patient; verify function of oxygen equipment; check compliance with oxygen therapy; verify compliance with medication regimen
Poor appetite	Depression, dyspnea, fever	Assess patient; examine medication schedule; review energy conservation techniques; contact physician

The plan of care is developed by the RCP based on the identification of the patient's problems or needs. It outlines the services the practitioner will provide in order to comply with the physician's plan of treatment, taking into account these problems and needs. The plan of care takes each problem or need, establishes a goal for the patient based on that problem or need, and identifies what the practitioner will do to assist the patient in achieving that goal. The plan of care for the patient who cannot remember how to use the medication for nebulizer treatments might be developed like this: problem 1—the patient cannot remember how much bronchodilator to use in his or her nebulizer; goal 1—the patient will use his or her medication as prescribed; action or service 1—provide the patient with unit-dose medication and set up treatment times after each meal and before bed.

Follow-up Care

Another aspect of the treatment plan is follow-up care. Depending on the nature of the patient's illness and the complexity of his or her needs, the patient may require a varying amount of follow-up care.

After the practitioner makes the initial evaluation and instructs the patient and caregivers on all devices prescribed by the physician, the RCP uses the plan of care to determine a follow-up schedule for the patient. Follow-up home visits allow the practitioner to reassess the patient, caregivers, and environment to determine whether the patient is responding to therapy and is complying with the physician's plan of treatment. The RCP also identifies goals that have been met and any new problems or areas of need. Depending on the complexity of the patient's problem and the equipment, the need for follow-up visits will vary. The plan of care for a patient just discharged home on a ventilator, for example, may call for home visits daily for 1 week, then weekly for 1 month, followed by monthly visits thereaf-

ter. Long-term stable patients may require only periodic visits for equipment maintenance, such as monthly, quarterly, or biannually.

It is ideal to completely reassess the patient during each follow-up visit, particularly when the home visits are done less frequently. It may be during a periodic visit that the patient is discovered to have an increase in pedal edema, sputum production, or depression (Table 17-3). Physical assessment and oximetry done on a patient who has recovered from pneumonia may reveal that the patient no longer needs oxygen therapy on a continuous basis. It may be determined during a follow-up visit that a patient is no longer able to care for himself or herself and needs someone to help. The physician should be notified of any significant findings and may prescribe a new plan of treatment. The new plan of treatment will, of course, require a new plan of care.

Equipment Maintenance

An important aspect of follow-up care is equipment maintenance. RCPs assess not only the patient, caregivers, and environment but also various types of medical equipment for appropriateness and proper function.

Each manufacturer of medical equipment has specific guidelines for periodic preventive maintenance. Home ventilators need filters changed and settings verified, and need to be removed from the patient's home for maintenance after a specified number of hours. Oxygen concentrators need to have their concentration and flow rates checked after a specified number of hours, and will also need to be removed periodically for more extensive maintenance. Liquid oxygen equipment needs to have flow rates verified as well as routine preventive maintenance. All electrically powered equipment should have an electrical safety check every 12 months.

Some routine maintenance can be performed by the patient or caregiver. External filters can be changed, nebulizers and humidifiers can be washed and disinfected, and tubings can be replaced. RCPs can perform many of the other routine maintenance procedures during their follow-up visits. This gives them the opportunity to check the patient's adherence to cleaning and maintenance procedures. RCPs should also check the hour meters that are placed on certain types of equipment like oxygen concentrators, ventilators, and CPAP machines to determine when scheduled maintenance is next due. These hour meters also give a good indication of patient compliance. Patients whose hour meters have not changed as much as expected are probably not using the equipment as prescribed. Noncompliance requires reinstruction in the use and necessity of the device to attain the treatment goal. The updated plan of care should reflect the noncompliance and reinstruction.

The RCP also evaluates the appropriateness of the equipment during these follow-up visits. The patient who will not disinfect his or her oxygen humidifier may need to have it removed, or the patient who cannot tolerate the noise his or her concentrator makes and therefore does not use it may require a liquid oxygen system. The patient who uses 50 ft of oxygen tubing on the oxygen system in order to move about the house may need reevaluation if gait problems develop. A CPAP patient with sleep apnea may need a different type of mask in order to obtain a better seal around the nose, or may need a change in pressure if he or she has gained or lost a significant amount of weight.

Summary

Assessment is an essential element of home care. The initial comprehensive assessment is done to evaluate the patient's clinical condition, his or her environment, and the ability of the patient and caregivers to provide appropriate care. Follow-up visits allow assessment of any new medical or technical problems and compliance of the patient with the treatment plan. In addition, progress toward the goals of therapy needs evaluation and documentation. The application of new technology to respiratory care equipment and the increasing number of pulmonary patients being cared for in the home have increased the demand for skilled home care RCPs.

REVIEW QUESTIONS

1. Which of the following is true regarding respiratory home care?
   a. its use is increasing
   b. it usually involves rudimentary forms of patient care and clinical expertise
   c. the technology required for respiratory home care lags behind hospital-based therapy
   d. it is mostly performed by on-the-job trainees

2. T F The type of patients receiving home respiratory care varies widely.

3. Which of the following is the most important factor in respiratory home care?
   a. treatment of physical disease
   b. treatment of psychological problems
   c. patient assessment skills
   d. management of physical and monetary resources

4. Which of the following would not be performed during a respiratory home care visit?
   a. arterial blood gas sampling and analysis
   b. mixed venous blood gas analysis
   c. collection of sputum samples
   d. sleep studies

5. T F JCAHO accreditation of home respiratory care has resulted in better patient care.

6. T F Respiratory therapists are frequently the only member of the home health care team.

7. Which of the following is (are) true regarding the initial home care evaluation?
   a. it may include diagnostic evaluation
   b. it is performed by a physician
   c. it involves evaluation of the patient only
   d. a and c

8. Which of the following is (are) true regarding the patient care plan?
   a. it is based on the initial evaluation
   b. it is a JCAHO requirement
   c. it is the same thing as the treatment plan
   d. a and b only

9. T F The plan of care is developed solely by the physician.

10. Which of the following would be a part of the environmental assessment?
    a. determining whether the person(s) with whom the patient lives is (are) willing to care for the patient
    b. determing whether home care equipment is functioning properly
    c. determining space requirements for ambulation and equipment
    d. a and c only

11. *Which of the following is a part of follow-up care?*

    a. *reducing care to minimize cost*

    b. *determing a treatment plan*

    c. *assessing the patient's compliance with the therapy*

    d. *all of the above*

REFERENCES

1. Kane NM: The home care crisis of the nineties, *Gerontologist* 29:1, 1989.
2. Balinsky W and Starkman JL: The impact of DRG's on the health care industry, *Home Care Manage Rev* 12:61, 1987.
3. Gilmartin ME: Mechanical ventilation in the home. In Gilmartin ME and Make BJ, editors: *Problems in respiratory care,* vol 1, ed 2, Philadelphia, 1988, JB Lippincott.
4. Dunne PJ, McInturff SL, Darr C: The role of home care. In Hodgkin JE, Connors GL, Bell CW, editors: *Pulmonary rehabilitation: guidelines to success,* ed 2, Philadelphia, 1993, JB Lippincott.
5. Home Care Advisory Panel, Department of Geriatrics: *Guidelines for the medical management of the home care patient,* Chicago, 1992, American Medical Association.
6. Dunne PJ: The role of the respiratory care practitioner in home care, *NBRC Horizons* 18:4, 1992.
7. *Accreditation manual for home care,* vol 1, *Standards,* Oakbrook Terrace, Ill, 1993, Joint Commission on Accreditation of Healthcare Organizations.
8. American Thoracic Society: Standards of nursing care for adult patients with pulmonary dysfunction, *Am Rev Respir Dis* 144:231–236, 1991.
9. Wilkins RL, Sheldon RL, Krider SJ: *Clinical assessment in respiratory care,* ed 2, St Louis, 1990, Mosby.
10. McCord M and Cronin-Stubbs D: Operationalizing dyspnea: focus on measurement, *Heart Lung* 21:167–179, 1992.
11. Kacmarek RM: Noninvasive monitoring of respiratory function outside of the hospital, *Respir Care* 35:719–727, 1990.
12. *Accreditation manual for home care,* vol 2, *Scoring guidelines,* Oakbrook Terrace, Ill, 1993, Joint Commission on Accreditation of Heathcare Organizations.
13. *Safety for older consumers: home safety checklist.* Washington DC, 1986. US Consumer Product Safety Commission.
14. Chmielinski MA: An educator's toolbox, *Home Health Care Dealer* 5:61–64, 1993.
15. McInturff SL: A model plan of care, *Home Health Care Dealer* 5:35–43, 1993.

Chapter 18

Pulmonary Rehabilitation Assessment

Gerilynn L. Connors and Kathleen V. Morris

LEARNING OBJECTIVES

Upon completion of this chapter, the reader should be able to accomplish the following:

1. *Identify the general purpose of pulmonary rehabilitation (PR) programs.*

2. *Identify the pathologic conditions and general evaluation criteria for acceptance into pulmonary rehabilitation programs.*

3. *Recognize the conditions for which a pulmonary rehabilitation program would be contraindicated.*

4. *Recognize the importance and methods of assessing the following in terms of pulmonary rehabilitation:*
   a. *medical history and symptoms*
   b. *physical examination*
   c. *medical lab testing*
   d. *exercise ability*
   e. *nutritional status*
   f. *quality of life*
   g. *activities of daily living (ADL)*
   h. *education*
   i. *patient outcome*

Chapter Outline

Patient Selection

Pertinent Medical History and Symptoms

Physical Symptoms

Physical Assessment

Medical Laboratory Testing

Exercise Assessment

Nutritional Assessment

Psychosocial and Quality of Life Assessment

Assessing Activities of Daily Living

Education Assessment

Home Care Referral Assessment

Assessment of Patient Outcomes

Summary

Chapter Overview

Pulmonary rehabilitation (PR) is a comprehensive treatment modality individualized to the patient's needs. PR includes patient assessment, training, exercise, psychosocial support, and follow-up.[1] Most important it

Table 18-1 Conditions Appropriate for Pulmonary Rehabilitation

Obstructive pulmonary disease
Chronic obstructive pulmonary disease (COPD)
Asthma
Asthmatic bronchitis
Chronic bronchitis
Emphysema
Bronchiectasis
Cystic fibrosis
Restrictive pulmonary disease
Interstitial fibrosis
Rheumatoid pulmonary disease
Collagen-vascular lung disorders
Pneumoconiosis
Sarcoidosis
Kyphoscoliosis
Rheumatoid spondylitis
Severe obesity
Poliomyelitis
Other conditions
Pulmonary vascular diseases
Lung resection
Lung transplantation
Occupational or environmental lung diseases

Reprinted with permission from Beytas L, and Connors GL: Organization and management of a pulmonary rehabilitation program. In Hodgkin JE, Connors GL, and Bell CW, editors: *Pulmonary Rehabilitation: guidelines to success*, ed 2, Philadelphia, 1993, JB Lippincott.

Table 18-2 Criteria to Be Evaluated in Selecting a Patient for Pulmonary Rehabilitation*

- Disease effect on patient's quality of life
- A decrease in physical activity
- Changes in occupational performance
- Dependence vs. independence in activities of daily living
- Disease effect on patient's psychosocial status (e.g., anxiety, depression, and such)
- Use of medical resources (e.g., hospitalizations, emergency room visits, and such)
- Presence of other medical problems
- Pulmonary function assessment
- Smoking history
- Patient motivation
- Patient commitment to time and active program participation
- Patient transportation needs
- Financial resources
- Patient's background

Reprinted with permission from Beytas L, and Connors GL: Organization and management of a pulmonary rehabilitation program. In Hogkin JE, Connors GL, and Bell CW, editors: *Pulmonary rehabilitation: guidelines to success*, ed 2, Philadelphia, 1993, JB Lippincott.
*Any patient with impairment due to lung disease who is motivated should be a candidate for pulmonary rehabilitation.

incorporates active participation of the patient as a focal point in the rehabilitation effort.

The first definition of PR was developed in 1974 by the American College of Chest Physicians' Committee on Pulmonary Rehabilitation. It states:

Pulmonary rehabilitation is an art of medical practice wherein an individually tailored multidisciplinary program is formulated which through accurate diagnosis, therapy, emotional support and education, stabilizes or reverses both the physio- and psychopathology of pulmonary diseases, and attempts to return the patient to the highest possible capacity allowed by his pulmonary handicap and overall life situation.[2]

This chapter addresses assessment of the pulmonary patient for PR. A thorough assessment of the patient is the cornerstone for developing an individualized and effective treatment program.

PR is not just a program for the end-stage patient with chronic obstructive pulmonary disease (COPD), nor is it simply therapeutic. PR is a necessity for patients with chronic lung disease and plays an important role in the prevention of lung disease through earlier screening and detection of pulmonary disease.[1,3] Programs focus on whole-person wellness, an awareness that rehabilitation incorporates the interactions between mind, body, and spirit.[4] Assisting the patient to develop awareness and control is an active growth process leading to good preventive self-care and symptom management. Involving the patient emphasizes the patient's role as the primary force in effecting his or her own progress.

Patient Selection

Patients with obstructive or restrictive lung disease and other specific conditions listed in Table 18-1 are appropriate candidates for PR.[5] In fact, any patient with impairment due to chronic lung disease can be a candidate for PR. The results of pulmonary function testing should not be used as the **only** criteria to determine patient eligibility for PR. The effects of the disease on the patient's functional ability and quality of life are more important criteria to consider. See Table 18-2 for the criteria to be evaluated in selecting a patient for PR.[5]

Permanent or temporary conditions that may be considered contraindications to pulmonary rehabilitation are severe psychiatric disorders such as dementia or organic brain syndrome, and unstable medical conditions such as congestive heart failure, acute cor pulmonale, substance abuse, metastatic cancer, significant liver dysfunction, or disabling stroke. Other issues to address during the initial assessment of the PR candidate are financial considerations and transportation.

The patient's motivation is another aspect for consideration when evaluating patients for PR. Does the patient feel pressure from his or her physician, spouse, or significant other to attend the PR program? Or is the patient self-motivated with a desire to improve functional ability and quality of life? Sometimes, patients will not be able to describe their reasons for attending a PR program, but they know they want a ray of hope. A skilled interviewer can assess the clients' needs and instill confidence in their ability to achieve change and see results. Establishing reasonable and achievable program goals can be the first step in building the patient's self-confidence, self-awareness, and symptom management skills. Provision of a supportive atmosphere stimulates increased interest and motivation.

Patients with severe disease are often unable to recognize their ability to improve over time. The increased work of breathing decreases the patients' functional level and creates limitations that alter quality of life. Many patients accept this as permanent. The idea of participating in an exercise program when they can hardly walk around the house may seem impossible to them. Constant feelings of shortness of breath result in anxiety and fear of activity.[6]

The interviewer can assist patients in improving their motivation and understanding of their perceived internal control and self-efficacy. Bandura[7] described these attributes as outcome and efficacy expectations. Outcome expectation is the belief that the recommended behavior will lead to a favorable outcome, while efficacy expectation is the belief that the behavior required to produce the outcome **can** be executed. It is important for the interviewer to discern the patient's efficacy and outcome expectations; the patient may accept that certain actions produce a particular outcome, but may question his or her ability to execute the action.

Throughout the PR program the instructors are aware of the clients' efficacy and outcome expectations and assist them in recognizing their ability to increase function—when, how, where, and for how long—both in the rehabilitation and home settings.

Pertinent Medical History and Symptoms

As discussed in Chapter 2, a thorough review of the patient's medical history and records builds the foundation for the assessment. Specific forms may be used for the PR assessment but are not necessary. Pertinent information for a complete PR medical history should include: history of pulmonary disease, other medical problems, exposure to pulmonary irritants, chemical addiction (nicotine, alcohol, etc.), and medication treatment. Table 18–3 gives the pertinent information to be gathered in the history taking.

"Other medical problems" need to be carefully evaluated.[8,9] These conditions have a direct effect on lung health, and since they are not pulmonary in nature, they are often overlooked. Regardless of how comprehensive the pulmonary rehabilitation program is, if these "other" conditions are not identified and treated, the patient will never reach his or her full rehabilitation potential. For example, orthopedic impairment will limit a patient's exercise potential and may require a modified exercise program. A patient

---

Table 18–3 Pertinent Information for a Complete Pulmonary Rehabilitation Medical History

History of pulmonary disease
Chief complaints
Childhood
Family
Other medical problems
Gastroesophageal reflux with chronic aspiration
Hiatal hernia
Sinusitis, rhinitis
Cardiovascular disease
Sleep disturbances
Orthopedic impairment
Neuromuscular problems
Exposure to pulmonary irritants
Occupational
Environmental
Recreational
Hobby
Chemical addiction
Nicotine (i.e., cigarette, pipe, cigar, chewing tobacco)
Alcohol
Caffeine
Other (i.e., cocaine, marijuana, etc.)
Medication treatment
Prescribed dose, frequency
Current use, dose, frequency
Over-the-counter medications used
Allergy

---

who presents with nasal or sinus drainage or esophageal reflux may aspirate the secretions, causing reflex bronchospasm.[10–13] Diabetic patients will need to understand the need for adjustment in their daily medication management regimen to compensate for increasing their exercise program. It is during the medical history that the "other" conditions are investigated with recommendations for testing and treatment to follow.

The interviewer must ask questions about the patient's past and current medication treatment program. This information will provide the basis for medication training to improve patient compliance. It is vital to know the components of the original medication prescription and actually how the patient is currently taking the medication. Often what is prescribed and how the patient takes the medicine are vastly different. Knowledge of any over-the-counter (OTC) medication the patient uses is also important. OTC medications taken for rhinitis, sinusitis, or allergy may affect the patient's physiologic responses to exercise. During the interview the patient should be asked to demonstrate how he or she uses the medication inhaler. This will also provide the caregiver with an understanding of the type of training the patient requires.

Physical Symptoms

The most common symptoms of lung disease, such as cough, sputum production, dyspnea, etc., have been covered in Chapter 2. Assessment of the "other" symptoms that may be present in the patient needing PR will be expanded on at this time.

Patient complaints of sneezing, nasal itching, nasal obstruction, increased nasal scretions, or postnasal drainage may be a sign of allergic rhinitis.[11] Headache, facial pressure, or congestion in the paranasal sinuses; pressure, itching, or popping in the middle ear; redness, discharge, or itching of the eyes; and generalized fatigue and malaise are all potential symptoms of allergic rhinitis.[11] Symptoms associated with sinusitis may be: fever, malaise, cough, sore throat, facial fullness, purulent nasal discharge, and pain.[10] The sinus pain may be located in the maxillary, frontal, ethmoidal, or sphenoidal areas.

Gastroesophageal reflux could lead to symptoms that cause the interviewer to suspect problems with the gastrointestinal tract, lungs, or heart.[12] Recurrent retrosternal burning that radiates up and down the chest or worsens on lying down or bending over, or pain with swallowing, is commonly seen with gastroesophageal reflux. Reflux may cause pulmonary symptoms that present as morning hoarseness, nocturnal cough, recurrent pneumonia (pulmonary infiltrates), or wheezing. Reflux may cause symptoms such as chest pain that suggest possible angina, but which in fact are due to esophageal reflux. The importance of assessing the "other" conditions cannot be overemphasized. Training the patient in the management of these is crucial in allowing the patient to reach full rehabilitation potential.

Physical Assessment

Physical examination in the PR setting is useful to detect the presence of any acute problem that may need treatment prior to starting the PR program. For example, the COPD patient with acute pneumonia will present with tachycardia, tachypnea, fever, and localized bronchial breath sounds. He or she needs acute care for the pneumonia before PR. In addition, physical examination helps determine the severity of the patient's chronic pulmonary problem, which is useful information when setting PR program goals and treatment.

The initial physical examination is done to assess heart rate and rhythm, respiratory rate and pattern, blood pressure, breathing pattern, breath sounds, body weight, presence of pedal edema, and use of accessory muscles. Other physical findings to note are neck vein distention, chest expansion, heart sounds, liver size, nasal septum deviation or blockage, and carotid and extremity pulses.

Physical examination findings are useful in following the effects of the PR program. Abnormalities may gradually subside when the PR program effectively improves the condition of the patient. As a result, periodic examination of the patient is done and the findings are documented in the patient record.

Table 18-4	Suggested Tests During Initial Evaluation of a Pulmonary Rehabilitation Candidate*
Spirometry pre/post bronchodilator	Exercise test with cutaneous oximetry and/or arterial blood gas analysis (simple or modified exercise test such as 6- or 12-min walk, Master's step exercise test, calibrated cycle ergometer, or motorized treadmill)
Lung volumes	
Diffusing capacity	
Resting arterial blood gas	
Chest radiograph	
Resting electrocardiogram	Complete blood count
	Basic blood chemistry panel

Adapted with permission from Connors GL and Hilling L, editors: *American Association of Cardiovascular and Pulmonary Rehabilitation: guidelines for pulmonary rehabilitation programs*, Champaign, Ill, 1993, Human Kinetics.
*It is acceptable to not repeat these tests if done within the 3 months prior to entering the pulmonary rehabilitation program or as determined by the pulmonary rehabilitation medical director.

Medical Laboratory Testing

Medical laboratory testing is an important component in patient assessment since clinical assessment alone is insufficient to detect, diagnose, or characterize lung disease. If the patient had recent testing done during a stable time, it may be unnecessary to repeat a specific test. The medical history and review of past records will indicate the tests that need to be done currently. The tests that may be needed during the initial evaluation of a PR candidate are shown in Table 18-4.[1] If "other" conditions have been discovered that would interfere with the rehabilitation process, additional tests may be considered: cardiovascular tests such as Holter monitoring, echocardiogram, or thallium exercise stress test; polysomnography; sinus radiographs; upper gastrointestinal series; and skin tests.

Exercise Assessment

Evaluation of the patient's exercise ability will allow a realistic and safe home exercise program to be developed.[14-17] The evaluation provides information about exercise-induced hypoxemia, whether supplemental oxygen with exercise training is needed, and the patient's cardiac response to exercise.[17] A simple exercise test is a 6- or 12-minute walk measuring the distance a patient covers in the specific time period. From this information a calculation of the patient's MET level and target heart rate (THR) is done. Monitoring vital signs before and after the walk and continuous oxygen saturation provide objective information regarding the patient's tolerance for exercise.

Determining the patient's upper extremity strength is also helpful when outlining the complete exercise program. Orthopedic problems, arthritis, balance, and gait abnormalities should also be evaluated to determine limitations to exercise.

An elaborate test, such as pulmonary exercise stress test (PEST), which measures expired gas volume to determine oxygen uptake ($\dot{V}O_2$) and minute volume ($\dot{V}E$), provides the most accurate measurement of metabolic work. PEST also provides a noninvasive determination of the anaerobic threshold, an important parameter of physical and cardiovascular fitness.

The specific exercise test chosen depends upon the individual patient goals and ability. The exercise assessment will set the foundation for the patient's exercise training program during rehabilitation and determine the home exercise prescription.

Nutritional Assessment

Inadequate nutrition plays a critical role in the morbidity and mortality of the patient with chronic lung disease.[18] Studies have associated increasing weight loss with severity of chronic airflow limitation. In one study it was found that 43% of emphysema patients studied showed evidence of significant malnutrition.[19] A significant increase in morbidity is associated with a weight loss that results in the patient weighing less than 90% of his or her ideal body weight.[19]

Nutritional assessment includes a diet and weight history, anthropometric measurements, visceral protein status, pulmonary function data, resting energy expenditure, and total caloric requirement calculation. The initial PR assessment should evaluate the need for a complete nutritional assessment by a dietitian. Excessive weight loss or gain or significant malnutrition suggests that a consultation with a dietician may be of value.

Reasons the pulmonary patient may experience weight loss are increased energy expenditure for the work of breathing; inadequate caloric intake due to fatigue and dyspnea; gastrointestinal symptoms related to medication, swallowing of air, or esophageal reflux; poor utilization of calories; and psychosocial factors such as depression, poverty, or poor eating and living arrangements. Medications can also deplete vitamins and minerals. Adequate fluid intake for secretion management, sodium restriction, reduction of gas-forming foods, a cholesterol-lowering diet, weight maintenance, and weight gain for the underweight or weight loss for the overweight patient are examples of nutritional goals. Other considerations include assessment of the patient's understanding of the dietary recommendations, ability to manage the plan, and willingness to comply. The extent of the nutritional evaluation is determined by each patient's needs.[20]

Psychosocial and Quality of Life Assessment

Quality of life assessment in patients with chronic lung disease is one of the most important and most difficult areas of the patient's evaluation. It includes major areas of dysfunction: dyspnea, fatigue, *mastery,* sleep disturbance, cognition, and various aspects of emotional dysfunction (anxiety, depression, frustration, anger, hostility, and embarrassment). The patient with chronic lung disease may present with mild to severe psychologic distress or emotional dysfunction requiring a thorough assessment and appropriate treatment.[21,22]

The most common psychologic distress of the patient with COPD is depression. Some investigations have found that 51% to 74% of patients with COPD suffer from depression.[21] During the assessment process the patient may characterize depression as a sleep disturbance, reduced appetite, decreased energy, reduced libido, feelings of hopelessness and pessimism, social withdrawal, sense of failure, poor concentration, and suicidal thoughts. Depression, if untreated, often results in the patient becoming socially isolated with decreasing physical activity.

Another symptom frequently reported is anxiety. During the assessment process the patient may exhibit anxiety with exaggerated body movement, rapid speech, palpitations, tachycardia, dyspnea, or sweating. Anxiety may exacerbate the physical symptoms of lung disease. For example, dyspnea is often worse in the presence of anxiety. Other emotional consequences of COPD reported are irritability, somatic preoccupation, dependency, frustration, sense of embarrassment, tension, anger, stress, denial, and fatigue.

Each pulmonary patient perceives differently the threat that illness has to all that is meaningful in his or her life. As the integrity of the body changes, so does the sense of well-being and wellness. In the patient suffering from lung disease the focus of life is changed from the use of energy to pursue physical activity, to the concentrated conservation of energy to struggle with routine daily activities. These patients lose independence and authority. Improvement in quality of life that is meaningful to the patient can best be measured through specific goal setting and evaluation. This encourages active participation by patients in the program and allows them to control outcomes. Exercise may enhance the psychological condition of the patient with COPD and may reduce anxiety, depression, and somatic symptoms.

Setting specific objectives followed by a plan of action and target date for achievement will assist the patient in measuring progress. Reinforcement, reassurance, and reassessment throughout the program assist in fulfillment of outcome expectations. Table 18–5 provides a sample plan of action. Referral of the patient for a complete psychological assessment with a psychologist, psychiatrist, or mental health professional may be necessary.

Assessing Activities of Daily Living

The ability of the patient to function independently in activities of daily living (ADL) needs to be assessed.

Table 18–5 *Sample Plan of Action*

Date	Objectives	Action*	Target Date	Comments
1/1	Upper extremity	10 reps, 0 weight	1/10	Able to do
1/17	Increase sets	10 reps, 2 sets, 0 weight	1/17	Without symptoms
		10 reps, 3 sets, 0 weight	1/24	No problems
1/31	Increase weight	10 reps, 3 sets, 1 lb.	1/31	No problems
		10 reps, 3 sets, 2 lb.	2/28	Too fatigued
		10 reps, 3 sets, 1 1/2 lb	3/14	No problems
		10 reps, 3 sets, 2 lb	3/31	No problems
4/1	Establish regular exercise routine 4–5 times per week	Sun-Mon-Wed-Thur-Fri	4/1	Rest Tues and Sat; best time to exercise, watching 6 PM news

*reps = repititions.

The ADL include a large variety of functions such as basic grooming, leisure activities, sexual performance, and work-related activities.[23] PR program content is designed to reduce and control the symptoms experienced by patients that lead to poor tolerance or avoidance of the ADL.

For example, the patient may be suffering from extreme dyspnea during hair grooming. This problem may be the result of poor arm muscle strength or endurance and the use of an inefficient breathing pattern during the activity. The caregiver should evaluate the patient's breathing pattern and oxygen saturation while performing the activity in question, looking for inefficient breathing patterns and desaturation. Breath holding; short gasps using the upper chest and accessory muscles; forced exhalation (not to be confused with pursed lips breathing); an irregular, jerky breathing pattern; unnecessary raising of the shoulders; throwing the head back slightly; paradoxical diaphragmatic movement; and asynchronous breathing represent possible inefficient breathing patterns and when present suggest the need for breathing retraining. Evaluation of the patient's upper extremities by an occupational therapist may need to be done to assess upper extremity range of motion, strength, endurance, sensation, and coordination.

Education Assessment

Researchers in the field of psychology have been the primary contributors to our understanding of how adults learn. Carl Rogers[24] was one of the most prominent researchers. He developed general ideas readily applicable to teaching self-care techniques to elderly adults.[24]

Adult learners only learn those things which they perceive important to their individual structure of self.[24] Information presented to the adult learner must be perceived as relevant by the learner. Caregivers working with patients in a PR setting will be called on to teach them about their illness and treatment. The caregiver must be able to explain to patients how the information presented is relevant to them. If this is not done, the majority of information presented will not be learned or will be soon forgotten.

Knowles[25] recognized that as one matures, one collects a vast reservoir of experience that affects future learning. Adult learners are usually problem-oriented and seek learning opportunities to solve problems with a desire to apply the new knowledge immediately.[25]

Adult learners have very individualized styles of learning. Each person has discovered through experience what works most successfully in his or her particular situation. Similarly, learners tend to have three ways of learning—through visual processes (seeing), auditory processes (hearing), and kinesthetic processes (doing).[4] At any particular time, the learner may use all three processes, but usually one is used more often than the others. The visual sense is important and most often used when trying to learn or understand new information.[4]

Learners who are visual picture things in their minds; they tend to read the newspaper rather than listen to the radio; read maps rather than ask for directions. Auditory learners tend to ask for directions or instruction; they learn best by having things explained verbally; they prefer listening to the radio rather than reading the newspaper. Learners who are kinesthetic learn best by doing things, by hands-on experience.

It makes good sense to establish the patients' best learning style and tailor educational programs accordingly. Participants who are visual will need materials to read and will learn by reading a patient handbook. Auditory learners will rely on lectures and audiocassette tapes, and kinesthetic learners will progress best by practicing the techniques learned.

In addition to assessing the participant's style of learning, the patient's knowledge of his or her lung disease and self-care techniques needs assessment.[26] Use of a simple pretest to assess knowledge allows the PR team to identify specific areas of weakness. The

Table 18–6	Protocol for Making an Educational Diagnosis of the Patient with Chronic Lung Disease
Assess learner characteristics	**Demographic and disease data**
	Age
	Sex
	Marital status
	Years of education completed
	Socioeconomic status
	Disease history
	Current disease status
	Sociopsychologic status
	Locus of control
	Health beliefs
	Cultural beliefs
	Degree of acculturation
	Level of self-efficacy
	Consider applicable learning theories
	Behavior modification
	Cognitive learning theory
	Process of valuing
Assess patient deficits	**Knowledge deficits**
	Anatomy and physiology of cardiopulmonary system
	Pathophysiology
	Medications
	Nutrition
	Emergency care
	Sexual activity
	Recreation/travel
	Community resources
	Home care
	Skill deficits
	Pursed lip breathing
	Postural drainage/clapping
	Use of inhalers
	Cleaning equipment
	Body mechanics
	Home modification

Adapted with permission from Hopp JW, and Neish CM: Patient and family education. In Hodgkin JE, Connors GL, and Bell CW, editors: *Pulmonary rehabilitation: guidelines to success,* ed 2, Philadephia, 1993, JB Lippincott.

patient's education and life experiences will influence their beliefs about health care and self-care techniques as well as influence their compliance during the PR program. In addition, visual or hearing defects need to be documented so care providers are aware of any special needs.

Following assessment of the patient's educational needs, the PR team can select the best instructional methods to apply: behavior modification, cognitive learning theory, process of valuing, or programmed learning.[26] Table 18–6 outlines the protocol for making an educational diagnosis. Each theory is effective when applied in the appropriate setting. Educating the elderly will be enhanced by praise in both the instructional and exercise segments of the PR program, regardless of the patient's individual learning style.[27,28] This is especially true in the case of the emotionally dependent elderly patient.[28]

Table 18–7	Evaluating Patient Outcomes

Changes in exercise tolerance
Pre- and post 6- or 12-min walk
Pre- and postpulmonary exercise stress test
Review of patient home exercise training logs
Strength measurement
Flexibility and posture
Performance on specific exercise training modalities (e.g., ventilatory muscle, upper extremity)
Changes in symptoms
Dyspnea measurements comparison
Frequency of cough, sputum production, or wheezing
Weight gain or loss
Psychologic test instruments
Other changes
Activities of daily living changes
Postprogram follow-up questionnaires
Pre- and postprogram knowledge test
Compliance improvement with pulmonary rehabilitation medical regimen
Frequency and duration of respiratory exacerbations
Frequency and duration of hospitalizations
Frequency of emergency room visits
Return to productive employment

Reprinted with permission from Beytas L, and Connors GL: Organization and management of a pulmonary rehabilitation program. In Hodgkin JE, Connors GL, and Bell CW, editors: *Pulmonary rehabilitation: guidelines to success,* ed 2, Philadelphia, 1993, JB Lippincott.

Home Care Referral Assessment

The fundamental objective of a PR program is to enable the patient to function at home with improved symptom management and increased ability to perform the ADL. The home care referral is not for every patient but will allow continued education, treatment, and reinforcement of the PR program.[29] See Chapter 17 for a comprehensive description of assessment in the home care setting.

Assessment of Patient Outcomes

A PR program is individualized to the patient's needs and reassessment is done concurrently during the program to meet those needs. The patient goals and objectives can be stated in outcome format. This will also comply with the Standards of the Joint Commission on Accreditation of Healthcare Organizations (JCAHO) for reporting of outcome measurements. Thorough PR assessments are labor-intensive, but improved patient outcomes at discharge validate the time spent. Table 18–7 lists the various areas to consider when evaluating patient outcomes.[5] The demonstrated outcomes of PR have been reported and a summary of the benefits can be found in Table 18–8.[30–32]

Summary

Pulmonary rehabilitation is a multidisciplinary program that is individualized to the patient's needs. Assess-

Table 18-8	Demonstrated Outcomes of Pulmonary Rehabilitation

Reduced hospitalizations and use of medical resources
Improved quality of life
Reduced respiratory symptoms (e.g., dyspnea)
Improved psychosocial symptoms (e.g., reversal of anxiety and depression and improved self-efficacy)
Increased exercise tolerance and performance
Enhanced ability to perform activities of daily living
Return to work for some patients
Increased knowledge about pulmonary disease and its management
Increased survival in some patients (i.e., use of continuous oxygen in patients with severe hypoxemia)

Reprinted with permission from Ries AL: Position paper of the American Association of Cardiovascular and Pulmonary Rehabilitation: scientific basis for pulmonary rehabilitation, *Cardiopulmonary Rehabil* 10:418–441, 1990. Published by JB Lippincott. Copyright 1990 by the American Association of Cardiovascular and Pulmonary Rehabilitation.

ment, patient training, exercise, psychosocial intervention, and follow-up are the components of PR. A training program alone or in conjunction with exercise is not PR. Assessment must be included. It is the most critical component of rehabilitation that sets the stage for individualizing the patient's program. Not every member of the rehabilitation team needs to assess every patient; however, if a patient deficit is determined, it must be addressed. COPD has an insidious onset developing over a 20- to 30-year period with a long asymptomatic period. If assessment and screening are done earlier in the disease process, prevention of the progressive disabling nature of lung disease may be possible.

REVIEW QUESTIONS

1. T   F   Pulmonary rehabilitation primarily involves treatment of acute and chronic lung disease.

2. Which of the following is (are) pathologic conditions for which pulmonary rehabilitation might be indicated?
   a. cystic fibrosis
   b. poliomyelitis
   c. rheumatoid spondylitis
   d. all of the above

3. Which of the following is not an evaluation criteria for acceptance into a pulmonary rehabilitation program?
   a. sputum gram stain
   b. smoking history
   c. arterial blood gases
   d. patient motivation

4. T   F   Metastic cancer would disqualify a patient who is trying to get into a pulmonary rehabilitation program.

5. Which of the following would be least pertinent in the pulmonary rehabilitation assessment of the patient's medical history?
   a. patient's hobbies
   b. illicit drug use
   c. number of siblings
   d. orthopedic fitness

6. T   F   Evaluation of exercise tolerance can involve the assessment of body mechanics.

7. Which of the following is not a typical goal of nutritional management in pulmonary rehabilitation?
   a. weight loss
   b. weight gain
   c. sodium reduction
   d. potassium reduction

8. Which of the following is the most common type of psychological distress in COPD patients?
   a. anger
   b. fear
   c. depression
   d. hostility

9. Which of the following is true regarding educational assessment in pulmonary rehabilitation?
   a. most patients are problem-oriented
   b. patients learn in the same manner
   c. relevance of the material to the task at hand is not important
   d. none of the above

10. Which of the following would not be a realistic outcome assessment for a patient with emphysema?
    a. enhanced activities of daily living (ADL)
    b. finding a cure for the disease
    c. increased survival
    d. decreased hospitalizations

REFERENCES

1. Connors GL and Hilling L, editors: *American Association of Cardiovascular and Pulmonary Rehabilitation: Guidelines for pulmonary rehabilitation programs,* Champaign, Ill, 1993, Human Kinetics.
2. Petty TL: *Pulmonary rehabilitation. Basics of RD,* New York, 1975, American Thoracic Society.
3. Bunch D: Pulmonary rehabilitation: the next ten years, *AARC Times* 12:54, 1988.
4. Morris K and Russo A: *P.A.T.H. Positive attitudes toward health: a handbook on pulmonary rehabilitation,* 1984, Seton Medical Center.
5. Beytas LJ and Connors GL: Organization and management of a pulmonary rehabilitation program. In Hodgkin JE, Connors GL, Bell CW, editors: *Pulmonary rehabilitation: guidelines to success,* ed 2, Philadelphia, 1993, JB Lippincott.

6. Connors GL, Hilling LP, Morris KV: Assessment of the pulmonary rehabilitation candidate. In Hodgkin JE, Connors GL, Bell CW, editors: *Pulmonary rehabilitation: guidelines to success,* ed 2, Philadelphia, 1993, JB Lippincott.

7. Bandura A: Self-efficacy: toward a unifying theory of behavior change, *Psychol Rev* 84:191, 1977.

8. Branscomb BV: Aggravating factors and coexisting disorders. In Hodgkin JE and Petty TL, editors: *Chronic obstructive pulmonary disease: current concepts,* Philadelphia, 1987, WB Saunders.

9. Connors GL, Hodgkin JE, Asmus RM: A careful assessment is crucial to successful pulmonary rehabilitation, *J Cardiopulmonary Rehabil* 8:435, 1988.

10. Brodovsky DM: Sinusitis. In Cherniack RM, editor: *Current therapy of respiratory disease,* ed 2, Toronto, 1986, BC Decker.

11. Druce HM and Kaliner MA: Allergic rhinitis. In Cherniack RM, editor: *Current therapy of respiratory disease,* ed 2, Toronto, 1986, BC Decker.

12. Nelson HS: Is gastroesophageal reflux worsening your patient's asthma?, *J Respir Dis* 11:827, 1990.

13. Proctor DF: Vasomotor rhinitis. In Cherniack RM, editor: *Current therapy of respiratory disease,* ed 2, Toronto, 1986, BC Decker.

14. Casaburi R and Wasserman K: Exercise training in pulmonary rehabilitation, *N Engl J Med* 314:1509, 1986.

15. Hodgkin JE: Exercise testing and training. In Hodgkin JE and Petty TL, editors: *Chronic obstructive pulmonary disease: current concepts,* Philadelphia, 1987, WB Saunders.

16. Ries AL: The role of exercise testing in pulmonary diagnosis, *Clin Chest Med* 8:81, 1987.

17. Ries AL, Farrow JT, Clausen JL: Pulmonary function tests cannot predict exercise-induced hypoxemia in chronic obstructive pulmonary disease, *Chest* 9:454, 1988.

18. Wilson DO and others: Body weight in chronic obstructive pulmonary disease. The National Institutes of Health intermittent positive-pressure breathing trial, *Am Rev Respir Dis,* 139:1435, 1989.

19. Angelillo VA: Nutrition and the pulmonary patient. In Hodgkin JE, Connors GL, Bell CW, editors: *Pulmonary rehabilitation: guidelines to success,* ed 2, Philadelphia, 1993, JB Lippincott.

20. Manicino JM, Donahoe M, Rogers RM: Nutritional assessment and therapy. In Casaburi R and Petty TL, editors: *Principles and practice of pulmonary rehabilitation,* Philadelphia, 1993, WB Saunders.

21. Emery CF: Psychosocial considerations among pulmonary patients. In Hodgkin JE, Connors GL, Bell CW, editors: *Pulmonary rehabilitation: guidelines to success,* ed 2, Philadelphia, 1993, JB Lippincott.

22. Kaplan RM, Eakin EG, Riese AL: Psychosocial issues in the rehabilitation of patients with chronic obstructive pulmonary disease. In Casaburi R and Petty TL, editors: *Principles and practice of pulmonary rehabilitation,* Philadelphia, 1993, WB Saunders.

23. Scanlan M, Kishbaugh L, Horne D: Life management skill in pulmonary rehabilitation. In Hodgkin JE, Connors GL, Bell CW, editors: *Pulmonary rehabilitation: guidelines to success,* ed 2, Philadelphia, 1993, JB Lippincott.

24. Rogers C: *Client centered therapy,* Boston, 1951, Houghton-Mifflin.

25. Knowles M. *The modern practice of adult education: andragogy vs pedagogy,* New York, 1970, Associated Press, pp 39–55.

26. Hopp JW and Neish CM. Patient and family education. In Hodgkin JE, Connors GL, Bell CW, editors: *Pulmonary rehabilitation: guidelines to success,* ed 2, Philadelphia, 1993, JB Lippincott.

27. Guyatt GH and others: Effect of encouragement on walking test performance, *Thorax* 39:818, 1984.

28. Pease RA: Praise elders to help them learn, *J Gerontol Nurs* 11:16, 20, 1985.

29. Dunne PJ, McInturff SL, Darr C: The role of home care. In Hodgkin JE, Connors GL, Bell CW, editors: *Pulmonary rehabilitation: guidelines to success,* ed 2, Philadelphia, 1993, JB Lippincott.

30. Clark CJ: Evaluating the results of pulmonary rehabilitation treatment. In Casaburi R and Petty TL, editors: *Principles and practice of pulmonary rehabilitation,* Philadelphia, 1993, WB Saunders.

31. Hodgkin JE: Benefits and the future of pulmonary rehabilitation. In Hodgkin JE, Connors GL, Bell CW, editors: *Pulmonary rehabilitation: guidelines to success,* ed 2, Philadelphia, 1993, JB Lippincott.

32. Ries AL: Position paper of the American Association of Cardiovascular and Pulmonary Rehabilitation: scientific basis of pulmonary rehabilitation, *J Cardiopulmonary Rehabil* 10:418, 1990.

ANSWERS TO REVIEW QUESTIONS

CHAPTER 1

1.	*b*	6.	*d*
2.	*c*	7.	*true*
3.	*a*	8.	*true*
4.	*b*	9.	*true*
5.	*false*	10.	*e*

CHAPTER 2

1.	*true*	7.	*c*
2.	*true*	8.	*c*
3.	*d*	9.	*true*
4.	*d*	10.	*d*
5.	*b*	11.	*b*
6.	*c*	12.	*b*

CHAPTER 3

1.	*true*	9.	*d*
2.	*c*	10.	*c*
3.	*b*	11.	*b*
4.	*false*	12.	*c*
5.	*true*	13.	*c*
6.	*b*	14.	*a*
7.	*true*	15.	*true*
8.	*b*		

CHAPTER 4

1.	*false*	17.	*c*
2.	*d*	18.	*b*
3.	*false*	19.	*true*
4.	*true*	20.	*a*
5.	*d*	21.	*b*
6.	*b*	22.	*a*
7.	*true*	23.	*false*
8.	*c*	24.	*c*
9.	*b*	25.	*c*
10.	*b*	26.	*false*
11.	*b*	27.	*true*
12.	*true*	28.	*d*
13.	*false*	29.	*true*
14.	*d*	30.	*false*
15.	*d*	31.	*d*
16.	*a*	32.	*d*

CHAPTER 5

1.	*b*	9.	*d*
2.	*false*	10.	*c*
3.	*false*	11.	*a*
4.	*d*	12.	*c*
5.	*c*	13.	*a*
6.	*a*	14.	*false*
7.	*true*	15.	*true*
8.	*c*	16.	*true*

17.	*d*	29.	*d*
18.	*b*	30.	*d*
19.	*b*	31.	*false*
20.	*c*	32.	*a*
21.	*b*	33.	*c*
22.	*a*	34.	*false*
23.	*d*	35.	*d*
24.	*d*	36.	*b*
25.	*c*	37.	*true*
26.	*b*	38.	*false*
27.	*c*	39.	*d*
28.	*true*	40.	*b*

CHAPTER 6

1.	*true*	22.	*d*
2.	*c*	23.	*true*
3.	*a*	24.	*false*
4.	*d*	25.	*a*
5.	*a*	26.	*true*
6.	*false*	27.	*b*
7.	*b*	28.	*d*
8.	*b*	29.	*c*
9.	*d*	30.	*false*
10.	*a*	31.	*a*
11.	*c*	32.	*a*
12.	*d*	33.	*c*
13.	*c*	34.	*a*
14.	*true*	35.	*d*
15.	*true*	36.	*a*
16.	*b*	37.	*c*
17.	*c*	38.	*true*
18.	*b*	39.	*false*
19.	*false*	40.	*d*
20.	*false*	41.	*c, c, c, b*
21.	*a*		

CHAPTER 7

1.	*false*	17.	*c*
2.	*b*	18.	*d*
3.	*c*	19.	*a*
4.	*d*	20.	*d*
5.	*true*	21.	*c*
6.	*false*	22.	*d*
7.	*a*	23.	*true*
8.	*b*	24.	*false*
9.	*a*	25.	*false*
10.	*d*	26.	*a*
11.	*true*	27.	*c*
12.	*c*	28.	*true*
13.	*d*	29.	*d*
14.	*b*	30.	*c*
15.	*true*	31.	*a*
16.	*true*		

CHAPTER 8

1.	false	16.	c
2.	false	17.	d
3.	c	18.	true
4.	true	19.	b
5.	b	20.	false
6.	d	21.	d
7.	a	22.	false
8.	b	23.	c
9.	d	24.	true
10.	true	25.	a
11.	d	26.	d
12.	c	27.	b
13.	c	28.	a
14.	d	29.	d
15.	true	30.	a

CHAPTER 9

1.	b	9.	b
2.	b	10.	c
3.	a	11.	b
4.	b	12.	d
5.	false	13.	a
6.	a	14.	b
7.	c	15.	c
8.	d		

CHAPTER 10

1.	d	11	d
2.	d	12.	c
3.	c	13.	b
4.	true	14.	a
5.	true	15.	c
6.	c	16.	b
7.	a	17.	a
8.	b	18.	d
9.	b	19.	b
10.	c	20.	d

CHAPTER 11

1.	false	13.	a
2.	d	14.	true
3.	a	15.	b
4.	b	16.	d
5.	false	17.	true
6.	d	18.	c
7.	b	19.	d
8.	true	20.	true
9.	d	21.	a
10.	c	22.	c
11.	true	23.	d
12.	b		

CHAPTER 12

1.	c	13.	false
2.	a	14.	b
3.	c	15.	b
4.	true	16.	true
5.	d	17.	c
6.	b	18.	true
7.	false	19.	d
8.	d	20.	true
9.	true	21.	d
10.	d	22.	b
11.	a	23.	d
12.	c		

CHAPTER 13

1.	a	11.	a
2.	b	12.	true
3.	true	13.	d
4.	false	14.	d
5.	b	15.	false
6.	c	16.	d
7.	d	17.	a
8.	true	18.	c
9.	a	19.	b
10.	d	20.	d

CHAPTER 14

1.	true	16.	a
2.	d	17.	true
3.	d	18.	d
4.	a	19.	b
5.	b	20.	false
6.	true	21.	c
7.	true	22.	b
8.	b	23.	a
9.	d	24.	c
10.	c	25.	d
11.	d	26.	true
12.	true	27.	d
13.	c	28.	a
14.	b	29.	true
15.	false	30.	c

CHAPTER 15

1.	true	9.	a
2.	true	10.	c
3.	d	11.	d
4.	c	12.	b
5.	d	13.	false
6.	d	14.	d
7.	d	15.	true
8.	b	16.	true

CHAPTER 16

1.	*b*	9.	*b*
2.	*b*	10.	*c*
3.	*true*	11.	*d*
4.	*false*	12.	*c*
5.	*true*	13.	*b*
6.	*false*	14.	*a*
7.	*a*	15.	*b*
8.	*d*		

CHAPTER 17

1.	*false*	6.	*true*
2.	*d*	7.	*d*
3.	*a*	8.	*c*
4.	*true*	9.	*a*
5.	*c*	10.	*b*

CHAPTER 18

1.	*a*	7.	*a*
2.	*true*	8.	*d*
3.	*c*	9.	*false*
4.	*b*	10.	*d*
5.	*true*	11.	*c*
6.	*false*		

Index

A

Abdomen
  examination of, 70
  movement of, paradoxical, in critically ill patient, 227, 229
Abdominal paradox, 58
Abortion, 196
Acid phosphatase (ACP), 90-91
Acid-base balance
  assessment of, 112-113, 118-119
    arterial blood bicarbonate in, 113
    base excess/base deficit in, 113
    hydrogen ion concentration in, 112
    partial pressure of arterial carbon dioxide in, 113
  disorders of, 114-115
    clinical recognition of, 114-118
    compensation for, limitations of, 116-117
    mixed, 117-118
Acidemia, 112
Acids, 112
Acidosis
  lactic, 115
  metabolic
    clinical recognition of, 115-116
    respiratory alkalosis and, 118
  respiratory, 114
    clinical recognition of, 114-115
    and metabolic, 117-118
    metabolic alkalosis and, 118
Acids, 112
Acquired immune deficiency syndrome (AIDS), CT scanning in, 154
Acrocyanosis in infants, 201
Activities of daily living (ADL) assessment of pulmonary rehabilitation, 379-380
Addison's disease, hyponatremia in, 88
Adventitious breath sounds, 63
Aerosol bronchodilators, pulmonary function testing before and after, 136
Afterload, pump function and, 284-285
Age
  chronologic, 196
  gestational, 196
  partial pressure of oxygen in arterial blood and, 106-107
  pulmonary function values and, 128
Air bronchogram, 159
Air conditioner, source and symptoms of, 20t
Airway(s)
  artificial, in critically ill patient, 224-225
  in assessing critically ill infant, 211
  assessment of, in critically ill patient, 223-225

Airway(s)—cont'd
  lower, obstruction of, clinical findings in, *228*
  obstruction of
    acute, physical signs of, 72
    chronic, physical signs of, 72-73
    in critically ill patient, 223-224
  upper
    obstruction of, clinical findings in, *228*
    resistance in, in infancy and childhood, 363
Airway pressures in ventilatory assessment in ICU, 254-257
Airway resistance (Raw)
  determining, 137-138
  in ventilatory assessment in ICU, 256
Alanine aminotransferase (ALT), 90
Alanine transaminase (ALT) in infant assessment, 207
Albumin, 92
  serum, in nutritional assessment, 348
Alkalemia, 112
Alkaline phosphatase (ALP), 90
  in infant assessment, 207
Alkalosis
  metabolic
    clinical recognition of, 116
    and respiratory, 118
    respiratory acidosis and, 118
  respiratory, 113
    clinical recognition of, 115
    metabolic acidosis and, 118
  ventilator-induced, 118
Allen test of collateral circulation, 107, *107*
Alphafetoprotein (AFP) as tumor marker, 93
Alveolar-arterial oxygen difference, 110
Alveolar-arterial oxygen tension, decreased oxygen transport and, 261
Alveolar-capillary membranes in gas exchange, 319
Ammonia, lung diseases associated with, 20t
Amplifier in invasive hemodynamic pressure monitoring system, 323-324
Amylase, 91
Anasarca, 29
Anatomic shunting, 107
Anemia, 84-85
Anemometers, mass flow, for lung volume measurement, 252
Anergy, 97
Angiography, pulmonary, 156, *157*
Anion gap, 89
Ankle swelling in pulmonary disorders, 29-30

Anode, 149
Anteroposterior (AP) view, 151-152
Antigen(s)
  carcinoembryonic, as tumor markers, 93
  oncofetal, as tumor markers, 93
Antimony, lung diseases associated with, 20t
Anxiety in clinical presentation, 38
Aorta, coarctation of, in infant, 204
Aortic pressure measurement, direct, 301, 303
Apgar scores, 197-198
Apical lordotic view, 150
Apnea
  in infants, 200
  sleep, 357-359
    obstructive, 358
      case study on, 364
      in infants and children, 363
    pulmonary function testing in, 142
    quantification of, 360
Apnea index, 360
Arrhythmia(s), 42
  sinus, 42
Arterial blood bicarbonate, 113
Arterial blood gases (ABG), 105, 107-108
  continuous intraarterial monitoring of, in ICU, 270
  in newborn assessment, 208, 209t
Arterial carbon dioxide, partial pressure of, 113
Arterial oxygen, partial pressure of, in clinical evaluation of oxygenation, 261
Arterial oxygen content, 109-110
Arterial pressure
  in critically ill patient, 239-242
  decreases in, 300
  increases in, 300
  mean, 301
  monitoring of, 299-303
    cannulation sites for, 300
    complications of, 300
    direct and indirect, disparities between, 299-300
    normal, 300
    waveforms for, 301
Arterial-alveolar tension ratio, decreased oxygen transport and, 261
Arterial-mixed venous oxygen content difference in critically ill patient, 266
Arteriotomy, 105
Artery(ies)
  pulmonary
    catheterization of, complications of, 313
    pulmonary artery catheter placement in, 312